# Instructor Curriculum Resource

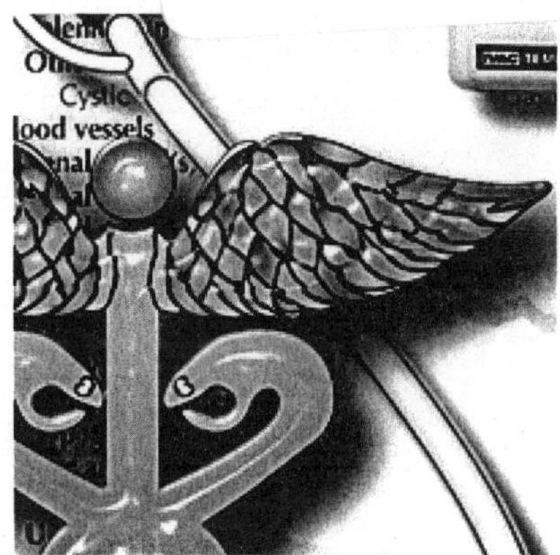

for

# The Medical Assistant: Administrative and Clinical

8th Edition

by Mary E. Kinn and Mary Ann Woods

---

Anne L. Lilly, RN, BSN, MVEd
Curriculum Consultant, Allied Health, Adult Education
Professor: Retired, Santa Rosa Junior College, Santa Rosa, CA
Medical Office Law and Ethics, Medical Insurance and Coding
Advanced Medical Terminology and Anatomy, Medical Office Procedures,
Immediate Past President: California Association of Medical Assistant Instructors
Member of The American Association of Medical Assistants

W. B. Saunders Company
*A Division of Harcourt Brace & Company*
The Curtis Center
Independence Square West
Philadelphia, PA 19106-3399

Instructor Curriculum Resource for
*The Medical Assistant,* 8th edition

ISBN 0-7216-7301-5



Printed in the United States of America

Last digit is the print number: 9 8 7 6 5 4 3 2 1

# Contents

# Acknowledgments

Thank you to my secretary and husband Pete, who copied manuscript, ran to the post office, proofread all the manuscript, cooked dinner and generally took care of everything, including me, while I wrote to meet deadline.

The publisher wishes to acknowledge the AAMA notice that the new, official curriculum document has not yet been finalized. "The language used for the curriculum content and competencies topics is adapted from the AAMA *Role Delineation Study: Occupational Analysis of the Medical Assisting Profession,* published by the American Association of Medical Assistants (AAMA), Chicago, IL. The AAMA does not endorse the language nor is the language the official, or taken from the official, AAMA medical assisting curriculum document."

# Preface

The Instructor Curriculum Resource is a supplement to the text, *The Medical Assistant*, 8th Edition and the *Student Mastery Manual* and the Virtual Medical Office Challenge CD-ROM, located on the inside book cover of the textbook. The Resource introduces and ties together a total learning system for you to successfully facilitate an educationally sound and effective learning experience for students. It is an educational tool to use in developing class materials using the system. It also contains the answers to all workbook activities. Both the beginning and experienced instructor will find many new and interesting theories presented within this Resource. The system is a result of an accumulation of applied theories and over 35 years of teaching experience.

Anne L. Lilly

# PART 1

# TO THE INSTRUCTOR

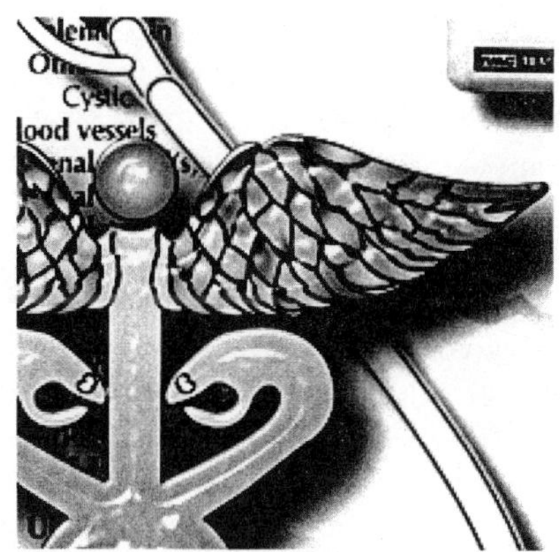

## A. THE TOTAL LEARNING SYSTEM

Instructors are always looking for a method to guarantee the educational process. They found quickly that there were no guarantees but that some strategies were more effective than others. Searching for successful strategies has been the focus of educational research from the early 1900's to today. In 1973, the AAMA developed a curriculum strategy based on both the original work of Blooms' *Taxonomy of Educational Objectives* and an analysis of the profession. This analysis was developed into a competency-based curriculum for entry level medical assisting practice. This curriculum was revised in late 1998 after a comprehensive role delineation study was conducted in 1996 and 1997. Many areas of competence remained the same or similar, but the study indicated the need for increased depth of knowledge and competence in performing tasks. Today, the AAMA, as a national certifying body, continues to set curriculum standards with the 1998 Curriculum of Content and Competencies necessary for achievement of entry-level competencies for medical assistants.

The Total Learning System is an educationally effective, technologically current approach to learning that meets the recommended AAMA Curriculum. It also meets the educational requirements for RMA preparation. It minimizes instructor and student busy-work and reflects the increased depth of knowledge recommended by the AAMA analysis. The system uses four components:

- The *8th Edition Textbook* includes content and performance objectives, and all content needed to perform the competencies listed in a basic entry-level Medical Assisting curriculum. The content and competencies of the text are specified in a grid in each chapter of the *Instructor Curriculum Resource.*
- A *Student Mastery Manual* provides learning activities from simple knowledge to complex evaluation. Exercises and activities are presented in a logical progression of learning within the chapters and throughout the manual. This allows students to demonstrate and use increasingly complex knowledge, and apply it in increasingly complex areas of competency applications in medical office situations. The procedures are formatted to provide objectives, evaluation and documentation for competency-based education.
- The *Saunders Virtual Office CD-ROM* will allow students to apply content and problem-solving competencies for required procedures within a realistic medical office setting. The *Student Mastery Manual* contains an introduction on using the CD-ROM, a description of the cases, the competencies for each case, and the forms the student needs to complete the cases. All this information is in Appendix C of the Mastery Manual.
- The *Instructor Curriculum Resource* explains and develops all Learning System components with Medical Assisting curriculum for certification and the necessary teaching strategies to make you an effective instrument for student learning and success. It contains
  - The Medical Assisting curriculum content and competencies for the chapter
  - A grid integrating textbook objectives, and the location in the textbook, Mastery Manual, or CD-ROM
  - Lesson plans
  - Internet, literature, and association resources
  - Mastery Manual answers

## B. COMPETENCY-BASED EDUCATION

- The 1998 AAMA Curriculum contains administrative, clinical, and transdisciplinary competencies for a Medical Assisting curriculum.
- These competencies are standards for entry-level job performance.
- Competencies need to be defined in certified Medical Assisting curriculum.
- The basis of competency-based education is using statements of educational objectives.
- Objectives directed to adults include development of instructional strategies in harmony with the demographics of the class.
- An appreciation of student demographics and characteristics is used in designing objectives to meet defined learning styles and learning stages.

### Designing Competency-Based Objectives

Does the instructor need to write objectives that are different from the text? Yes!

- Textbook objectives may not state specific levels in the learning process, as lesson plans require.
- Most textbook objectives are broad and are really statements of long-term outcomes called terminal performance objectives.
- While these objectives may deal with behaviors, they often are not specific enough to provide all the standards necessary for competency-based objectives.
- Most objectives in a medical assistant text may be used with some modification so that each objective contains the entire and specific standards of competency-based objectives.
- Objectives designed to teach adults are quite different from those addressed to children or special education students.
- Medical assistant learning objectives should clarify exactly the minimum knowledge and skills that must be achieved by all the students.

### Essential Components of Competence Objectives

Competency-based objectives contain three parts.

1. **The task or behavior.** This indicates what will happen and what level of learning order is required. Behavior must be observable and measurable. This requires an action verb. Passive nonmeasurable verbs such as *knows* or *understands* are not valid objectives. Bloom originally described both learning order and writing objectives in his *Taxonomy of Educational Objectives.* Educators have since developed many action verbs that allow instructors to describe exactly the behavioral level in the learning order that is expected of the student.

   Table I-1, p. 3, contains the levels in the learning order as described by Bloom, short descriptions of the levels, and some action verbs. These will help to write and clearly state objectives specific to your lessons.
2. **The conditions or setting.** This includes surroundings or conditions within which the student is expected to perform the task. Conditions are necessary to describe a variety of settings. Conditions may include the equipment to be used or the setting.
3. **The evaluation or standard.** This tells student and evaluator how well a behavior must be performed. A cognitive objective may require 75% accuracy, whereas a performance objective may require 100% accuracy. Evaluation may include time, distance, number of repetitions, etc.

Examples:

The student will correctly identify the contaminated items in a picture (task) with 90% accuracy, or will identify 9 of 10 items (standards). Upon the completion of this lesson or in the laboratory (conditions)

OR

The student will choose the correct method of taking a temperature on five patients when given sufficient information by the instructor.

**All procedures in the Mastery Manual include the task, conditions, and standards.**

**Table I-1 Levels of Learning***

| LEVEL | DESCRIPTION | ACTION VERBS |
|---|---|---|
| **Cognitive Area** | | |
| 1. Knowledge | Memorizing materials, recognition, or recall | To define, recognize, list, match, repeat, name, identify, select, distinguish, label |
| 2. Comprehension | Understanding, getting the meaning of it , reorganizing | To give examples, explain, illustrate, restate, demonstrate, interpret, describe, summarize, discuss, change, transform |
| 3. Application | Using newly learned materials in a different format—from concrete to abstract and reverse | To apply, organize, restructure, calculate, operate, practice, classify, solve, choose, generalize, transfer, demonstrate |
| 4. Analysis | Breaking materials down into component parts, identify the relationships of each | To compare, differentiate, diagram, distinguish, describe, classify, analyze, contrast, experiment, debate, question, examine |
| 5. Synthesis | Combining elements and parts to form a new total part | To plan, solve, design, combine |
| 6. Evaluation | Making judgments about the value of something from self-produced ideas | To judge, consider, critique, conclude, evaluate, select, score, assess, revise, rate, measure |
| **Affective area** | | |
| values, feelings, attitudes | Receiving | To accept, choose, listen, select |
| | Responding | To approve, tell, volunteer, recite, help |
| | Valuing | To choose, share, support, join, appreciate |
| | Organizing | To formulate, defend, relate |
| | Characterizing | To discriminate, behave, serve, verify |
| **Psychomotor area** | | |
| Requires cognitive applications—use action verbs from list | Learning involves doing at differing levels of cognition | To imitate, manipulate, be precise, articulate<br>Each verb listed denotes a more complex performance |

*Data from Bloom's *Taxonomy of Educational Objectives*

## C. INSTRUCTIONAL STRATEGIES FOR TEACHING THE ADULT LEARNER

### 1. Instructors become more effective when they:

- understand why students are in class
- understand how adults prefer to learn
- use teaching techniques to those characteristics
- use the above knowledge incorporated into a lesson plan.

Using these strategies makes learning more enjoyable to students and instructing much easier and more rewarding. They allow instructors the greatest chance of success in motivating students and helping students to master the materials.

### 2. Adult motivations for education—why students are in class

- Adults decide to obtain learning experiences usually to cope with specific life-changing events. Use surveys to address student goals, life events, and motivational factors.
- Adults are goal orientated. For most adults learning alone does not bring the reward they are seeking. The reward comes with goal achievement such as placement in a position, advancement in a job, or entry into a higher level of schooling.
- Adults are motivated by the usefulness of material to be learned.
- Increasing or maintaining self-esteem is a strong motivator for entering a class.
- Adults are very responsive to learning experiences in their teachable moments: i.e., close to a promotion, changes in responsibility, possibility of advancement, increased salary.
- Adults cannot be threatened, tricked, or conned into learning.

### 3. Use Adult Learner Characteristics—to write objectives, design lesson plans, and plan classroom activities

#### a. Adults have expectations

- More impatient in proceeding directly to learning and performance objectives
- Much less tolerant of busywork
- Have more compelling responsibilities competing with their education time

*Objectives:*

- Valid objectives contain behavior, controlling factors, and evaluation.
- Let the learner know exactly what is expected.
- Be specific in behavior and direct each to only one behavior.
- Relate directly to material to be learned.

*Lesson Plan Design:*

- Write LEARNER OBJECTIVES for each lesson.

*Classroom:*

- Put learner objectives up at beginning of class.
- Ask for other objectives from students.
- Find out what they need to learn by a short survey.
- Teach to the objectives.

#### b. Adults need to be able to integrate new ideas with what they know

- They have greater difficulty in remembering isolated facts.

*Objectives:*

- Write sequential objectives; build on previous knowledge.

*Lesson Plan Design:*

- Start a lesson that refers to previous learning and life experiences.
- Refer back to previous objectives and knowledge.
- Explain how you intend to integrate knowledge.

*Classroom:*

- Start class with reminder of past lesson or life experience that will get students' attention. This is the opening "GRABBER" that tells the student "this will be a worthwhile time."
- Create activities to help learner organize and store knowledge with previous material.
- Sell students on value of information. Straightforward is the preferred style.
- Obtain student comments about lesson and learner class experience.

#### c. Information that conflicts with what is known or believed is integrated more slowly and requires a new learning cycle for adults

- Less willing to adopt new ways
- More rigid in thinking, like set patterns of behavior regarding right, wrong, fact, fiction
- Have more experience living and relate new facts to life experiences

*Objectives:*

- Write objectives that measure specific level of learning required

*Lesson Plan Design:*

- Lessons need to be designed to obtain responses that show the students' present level of knowledge. A *pretest* will do this for the instructor. A pretest can be very informal or written. Include phases of the learning cycle: (experiencing, examining, explaining, applying) when writing objectives and lesson plans.

*Note:* The learning cycle will be explained in the next part.

*Classroom:*

- When opinions are presented such as in law, ethics, or discussing the medical assistant's role, obtain feedback from students to find out whether student concepts and ideas are in conflict with instructor.
- Protect minority opinion and make connections between opinions and ideas.
- Provide a *lesson plan* that covers all phases of the learning cycle when presenting new concepts.
- Encourage brainstorming to gather a large variety of potential solutions to problems.

## d. Adult learners prefer single-concept, single-theory lessons that focus heavily on the application of content to current problems or needed skills

*Objectives:*

- Objectives all should relate to one skill or concept; i.e., "List 10 men and 5 women influential in the history of medicine," rather than, "Know the important people in the history of medicine."

*Lesson Plan Design:*

- Within a *lesson,* present ideas one at a time and refer to the objective being covered.
- Summarize the lesson with review materials to conclude your presentation, and then give an oral or written posttest.

*Classroom:*

- Minimize competing intellectual demands. One subject at a time makes it easier for students.

## e. Fast-paced, complex, or unusual learning tasks interfere with learning the concepts and data

- Give students time between learning theory and performing tasks.
- Talk slowly. Students require a longer time to perform physical and mental tasks.

*Objectives:*

- Keep theory and performance objectives in separate lessons.
- Introduce in sequential order.
- Allow students to comprehend before applying.

*Lesson Plan Design:*

- Keep *lesson* formats similar.
- Do not be too innovative.
- Be consistent with expectations.

*Classroom:*

- Anchor new lessons to concepts in life experiences and values sets.
- Stick to objectives and lesson plan. Unexpected changes in lessons or tests may produce anxiety that interferes with performance.

## f. Adults tend to be slower in some psychomotor learning tasks

- Adults compensate by being more accurate and make fewer trial and error ventures.

*Objectives:*

- Objective needs to allow for time and accuracy.

*Lesson Plan Design:*

- Present performance lesson at a pace that permits mastery.
- Provide for demonstration and practice time immediately afterward.
- First instructor demonstration must be 100% accurate.

*Classroom:*

- Use repetition and audio-visual aids.
- Use practice opportunities with the instructor present.
- Encourage students to begin with exact imitation of demonstrated task.
- Watch students manipulate objects and require perfect precision.
- Build one skill upon the other to coordinate a series of habitual acts.

## g. Adults require physical comfort to maximize learning

- Students in their 40's and above have slower responses in sight, hearing, mobility, and dexterity. It is difficult to learn when tired or distracted

*Objectives:*

- May address comfort in objective, such as "Today students who have difficulty seeing will sit in front of the room."

*Lesson Plan Design:*

- Plan for lessons in multiples of 50 minutes.

- Skills are demonstrated and return demonstrated in front of instructor in order to allow for immediate learning and developing of psychomotor skills.
- Prevent students from practicing incorrect techniques.

*Classroom:*

- Provide breaks every 50 minutes. If that is not possible, plan a moving activity related to the lesson.
- Place interesting activities for first hour after lunch if possible.
- Keep classroom lights on.
- Provide a well-ventilated class and a quiet atmosphere to accommodate for restricted powers of adjustment to temperature change, noise,or visual distractions.
- In the laboratory have sufficient equipment so the students can practice while the instructor is scheduled to be present. When basic technique is correctly performed, students may practice alone or with others.

### h. Adults prefer self-directed and self-designed learning projects by a margin of more than 5 to 1 over group learning experiences led by instructors

*Objectives:*

- Write self-directed and -designed learning objectives.
- Example: Design a short project that will allow the student to learn and apply the stated objectives listed below.

*Lesson Plan Design:*

- Provide lessons in a variety of formats and learning activities.
- Introduce group activities slowly and do not use them too frequently.
- Obtain comments on student receptiveness.
- Provide programmed instruction, books, computer, television, and independent activity.
- Provide clear, measurable learner objectives.
- Ask for student opinions and experiences during lessons to keep them involved.

*Classroom:*

- Provide competent, adequate direction to prevent frustration during self-directed activity.
- Instructor must be available for direction and individual learning.
- Lectures and seminars increase the success of self-directed activities.

### i. Adults tend to take errors personally and are more likely to let them affect self-esteem

Self-esteem is on the line when adults are asked to try new behaviors or answer questions in front of peers. They take fewer risks. They may misinterpret personal or judgmental comments. Going to school is voluntary and a sacrifice. They expect to be treated with respect. They suffer more from being deprived of success. Adults need ideas accepted even if it is not the right answer. And don't forget that they come from different cultures and heritage. Instructors need to understand the beliefs of cultures in the class; i.e., Hawaiian, Vietnamese, and European versus the usual American students.

*Objectives:*

- Write objectives that address an accomplishment in the class.
- Examples: Students list three items learned in class today. Students indicate which objectives they have met by the end of class period.

*Lesson Plan Design:*

- A *posttest* designed to reinforce learner objectives allows for great success. Posttest at least weekly. Base major tests on objectives and posttests.
- Ask an evaluation question about the class presentation on the test.

*Classroom:*

- Use open-ended questions to draw out learners.
- Instructors need to acknowledge all responses in a positive manner.
- Keep pontificating to a minimum.
- Ask students "why?" Use short written posttests.
- Use volunteers to answer questions whenever possible.
- Discuss improvement needs in private.

### j. Adults have the same learning preference styles as younger people.

When you see a child whose dominant learning style is tactile, it will be the same when 60!

*Objectives:*

- Have all students take a short survey, as it will reinforce known styles.
- Students share what works for them with their style of learning.

*Lesson Plan Design:*

- Give students a learning preference survey. There are many forms available. A common form is the Barsch Learning Preference Survey. Learning style surveys may be obtained from guidance counselors or special education instructors.

- Develop auditory, visual, and tactile teaching techniques (learning styles).
- Use a lesson plan format that incorporates these techniques.

*Classroom:*

- Design the lesson plan to present materials and information in all learning styles to allow all students to learn. Learning styles are included in the next part.

**Table I-2 Student Learning Styles Integrated to Classroom Learning Experiences**

| TACTILE | AUDITORY | VISUAL |
|---|---|---|
| 1. Allow students to give each other return demonstrations | 1. Read aloud steps for demonstration | 1. Use checklist for return demonstrations |
| 2. Demonstrate as often as possible | 2. Read summary or outline of materials aloud | 2. Sit where student can see visuals |
| 3. Assign computer programs | 3. Face students while talking | 3. Point to topic you are talking about |
| 4. Students work in pairs and teach each other | 4. Give oral instructions | 4. Walk back and forth to keep students' attention |
| 5. Ask students to write for you on board | 5. Provide acronyms for memory aids | 5. Put up charts, graphics, etc. |
| 6. Have students write questions for instructor | 6. Encourage students to tape-record lectures | 6. Have students close eyes and visualize |
| 7. Ask students to take notes, write objectives, or outline chapter | 7. Encourage students to study in a group | 7. Use overhead projectors for lesson plan |
| 8. Encourage students to study while moving | 8. Take turns leading groups | 8. Put objectives on chart or projector |
| 9. Games requiring set-up or placement of objects | 9. Verbally review objectives. | 9. Video tapes, surgeries, demonstrations |
| | 10. Word spelling or object identification activities | 10. Have student design transparencies |

## D. STYLES AND STAGES IN LEARNING EXPERIENCES

### 1. Styles

When instructors address teaching activities to all the learning styles, students have more success. The learning styles are visual, auditory, and tactile. Students usually have a dominant and secondary learning style. Be wary of teaching to your learning style rather than the students'. A list of learning styles follows with activities and techniques the instructor may employ. These techniques are integrated into the sample *Lesson Plan Form* presented on pages 10 and 11. Table I-2 demonstrates the use of various activities that can be used in the classroom by the instructor to meet student learning styles.

### 2. Stages

The term *learning stages* refers to the process a student must go through to reach each level of learning as described by Bloom in Table I-1. The stages help shape an effective and dynamic interactive lesson plan and incorporate all learning levels necessary for student competence. These stages are:

- EXPERIENCE: Personal involvement with specific happenings or experiences allows for understanding and memorization of materials. See Table I-2, Learning Styles.
- EXAMINATION: The student examines the experience with thoughtful inspection that allows comprehension or grasping the meaning.
- EXPLANATION: The student is able to explain and draw logical conclusions using theoretical concepts. This process requires building on previous learning levels to apply and analyze concepts.
- APPLICATION: This includes drawing conclusions through practical study. Here the student synthesizes and evaluates in drawing conclusions. These conclusions guide one's decisions and actions. The student is now ready to begin the next learning level or proceed with new materials.

Use these stages in a sequential manner to provide activities that develop the level of knowledge and competence described in the lesson objectives.

Table I-3 integrates classroom learning stages and includes learning style activities for each stage. Notice the letters A, V, and T after the listed classroom activities. V = visual, A = auditory, and T = tactile. These letters indicate the student learning style the activity is addressing.

**Table I-3 Learning Stages Integrated into Classroom Activities and Learning Styles**

| 1. Specific Happenings or Experience | 2. Thoughtful Inspection or Examination | 3. Theoretical Concepts or Explanation | 4. Practical Study—Application |
|---|---|---|---|
| a. Laboratories —VAT<br>b. Skill practice—VAT<br>c. Observations or transparencies—VT<br>d. Text reading—V<br>e. Simulations—VAT<br>f. Games/puzzles—VT<br>g. Field work—VAT<br>h. Films—VA<br>i. Readings—V, or aloud—A<br>j. Recall experience—A | a. Logs —T<br>b. Journals —VT<br>c. Discussion—A<br>d. Brainstorming/lists—AT<br>e. Thought questions—A<br>f. Rhetorical questions—A<br>g. Draw pictures—VT<br>h. Design an illustration or graph—VT<br>i. Note taking—VT | a. Simulations/ Role play—VAT<br>b. Papers—VT<br>c. Laboratory—VAT<br>d. Projects—AT<br>e. Homework—VAT<br>f. Make a videotape for hearing impaired—A<br>g. Make a model of anatomy—V T<br>h. Draw pictures—VT | a. Lecture —VAT<br>b. Clinical study—VT<br>c. Explain a procedure on tape—AT<br>d. Make tape for blind person—A<br>e. Describe something to another—A T<br>f. Model building—VT<br>g. Field work—VAT<br>h. Analogies—A<br>i. Other |

## E. IMPLEMENTING THE TOTAL LEARNING SYSTEM

### 1. Using the *Instructor Curriculum Resource*

Each chapter in *Instructor Curriculum Resource* contains the following topics, with corresponding numerical headings for each chapter.

- CHAPTER HEADING—An introductory paragraph addressed to the instructor
- USING THE LEARNING SYSTEM

1. MEDICAL ASSISTING ENTRY-LEVEL CURRICULUM FOR COMPETENCY

   These are included for the instructor to review with and correlate with textbook objectives. When there is a guest lecturer, these items should be reviewed with the lecturer, as this clarifies materials the students need. These items may be reviewed again at the end of the chapter so that the students integrate textbook objectives with knowledge, performance, and competence. In many cases these items are repeated in chapter lesson plans. This indicates that instructors need to increase depth of knowledge and application for these areas.

2. MEDICAL ASSISTING ENTRY-LEVEL CURRICULUM INTERFACE

   A. *Grid to use the Total Learning System:* This indicates locations of Learning System components (*Instructor Curriculum Resource* lesson plans, textbook, Mastery Manual, and CD-ROM) with textbook objectives and medical assisting curriculum for each lesson. A sample grid is shown below.

| TEXTBOOK OBJECTIVES | LEARNING SYSTEM LOCATION | MA CURRICULUM |
|---|---|---|
| Cognitive | | Content |
| 1. Define and spell terms in Vocabulary | • Manual Part 1-A | • Applications of medical terminology |
| 2. Describe four important features of an appointment book | • Text p. 122<br>• Lesson plan<br>• Manual Part B<br>• CD-ROM Admin. | • Risk management<br>• Basic medical office functions |
| 3. List and explain three basic guidelines to follow in scheduling appointments | • Lesson plan content<br>• Text pp. 122, 124, 125<br>• Manual Parts B & C | • Basic principles and mental health<br>• Recognize and respond to verbal and nonverbal communications<br>• Adaptations for individual needs |

3. RESOURCES

   This section will have a number of Internet links for the instructor to check out. These sites are just the tip of the iceberg and will lead the instructor to some wonderful educational and instructional tools. There are also some video resources, books, and periodicals.

4. LESSON PLAN

   TIME—Includes suggested lecture & lab hours

   The same as suggested in Table I-5, p. 16, Program Guide, to meet certifying needs. Each chapter has a lesson plan that follows the same format and is discussed in Part F, Developing the Lesson plan.

5. MASTERY MANUAL CHAPTER ANSWERS WILL BE HERE/EXPLANATION OF MASTERY MANUAL USE

   **Part 1 Content Mastery**
   The answers to the six levels of knowledge for all activities are placed here. Some answers are in chart form and are available as Transparency Masters. Mastery Manual activities are designed to meet textbook objectives and Medical Assistant content and competencies. They are not taken from the textbook.

   - Part 1 activities should be completed before the CD-ROM is used. These activities are best assigned after chapter readings and discussion.
   - The activities are designed to be completed after the student has studied the material. The answers should not be copied from the textbook.
   - There are a variety of activities to cover student learning styles.
   - The activities address learning competencies at differing levels in the learning process as described in Tables I-2 and I-3.
   - The activities assist students to meet chapter objectives and curriculum content.
   - Choose the activities according to learning levels desired by the Medical Assistant program. Adult education programs may want students to *know, comprehend,* and *apply* learning. Vocational and AS degree programs, with CAAHEP or other accreditation, may require the student to use learning in the other domains. This includes the ability to analyze, synthesize, and evaluate.

   Part 1 requires the student to use knowledge at six increasingly complex levels. These levels always follow the same lettering format in the Mastery Manual.

   **Part 2 Competency Challenge**

   - This part provides for development of competencies for the Medical Assistant curriculum. Many competencies may be achieved using the CD-ROM and Procedures. All procedures have activities in the Mastery Manual. Have students complete Part 1 before beginning this part.
   - Students are directed to the CD-ROM with ⊕ symbol and appendices with ▲ symbol.
   - Procedures adapted from textbook are located at the end of the Mastery Manual chapters. All contain competency objectives with accompanying tasks, standards, and conditions and a check-off list for evaluation.
   - Competencies in this part are often developed from the psychomotor domain by demonstrating procedures and manipulating objects.
   - Some activities require use of the affective domain by requiring responding, valuing, and organizing thoughts and ideas.
   - The activity may be an isolated application or a continuing part of one of four case studies used throughout the Mastery Manual and CD-ROM.
   - The Instructor Resource provides guidance for these studies in each chapter.
   - Forms are in Mastery Manual chapters or Appendix C and may be copied for student use.
   - It is hoped that these clinical studies will help the student relate to both the normal and unusual events that occur in a medical office or clinic setting.

   **Part 3 Clinical Applications**
   Many situations presented here will be related to legal, ethical, or patient education applications that the student and instructor can discuss. They help students develop understanding of potential situations and plan outcomes.
   **An Examaster testbank file** is available. It may be obtained free of charge when the *Total Learning System* is ordered.

## 2. General Use of the *Student Mastery Manual*

The *Student Mastery Manual* and *Saunders Virtual Medical Office CD-ROM* comprise the package. Both learning tools allow students to complete all the textbook objectives and the curriculum Content and Competencies of Medical Assisting accrediting bodies. The *Student Mastery Manual* is designed to complement the 8th Edition Textbook of Kinn and Woods, *The Medical Assistant, Administrative and Clinical.*

When used as prescribed, the Total Learning System will allow the instructor to:

- Develop and use educationally sound strategies
- Write competency-based theory and performance objectives
- Develop lesson plans which meet all the components described in this part
- Use the Learning System chapter by chapter
- Provide answers to the activities in the *Competency Manual*
- Include overhead talking points for all chapters
- Provide Instructor Resources
- Bring mastery to the student, which ultimately results in better patient care

## F. THE DEVELOPMENT OF A LESSON PLAN

A lesson plan is as simple or complex as an instructor requires. It is usually a guide for the instructor to conduct a 50-minute class. It does not contain all the information presented in class. Instructors with longer classes can design a lesson for each 50-minute part. A simple lesson plan includes those items that allow a class to be conducted with form and direction.

A sample lesson plan form with the developmental steps follows.

- The sample lesson plan simply guides the instructor in constructing the finished product.
- Each part of the plan is explained.
- Examples of adult characteristics to be used in developing objectives are given. Some sample objectives for the content are given.
- The content outline contains adult characteristics and a brief content outline for a skill theory and performance class of 100 minutes. This is very brief and would require extra notes.
- Notice the variety of learning strategies, styles, and stages that are listed on the right-hand side of the plan.
- Note the sequential order of the learning stages in the materials presented.
- Use of the lesson plan will ensure the students learn what is expected.

A blank lesson plan form is included in Table I-4, pp. 13-14, and in Appendix D. The blank lesson plan may be reproduced as necessary to use in this course.

**SAMPLE LESSON PLAN FORMAT: Includes adult characteristics and instructor use**

**LESSON PLAN**

**TOPIC:** Only one per lesson **TIME:** Usually 50 minutes

**LESSON #:** This is used for a series of lectures with the same overall topic

**OPENING:** This may be a joke, an action such as a loud conversation, handing students something as they enter class, or standing silently until all students realize nothing is happening.

**PRETEST:** Keep simple, meet an objective, find knowledge level or values

- Adult characteristic—Information that conflicts with what is known or believed is integrated more slowly and requires new learning cycle for the adult.
- Ask student to write what is known about next day's lesson.
- Use words such as who, what, where, when, how, and why.

**LEARNER OBJECTIVES** (Write at least 1 Per ½ HOUR) **TIME:** Usually 5 minutes to review

- Adult characteristic—Adults have expectations.
- Learners prefer single-concept, single-theory lessons.
- Use the action verbs necessary to describe exactly what instructor wants students to learn.

Some action verbs are located in the blank lesson plan (Table I-4). Many more are in Table I-1. Other action verbs may be found in the references at chapter end.

- Put up objectives whether they are more specific than the textbook objectives or from the 8th Edition Textbook chapter.

Sample objectives are:
— will take notes during demonstration
— will repeat or write the five essential steps in skill #
— will practice the skill immediately after demonstration
— will read each step aloud before completing and proceeding to the next step

*Post objectives on overhead, in syllabus, or on flip chart for each class and read aloud.*

**CONTENT OUTLINE:** Choose activities from previous tables and sample blank lesson plan.
Adult characteristic—Adults need to be able to integrate new ideas with what they know.
Tie in previous knowledge with today's lesson.
*For example: to demonstrate a skill after theory remember that:*

- Fast-paced, complex, or unusual learning tasks interfere with learning the concepts and data.
- Present data in a singular and organized fashion, with visual, explanation, and provide time to examine and question.
- Follow the outlines in lesson plan and fill in where necessary.

Remember, adult characteristics are:

- Adults tend to be slower in some psychomotor learning tasks.
- Allow ample supervised practice before independent practice.
- Allow practice immediately after demonstration and watch each student.

**ASSIGNMENT EXAMPLES**
Independent skill practice. Check off next scheduled lab.
Read next chapter in 8th Edition Textbook and complete standard chapter assignment.

**POSTTEST:** Choose from objectives, Examaster, give oral and written directions—5 minutes

**LEARNING EQUIPMENT NEEDED**
Here list transparencies, forms, activity supplies, clinical supplies

**NOTES:**

**Analyze and evaluate your lesson plans using the standards below**

- Are adult characteristics included in the plan?
- Does it include at least one activity in sequential order from each of the learning stages listed earlier?
- Does it include a variety of learning styles discussed earlier?
- What do you see as the highest educational level reached in this lesson according to Table I-1? Is this the level the instructor desired?

If the answers are yes, then the lesson meets the objectives and provides a sound educational format and learning experience.

Good luck with your medical assisting instructor experiences as you use the Total Learning System with the medical assistant *Student Mastery Manual.*

**SAMPLE** —100-minute class lecture and laboratory combined **#Minutes in bold**

1. Show a film on the skill **10 min.**
2. Discuss and identify essential components **10 min.**
3. List purpose, problems, techniques, patient considerations, Medical Assistant role **10 min.**
4. Identify behavior, circumstances, evaluation, and grading system for skill **5 min.**
5. Demonstrate the skill in small groups of ten or less so that all may see psychomotor activities needed. **10 min each 20 min.**

**55 min. End first hour Class break for 10 minutes**

Reassemble for second 55-minute period

1. Break students into groups of two, read procedure, and proceed with practice.
2. One student reads aloud while other follows steps.
3. Observe each student before allowing independent practice and give individual technique Instruction. **55 min. End second hour**

**End lesson; total time 100 minutes**

**SUMMARY:** Successful instructional strategies include:

- Planning lessons using adult learning characteristics throughout.
- Writing and using competency-based objectives in instruction.
- Using the learning styles in designing lesson content and activities.
- Planning activities from each stage of the learning cycle.
- Developing a lesson plan using the knowledge above.

**Table I-4 BLANK LESSON PLAN**

**LESSON PLAN**

TOPIC ____________________ TIME ____________________

LESSON # ____________________

OPENING: ________________________________________

________________________________________

PRETEST

________________________________________

________________________________________

CONTENT OBJECTIVES ( At least 1 PER 1/2 HOUR) TIME ____

________________________________________

________________________________________

________________________________________

________________________________________

________________________________________

________________________________________

________________________________________

________________________________________

Post objectives on overhead, in syllabus, or on flip chart for each class
Read aloud

CONTENT OUTLINE *Activities:* Choose from list to right TIME ____

________________________________________

________________________________________

________________________________________

________________________________________

________________________________________

________________________________________

________________________________________

________________________________________

________________________________________

**Action verbs for writing objectives**

*Knowledge*—define, match repeat, select

*Comprehension*—express, explain, restate, discuss, demonstrate, describe

*Application*—organize, solve, transfer, classify, choose, illustrate, practice

*Analysis*—distinguish, compare, list, subdivide, contrast, debate

*Synthesis*—design, plan, solve

*Evaluation*—judge, assess, compare, critique, rate

*Classroom Activities*—
Use list below and provide for student learning styles (VAT) and stages (#1-4)

1. *Experiencing*
   a. Laboratories—VAT
   b. Skill Practice—VAT
   c. Observations/transparencies—VT
   d. Games/puzzles —V T
   e. Text reading—V
   f. Simulations—VAT
   g. Field work—VAT
   h. Films—VA
   i. Readings—V, aloud—A
   j. Recall experience—A
   k. Taking notes —VT
2. *Examination*
   a. Logs—T
   b. Journals—VT
   c. Discussion—A
   d. Brainstorming/Lists—AT
   e. Thought questions—A
   f. Rhetorical questions—A
   g. Drawing pictures—VT
   h. Designing or graphing—VT

*Table continues on following page*

ASSIGNMENT

POSTTEST: choose from objectives, give oral and written directions

LEARNING EQUIPMENT NEEDED
LIST transparencies, forms, activity supplies, clinical supplies

3. *Explanation*
   a. Simulations/role play—VTA
   b. Papers & Homework—VT
   c. Laboratory & Projects—VAT
   d. Making videotape for hearing impaired—A
   e. Making a model of anatomy—VT
   f. Drawing pictures—VT

4. *Application*
   a. Lecture—VAT
   b. Case study—VT
   c. Explaining procedure on tape to person—AT
   d. Making tape for blind person—A
   e. Describing something to another—AT
   f. Model building—VT
   g. Field work—VAT
   h. Analogies—A

**NOTES:**

## G. COURSE SYLLABUS

### 1. Organization of the Course

The hours in Table I-5 are suggested times to cover materials in an accredited curriculum. Lecture hours are designated as contact hours in which the instructor uses various learning styles and explains the concepts in the chapters. A variety of discussion techniques may be used including guests, question and answer, student presentations, group activities, and problem solving or straight lecture. Designated laboratory hours are intended to be the time for competency applications including practice time for procedures, demonstration of procedures, individualized instruction, films, completing the CD-ROM or competency manual activities, field trips, procedural evaluations, and the like. Laboratory hours may be located in a school medical laboratory, the classroom, a computer laboratory, or in the field. Often, when accounting for instructional hours as a percentage of faculty workload, one lecture hour equals three laboratory hours of instructional time. Other programs consider lecture and lab hours the same, and class may be easily planned in this manner. This syllabus meets both criteria.

The 8th Edition Textbook is designed to be completed by students in two 17-week semesters of 9 months, or in 900+ hours including lecture, laboratories, and externship. Depending upon program needs and design, the 8th Edition Textbook may be used in a variety of ways. Options include breaking the 8th Edition Textbook into different courses to develop different areas of Medical Assisting. A basic receptionist course would include the material in Unit 1, an Administrative Medical Assistant course would include Units 1 and 2, and a Clinical Medical Assistant course would include Units 1 and 3. The first Unit might be taught as a core course concurrent with Units 2 or 3.

## 2. Content and Instructional Hours

### Table I-5 Suggested Times to Cover Materials

| MATERIAL | LECTURE HOURS | LABORATORY HOURS |
|---|---|---|
| **UNIT ONE: PROFESSIONALISM, LEGAL CONCEPTS, COMMUNICATION SKILLS** | | |
| 1. Introduction to Medical Assisting | 2 | 3 |
| 2. Medical Assisting Externship and Preparing to Find a Position | 2 | 3 |
| 3. A Brief History of Medicine | 2 | 3 |
| 4. Medical Practice Systems | 2 | 3 |
| 5. Medical Ethics | 3 | 9 |
| 6. Medicine and the Law | 3 | 9 |
| 7. Interpersonal Skills and Human Relations | 3 | 9 |
| 8. Patient Reception | 3 | 9 |
| 9. Telephone Techniques | 3 | 9 |
| 10. Appointment Scheduling and Time Management | 3 | 9 |
| **TOTAL HOURS FOR UNIT ONE** | **26** | **66** |
| **UNIT TWO: ADMINISTRATIVE CONTENT AND COMPETENCIES** | | |
| 11. Correspondence and Mail Processing | 3 | 9 |
| 12. Dictation and Transcription | 3 | 9 |
| 13. The Computer in Medical Practice | 3 | 9 |
| 14. Filing Methods and Record Keeping | 3 | 9 |
| 15. Health Information Management | 3 | 9 |
| 16. Professional Fees and Credit Arrangements | 3 | 12 |

| MATERIAL | LECTURE HOURS | LABORATORY HOURS |
|---|---|---|
| 17. Managing Practice Finances | 3 | 12 |
| 18. Banking Services and Procedures | 3 | 12 |
| 19. Billing and Collections | 3 | 12 |
| 20. Health Insurance and Managed Care | 3 | 12 |
| 21. Coding and Claims Processing | 3 | 12 |
| 22. Library, Research, Travel, and Meetings | 3 | 3 |
| 23. Facility Environment | 3 | 3 |
| 24. Management Responsibilities | 3 | 6 |
| **TOTAL HOURS FOR UNIT TWO** | **66** | **138** |
| **UNIT THREE: CLINICAL SKILLS—CONTENT AND COMPETENCIES** | | |
| 25. Patient Assessment | 3 | 12 |
| 26. Infection Control | 3 | 12 |
| 27. Vital Signs and Anthropometric Measurements | 3 | 12 |
| 28. Assisting with Primary Physical Examinations | 3 | 12 |
| 29. Assisting in Cardiology | 3 | 12 |
| 30. Assisting with Pulmonary Procedures | 3 | 12 |
| 31. Assisting in Otorhinolaryngology | 3 | 12 |
| 32. Assisting in Gastroenterology | 3 | 12 |
| 33. Assisting in Gynecology and Obstetrics | 3 | 12 |
| 34. Assisting in Pediatrics | 3 | 12 |
| 35. Assisting in Neurology | 3 | 12 |

*Table continues on following page*

| | | |
|---|---|---|
| 36. Assisting in Dermatology | 3 | 12 |
| 37. Assisting in Orthopedic Medicine | 3 | 12 |
| 38. Assisting in Urology and Male Reproduction Procedures | 3 | 12 |
| 39. Assisting in Elder Care | 3 | 12 |
| 40. Assisting with Office Emergency Procedures | 3 | 12 |
| 41. Assisting with Diagnostic Imaging and Therapeutic Modalities | 3 | 12 |
| 42. Clinical Laboratory | 3 | 12 |
| 43. Urinalysis | 3 | 12 |
| 44. Venipuncture | 3 | 12 |
| 45. Assisting in Hematology and Serology | 3 | 12 |
| 46. Assisting in Microbiology | 3 | 12 |
| 47. Nutrition and Exercise | 3 | 12 |
| 48. Applying the Principles of Pharmacology | 3 | 12 |
| 49. Administering Medications | 3 | 12 |
| 50. Preparing for Surgery | 3 | 12 |
| 51. Surgical Methods | 3 | 12 |
| 52. Assisting with Surgical Procedures | 3 | 12 |
| **TOTAL HOURS FOR UNIT THREE** | **84** | **356** |
| **UNIT FOUR EXTERNSHIP** | | **200** |
| **TOTAL PROGRAM HOURS** | | **936** |

### 3. Competency Evaluating and Grading

#### a. Instructors use different strategies when grading

Adult learners:

- prefer to be graded on completing work and activities
- do not like to have the greatest percentage of the grade related to testing
- want grading standards to judge their performance.

Grades may be assigned points or given in percentages. In either case, typically 25% of the grade would be on performance competencies in the laboratory, 25% on *Competency Manual* and CD-ROM activities, and 50% on testing, including quizzes and examinations. It is important to be consistent with program and school policy when grading.

#### b. Students need pass/fail standards in relationship to test grades and laboratory performance

Using the grading method mentioned above it is possible to pass the course with Ds on tests. Instructors may prevent this by limiting the number of Ds that may be obtained or having a minimal passing standard for the final examination. Often schools have competency standards for procedures to prevent students who consistently perform poorly from passing the course. Consistently poor performance is an indication of overall weakness. It is not in the best interest of the student or patient to pass with consistently poor performance in theory or competency. All standards need to be in writing.

#### c. Strategies for developing laboratory grading and evaluation standards

- The teaching-learning process in the Procedure Skills Laboratory includes demonstration, practice, and testing (check-off). Students are expected to participate fully in all components of this process.
- Failure to perform at a satisfactory level in Procedure Skills testing will result in required repeat of practice and testing (check-off). The testing session may be terminated if there is sufficient evidence that the student is not prepared for the test.
- Three separate testing sessions per skill will be permitted including the initial skills test and two repeats.
- No more than one skills testing session will be conducted in any one day.
- If the skills test is not satisfactorily passed within the testing session limit, the student will fail the course.
- There will be a limit of three repeat check-off sessions necessary to successfully pass the skill. The student may repeat only ___ number (Instructor: set standards) of skills three times. If this number of three repeats is achieved, all subsequent skills must be completed within two attempts. Failure to successfully complete any subsequent skills after notification of reduced repeat status will result in a course failure. This policy is based upon the belief that the unlimited repeated failures will result in medical assistant candidates of questionable aptitude.
- Deadline dates for the completion of repeat skills testing will be established by the instructor. Failure to meet deadline dates will result in a performance grade of 0 for that skill.

#### d. Procedure Competency Standards and Evaluation

1) Standards for PROCEDURE COMPETENCY EVALUATION FORM

ABOVE EXPECTED PERFORMANCE LEVEL = **AEL** **VALUE 3 POINTS**

- Meets Competency Objective Statement of task, conditions, and standards.
- The quality of performance is *above* the expected level of achievement.
- Requires less than expected amount of guidance for stated level of achievement.
- Has professional dress and demeanor.
- Competence is completed at time and place specified by instructor.

AT EXPECTED LEVEL = **EL**
**VALUE 2 POINTS**

- Meets Competency Objective Statement of task, conditions, and standards.
- The performance is at the expected level of achievement on *first attempt*.
- Requires the expected amount of guidance for stated level of achievement.
- Has professional dress and demeanor.
- Competence is completed at time and place specified by instructor.

AT EXPECTED LEVEL = **EL**
**VALUE 1 POINT**

- Meets Competency Objective Statement of task, conditions, and standards on *second or third attempt*.
- The quality of performance is at the expected level of achievement.
- Requires the expected amount of guidance for stated level of achievement.

- No more than *two repeats* to achieve competence.
- Has professional dress and demeanor.

BELOW EXPECTED LEVEL = **BEL**
**VALUE 0 POINTS = UNSATISFACTORY**

- The quality of performance is below the expected level of achievement for Competency Objective Statement of task, conditions, and standards.
- Requires *more than* the expected amount of guidance for stated level of achievement.
- Exceeded allowed number of attempts or did not repeat in a timely fashion.
- Does not have professional dress and demeanor.

Grade = Total number possible points for each procedure by # procedures = 100% of procedure points. The passing criteria and professional behavior components are left to instructor. Suggested criteria is 80% to performance; 20% to professionalism.

2) Procedure Competency Evaluation Form

The procedures listed for evaluation are those contained in the textbook and Mastery Manual. Other performance competencies contained in the objectives are identified in each chapter interface grid in this resource.

The form on the following pages is designed to meet grading standards as explained above. The forms are separated according to Units I and II. Unit III forms are separated according to sections for ease in grading. Suggested grading scales are included. Each Mastery Manual has these forms as Appendix A.

## H. PROCEDURE COMPETENCY LIST AND EVALUATION FORMS

### Procedure Competency Evaluation Form

| **UNIT I PROFESSIONALISM** GRADING STANDARDS ⇒<br><br>**PROCEDURES in Text & Mastery Manual** ⇓ | AEL = 3 points Above expected performance level first attempt = A **POINTS** ⇓ | EL = 2 points At expected performance level with first attempt =B **POINTS** ⇓ | EL = 1 point At expected performance level after 2 or 3 attempts = C **POINTS** ⇓ | BEL = 0 points More than 3 attempts = below expected performance **POINTS** ⇓ |
|---|---|---|---|---|
| 2-1 Preparing resume | | | | |
| 2-2 Answering help wanted ad | | | | |
| 8- 1 Preparing charts | | | | |
| 8-2 Registering patient | | | | |
| 8-3 Professional image | | | | |
| 9-1 Answering telephone | | | | |
| 9-2 Place outgoing calls | | | | |
| 10-1 Preparing appointment book | | | | |
| 10-2 Scheduling new patients | | | | |
| 10-3 Scheduling diagnostic tests | | | | |
| **TOTAL POINTS FOR UNIT I 10 PROCEDURES** | **A = 27-30** | **B = 24-26** | **C = 20-23** | **D = 19** |
| Additional procedures | | | | |
| | | | | |
| | | | | |
| Total points for instructor-added procedures | | | | |

| **UNIT II ADMINISTRATIVE COMPETENCIES** GRADING STANDARDS ⇒ **PROCEDURES in Text & Mastery Manual** ⇓ | AEL = 3 points Above expected performance level first attempt = A **POINTS** ⇓ | EL = 2 points At expected performance level with first attempt = B **POINTS** ⇓ | EL = 1 point At expected performance level after 2 or 3 attempts = C **POINTS** ⇓ | BEL = 0 points More than 3 attempts = below expected performance **POINTS** ⇓ |
|---|---|---|---|---|
| 11-1 Composing business correspondence | | | | |
| 11-2 Writing instruction sheets | | | | |
| 12-1 Transcribing machine dictation using typewriter | | | | |
| 12-2 Transcribing machine dictation using computer or word processor | | | | |
| 13-1 Operating a computer | | | | |
| 14-1 Initiating a new patient file | | | | |
| 14-2 Color coding patient files | | | | |
| 14-3 Filing supplemental materials | | | | |
| 15-1 Performance—Initiating a medical record according to Procedure 8-1 | | | | |
| 16-1 Explaining professional fees | | | | |
| 16-2 Making credit arrangements with a patient | | | | |
| 17-1 Posting service charges and payments using pegboard | | | | |
| 17-2 Accounting for petty cash | | | | |
| 18-1 Writing checks in payment of bills | | | | |
| 18-2 Preparing a bank deposit | | | | |
| 18-3 Reconciling a bank statement | | | | |
| 19-1 Preparing monthly billing statements | | | | |
| 19-2 Collecting delinquent accounts | | | | |
| 21-1 Completing insurance forms | | | | |
| 21-2 Making Medicare electronic submissions | | | | |
| 22-1 Making travel arrangements | | | | |
| 22-2 Arranging a group meeting | | | | |

*Table continues on following page*

| PROCEDURES in Text & Mastery Manual ⇓ | AEL = 3 points Above expected performance level first attempt = A POINTS ⇓ | EL = 2 points At expected performance level with first attempt = B POINTS ⇓ | EL = 1 point At expected performance level after 2 or 3 attempts = C POINTS ⇓ | BEL = 0 points More than 3 attempts = below expected performance POINTS ⇓ |
|---|---|---|---|---|
| 23-1 Establishing and maintaining a supply inventory system | | | | |
| **TOTAL POINTS FOR UNIT II 23 PROCEDURES** | **A = 62-69** | **B = 49-61** | **C = 35-48** | **D & F = below 35** |
| Additional procedures | | | | |
| | | | | |
| | | | | |
| | | | | |
| | | | | |
| | | | | |
| | | | | |
| Total points for instructor-added procedures | | | | |

| **UNIT III CLINICAL PROCEDURES** GRADING STANDARDS ⇒ **PROCEDURES in Text & Mastery Manual** ⇓ | AEL = 3 points Above expected performance level first attempt = A **POINTS** ⇓ | EL = 2 points At expected performance level with first attempt = B **POINTS** ⇓ | EL = 1 point At expected performance level after 2 or 3 attempts = C **POINTS** ⇓ | BEL = 0 points More than 3 attempts = below expected performance **POINTS** ⇓ |
|---|---|---|---|---|
| **Section 7**—Fundamental principles of patient care | | | | |
| 25-1 Obtaining a medical history | | | | |
| 26-1 Handwashing for assisting with medical procedures | | | | |
| 26-2 Sanitizing of instruments | | | | |
| 26-3 Wrapping instruments and supplies for steam sterilization | | | | |
| 26-4 Using the steam autoclave | | | | |
| 27-1 & 2 Obtaining an oral temperature using a glass or electronic thermometer | | | | |
| 27-3 Obtaining an aural temperature using the tympanic system | | | | |
| 27-4 & 27-5 moved to pediatrics chapter | | | | |
| 27-6 Obtaining an axillary temperature | | | | |
| 27-7 and 27-8: Assessing the patient's pulse and determining respirations | | | | |
| 28-9 Determining a patient's blood pressure | | | | |
| 28-10 Measuring a patient's height and weight | | | | |
| **Total points section 7 12 procedures** | **A = 33-36** | **B = 29-32** | **C = 25-28** | **D or F =below 25** |
| **Section 8**—Protocols of patient care | | | | |
| 28-1 Assisting with a physical exam | | | | |
| 29-1 Performing a multichannel ECG | | | | |
| 29-2 Applying the Holter monitor | | | | |
| 30-1 Administering Mantoux tuberculin skin test | | | | |
| 30-2 Performing volume capacity spirometric test | | | | |
| 30-3 Collecting a specimen by swab for throat culture | | | | |

*Table continues on following page*

| PROCEDURES in Text & Mastery Manual ⇓ | AEL = 3 points Above expected performance level first attempt = A POINTS ⇓ | EL = 2 points At expected performance level with first attempt = B POINTS ⇓ | EL = 1 point At expected performance level after 2 or 3 attempts = C POINTS ⇓ | BEL = 0 points More than 3 attempts = below expected performance POINTS ⇓ |
|---|---|---|---|---|
| 30-4 Obtaining a sputum specimen for culture | | | | |
| 31-1 Measuring distance acuity using the Snellen chart | | | | |
| 31-2 Assessing color acuity | | | | |
| 31-3 Irrigating a patient's eyes | | | | |
| 31-4 Instilling eye medicine | | | | |
| 31-5 Irrigating the patient's ear | | | | |
| 31-6 Instilling medicated otic drops | | | | |
| 32-1 Assisting with the colon examination | | | | |
| 32-2 Stool specimen collecting | | | | |
| 32-3 Inserting a rectal suppository | | | | |
| 33-1 Assisting with examination of a female | | | | |
| 33-2 Teaching the patient breast self examination | | | | |
| 33-3 Preparing the patient for cryosurgery | | | | |
| 33-4 Establishing the EDD using Nägele's rule and the lunar method | | | | |
| 34-1 Measuring circumference of infant's head | | | | |
| 34-2 Obtaining pediatric vital sign and vision screening | | | | |
| 34-3 Preventative wrapping of a child | | | | |
| 34-4 Applying a urinary collection device | | | | |
| 34-5 Determining temperature using the rectal method | | | | |
| 35-1 Preparing the patient for an EEG | | | | |

| PROCEDURES in Text & Mastery Manual ⇓ | AEL = 3 points Above expected performance level first attempt = A POINTS ⇓ | EL = 2 points At expected performance level with first attempt = B POINTS ⇓ | EL = 1 point At expected performance level after 2 or 3 attempts = C POINTS ⇓ | BEL = 0 points More than 3 attempts = below expected performance POINTS ⇓ |
|---|---|---|---|---|
| 36-1 Obtaining wound exudate for culture | | | | |
| 37-1 Assisting with cast application | | | | |
| 37-2 Applying a triangular arm sling | | | | |
| 37-3 Applying an ice bag | | | | |
| 38-1 Catheterizing a female patient | | | | |
| 38-2 Catheterizing a male patient using a straight catheter | | | | |
| 38-3 Teaching testicular self examination | | | | |
| 39-1 Assisting visually impaired elderly | | | | |
| 40-1 Performing CPR | | | | |
| **Total points section 8 35 procedures** | **A = 95-105** | **B = 76-94** | **C = 53-75** | **D = below 53** |
| **Section 9**—Understanding and performing diagnostic orders and tests | | | | |
| 41-1 Assisting with an x-ray examination | | | | |
| 41-2 Assisting with ultrasound therapy | | | | |
| 42-1 Using a microscope | | | | |
| 43-1 Assessing urine for color and turbidity | | | | |
| 43-2 Measuring specific gravity using a urinometer | | | | |
| 43-3 Testing urine with chemical reagent strips | | | | |
| 43-4 Testing urine for glucose using Clinitest tablets | | | | |
| 43-5 Testing urine for protein using the SSA precipitation test | | | | |
| 43-6 Analyzing urine microscopically | | | | |

*Table continues on following page*

| PROCEDURES in Text & Mastery Manual ⇓ | AEL = 3 points Above expected performance level first attempt = A **POINTS ⇓** | EL = 2 points At expected performance level with first attempt = B **POINTS ⇓** | EL = 1 point At expected performance level after 2 or 3 attempts = C **POINTS ⇓** | BEL = 0 points More than 3 attempts = below expected performance **POINTS ⇓** |
|---|---|---|---|---|
| 43-7 Collecting a clean catch specimen for culture or analysis | | | | |
| 43-8 Performing a pregnancy detection test | | | | |
| 44 -1 Collecting venous blood sample using the syringe method | | | | |
| 44-2 Collecting a venous blood sample using the evacuator method | | | | |
| 44-3 Performing butterfly draw using hand vein | | | | |
| 44-4 Collecting a capillary blood sample | | | | |
| 45-1 Performing a microhematocrit | | | | |
| 45-2 Obtaining a hemoglobin count | | | | |
| 45-3 Filling a unopette | | | | |
| 45-4 Charging a hemacytometer | | | | |
| 45-5 Counting cells in the Neubauer ruled hemacytometer | | | | |
| 45-6 Preparing a smear stained with Wright stain | | | | |
| 45-7 Performing a differential examination of a smear | | | | |
| 45-8 Determining a sedimentation rate by the Wintrobe method | | | | |
| 45-9 Determining cholesterol level using a ProAct testing device | | | | |
| 45-10 Performing a blood glucose Accu-Chek test | | | | |
| 45-11 Determining ABO group using a slide test | | | | |
| 45-12 Determining Rh factor using the slide method | | | | |
| 46-1 Inoculating a blood agar plate for strep throat culture | | | | |
| 46-2 Streaking plates for quantitative cultures | | | | |

| **PROCEDURES in Text & Mastery Manual** ⇓ | AEL = 3 points Above expected performance level first attempt = A **POINTS** ⇓ | EL = 2 points At expected performance level with first attempt = B **POINTS** ⇓ | EL = 1 point At expected performance level after 2 or 3 attempts = C **POINTS** ⇓ | BEL = 0 points More than 3 attempts = below expected performance **POINTS** ⇓ |
|---|---|---|---|---|
| 46-3 Preparing a direct smear or culture smear for staining | | | | |
| 46-4 Staining a smear with Gram stain | | | | |
| 46-5 Performing a rapid strep test | | | | |
| 46-6 Performing a cellulose tape collection for pinworms | | | | |
| 46-7 Mono-Test for infectious mononucleosis | | | | |
| **Total points section 9 34 procedures** | **A = 92-102** | **B = 82-91** | **C = 72-81** | **D = below 72** |
| **Section 10**—Advanced clinical care techniques | | | | |
| 47-1 Reading food labels | | | | |
| 47-2 Determining fat fold measurements | | | | |
| 48-1 Calculating the correct dosage for administration | | | | |
| 48-2 Calculating the correct dosage for administration using two systems of measurement | | | | |
| 48-3 Calculating the correct dosage for child when only adult measurement available | | | | |
| 48-4 Calculating the correct dosage for administration using body weight | | | | |
| 49-1 Filling a syringe | | | | |
| 49-2 Giving an intramuscular injection | | | | |
| 49-3 Giving a Z-tract intramuscular injection | | | | |
| 49-4 Giving a subcutaneous injection | | | | |
| 49-5 Giving an intradermal injection | | | | |
| 50-1 Identifying surgical instruments | | | | |
| 51-1 Hand washing for assisting with surgical procedures | | | | |

| **PROCEDURES in Text & Mastery Manual** ⇓ | AEL = 3 points Above expected performance level first attempt = A **POINTS** ⇓ | EL = 2 points At expected performance level with first attempt = B **POINTS** ⇓ | EL = 1 point At expected performance level after 2 or 3 attempts = C **POINTS** ⇓ | BEL = 0 points More than 3 attempts = below expected performance **POINTS** ⇓ |
|---|---|---|---|---|
| 51-2 Gloving using the open glove method | | | | |
| 51-3 Gowning with a sterile gown | | | | |
| 51-4 Gloving using the closed glove technique | | | | |
| 52-1 Transferring sterile instruments | | | | |
| 52-2 Pouring a sterile solution into a container on a sterile field | | | | |
| 52-3 Preparing a patient's skin for surgery | | | | |
| 52-4 Opening a sterile pack that will serve as a sterile field | | | | |
| 52-5 Opening a sterile pack to add contents to sterile field | | | | |
| 52-6 Adding sterile items in a peel-back wrapper to a sterile field | | | | |
| 52-7 Assisting during a minor surgical procedure | | | | |
| 52-8 Assisting with suturing | | | | |
| 52-9 Removing sutures | | | | |
| **Total points section 10 21 procedures** | **A = 68-75** | **B = 60-67** | **C = 52-59** | **D = below 52** |
| **Total points all procedures** Total number procedures 155 | **A = 432-480** | **B = 384-431** | **C = 336-430** | **D = 288-335** |
| Additional procedures | | | | |
| 25 developing patient teaching plans | | | | |
| | | | | |
| | | | | |
| | | | | |
| | | | | |
| | | | | |
| Total points instructor-added procedures | | | | |

## References

### Internet sites

Curriculum ideas and activities : **http://www.microsoft.com/education/hed/faculty/curric.htm**
Community College page: **http://www.microsoft.com/education/hed/ccpage.htm**

### Books and Pamphlets

Barsch J: Barsch Learning Style Inventory, 1980.

Diamond RM: *Designing and Assessing Courses and Curricula: A Practical Guide.* Jossey-Bass Higher and Adult Education Series, 1997.

Dirkx JM, et al.: *Guide for Planning and Implementing Instruction for Adults: A Theme-Based Approach.* Jossey-Bass Higher and Adult Education Series, 1997.

Kolb DA: *Experiential Learning: Experience as the Source of Learning and Development.* Englewood Cliffs, NJ, Prentice-Hall, 1984.

Krathwohl D, Bloom BS: *Taxonomy of Educational Objectives, Handbook 1: Cognitive Domain.* United Kingdom, Longman Group, 1984.

Langenbach M: *Curriculum Models in Adult Education,* Krieger Publishing Co., 1993.

Mager R: *Preparing Instructional Objectives.* Palo Alto, Fearon Publishers, 1963.

Steenburgen-Gelb F: *A Practical Guide to Writing Goals and Objectives.* Academic Therapy Publications, 1981.

Svinicki M, Dixon R: "The Kolb Model Modified for Classroom Activities," *College Teaching* 1987; 35 (4).

Walker DF: *Curriculum and Aims.* Thinking About Education Series, Jonas F. Soltis, Paperback, 1987.

# PART 2

## APPLYING THE TOTAL LEARNING SYSTEM BY CHAPTER

# 1

# Introduction to Medical Assisting

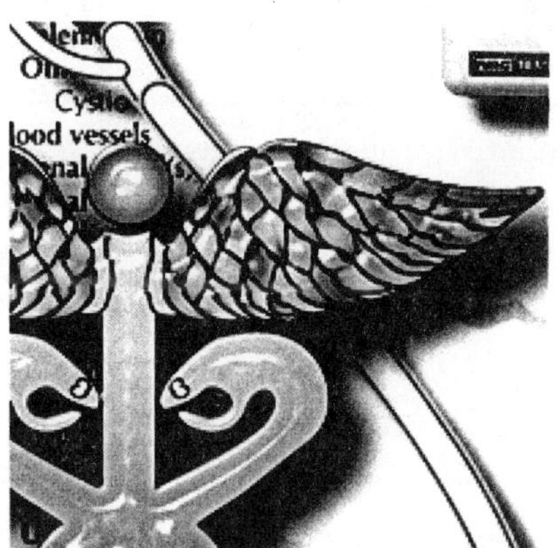

This is probably the first day of class for the students. They will give their complete attention. Their anxiety levels are high and the instructor can use this opportunity to start out by planning an introduction that is helpful to the students. Many students have no idea how they learn or how to study to their strengths. This is an opportunity to administer a learning style survey. Obtain one through counselors or the special education division of your school. The survey may be brief and should include materials to guide the instructor in suggesting study techniques directed to particular learning styles. Students are grateful for this help. Enthusiasm, confidence, and motivation to succeed are immediately enhanced.

## USING THE LEARNING SYSTEM

### 1. MEDICAL ASSISTANT ENTRY-LEVEL CURRICULUM

CONTENT Relate to objectives on Textbook p. 3 and Chapter 1 Mastery Manual.

- Personal attributes
- Project a professional manner and image
- Job readiness
- Workplace dynamics
- Allied health professions and credentialing

Review the above content using the following grid and explain how students develop knowledge in these areas and how these items lay the foundation for medical assistant education. Presume these are the students' first introductions to professional and ethical concepts. Explain that these items will be reinforced for the entire length of the program. Students will be evaluated on these items in the externship program.

### 2. MEDICAL ASSISTANT ENTRY-LEVEL CURRICULUM INTERFACE

| TEXTBOOK OBJECTIVES | LEARNING SYSTEM LOCATION | MA CURRICULUM |
|---|---|---|
| **Cognitive** | | **Content** |
| 1. Identify 10 career opportunities available to a trained MA | • Text p. 4–5<br>• Manual Part 1-A | • Job readiness<br>• Allied health professions and credentialing |
| 2. List five personality traits that are beneficial to the successful MA | • Text p. 8<br>• Lesson plan<br>• Manual Part 1-C | • Personal attributes<br>• Project a professional manner and image |

*chart continues on following page*

| TEXTBOOK OBJECTIVES | LEARNING SYSTEM LOCATION | MA CURRICULUM |
|---|---|---|
| **Cognitive** | | **Content** |
| 3. Identify at least five general knowledge areas in which the medical assistant should be proficient | • Manual Part 1-C | • Personal attributes<br>• Project a professional manner and image<br>• Job readiness<br>• Workplace dynamics<br>• Allied health professions and credentialing |
| 4. Differentiate administrative and clinical MA responsibilities | • Manual Part 1-D & 1-E | • Job readiness<br>• Workplace dynamics |
| 5. Describe MA training programs available | • Text p. 6<br>• Lesson plan | • Job readiness<br>• Workplace dynamics<br>• Allied health professions and credentialing |
| 6. Name four professional organizations that provide educational opportunities and certification examinations | • Text pp. 10–11<br>• Manual Part 1-F and Part 3 | • Project a professional manner and image<br>• Job readiness<br>• Allied health professions and credentialing |

## 3. RESOURCES

Learning style questionnaires available for purchase include:

- Learning style inventory by Kolb
  McBer and Company, 116 Huntington Ave, Boston, MA 02116 617-437-7080
- The Learning Tape Measure
  Excel Inc, 23385 Old Barrington road, Barrington, IL 60010 847-382-7272
- Barsch Learning Style Survey @ amazon.com

Assigning topics and using the Internet is one of the easiest ways to allow students to become computer comfortable. Re-entry students particularly respond well to these exercises. Internet and computer time is available at public libraries, adult education schools, college libraries, and some businesses.

See Mastery Manual answers in Section 6, Part 1-F for sites specific to this chapter.

## 4. LESSON PLAN TIME 2 hours lecture, 3 hours lab

**Opening:** Greet students at the door this first day of class. Introduce self; be sure to include instructional qualifications. Have students introduce themselves. After Chapter 1, always assign students to study, outline, and record chapter highlights to prepare them for the lesson to be discussed in the next class.

Approx. 30 min.

**Pretest:** Instructional skills survey.
Obtain from school or resource list. When completed, review the learning styles and activities in Table I-2, p. 7 from the Introduction. Use these activities as suggestions for all students. Obtain a show of hands regarding student understanding of where Medical Assistants are employed, length of training, credentialing, etc.

Approx. 30 min.

**Objectives:** Compare content with the objectives, which cover all learning levels. Explain use of the Mastery Manual. Cover use of the Mastery Manual "Parts" and instructor expectations. Explain use of the Mastery Manual in the Total Learning System.
Discuss the differing levels of learning as noted in Part 1 of each chapter. Explain use of the CD-ROM for this program. There is no specific application in the CD-ROM for Chapters 1, 2, or 3. This will allow the instructor to arrange for access to a CD-ROM-equipped computer on campus, through the public library, or for personal use. Most students will be able to complete these activities as assigned. Instructors should complete all CD-ROM activities before assigning to students.

Approx. 10 min.

**Content:** Use the textbook objectives to review all content and then have students complete Mastery Manual Part 1 within the class.

Approx. 30 min.

This chapter is easy to grasp, and use of the Manual covers all the textbook objectives. Use the learning time to complete Chapter 1, Part 1. Use the lab time to complete and discuss Parts 2 and 3. This will stimulate lively discussion and begin to develop ethical concepts. Have students identify, using the telephone book, potential employers, and types of health care services that may use the MA.

**Assignment:** Read and study Chapters 1 and 2. Write answers to Textbook items for both chapters. Write on board before class. Call students by first name at least three times to memorize names ASAP.

**Posttest:** Hand out two objective statements and have students complete and turn in.

Approx. 10 min.

**Total time 110 minutes**

## 5. MASTERY MANUAL ANSWERS

### PART 1 CONTENT MASTERY

This Part addresses the levels in the learning process as presented earlier in the curriculum guide. The learning levels are listed with the answers below.

#### A. Learning Level: Knowledge

Responses show materials have been memorized. All matching exercises give students definitions from Textbook p. 4. Towards the end of various courses students should be able to write their own accurate definitions. Answers: Text p. 4 or below.

1. c; 2. e; 3. h; 4. g; 5. i; 6. a; 7. j; 8. b; 9. d; 10. f

#### B. Learning Level: Comprehension

Reponses indicate student understands some of the concepts. Obviously, not all concepts are covered here. Many are covered in the testbank or as students use CD-ROM ⊕. As students complete activities in the future, note dress and manner of some of the medical assistants in the CD-ROM.

Answers:

1. There is no mandatory retirement for medical assistants. It depends upon office policy.
2. Most physicians have more than one medical assistant.
3. Facilities tend to hire trained persons, especially in a medical office. Many insurance companies now require certified medical assistants.
4. Job turnover getting higher but still very stable.
5. Everyone needs training in CPR, especially anyone working in a medical facility.

#### C. Learning Level: Application

Answers: Proficiency in 1, 3, 4, 7, 8, 9

#### D. Learning Level: Analysis

Answers:
Adminstrative areas are 2, 3, 5, 6, 7

Clinical areas are 1, 4, 8, 9, 10

Other competencies are listed in the chapter under heading titled DUTIES

#### E. Learning Level: Synthesis

Student is judging materials. Answers will be individual to each student. This activity is directed toward helping students evaluate competencies based on the knowledge they had before entering the program and what they perceive as important today. This will give you, the instructor, the ability to discuss perceptions and clarify student reasoning as needed. Remember, adults find it difficult to change preconceived ideas.

#### F. Learning Level: Evaluation

This activity serves to bring in other sources to explain the profession. In a fun and exploratory manner, it helps students begin to use computer technology. Obtaining Internet sites may be limited to a few students depending upon computer, modem, and Internet access. Many school libraries provide access, and you may be able to take students as a group to start them on their Internet adventure.

All sites unless otherwise designated begin: http://www.

1. This site will lead you to others:
http://sc1.switchboard.com/SideClick/1/navsp.asp?MEM=1

2. This site will lead students to national health related associations:
http://www.ama-assn.org/med_link/nation.htm.

www.chaospro.com/wssma/cma.html [Certifying information site]

3. Specific association sites include the following sites:
www.aama-ntl.org/dedicate/htm [AAMA site:]

www.cmaa-ca.org [California organization site:]

http://www.aapc-natl.org/ [AAPC site]

## PART 2 COMPETENCY CHALLENGE

While there are no specific competencies in the chapter, the development of professional attitudes may lead to professional dress and image. Be sure to discuss these ideas in lab time and encourage students to express thoughts. Differentiate thought and behavior versus feelings. These problem-solving incidents reinforce the significant ideas and content included in the chapter. They also carry the student into affective areas of thinking where values can be discussed. The goal is to raise the student's level to evaluate, think, and judge on an ethical level regarding discretion and professionalism.

Situation A: This is not discrete behavior

Situation B: Polly is not exhibiting professional behavior. She needs to be less "flashy" and to work with the team.

## PART 3 CLINICAL APPLICATIONS

According to the 8th Edition Textbook, professionalism is demonstrated by a trained person who is certified, has a pleasant and positive attitude, is courteous, empathetic, discreet, well groomed, takes initiative and responsibility, and is sensitive to ethnic diversity. Lastly, professionals voluntarily take part in continuing education. Professionalism in the person trained on the job (OJT) is not easily determined. Certainly, according to the book it does not meet the criteria. But today there are many persons who do meet the standards as the physician has educated them very well and they are certified by the AAMA. It would depend upon many variables, but probably it is not for anyone but the supervisor or physician to judge and act upon.

# 2

# Medical Assisting Externship and Preparing to Find a Position

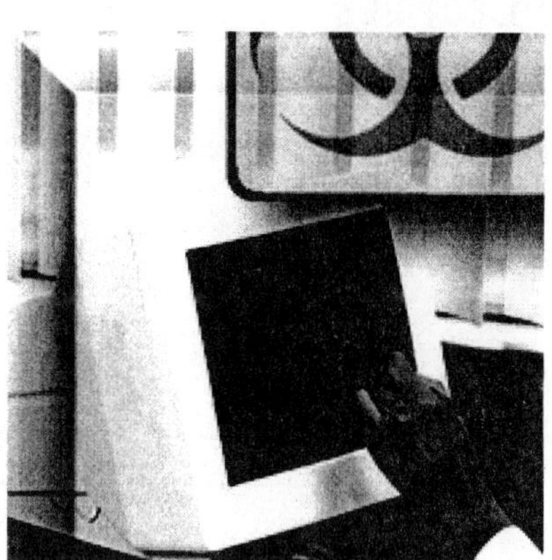

In a vocational education program, success is measured by the students' ability to obtain employment. The activities in this chapter allow you to prepare students for externship expectations. Usually your program will have an externship packet with student guidelines, medical office procedures, confidentiality statements, task records, and immunization and evaluation forms. Students usually complete resume writing toward the end of the externship. An introduction to the externship and importance of resume preparation is sometimes covered early in the course and more thoroughly before completion.

## USING THE LEARNING SYSTEM

### 1. MEDICAL ASSISTANT ENTRY-LEVEL CURRICULUM

CONTENT

- Apply knowledge
- Develop professional attitudes
- Job readiness

COMPETENCIES

- Developing professional attitudes
- Interacting with other health care professionals
- Interacting with patients
- Performing administrative procedures
- Performing clinical procedures

### 2. MEDICAL ASSISTANT ENTRY-LEVEL CURRICULUM INTERFACE

| TEXTBOOK OBJECTIVES | LEARNING SYSTEM LOCATION | MA CURRICULUM |
|---|---|---|
| **Cognitive** | | **Content** |
| 1. Define and spell terms in the Vocabulary | • Text p. 14<br>• Manual Part 1-A | • Apply knowledge<br>• Job readiness |
| 2. List five personality traits that are beneficial to the successful MA | • Text p. 8<br>• Manual Part 1-B | • Job readiness<br>• Developing professional attitudes |

*Chart continues on following page*

| TEXTBOOK OBJECTIVES | LEARNING SYSTEM LOCATION | MA CURRICULUM |
|---|---|---|
| Cognitive | | Content |
| 3. Briefly explain four responsibilities of the student during externship | • See content list<br>• Text p. 15<br>• Manual Part 1-B | • Apply knowledge<br>• Interacting with other health care professionals<br>• Interacting with patients<br>• Performing administrative procedures<br>• Performing clinical procedures |
| 4. Describe the responsibilities of an externship office | • Text p. 15<br>• Manual Part 1-B | • Job readiness<br>• Workplace dynamics |
| 5. Explain how a student will benefit from externship experience | • Text p. 15<br>• Manual Part 1-B | • Job readiness<br>• Workplace dynamics<br>• Interacting with other health care professionals<br>• Developing professional attitudes |
| 6. List the three steps in applying for a position | • Text p. 16<br>• Manual Part 1-B | • Developing professional attitudes<br>• Interacting with other health care professionals |
| 7. Identify the five essential parts of a personal inventory | • Manual Part 1-B<br>• Manual Part 2-1 | • Job readiness<br>• Developing professional attitudes |
| 8. List seven basic items that should be included in every resume | • Text p. 19<br>• Manual Part 2<br>• Procedure 2-1 | • Job readiness<br>• Interacting with other health care professionals |
| 9. Specify five items that must not be inserted in a resume | • Text p. 19<br>• Manual Part 1-B-4 | • Job readiness<br>• Developing professional attitudes |
| 10. Cite five sources of leads for employment as a medical assistant | • Text p. 19<br>• Manual Part 1-F | • Job readiness<br>• Interacting with other health care professionals |
| 11. List three avenues of evaluation that an interviewer may use in selecting an employee | • Text p. 20 | • Interacting with other health care professionals<br>• Job readiness<br>• Developing professional attitudes |

| PERFORMANCE OBJECTIVES | All completed in Part 2 and 3 of Mastery Manual | COMPETENCY |
|---|---|---|
| 1. Prepare a personal inventory | • Text p. 16<br>• Mastery Manual Part 2 | • Applying knowledge<br>• Developing professional attitudes<br>• Interacting with other health care professionals<br>• Interacting with patients<br>• Job readiness |
| 2. Prepare two examples of a resume | • Procedure 2-1<br>• Mastery Manual Part 2 | |
| 3. Demonstrate a telephone request for an interview | • Lab demonstration | |
| 4. Write a letter in response to a newspaper Help Wanted ad | • Mastery Manual Part 2<br>• Procedure 2-2 | |
| 5. Compose a follow-up letter of thanks after an interview for a position | • Mastery Manual Part 2 | |

## 3. RESOURCES

Collect samples of resumes from re-entry or career search departments.
Local employment development or state job training agency may provide a speaker.
Professional Medical Assistant May/June 1998

www.monster.com **The Monster Board 1-800-666-7837**

www.healthopps.com **Health Opps 1-800-293-2700**

www.medsearch.com **Medsearch 1-800-899-7058**

## 4. LESSON PLAN TIME 2 hours lecture, 3 hours lab

**Opening:** This depends upon whether the class is covered early in the program or near time of externship experience and completion. It is suggested that this be covered as close to the actual experience as possible. Seminar as part of the externship is an excellent time to complete resume writing. If reviewed early in the course, only have students do activities in Part 1, items A and B and leave the remainder until later. These items cover basic theory. The others are for use when they can be applied in a timely manner.

**Pretest:** Find out how many have had OJT or written a resume

**Objectives:** Post them prominently and review

**Content:** Lesson 1, 2 hr—Go through the objectives and questions with the students. This chapter covers the latest techniques on resume writing. Review the content and competency Transparency Master #1 items, explaining their use in the medical office. Have students orally answer Textbook memory joggers. If you have an externship policy and procedure manual, this is a good time to distribute it to students. Talk to students about attendance and its importance, especially when it comes to letters of recommendation.
Lesson 2 (lab), 2 hr—Have a guest lecturer to help students put together a beginning resume.
Lesson 3 (lab), 1 hr—Finalize resume.

**Assignment:** Lesson 1—Complete personal data sheet for resume writing class.
Lesson 2 (lab)—Type resume for last hour of lab.

**Posttest:** Take each student through an interview process as an extracurricular activity. Sometimes externship sites will assist with this activity. Other times colleagues in the school may conduct one or two interviews for students. The object is to obtain comments on student interview skills and give suggestions for improvement.

**Absent students:** Speak to students as soon as they return. Ask if they are well. Remind them to check with another student to see what was missed and to check syllabus for assignments. Speak to all students about makeup policy for quizzes and tests.

**Notes:**

## 5. MASTERY MANUAL ANSWERS

### PART 1 CONTENT MASTERY

This Part addresses the levels in the learning process as presented earlier in the curriculum guide. The learning levels are listed with the answers below.

#### A. Learning Level: Knowledge

1. d; 2. h; 3. e; 4. a; 5. i; 6. g; 7. c; 8. j; 9. f; 10. b

#### B. Learning Level: Comprehension

1. Benefits to student—may obtain job, learns exactly what is expected in working world, learns deficits and areas to improve, may be able to educate office employees with new techniques.

   Responsibilities of student—Professional appearance and behavior, report at specified days and times, expect supervision, sign confidentiality and privacy statement.
2. Responsibilities of the externship office to the student in externship—must agree to complete student evaluation, agree to provide student with opportunity to complete required skills, not use as an extra free employee, provide constant supervision.
3. a-d—These are really self-explanatory to the instructor.
4. Photograph, names of spouse or children, place of birth, religious preference, age, marital status, references, reason for leaving position, previous salary

#### C. Learning Level: Application

The questions to ask oneself before applying for a job are:
How did I perform in my externship experience? What are my strengths and weaknesses? What type of work do I want? Where can I function best? Am I a team player? How do I handle stress and fast pace? Do I prefer clinical or administrative work? Do I like small groups or large? Do I like family practice or specialty? How important are salary, hours, location? What are my minimum desires?
Employer considerations are: Is my application complete? Do I look professional? Do I function well with others as part of a team? Do I take criticism personally? How did I function as a student on the job?

The answers are variable according to the student.

#### D. Learning Level: Analysis

Distinguish working conditions and opportunities between a family practice and a specialty office. Students will need help with this from instructor and their current perceptions of the way things are in these offices. Answers will vary according to region and experience.

#### E. Learning Level: Synthesis

Steps in applying for a job should be orderly and include:
a. Decide type of position; b. write sample resume; c. write sample cover letter, d. set time lines and date for availability; e. write questions to ask employer; f. look for advertised positions; g. finalize and send resume and cover letter.

#### F. Learning Level: Evaluation

The students need to complete this exercise before completion of the Medical Assistant program.

## PART 2 COMPETENCY CHALLENGE

As instructors, it is our responsibility to have students prepare themselves for the local job market. After students prepare their data sheet is a good time to have someone come from the school employment or re-entry office to help students with a basic resume design format and help students prepare their resumes. Have students bring in a newspaper and hand write the inquiry letters in class. They may then complete them on computer.

## PART 3 CLINICAL APPLICATIONS

1. Is it ethical? This can be an enthusiastic discussion as you lead students through the problem-solving process outlined in Chapter 4, Part 3. As instructors, it is interesting to keep notes on the results each year.

   When students can compare what they need to learn to do a real analysis of the job, it increases motivation and enthusiasm for learning. If the students do not feel competent at this time, it is time for them to problem solve and plan strategies to reach mastery. Often we can pass a test, yet not feel competent to do a job. Volunteering in the medical field is a good way to develop competence.

   This is the first chapter with procedures written with Competency Objectives. It is suggested that you have all the students complete the personal data sheets at home and then work on the resume in a lab or class setting.

2. When you go to fill out a job application, what items should you take with you?

   Black pen, index card with dates of schooling, experiences, words easily misspelled, resume, references, letters of recommendation, Wite-Out.

# 3

# A Brief History of Medicine

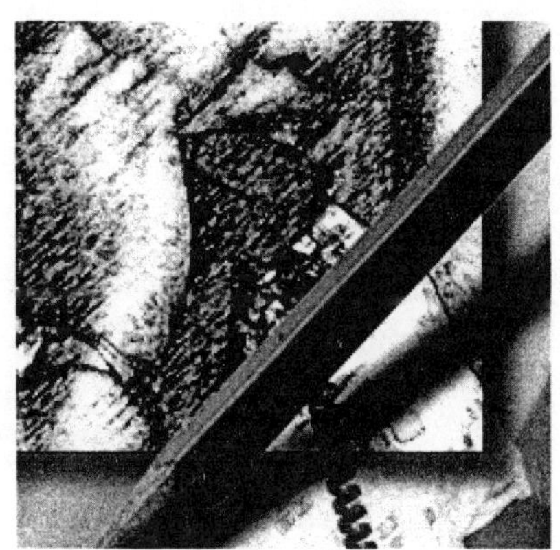

This chapter is covered as a matter of interest and appreciation to the student. Appreciation of history in one's subject develops perspectives in working as a team member, developing ethical standards, and promoting lifelong learning. The exercises cover all the chapter objectives in a variety of forms. Part 1 activities are self-explanatory and are objective-oriented. Part 2 and 3 exercises require critical thinking, using judgment, and forming values. It is hoped that they will enlighten the student to the value of lifelong learning and the necessity to be aware of changes in modern medicine.

## USING THE LEARNING SYSTEM

### 1. MEDICAL ASSISTANT ENTRY-LEVEL CURRICULUM

CONTENT

- Hereditary, cultural, and environmental influences on behavior
- Adaptations for individual's needs
- Word building and definitions
- Applications of medical terminology

### 2. MEDICAL ASSISTANT ENTRY-LEVEL CURRICULUM INTERFACE

| TEXTBOOK OBJECTIVES | LEARNING SYSTEM LOCATION | MA CURRICULUM |
|---|---|---|
| **Cognitive** | | **Content** |
| 1. Define and spell terms in the Vocabulary | • Text pp. 26-27<br>• Manual Part 1-A | • Word building and definitions<br>• Applications of medical terminology |
| 2. Identify two ancient mythologies that contributed a major part of medical terminology | • Text p. 27<br>• Manual Part 1-B | • Word building and definitions<br>• Applications of medical terminology |
| 3. Distinguish between and describe the two medical symbols in general use today | • Text p. 28<br>• Lesson plan | • Hereditary, cultural, and environmental influences on behavior |

*Chart continues on following page*

| TEXTBOOK OBJECTIVES | LEARNING SYSTEM LOCATION | MA CURRICULUM |
|---|---|---|
| **Cognitive** | | **Content** |
| 4. Name the oath that has been given to new physicians for more than 2,000 years | • Text p. 15<br>• Lesson plan | • Hereditary, cultural and environmental influences on behavior |
| 5. Name the most famous medical school at the end of the 19th century | • Text p. 3<br>• Lesson plan | • Hereditary, cultural, and environmental influences on behavior |
| 6. Name the 20th century educator who played a major role in developing U.S. medical education | • Text p. 30<br>• Lesson plan | • Hereditary, cultural, and environmental influences on behavior |
| 7. Identify the important discovery made by W. Harvey and substantiated 200 years later | • Text p. 31<br>• Manual Part 1-C | • Hereditary, cultural, and environmental influences on behavior |
| 8. Name the 18th century English surgeon declared the Founder of Scientific Surgery (John Hunter) | • Text p. 32 | • Hereditary, cultural, and environmental influences on behavior |
| 9. Name the Hungarian physician who earned the title "Savior of Mothers" | • Text p. 37<br>• Manual Part 1-B & 1-C | • Hereditary, cultural, and environmental influences on behavior |
| 10. List the names of five 19th-century women who contributed significantly to medical history | • Text pp. 36-37<br>• Manual Part 1-B & 1-C | • Hereditary, cultural, and environmental influences on behavior |
| 11. Name the surgeon who performed the first human heart transplant | • Text p. 3<br>• Lesson plan | • Hereditary, cultural, and environmental influences on behavior |
| 12. Name two agencies of the United States Department of Health and Human Services that play an important role in the advancement of health in the U.S. and the world | • Text p. 39<br>• Manual Part 3 | • Hereditary, cultural, and environmental influences on behavior |

## 3. RESOURCES

www.healthatoz.com **Go to the History of Medicine link**

- See Part 1-E for other Internet sites
- *Companion Encyclopedia of the History of Medicine,* Pay Porter, William F. Bynum, Editors. Routledge Companion Encyclopedia, 1994.
- Porter R: *The Greatest Benefit to Mankind: A Medical History of Humanity.*
- Gordon R: *The Alarming History of Medicine/Amusing Anecdotes from Hippocrates to Heart Transplants.* St Martin's Press, 1994.
- Vogel VJ: *American Indian Medicine* (Civilization of the American Series, Vol 95), University of Oklahoma Press, Reprint edition, 1990.
- Stevens R: *American Medicine and the Public Interest*, University of California Press, Updated edition, 1998.

## 4. LESSON PLAN TIME 2 hours lecture, 3 hours lab

**Opening:** Ask students what history means to them. How many history courses have they taken?

**Pretest:** Can students name a person who discovered something to do with medicine?What did they discover? Did students know about this person before reading the chapter? Are students aware there were only 137 cases of measles in the United States in 1996? It is soon to be eradicated and history will be made.

**Objectives:** Transparency Master 3-1
Use the 8th Edition Textbook. Write one affective objective. Use action verbs from Introduction.
Relate action verb to role delineation item. Objective may deal with perceptions, e.g., medical history being made today, smallpox eradicated, human genome project taken on by biotech firm and may be completed in 2001. How will these affect history?

**Content:**
Follow textbook outline and discuss the 8th Edition Textbook objectives using the Mastery Manual. Did students successfully complete Part 1 with instructor? The Mastery Manual Exercises meet most objectives. Complete Parts 2 and 3 in lab.

**Assignment:** For next chapter read, complete questions, be prepared to answer Mastery Manual Part 1 items. Know terms and definitions. Make flash cards for all chapters to date and put in alphabetical order; term on front, definition on back. Break all terms into medical parts when able.

**Posttest:** Use objective statements as questions. Have students list two important points discussed or use the Examaster testbank.

## 5. MASTERY MANUAL ANSWERS

### PART 1 CONTENT MASTERY

#### A. Learning Level: Knowledge

1. f; 2. i; 3. a; 4. h; 5. j; 6. c; 7. b; 8. e; 9. g; 10. d

catheterization: putting a tube into body cavities or hollow organs
chemotherapy: treatment of disease using chemicals

#### B. Learning Level: Comprehension

1. e; 2. h; 3. a; 4. b; 5. j; 6. f; 7. i; 8. d; 9. c; 10. g

#### C. Learning Level: Application

| Discoverer | Anatomy | Disease | Surgeries | Medical Rx | Sterilization |
|---|---|---|---|---|---|
| **Erlich** | 1900s | | | | |
| **Harvey** | 1600s | | | | |
| **Rush** | | 1700s | | | |
| **Koch** | 1800s | | | | |
| **Lister** | | | | | 1800s |
| **Reed** | 1900s | | | | |
| **Salk** | | | | 1900s | |
| **Long** | | | 1800s | | |

#### D. Learning Level: Analysis

Look at the stage of medicine today and imagine that these persons had not lived to make the discoveries they did. Students will contemplate the individual effects each pioneer has had on the overall scope of medicine. Would someone else have soon discovered the form of vaccination? Was his association of the maid's disease happenstance, and would another have tested in the same way? It doesn't seem so with today's medical research and experimentation requirements. We might not be as advanced as we are today in immunizations. Reassure students that there are no correct answers.

#### E. Learning Level: Synthesis

Some interesting Internet sites to give to the students are:

- www./yahoo.com/Health/Medicine/ **History is full of medieval medicine, people**
- www.pbs.org **This interesting site leads to people of the century and science and technology developments. An excellent resource.**
- www.historychannel.com **Many subjects and "This day in history"**
- http://www.asap.unimelb.edu.au/hstm/hstm_ove.htm **A link to the virtual library of Health, Science and Medicine**
- http://www.imss.org **This is the International Museum of Surgical Science and has lots of information on surgical breakthroughs. It also has an interactive page that allows one to be a patient in the 1800s**

## F. Learning Level: Evaluation

This area is all personal opinion, reasoning, and critical thinking. Developing Consensus is an interesting exercise, which enhances the concept of teamwork, as discussed in Chapter 1. It need not be used to stifle opinion or learning.

## PART 2 COMPETENCY CHALLENGE

There are no performance competencies in this chapter, however, discussion of Part 2 brings history into today's applications. This activity allows the adult learner to realize the need of these discoveries in a healthy society. A short discussion will increase appreciation of history and may heighten awareness of rapid changes in medicine, as well as reinforcing the need for lifelong education.

## PART 3 CLINICAL APPLICATIONS

There are many implications for today's medicine:

- genetic testing
- abortion for choosing baby's gender
- turning down patients for lack of insurance
- computer access to private information
- changing roles of health personnel

# 4

# Medical Practice Systems

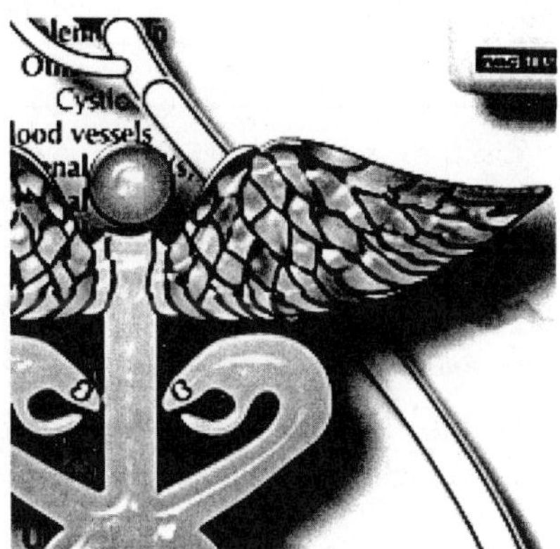

This chapter is directed to appreciating the development of medicine and its application to medical care today. Specialization has become increasingly complex, and the family practitioner has had a resurgence that requires more multiskilled personnel than ever before. The information in this chapter forms a foundation for the medical assistant to understand some of the business and financial practices of the medical office and specific types and uses of health delivery. You will begin to understand the way a medical assistant works with physicians and patients.

## USING THE LEARNING SYSTEM

### 1. MEDICAL ASSISTANT ENTRY-LEVEL CURRICULUM

CONTENT

- Applications of medical terminology
- Legal guidelines/requirements for health care
- Hereditary, cultural, and environmental influences on behavior
- Adaptations to individual needs
- Allied health professions and credentialing
- Job readiness

### 2. MEDICAL ASSISTANT ENTRY-LEVEL CURRICULUM INTERFACE

| TEXTBOOK OBJECTIVES | LEARNING SYSTEM LOCATION | MA CURRICULUM |
|---|---|---|
| **Cognitive** | | **Content** |
| 1. Define and spell terms in the Vocabulary | • Text p. 42<br>• Manual Part 1-A | • Applications of medical terminology |
| 2. Name the system of medical care delivery that has brought about a significant change in medical practice in the past decade | • Text p. 43<br>• Manual Part 2 | • Applications of medical terminology<br>• Hereditary, cultural, and environmental influences on behavior |
| 3. State the principal difference between the training of the M.D. and the D.O. | • Text pp. 44-45<br>• Manual Part 1-B | • Hereditary, cultural, and environmental influences on behavior<br>• Applications of medical terminology<br>• Legal guidelines/requirements for health care |

*Chart continues on following page*

| TEXTBOOK OBJECTIVES | LEARNING SYSTEM LOCATION | MA CURRICULUM |
|---|---|---|
| **Cognitive** | | **Content** |
| 4. List the three medical practice business structures discussed in the chapter | • Text p. 42<br>• Lesson plan | • Hereditary, cultural, and environmental influences on behavior<br>• Legal guidelines/requirements for health care |
| 5. Name and compare two principal methods of paying for medical care | • Text p. 43<br>• Manual Part 2 | • Hereditary, cultural, and environmental influences on behavior<br>• Legal guidelines/requirements for health care |
| 6. Identify 10 or more allied health occupations that might be represented in a medical practice | • Text p. 48<br>• Table 4-2<br>• Manual Part 1-F | • Hereditary, cultural, and environmental influences on behavior<br>• Adaptation to individual needs<br>• Allied health professions and credentialing |

## 3. RESOURCES

**The** history channel.com **and** yahoo.org/history **sites have some very interesting learning items. Internet sites for the students to use include:**

http://www.ama.org/

http://www.yahoo.com/health/

www.math.ubc.ca/Latin dictionary:

www.aama-ntl.org

State laws regarding the practice of medicine; California—Business and Professions Code

*The Professional Medical Assistant,* AAMA, Chicago, IL. Issues March/April 1994, Nov/Dec 1994

American Association of Medical Assistants 1-800-ACT-AAMA

State and federal laws regarding MA practice

## 4. LESSON PLAN    TIME 2 hours lecture, 3 hours lab

**Opening:** Hold up telephone book; read some of the specialties listed.

**Pretest:** Give the students a quick spelling test of the words in Vocabulary as the pre-test.

**Objectives:** This is a chapter where you can experiment writing one or two objectives specific to content items and then choose the chapter objectives you want students to meet.

**Content:** Follow content outline in textbook. Define each term in the outline very simply. Critical thinking activity 2 in textbook can be used to grasp an understanding of medical payment systems. Ensure students understanding that an HMO is a form of managed care. Explain the medical assistant role today. Begin discussions of type of care with which the MA can assist. Emphasize that the CMA examinations will address these items. Have students close texts. Review *orally* all the activities in Part 1 to cover chapter objectives and MA content requirements. Obtain feedback as to the importance or relevance of this information to students. Emphasize legal importance of business structure and delivery of care. Discuss legal limitations on various types of licensure, certification, etc. Oral review of all Mastery Manual items in Part 1 completes all chapter objectives through the learning cycle. Work through the difficult items together with students. Parts 2 and 3 are short, but they start students thinking.

**Lab:** Use lab time to orient students to the CD-ROM ⊕ . Case One ⊕ has a referral to a specialist.

**Assignment:** Next chapter, study, read, outline, or write answers to questions and be prepared to discuss critical thinking items.

**Posttest:** Vocabulary and spelling or Part 2 might serve as posttest.

## 5. MASTERY MANUAL ANSWERS

### PART 1 CONTENT MASTERY

### A. Learning Level: Knowledge

1. Dermatology 2. Allergy 3. Geriatrics 4. Neurology 5. Otorhinolaryngology 6. Psychiatry 7. Orthopedist or Physical Medicine 8. Pathology 9. Ophthalmology 10. Cardiothoracic surgeon

### B. Learning Level: Comprehension

| | **Medical doctor** | **Doctor of osteopathy** | **Chiropractor** | **Podiatrist** |
|---|---|---|---|---|
| **Initials of degree** | M.D. | D.O. | D.C. | D.P.M. |
| **Treatment allowed** | All medical disorders and surgeries. Must have specialty designation | Same as M.D. All branches of medicine and surgery | Manipulation of back only; physical therapy; no surgery | On feet only; certain specified surgeries, bunions, nails |
| **Prescriptions allowed** | All | All | Medications to treat disorders of back | None |

Check with your state licensing agency for prescription accuracy.

## C. Learning Level: Application

Student is able to include personal experience and opinion while applying new textbook knowledge learned about specialties. This is an opportunity to clarify specialty practice concepts.

## D. Learning Level: Analysis

Note: Tabers Cyclopedic Medical Dictionary allows for -ology or -ogy as complete suffixes. Either may be used. These word are split as combining forms.

| | |
|---|---|
| 1. Rheumato/logy | Gr. Rheumatismos/acute or chronic inflammation of joints/watery accumulation/ the study of |
| 2. Radio/graph/er | x-rays/ written/one who/ person who takes x-rays |
| 3. Ped/iatr/ics | children/ the treatment of/ pertaining to |
| 4. Uro/logy | urine/ the study of formation / diagnosis, treatment |
| 5. An/esthesiol/ogy | no/not/ sensation/ the study of |
| 6. Pulmon/olog/ist | lung/ the study of/ specialist |
| 7. Orthot/ist | straight/ specialist person who straightens bone and muscle deformities using external devices |
| 8. Cyto/ techno/logist | cell/work on/ special study |
| 9. Electro/neuro/diagnosti/cian | electric/ nerves/complete knowledge/ specialist |
| 10. Respirator/y Techn/ologist | breathing/act of /special study/ one who specializes in the study of |

## E. Learning Level: Synthesis

Types of health care support personnel may include

MA, or Medical Assistant—all treatments directed by M.D. unless excluded by law

Clinical Laboratory Technician—taking blood and performing laboratory tests. Some states allow the MA to perform part or all of this function

PA—treating patients and prescribing medications

RAD—taking x-rays

Surgical Technician—assisting at office surgeries

NP—specialists in nursing practice—assess, diagnose, and treat patients within scope of license

Students need to become aware of the scope of practice of all health care workers. This helps students to become aware of others' scope of practice in the medical office.

## F. Learning Level: Evaluation

This activity is designed to help students evaluate the different practices by discussing the various needs of each. The instructor can review the different specialties in a general way. Registration procedures are similar. Physical examination concentrates on the specialty area in great depth; the patient history taken is very extensive. Billing uses similar procedures but very complex terms relative to the specialty. Back office equipment is different for each specialty. Family practice may have one major piece of equipment for each specialty; e.g., an ECG machine but not Doppler or echocardiography equipment.

## PART 2 COMPETENCY CHALLENGE

The important points relate to the patient's right to the best care, best diagnosis, and the ethical reasoning of a family care physician realizing the patient's need for specialty expertise. Physicians may be able to do the same tasks but not interpret completely.

## PART 3 CLINICAL APPLICATIONS

A. Unethical. A specialist should treat only for the referred problem. The situation is hard to monitor except by an insurance carrier who might deny payment.

B. It is important to stress that patients have a right to know who is touching their body and the educational and professional level of the worker. It is deceitful to not wear a name tag . Most patients believe the persons in white are nurses caring for them, not other allied health persons. Most patients still think all nurses have the same preparation and degree.

# 5

# Medical Ethics

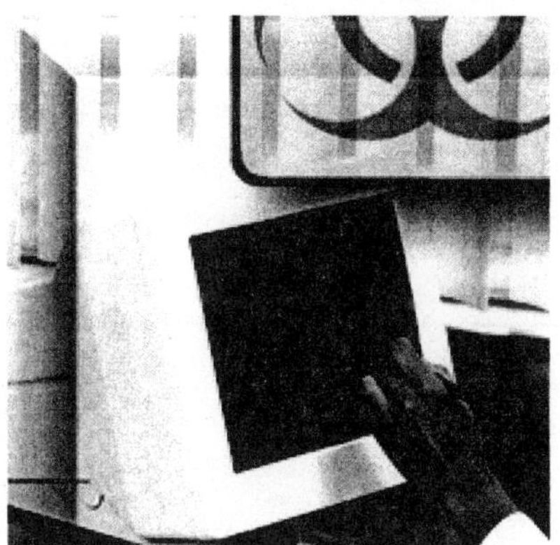

Ethics are complex, but basic principles remain fairly constant. It is important to understand the medical assistant's role in medical ethics. Students need to understand the following concepts:

- Ethics are directed toward the highest good and frequently require more of us than the law requires.
- Patient decisions are not a matter of judgment or conversation.
- The medical assistant has to honor the patient and leave medical decisions to the physician and patient.

You can teach students to solve ethical problems. Ethics in business, as in the medical office, asks that we do no harm, respect a person's right to make choices, promote the good of the office, and provide assistance to those in need. Whenever the medical assistant has contact with another or performs a service, ethical behavior will be considered the standard.

## USING THE LEARNING SYSTEM

### 1. MEDICAL ASSISTANT ENTRY-LEVEL CURRICULUM

CONTENT

- Medical ethics and related issues
- Basic principles of psychology
- Adaptations for individual's needs
- Practice within the scope of education, training, and personal capabilities

COMPETENCIES

- Identify and respond to issues of confidentiality
- Explain general office policies

All items are listed because they have ethical applications. These applications can be taught to students by raising consciousness of these issues and expecting ethical behavior in lecture and laboratory. After using Part 1 to meet the Textbook objectives, much of the rest of the Mastery Manual attempts to foster discussion of the medical assistant's ethical obligations and restrictions as stated in Objective 10.

## 2. MEDICAL ASSISTANT ENTRY-LEVEL CURRICULUM INTERFACE

| TEXTBOOK OBJECTIVES | LEARNING SYSTEM LOCATION | MA CURRICULUM |
|---|---|---|
| **Cognitive** | | **Content** |
| 1. Define and spell terms in the Vocabulary | • Text p. 51<br>• Manual Part 1-A | • Applications of medical terminology |
| 2. Differentiate between the terms *ethics* and *etiquette* | • Text p. 51 | • Medical ethics and related issues<br>• Basic principles of psychology<br>• Adaptations for individual's needs |
| 3. Identify the earliest written code of ethical conduct for medical practice | • Text pp. 51-52<br>• Manual Part 1-A & 1-C | • Medical ethics and related issues<br>• Basic principles of psychology |
| 4. Name the ancient Greek oath that remains an inspiration to physicians today | • Text p. 51<br>• Manual Part 1 | • Medical ethics and related issues |
| 5. Identify a code that was an example for the AMA Principles of Medical Ethics | • Text p. 52<br>• Manual Part 1-A | • Medical ethics and related issues |
| 6. State a significant reason for the 1980 revision of the AMA Principles | • Text p. 52<br>• Manual Part 1 | • Medical ethics and related issues<br>• Adaptation for individual needs |
| 7. State the maximum penalty that a medical society can impose upon a member for unethical conduct | • Text p. 53<br>• Manual Part 1 | • Medical ethics and related issues<br>• Adaptations for individual's needs |
| 8. Discuss what information about a patient may be released and to whom. | • Text pp. 55-56<br>• Manual Part 1-D | • Medical ethics and related issues<br>• Basic principles of psychology<br>• Adaptations for individual's needs<br>• Practice within the scope of education, training, and personal capabilities<br>• Identify and respond to issues of confidentiality<br>• Explain general office policies |

| TEXTBOOK OBJECTIVES | LEARNING SYSTEM LOCATION | MA CURRICULUM |
|---|---|---|
| **Cognitive** | | **Content** |
| 9. Discuss the application of ethics in dealing with fees and charges | • Text pp. 56-58<br>• Manual Part 1-D | • Medical ethics and related issues<br>• Basic principles of psychology<br>• Adaptations for individual's needs<br>• Practice within the scope of education, training, and personal capabilities<br>• Identify and respond to issues of confidentiality<br>• Explain general office policies |
| 10. Discuss the MA ethical obligations and restrictions | • Text p. 59, Fig. 5-4<br>• Manual Part 3 | • Medical ethics and related issues<br>• Basic principles of psychology<br>• Adaptations for individual's needs<br>• Practice within the scope of education, training, and personal capabilities<br>• Identify and respond to issues of confidentiality<br>• Explain general office policies |

## 3. RESOURCES

Journal: *Medical Ethics*
Purtillo, R. *Ethical Dimensions in the Health Professions,* 2nd Ed. Philadelphia, W.B. Saunders, 1993
Medcom/Trainex videos— "Advance directives" and "The right to die" PO Box 6003, 6060 Phyllis Drive, Cypress, California 90603 1-800-877-1443
Internet sites for medical ethics
http://www.expomed.com/ethics.htm **An interactive role-playing site for medical ethics issues**
www.yahoo.com **Medical ethics search: search criteria = ethics, medical**
There are about 40 more links here, usually to medical ethics questions, but some apply to office practice.

## 4. LESSON PLAN TIME 3 hours lecture, 9 hours lab

**Opening:** Try discussing Objective 2, or better yet, set up a situation with a student and be rude to her as an attention-getting role play. Then discuss what you did and how students felt observing the scene.

**Pretest:** Ask, "Who understands the meaning of ethics?" Explain textbook application.

**Objectives:** Review 8th Edition Textbook objectives and write two of your own, such as:

1. Students will name steps in decision making and give examples of their personal use of these steps.
2. Students will evaluate the handling of two clinical situations requiring decision making.

**Content:**

1. Put up a chart of the objectives and have students answer or discuss each.
2. Review Curriculum Content and extract an ethical situation pertaining to each.
   - Medical ethics and related issues. Confidentiality is critical.
   - Basic principles of psychology. When we understand psychology we can practice ethics with ease. We learn how to tactfully say, "Mind your own business."
   - Adaptations for individual's needs. We tell patients only information pertinent to them.
   - Practice within the scope of education, training, and personal capabilities. We do not give false assurances.
   - Identify and respond to issues of confidentiality. Do not discuss patients with friends, family, or staff (unless it's the physician).
   - Explain general office policies. Prepare patients for services, fees, etc. before they are given care.
3. Laboratory: Complete Parts 2 and 3 of Mastery Manual in lab. This gets students to the meat of ethics and raises cognitive evaluation skills quickly. Students really enjoy these activities.
4. One possible activity is to break students into groups of 4 to 5. When they discuss the situations, have each student write her personal opinion, and how it should be ethically handled, and then have the group come to a consensus on the best solution to the dilemma. This gives practice in teamwork dynamics.
5. Have group write any ethical dilemma and role play it. Have other groups offer opinions and suggestions.

**Assignment:** Complete Mastery Manual activities in Part 1. Read, study answer questions in next chapter.

**Posttest:** Use questions from testbank.

## 5. MASTERY MANUAL ANSWERS

### PART 1 CONTENT MASTERY

#### A. Learning Level: Knowledge

1. j; 2. g; 3. a; 4. e; 5. i; 6. h; 7. d; 8. b ; 9. f; 10. c

## B. Learning Level: Comprehension

Explanation of false statements

1. Physicians may take or reject any patient they desire as long as they do not discriminate regarding race or religion. Pediatric practices limit patients' ages. Other practices limit practice to specialties.
2. Standards apply to all.
3. Ethics require that everyone have access to the same care, but they do not require everyone to have the same care. This standard is currently developing and some ethicists ask that everyone receive the same minimum care.
4. Pregnant women who have a history of family disease and disorder may obtain genetic counseling, but it is not an ethical standard or a right.
5. The ethical principle of confidentiality applies to all areas of patient care. This principle is so important that it now has legal applications.

## C. Learning Level: Application

1. Current opinions are contained in The AMA Principles of Medical Ethics (annotated 1996-1997). These are the issues facing physicians today. Physicians violating these standards may be expelled from the medical society.
2. It was revised in 1980 to clarify and update language and balance standards. The current opinions further clarify the principles and are updated more frequently.
3. The earliest written code is the Code of Hammurabi, written by the Babylonians. The Hippocratic Oath is much better known today.

## D. Learning Level: Analysis

Decide whether the following behaviors concern etiquette or ethics and give your reasons.

1. Professional courtesy: an etiquette decision only. This is neither good nor bad
2. Ghost surgery: ethical decision—dishonest
3. Charging interest fees: etiquette
4. Medical assistant giving advice: ethical and legal
5. Releasing information: ethical and legal
6. Patient asks to see chart: ethical

**E** and **F** are personal opinion responses. Answers may be based on AAMA code of ethics and also on physician's current opinions.

## PART 2 COMPETENCY CHALLENGE

A. The three situations will bring many responses.

For Miss Gonzalez-Soler, the medical assistant needs to find out why she does not want to or cannot follow the diet. There is some type of barrier.

B. The insurance company must send a written request. There is no way the medical assistant can let information out unless the requesting party puts it in writing and the patient has agreed to the release of information.

## PART 3 CLINICAL APPLICATIONS

▲ See Appendix B in this guide.

Explain that the steps in decision making are necessary to help the student evaluate, judge, and consider ethical situations.

A. This model is an adaptation of the basic problem-solving model

1. State the problem as clearly as possible; an objective statement—neutral
2. Gather information; facts of situation, what caused problem
3. Identify ethical consideration or problem involved
4. Identify available solutions and the problems associated with each. Answer for each solution: what will be accomplished, does this have a positive benefit, can this apply to all situations, will it stand public scrutiny?

Select the best solution and implement the decision.

B. Review the Fundamental Elements from text p. 59 and Bill of Rights p. 60 with students. Relate these to medical assistant practice and responsibilities.

# 6

# Medicine and the Law

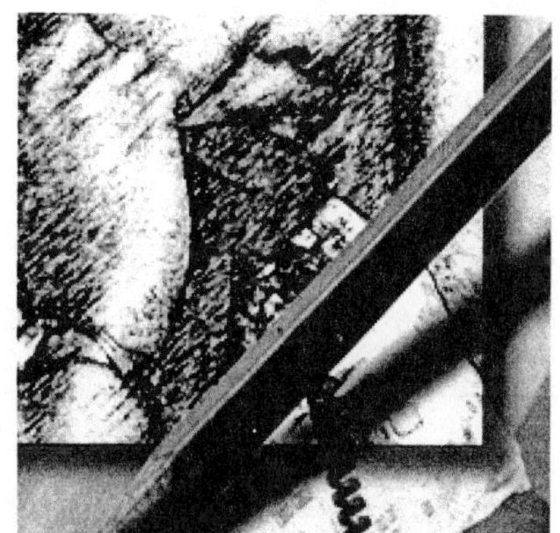

As medical assistant instructors, we have the responsibility to know the medical assistant's scope of practice and laws of our state regarding the practice of medicine. The lawyer for the local medical society can usually assist in explaining certain regulations and may provide you with copy of a legal handbook given to physician members. The medical assistant needs awareness of all the legalities surrounding medical practice. As an agent for the physician the medical assistant is involved in treating patients within legal limits of both criminal and civil laws, filing legal reports, and constantly living under the threat of malpractice suits. The medical assistant has great responsibility in assisting the physician with all legal requirements of practice and in preventing malpractice claims because of medical assistant actions.

## USING THE LEARNING SYSTEM

### 1. MEDICAL ASSISTANT ENTRY-LEVEL CURRICULUM

CONTENT

- Legal guidelines and requirements for health care
- Risk management

COMPETENCIES

- Identify and respond to issues of confidentiality
- Perform within legal and ethical boundaries
- Document appropriately
- Perform risk management procedures

### 2. MEDICAL ASSISTANT ENTRY-LEVEL CURRICULUM INTERFACE

| TEXTBOOK OBJECTIVES | LEARNING SYSTEM LOCATION | MA CURRICULUM |
|---|---|---|
| **Cognitive** | | **Content** |
| 1. Define and spell the terms listed in the Vocabulary | • Text p. 63<br>• Manual Part 1-A | • Medical terminology applications<br>• Perform within legal and ethical boundaries |
| 2. State the purpose of medical practice acts and how they are established | • Text p. 64 | • Legal guidelines and requirements for health care<br>• Risk management<br>• Perform within legal and ethical boundaries |

*chart continues on following page*

| TEXTBOOK OBJECTIVES | LEARNING SYSTEM LOCATION | MA CURRICULUM |
|---|---|---|
| **Cognitive** | | **Content** |
| 3. List the three methods by which licensure may be granted | • Text p. 65 | • Legal guidelines and requirements for health care<br>• Risk management<br>• Perform within legal and ethical boundaries |
| 4. List the general categories of cause for revocation or suspension of a license | • Text p. 65 | • Legal guidelines and requirements for health care<br>• Risk management<br>• Perform within legal and ethical boundaries |
| 5. Explain the difference between *criminal* and *civil* law | • Text p. 65<br>• Manual Part 1-B | • Legal guidelines and requirements for health care<br>• Perform within legal and ethical boundaries |
| 6. Define a contract and explain its importance in a health care facility | • Text pp. 65-66<br>• Manual Part 1-B | • Risk management<br>• Legal guidelines and requirements for health care<br>• Perform within legal and ethical boundaries |
| 7. Outline the correct way for a physician to terminate the physician-patient relationship | • Text p. 66<br>• Lawyer discussion | • Legal guidelines and requirements for health care<br>• Risk management<br>• Perform within legal and ethical boundaries |
| 8. State the four "Ds of Negligence" as published by the American Medical Association | • Text p. 68<br>• Lawyer discussion<br>• Manual Part 1-A | • Legal guidelines and requirements for health care<br>• Risk management<br>• Perform within legal and ethical boundaries |
| 9. Briefly describe the arbitration procedure and identify three advantages | • Text p. 71<br>• Lawyer discussion | • Legal guidelines and requirements for health care<br>• Risk management<br>• Perform within legal and ethical boundaries |
| 10. List the six components of informed consent | • Manual Part 1-C<br>• Lawyer discussion | • Legal guidelines and requirements for health care<br>• Risk management<br>• Perform within legal and ethical boundaries |

| TEXTBOOK OBJECTIVES | LEARNING SYSTEM LOCATION | MA CURRICULUM |
|---|---|---|
| Cognitive | | Content |
| 11. Explain the purpose of Good Samaritan Acts | • Lawyer discussion | • Legal guidelines and requirements for health care<br>• Risk management<br>• Perform within legal and ethical boundaries |
| 12. State two restrictions imposed on physicians by the Anatomical Gift Act | • Lawyer discussion | • Legal guidelines and requirements for health care<br>• Risk management<br>• Perform within legal and ethical boundaries |
| 13. Explain the medical assistant's role in claims prevention | • Lesson 2 instructor<br>• Text pp. 77-78<br>• Manual Parts 1-C, 1-D, 3 | • Legal guidelines and requirements for health care<br>• Risk management<br>• Perform within legal and ethical boundaries |

## 3. RESOURCES

a. Because students often minimize the impact of legal issues on the office, the chapter needs to reinforce their importance. Instructors will need to obtain state laws for all areas, particularly abuse reporting, communicable disease reporting and forms, treatment of minors, medical waste disposal, public health reporting requirements, state tax, and business laws.

b. Collect samples of forms from physician offices and hospitals to show to students.

c. Title 22 and other federal regulations show regulations pertinent to hospitals, clinical labs, etc.

Some interesting Internet sites pertinent to legal topics include:
http://www.legalethics.com/pa/fed/legis.htm
http://www.freeadvice.com
http://consumerlawpage.com **Articles, brochures, and more links**

## 4. LESSON PLAN    TIME 3 hours lecture, 9 hours lab

**Opening:** Introduce lawyer for Lesson 1. Plan for 2 to 3 hours.
Lesson 2: Ask students about personal experiences with reporting child abuse. Develop into subject about determining when and to whom to report.
**Note:** The student needs to acquire quite a bit of theory from this chapter. It needs to be first read and then discussed. The objectives the instructor will test must be clearly stated. It is best to review the chapter, assign the Mastery Manual, and then review the Mastery Manual in the labs. Use a lawyer to cover this material if possible. The lawyer for the local medical association may be willing to speak to the students.

**Pretest:** Omit for Lesson 1. Lesson 2, write 3 things learned from lawyer regarding MA practice.

**Objectives:**
**Lesson 1:** Some chapter objectives are not covered in the Mastery Manual. All objectives should be covered in the lawyer's discussion. Students must cover objectives to meet MA content requirements. It would be prudent to have the lawyer cover these topics and the items listed below in content.
Post the objectives as you and the lawyer have defined them. Make an outline of the topics to be discussed and incorporate them into objectives. Tell the guest you will have them posted to keep the subject on track.
**Lesson 2:** Write your own objectives directed to interactive learning experiences that the student can use to choose, respond, appreciate, formulate, and defend ethical and legal behaviors.

**Content:**
**Lesson 1:** This may be a lecture or discussion format. Suggested topic outline for lawyer includes materials from all objectives and especially 3, 4, 9, 11, 12, and 13 textbook objectives. Include the following topics: legal disclosures, federal regulations, common reasons for malpractice suits, confidentiality issues, legal treatment of minors, medical record requirements, computer security, treatment of personnel records, and telephone security.
**Lesson 2:** Have students give feedback on lawyer visit. Pick learning style activities from sample lesson plan to allow students to review the materials below. The goal is to raise consciousness above minimally legal behaviors to the practice of highly ethical reasoning and behaviors.
- Clarify legal concepts and medical assistant responsibilities
- Review specifics of state regulations, legal disclosures, and forms
- Review basic OSHA regulations and the Controlled Substances Act
- Discuss all Mastery Manual activities in class

**Laboratory hours:** Review the Mastery Manual for the objectives not covered by lawyer. Have students complete all Mastery Manual parts.
- Discuss with students what questions a prospective employer might ask a student to test the MA's understanding of state law and MA practice. Why is this knowledge important to an employer?
- Have students practice obtaining signed consents for procedures from classmates.
- Have students write a script for informed consent.
- Go on a field trip to small claims court. Get copies of forms that need to be served and spend at least 2 hours observing. Have students write a paper on the legal process. Can this information help them in the physician office?

**Assignment:** After lawyer presentation, require students to complete Mastery Manual Part 1 by next lab.

**Posttest:** Use Examaster testbank of issues addressed by lawyer and textbook memory joggers.

## 5. MASTERY MANUAL ANSWERS

### PART 1 CONTENT MASTERY

### A. Learning Level: Knowledge

1. f; 2. i; 3. e; 4. a; 5. g; 6. j; 7. b; 8. c; 9. h; 10. d

11. Civil law; administrative
12. Tort law
13. Malpractice
14. Duty—to patient, was contract legal
    derelict in duty—did physician meet the standard of care
    direct cause—resulted directly from treatment or lack thereof
    damages—did result to the patient

### B. Learning Level: Comprehension

1. Types of contracts—express (verbal) and implied
2. The components of legal contracts—offer & acceptance, legal subject matter, legal capacity, consideration
3. Importance of a contract in a health care facility—many procedures require consent and are covered by law as contracts; just seeing the patient makes a legal contract with rights and responsibilities for all personnel
4. Response will vary depending on the individual's experiences
5. A crime is punishable by jail; a tort is settled civilly as a suit

### C. Learning Level: Application

1. Missing components are: why the procedure should be done and the expected benefits of the proposed treatment
2. State the medical assistant's role in obtaining informed consent.

   The medical assistant asks the patient if the physician has explained all the components of informed consent. Then the medical assistant is merely a witness to the signature. The medical assistant is not a witness to the informed consent. It is best to have the person explaining the procedure obtain the consent.

### D. Learning Level: Analysis

List the major categories in which the OSHA regulations are contained.

1. Hazard communications
2. An exposure plan
3. Medical waste management plan
4. Housekeeping plan
5. Personal protective measures
6. General safety precautions
7. Fire safety plan
8. Staff development plan

### E. Learning Level: Synthesis

Reports usually go to the local public health department, which is a division of the USPHS. The reports are forwarded to the CDC.
Child abuse reporting does include the medical assistant because most states require health care workers to report suspected abuse.

### F. Learning Level: Evaluation

What legal requirements must the facility complete before you start work?
The first of three Hepatitis B injections and OSHA training as stated in the training plan.

## PART 2 COMPETENCY CHALLENGE

Peter Pepper has three teen-age children who have also been seen in the clinic. The oldest, Peter, Jr., is 16. He makes an appointment to be seen. When he checks in with the receptionist, she asks if his mom OK'd the visit. He says his visit is "private." The receptionist sets up the charge slip and sends it back with the chart. The physician treats him for a sexually transmitted disease.

1. Who is responsible for the bill?

   Mr. Pepper, but this is a real problem. If it is sent to Dad, he will know Pete was in and ask him about it. If insurance is used, Dad will get an EOB and still find out about Pete's visit.
2. Can Pete, Jr., authorize his own care?

   For STD, yes.
3. Who pays for the medication prescribed?

   Mr. Pepper, but Pete, Jr., probably will want to avoid telling his dad.
4. Does the parent have right to access the records?

   No.

## PART 3 CLINICAL APPLICATIONS

List one legally sound behavior for the listed items below. Completion will demonstrate an understanding of your ability to apply these objectives to your practice.

Example: Demonstrate initiative and responsibility.
Put a consent form with the patient's chart when a procedure is scheduled.

1. Do not promise a cure, but empathize; don't diagnose or prescribe.
2. Keep records of what was done and why. Send letter and payments as directed.
3 Use discretion in telephone and office conversations.
4. Do not perform a procedure if you are not trained. Ask for training.
5. File disclosure reports as required.
6. Always check with physician before releasing any information.
7. Do not perform tasks outside of your training or those prohibited by your office policy.
8. Keep toxic substances out of reach and clearly labeled.
9. Explain policies and procedures with brochures before patient sees physician.
10. Provide reports to financial firms every month.
11. Always wash hands between patients and when entering or leaving the office.
12. Make sure tests are accurate by carrying out quality control procedures. Have check-off lists.

# 7

# Interpersonal Skills and Human Relations

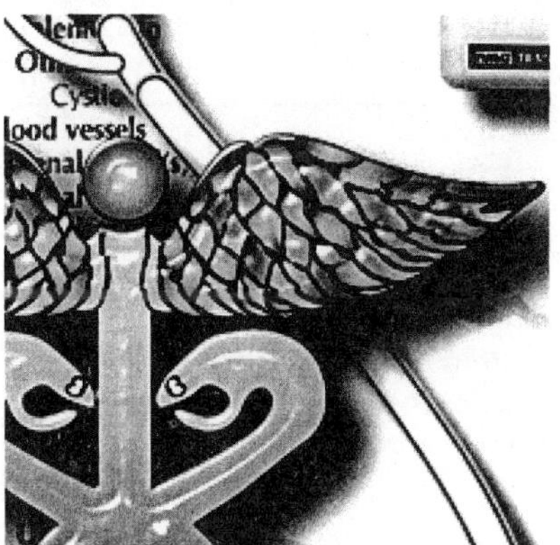

This chapter introduces the student to the concept of effective communications and the student's ability to develop those skills. It also reinforces the role of communication dynamics in understanding and applying information about demeanor, cultural differences, patient care, and teamwork. Through the learning system, students will be able to comprehend the material, apply many of the concepts, and evaluate their personal skills and behaviors. As instructors, it is important to reinforce that happy patients neither sue nor complain. The Mastery Manual meets all the Textbook objectives and MA entry-level curriculum.

## USING THE LEARNING SYSTEM

### 1. MEDICAL ASSISTANT ENTRY-LEVEL CURRICULUM

CONTENT

- Basic principles of psychology
- Mental health and applied psychology
- Principles of verbal and nonverbal communication
- Recognition and response to verbal and nonverbal communications
- Workplace dynamics

COMPETENCIES

- Recognize and respond to verbal and nonverbal communications
- Receive, organize, prioritize, and transmit information
- Instruct individuals according to their needs
- Explain general office policies
- Recognize and respond to oral communications

Review these at the start to enhance awareness and again at the end of the chapter.
In Part 3, discuss applications to patient communication. See the Role Delineation Study for even more specific lists.

## 2. MEDICAL ASSISTANT ENTRY-LEVEL CURRICULUM INTERFACE

| TEXTBOOK OBJECTIVES | LEARNING SYSTEM LOCATION | MA CURRICULUM |
|---|---|---|
| **Cognitive** | | **Content** |
| 1. Define and spell the terms in the Vocabulary | • Text p. 81<br>• Manual Part 1-A | • Basic principles of psychology |
| 2. State the factors that most influence the formation of a first impression | • Text p. 82<br>• Manual Part 1-C | • Basic principles of psychology<br>• Mental health and applied psychology |
| 3. List three distinct steps in communicating with the patient | • Text pp. 82-83<br>• Manual Part 1-A | • Mental health and applied psychology<br>• Principles of verbal and nonverbal communication<br>• Recognize and respond to verbal and nonverbal communications |
| 4. Name the three components of listening | • Text pp. 82-83<br>• Manual Part 1-D | • Principles of verbal and nonverbal communication |
| 5. List four possible barriers to communication | • Text pp. 83-84<br>• Manual Part 1-B | • Principles of verbal and nonverbal communication |
| 6. Briefly describe the paths of communication | • Text p. 84<br>• Manual Part 1-D | • Principles of verbal and nonverbal communication<br>• Recognize and respond to verbal and nonverbal communications |
| 7. List seven rules of good team cooperation | • Text p. 87<br>• Manual Part 2 | • Principles of verbal and nonverbal communication<br>• Workplace dynamics |
| 8. List and briefly describe the three styles of management | • Text p. 88<br>• Manual Part 1-F | • Workplace dynamics |
| | | **Competencies** |
| 9. Explain the meaning of being a patient advocate | • Text p. 89<br>• Manual Part 3 | • Respond to and initiate written communications<br>• Recognize and respond to verbal and nonverbal communications<br>• Receive, organize, prioritize, and transmit information<br>• Instruct individuals according to their needs<br>• Explain general office policies |

## 3. RESOURCES

Purtillo, R. *Health Professionals and Patient Interaction,* 5th edition, Philadelphia, W. B. Saunders, 1996.

**"Communication Skills," American Journal of Nursing, Videos. 555 West 57th St., New York, NY 10019-2961 1-800-225-5256.** www.ajn-ntl.org

**HRDQ Company—Specializing in communication training materials. Check for affordable games and activities for lab. 2002 Renaissance Blvd #100, King of Prussia, PA 19406-2756 1-800-633-4533.** www.hrdq.org

http://www.yahoo.com/Social Science/Communications **A general site with many links to specific communication topics**

http://www.yahoo.com/Social_Science/Communications/Intercultural_Communication/

http://search.excite.com/search.gw?search=communication+techniques+interpersonal+powerful+&tsug=2&csug=10&sorig=rpage **This site has many book references**

www.amazon.com **Search for topic "communication"**

## 4. LESSON PLAN **TIME 3 hours lecture, 9 hours activities**

**Opening:** Tape each student's non-dominant hand to his or her side and have the students stay in first hour of lecture with this disability.

**Pretest:** Have students take out a piece of paper and write all the physical barriers to communication they know. List some on the board.

**Objectives:** Use Textbook objectives plus these suggested affective objectives.

1. Select a personal communication behavior that needs improvement and write goals to change this behavior.
2. Plan responses to indicate phases of listening.
3. Choose and demonstrate a teamwork exercise and evaluate its effectiveness.
4. Examine three different cultures and examine their influence on medical office communications.

**Content:**
**Lesson 1:** Review, discuss, and have students give examples of personal experiences relating to the 8th Edition Textbook objectives. This material is easy to read, thought provoking, and very current. Students might read the chapter and write the answers to the objectives before starting discussion. The focus may be spent on having active participation throughout the lesson in both verbal and nonverbal communication forms.
**Lesson 2:** Lab—Complete as many of the activities in the Mastery Manual and CD-ROM as the time allots. In the CD-ROM review communication items and point to observing, listening, and response phases of communication. Other lab exercises might include:

1. Have a student choose a physical barrier and let another role-play a communication activity. If you can write them down beforehand, all students may try this. Provide questions for evaluation. What was hard to communicate? What new appreciation does student have for problems? How will student respond in future?
2. Using Part 1-E as a basis for the activity, have students role-play communication techniques with a barrier relating to each of the specific cultural traditions identified.

*Chart continues on following page*

3. Students go to any library and find a reference on communication. Make a list from the book of five effective methods of communication. Cite the pages and source. Discuss them in lab. Also list poor communication styles.
4. Observe a communication at home or someplace else. Write a brief description of what happened, including positive and negative observations and communications.
5. Play medical Pictionary or other game of nonverbal communication. Have students write their strong points and weak points in communication.
6. CD-ROM ⊕ See the Administrative Sections on reception telephone skills, correspondence, and taking a history. Point out communication styles on the CD-ROM ⊕ . Evaluate communication skills seen on the CD-ROM ⊕ . These activities are designed for mastery of the MA curriculum and associated textbook objectives.

**Assignment:**
Before Lesson 1: Have students write a one-page paper on the most important concept in the chapter and why it is so important.
Before Lesson 2: Complete Mastery Manual activities in Part 1.

**Posttest:**
Lesson 1: Student writes what he has learned about physical disabilities. Expect at least five responses.
Lesson 2: Questions from Examaster testbank or questions from objectives.

## 5. MASTERY MANUAL ANSWERS

### PART 1 CONTENT MASTERY

#### A. Learning Level: Knowledge

1. e; 2. f; 3. g; 4. h; 5. i; 6. j; 7. d; 8. c ; 9. b; 10. a
11. observation, listening, response

#### B. Learning Level: Comprehension

1. Empathy is an intellectual awareness or understanding of the feeling, whereas sympathy is a feeling or projecting relationship. Empathy is objective. Sympathy is judgmental.
2. Barriers are physical impairment, language, bias, discrimination, and personal prejudice.

Students might complete one role-play. Students who recognize the results of ineffective verbal and nonverbal communications are communicators that potentially may be very effective with patients.

#### C. Learning Level: Application

| **Behavior** | **Positive** | **Negative** |
|---|---|---|
| **Facial expression** | Smile | Grimace, frown |
| **Touching** | Hand shake<br>Assist onto examination table if necessary | Hand on arm or leg |
| **Stance** | Stand straight and listen | Hands on hips<br>Slouched and tired |
| **Hand gesture** | Wave hello, goodbye with eye contact | Dismissive gesture |

2. Other factors influencing first impressions include tone of voice, eye contact, grooming, and physical appearance.

## D. Learning Level: Analysis

There are various responses that are correct. Students should give examples of the responses they believe are appropriate to guide their thinking. Students with different cultural backgrounds may give varying answers.

## E. Learning Level: Synthesis

This is probably one of the most important exercises to complete in class. It allows students to use knowledge and apply it in communications with more people of different heritage.

## F. Learning Level: Evaluation

Autocratic personality style answers 7 or more as "usually"
Democratic style answers 7 or more as "sometimes"
Laissez-faire style answers 7 or more as "hardly ever"

Application: when a person is autocratic in her own personal style, she will carry those behaviors into the work setting. If one is autocratic, one needs to lighten up and learn coping skills. If your personal style is laissez-faire and the manager is autocratic, one needs to become more attentive and accountable. The easiest to be and work with are democratic communication and personality types.

## PARTS 2 AND 3

Students complete together in lab and have some roundtable discussions.

# 8

# Patient Reception

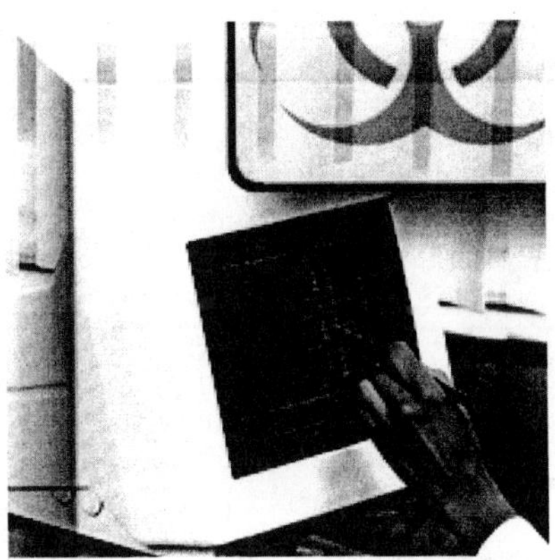

Activities in the Mastery Manual and CD-ROM meet chapter objectives and enhance student understanding of theMedical Assistant Curriculum Content and competencies. Students often tend to minimize reception functions, yet in "the real world," the professional will verify that this initial introduction for new and established patients sets the tone for the entire visit. In this chapter students need to understand the concept of customer service. Activities involve the student in using the levels of learning and in developing affective recognition of personal beliefs and behaviors. This awareness may lead to increased reasoning and application of ethical considerations.

## USING THE LEARNING SYSTEM

### 1. MEDICAL ASSISTANT ENTRY-LEVEL CURRICULUM

CONTENT

- Basic medical office functions
- Basic principles of psychology
- Mental health and applied psychology
- Document appropriately
- Project a professional manner and image

COMPETENCIES

- Instruct individuals according to their needs
- Explain office procedures and policies

Review with the student the use of these items in the medical office. For instance, the first person in the office is expected to pull patient charts for the day. Often the last person in the evening types or prints the appointment schedule. As you review the content involved, all the items will be discussed.

## 2. MEDICAL ASSISTANT ENTRY-LEVEL CURRICULUM INTERFACE

| TEXTBOOK OBJECTIVES | LEARNING SYSTEM LOCATION | MA CURRICULUM |
|---|---|---|
| **Cognitive** | | **Content** |
| 1. Define and spell the terms in the Vocabulary | • Text p. 91<br>• Manual Part 1-A | • Basic medical office functions |
| 2. List six considerations in keeping a reception room comfortable for patients | • Text pp. 91-92<br>• Manual Part 1 -C | • Basic principles of psychology<br>• Mental health and applied psychology |
| 3. State two reasons for checking supplies at the beginning of each day | • Text pp. 92-93<br>• Manual Part 1-C-2 | • Basic medical office functions<br>• Document appropriately |
| 4. Identify and discuss the importance of three components of greeting arriving patients | • Text p. 93<br>• Manual Part 2 | • Project a professional manner and image |
| 5. Instruct new patient about providing personal data for the records and completing a registration form | • Text pp. 95-96<br>• Manual Part 1-B | • Document appropriately<br>• Project a professional manner and image<br>• Instruct individuals according to their needs<br>• Explain office procedures and policies |
| 6. List three actions a medical assistant might take to reduce stress caused by a delayed schedule | • Text p. 97<br>• Manual Part 1-D | • Instruct individuals according to their needs |
| 7. Discuss ways a medical assistant might help a physically impaired, uncomfortable or ill patient | • Text p. 87<br>• Manual Part 1-D | • Project a professional manner and image<br>• Instruct individuals according to their needs |
| 8. Suggest a way to successfully handle an angry patient | • Text p. 96<br>• Manual Part 1-F | • Project a professional manner and image<br>• Instruct individuals according to their needs |
| **Performance** | | **Competencies** |
| 1. Follow correct procedure for preparing patient charts for the day's appointments | • Text p. 93<br>• Procedure 8-1 | • Document appropriately<br>• Instruct individuals according to their needs<br>• Explain office procedures and policies |

| TEXTBOOK OBJECTIVES | LEARNING SYSTEM LOCATION | MA RECOMMENDED CURRICULUM |
|---|---|---|
| **Cognitive** | | **Competencies** |
| 2. Complete a new patient's registration form | • Text p. 94<br>• Procedure 8-3<br>• Manual Part 12<br>• Transparency Master 8-2 | • Document appropriately<br>• Instruct individuals according to their needs<br>• Explain office procedures and policies |
| 3. Demonstrate how the medical assistant maintains a professional appearance | • Extra procedure not in textbook—use for evaluation of professional image in lab and externship | • Project a professional manner and image |

## 3. RESOURCES

- Articles from the Professional Medical Assistant Magazine from the AAMA.
- Better Business Bureau has literature on customer service.
- Chamber of Commerce will come and talk to students about receiving new clients. Their entire focus is on greeting newcomers and business to the city.
- *The Doctor's Office*—Publication on all facets of the office. Subscription is less than $100.

ALL SITES BEGIN WITH **http://**

www.yahoo.com/Business and Economy/Companies/Corporate Services/Public Relations
**A site for access to links with hints for working with the public**

www.prsa.org/ **Public Relations Society of America**

## 4. LESSON PLAN **TIME 3 hours lecture, 9 hours lab**

**Opening:** This is a real attention-getting device: Start class by ignoring students for 1 minute. Turn your back and do not acknowledge. Then ask students how they felt when they were ignored. Relate students' feelings to patients' feelings when they are not acknowledged.

**Pretest:** Ask what is needed to greet people effectively. Write those actions on the board or overhead projector.

**Objectives:** Review objectives with students, explain how activities meet objectives

**Content:**
Review points as related to AAMA curriculum and objectives in grid. Use the Mastery Manual and complete all activities.
The reception room
  Features of the area—clean, restful, adequate seating, lighting, good ventilation, comfortable temperature, other amenities
Preparing for patient arrival
  Know your patients, review and replenish charts
Greeting the patient
  Name the qualities you (student) want when going to a physician's office
  Eye contact, acknowledgment, introduce self if patient or you are new, greet patients by name, tell patients what to expect, signing in is a loss of privacy unless list is kept away from patients
Introductory procedures—Registration, Patient history, pp. 95-96
  Pass out registration forms and have students fill out on themselves.
  Then critique for lack of information or problem areas.
Consideration for patients' time
  If wait will be longer than 10 min., let patient know
Assisting the patient when needed
Special needs patients
  Escorting and instructing
  Handling complaints
  Learn to effectively handle potential problems—talkers, children, anger, relatives
Friendly farewell
Legal Confidentiality—establish friendly atmosphere; happy patients do not sue.
Ethics—When you register a patient known to you, you must not intermingle professional and personal relationship.

**Lab activities:**

1. Complete Part 2 and 3 of Mastery Manual. Students will need access to ⊕ CD-ROM to complete.
2. Use Procedure 8-1 and the forms for patients' charts from ▲ Appendix B. Have students purchase folders so that they have at least 20 per student. They will need to tear out the chart forms and make copies of them for this activity and the activities in Chapter 14. When students have the equipment, have them put chart and forms together and number them 1 to 20. Students need some way to hold the forms in the charts. Have a place to store charts if possible.
3. Have students fill out registration form for another classmate following Procedure 8-2.
4. The procedure for professional dress is placed here for you to use to establish standards in the lab and to grade students. It may be modified according to school requirements.

**Assignment:** Study next chapter and define the vocabulary.

**Posttest:** Write the eight steps in preparing patient charts for the day.

## 5. MASTERY MANUAL ANSWERS

### PART 1 CONTENT MASTERY

#### A. Learning Level: Knowledge

1. c; 2. f; 3. j; 4. i; 5. g; 6. b; 7. e; 8. a; 9. h; 10. d

#### B. Learning Level: Comprehension

1. Responsible party
2. a. 6; b. 8; c. 2; d. 1; e. 3; f. 7; g. 5; h. 4

#### C. Learning Level: Application

1. This application allows students to set their standards for dress in the laboratory and the medical office. With a discussion, the instructor and class often reach consensus and everyone is required to meet those standards of professional dress and conduct. All students benefit from this activity due to the broad range of cultures. The instructor can then evaluate the student according to the peer-developed standards, which are usually in line with those of the program.
2. When all the listed information is missing, it usually means supplies were not checked and restocked at the beginning of the day. The medical assistant *does not assume* someone else resupplied the area and must ensure the patient charts and rooms are ready.

#### D. Learning Level: Analysis

1. The instructor has a variety of responses. Other suggested responses may include
   a. Thank you for checking in, Mr.____. If you will take a seat I will have the medical assistant call you ASAP.
   b. Bring children to desk and ask them to do something such as straighten papers, color with book, or read a book to you "to soothe you" while you work.
   c. Simply state that as much as you wish you could answer them, patient confidentiality does not allow you to do so.
   d. Check the reception area and give items to patient on the way out or have a lost and found area and just put leftovers there at day's end. Give items away every three months.
   e. Ask if you may escort him to an empty seat while waiting for the physician. If you know you have blind or other disabled patients, you may get books on tape or large print books. Also, these patients should not be kept waiting excessively long as usually another person brings them to the doctor. Consideration is the key.

#### E. Learning Level: Synthesis

Explain why the others are not essential. ** Indicates essential items

- Cleanliness **
- Dust free—nothing can be dust free
- Restful colors **—relaxing to patients
- Benches and metal chairs**—uncomfortable, makes for lots of complaints
- Regulated temperature **—allows patients to be comfortable
- Lighting to read by **
- Recent magazines **—distracts patients from worry or pain
- Professional journals not appropriate for lay audience
- Coffee machine—patients may be NPO; hot liquids are dangerous to children
- Rugs—dangerous and slippery unless wall to wall. Disabled people may have a hard time on wall-to-wall carpet.

## F. Learning Level: Evaluation

List five behaviors or surroundings you expect as a patient when you go to a medical office. Prioritize them in order of personal importance to you.
Instructor: Evaluate student responses as related to what the medical office can reasonably provide and MA responsibilities. Stress the need to put aside personal life and be professional.

## PART 2 COMPETENCY CHALLENGE

⊕ ▲ Provide CD-ROM access so that student may complete the interactive patient registration. Use form from Mastery Manual Appendix B.

A. ⊕ Use the CD-ROM and complete the activity for registering a new patient. All the information will be provided for you. Use Appendix B for patient chart forms. Copy and complete the forms as you work with the CD-ROM scenario.

B. ▲ Use the patient case studies in Appendix A as examples of patients to be greeted for the day. In the classroom, role-play greeting these patients, answering their concerns, and getting them comfortably settled in the reception area while waiting to see the physician. Your instructor will guide a discussion of each situation.

C. Prepare charts for all the patients described in Appendix A. Your instructor will provide you with the charts or you may buy them at an office supply store. Use Procedure 8-1, Preparing Charts for Scheduled Patients, as a guide. When you have the charts prepared, place the patient's name on a label on the chart. In a subsequent chapter you will learn to complete the label according to a filing system, collate, and organize these files. Put copies of all the chart forms in each patient's chart. You will work with these forms in later chapters.

D. Use Procedure 8-2, Registering a New Patient, and complete a new patient registration form for yourself. The form is in Appendix B. Be sure to copy the form you will need about 20 of these as you complete competencies in this manual.

## PART 3 CLINICAL APPLICATIONS

These items include personal opinion for discussion and ethical consideration of chapter topics.

1. Discuss the ethical concepts around negative attitudes; lack of daily cleaning in the reception area; wearing heavy perfume; having hair hanging in the face; not shaving daily or having an untrimmed beard.
2. Are today's standards too rigid?
3. If an office does not have a dress code, are jeans or other casual wear acceptable?
4. How would you feel if you had the following office mates? Why?
   a. A skinny MA with pocked face and old, clean uniforms
   b. A heavy physician's assistant who looked very unkempt
   c. A very heavy medical assistant who was always neat, pleasant, and friendly
   d. A loud, boisterous, curt MA

# 9

# Telephone Techniques

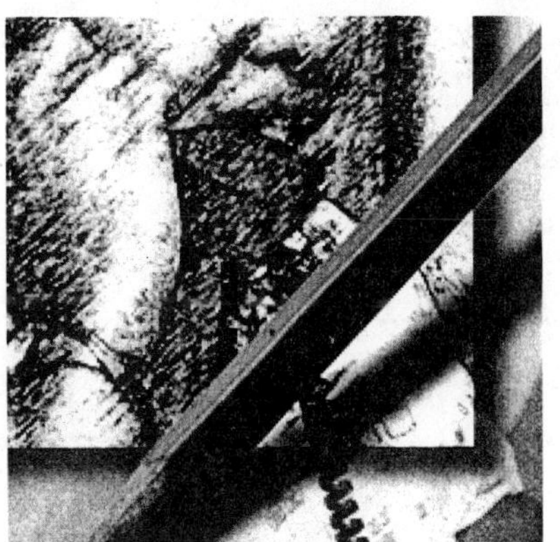

Using the telephone correctly is such an important part of the medical assistant's activity that sufficient time must be reserved and adequate emphasis placed on practicing good telephone form. A trainer telephone is the best equipment to have. Often it may be borrowed from the local telephone company. A guest speaker may bring some equipment and have a training session. Portable handsets may also be used. It is important that students do not play at this activity. After sufficient practice, some role-play with tape recording of Part 2 activities will help the students realize how much practice and skill answering the telephone requires. Developing this skill encompasses the main standard from the Role Delineation Study: that is, to receive, organize, prioritize, and transmit information. All the items listed below are an integral part of this skill, and students need to develop an awareness of the degree of difficulty required to be effective in answering the telephone in the medical office.

## USING THE LEARNING SYSTEM

### 1. MEDICAL ASSISTANT ENTRY-LEVEL CURRICULUM

CONTENT

- Applications of medical terminology
- Legal guidelines and requirement for care
- Adaptations for individual needs
- Risk management
- Mental health and applied psychology

COMPETENCIES

- Perform telephone and in-person screening
- Demonstrate telephone techniques
- Recognize and respond to verbal and nonverbal communication
- Perform risk management procedures
- Respond to and initiate written communications

## 2. MEDICAL ASSISTANT ENTRY-LEVEL CURRICULUM INTERFACE

| TEXTBOOK OBJECTIVES | LEARNING SYSTEM LOCATION | MA CURRICULUM |
|---|---|---|
| **Cognitive** | | **Content** |
| 1. Define and spell the terms in the Vocabulary | • Text p. 100<br>• Manual Part 1-A | • Applications of medical terminology |
| 2. Discuss the importance of telephone communications | • Text p. 101<br>• Manual Part 1-B | • Adaptations for individual needs<br>• Risk management<br>• Mental health and applied psychology |
| 3. List ways that the MA can develop a pleasing telephone personality | • Text pp. 102-103<br>• Manual Part 1-C | • Adaptations for individual needs<br>• Risk management |
| 4. Cite seven items to be included in taking a complete telephone message | • Text p. 106<br>• Manual Part 1-D | • Legal guidelines and requirement for care<br>• Risk management |
| 5. Identify 10 kinds of telephone calls the MA should be able to handle successfully | • Text pp. 107-110<br>• Manual Part 1-F | • Legal guidelines and requirement for care<br>• Risk management |
| 6. Identify six kinds of telephone calls that will need to be referred to the physician for response | • Text pp. 110-112<br>• Manual Part 1-F | • Legal guidelines and requirement for care<br>• Adaptations for individual needs<br>• Risk management |
| 7. Explain what is involved in monitoring telephone calls | • Text p. 111<br>• Manual Part 1-E | • Legal guidelines and requirement for care<br>• Risk management |
| 8. Explain what is meant by preplanning a call | • Text p. 115<br>• Manual Part 1-F | • Legal guidelines and requirement for care<br>• Risk management |
| 9. Explain the ways an operator-answered telephone answering service can benefit a medical practice | • Text pp. 114-115<br>• Manual Part 1-E | • Legal guidelines and requirement for care<br>• Risk management |
| | | **Competencies** |
| 1. Demonstrate the appropriate method of placing and receiving telephone calls | • Text pp. 103-104<br>• Manual Part 2<br>• Procedure 9-1<br>• Procedure 9-2 | All of the following statements apply to Nos. 1 through 5<br>• Perform telephone and in-person screening<br>• Demonstrate telephone techniques |

| TEXTBOOK OBJECTIVES | LEARNING SYSTEM LOCATION | MA CURRICULUM |
|---|---|---|
| **Cognitive** | | **Competencies** |
| | | • Recognize and respond to verbal and nonverbal communication<br>• Perform risk management procedures |
| 2. Using a multiple-line telephone, demonstrate the correct handling of two incoming calls, one of which must be transferred to another person | • Manual Part 2<br>• Procedure 9-1 | All above statements apply<br>• Respond to and initiate written communications |
| 3. Correctly record a telephone message from a laboratory facility reporting test results on a patient | • Manual Part 2<br>• Procedure 9-1 | All above statements apply<br>• Respond to and initiate written communications |
| 4. Respond to a call from a pharmacist regarding a request for a prescription refill, demonstrating appropriate precautions and completing necessary information | • Manual Part 2<br>• Procedure 9-1 | All above statements apply<br>• Respond to and initiate written communications |
| 5. Using a list of local social service agencies, respond to telephone calls for emergency treatment (at a poison or burn center) and for nonemergency services (at a facility for disabled children or a cancer-screening center) | • Manual Part 2<br>• Procedure 9-1 | All above statements apply |

## 3. RESOURCES

http://www.scheduling-medical.com/patcom.html = **Access to sample automated patient telephone reminder function**
http://av.yahoo.com/bin/query?p=telephone+guidelines&hc=0&hs=0 = **Links to hundreds of sites for telephone guidelines and use in a variety of settings**
AAACN has published *Standards for Telephone Triage. . .* They can be reached at aaacn@mail.ajjcom or www.iNurse.com/~AACN—**This association is for nurses, but is applicable for triage standards**
*Telephone Courtesy and Customer Service*, Lloyd Flinch Crisp Publications
Friedman, N: *Telephone Skills from A to Z*, Crisp Publishers, 1200 Hamilton Court, Menlo Park, CA 94025-1427 1-800-442-7477.
Loudin, A: *Putting an Automated System to Work*, PMA, May/June 1998.
Equipment needed includes message slips from Mastery Manual and extras and telephone system for students to complete competency activities.

## 4. LESSON PLAN TIME 3 hours lecture, 9 hours lab

**Opening:** An effective opening is to use a cellular telephone and demonstrate an effective and an ineffective telephone conversation with a patient. Have a patient on the line and make notes. Have a student try it. Ask students to identify problems.

**Pretest:** Ask students what you did that made the call effective, and what detracted from effectiveness. How do they feel about using the telephone? Who is comfortable, who is not? The comfortable telephone users are usually the verbal learners. Pair them with auditory learners. They will help each other grow.

**Objectives:** Explain how the objectives tie in with MA entry level competencies.

**Content:** Outline
GENERAL GUIDELINES
Your Telephone Personality
Confidentiality
Holding the Telephone Handset Correctly
Developing a Pleasing Telephone Voice
How Is Your Diction?
INCOMING TELEPHONE CALLS—points for consideration
Personal Calls
Answering Promptly
Personalizing the Call
Identifying the Facility and Yourself
Identifying the Caller
Offering Assistance
Screening Incoming Calls
Minimizing Waiting Time
Transferring a Call
Answering a Second Call
Ending a Call
TECHNIQUES FOR TAKING A TELEPHONE MESSAGE
Be Prepared
Information Required
Transmitting and Recording the Message
Taking Action
INCOMING CALLS THE MEDICAL ASSISTANT CAN HANDLE
New Patient and Return Appointments
Inquiries About Bills
Inquiries About Fees
Requests for Insurance Assistance
X-ray and Laboratory Reports
Satisfactory Progress Reports from Patients
Routine Reports from Hospitals and Other Sources
Office Administration Matters
Requests for Referrals
Prescription Refills
INCOMING CALLS THAT REQUIRE TRANSFER TO THE PHYSICIAN OR CALL-BACK
Calls from Other Physicians—Immediate transfer to M.D.
Patients Who Will Not Reveal Symptoms—Leave written message for M.D. to call back
Unsatisfactory Progress Reports—Leave written message for M.D. to call back
Requests for Test Results—Leave written message for M.D. to call back

Third Party Requests for Information—Information or permission from patient
Complaints About Care or Fees—Leave written message for M.D. to call back
Unidentified Callers—Have patient write personal letter
Calls from Family and Friends—Leave written message for M.D.
OCCASIONAL SITUATIONS
Messages for Correction
Angry Callers—Empathize, empathize, empathize and ask, "What can I do for you?"
Monitoring Calls
Requests for House Calls—Depends upon physician practice. Follow guidelines
Responding to Emergency Calls—Emergency calls go directly to M.D. if protocols are not written
Triage Guidelines—Must be written before any advice can be given
Written protocol for urgent and emergent problems
ROUTINE BUT TROUBLESOME CALLS
Appointment Changes
Statements
Prescription Refills
Physician "Shopping"
Unauthorized Inquiry
TELEPHONE ANSWERING SERVICES (discuss advantages and disadvantages)
Operator-Answered Services
Electronic Answering Devices
Voice Mail
Automatic Routine
PLACING OUTGOING CALLS
Preplanning the Call
Placing the Call
Long Distance Service
Time Parts
Dialing Direct
Operator-Assisted Calls
International Service
Wrong Numbers
Conference Calls

**Assignment:** Before lecture and discussion, students need to read and study the entire chapter. Ask students to make flash cards of all the little boxes of hints in the chapter, e.g., Tips on developing a pleasing telephone voice. Lesson 2 will be completion of all Mastery Manual activities. Students need to plan calls and prepare by practicing procedures at home. Have telephones set up and give out simple scripts to practice situations. Students need as much lab time as possible. Arrange for students to go to various offices and observe other MAs answering the telephone.

**Posttest:** Give a short theory test after Lesson 1.

## 5. MASTERY MANUAL ANSWERS

### PART 1 CONTENT MASTERY

### A. Learning Level: Knowledge

1. d; 2. f; 3. a; 4. j; 5. h; 6. b; 7. i; 8. c ; 9. g; 10. e

### B. Learning Level: Comprehension

Incoming calls from: Patients calling for appointments or advice; emergencies; physician referrals; laboratories reporting test results; new patients asking for appointment

### C. Learning Level: Application

Warm, friendly smile, confident, courteous, tactful, speak slowly and distinctly

### D. Learning Level: Analysis

1. Information forgotten is: where the treadmill was performed and patient's home number
2. Review the components of a message.

### E. Learning Level: Synthesis

1. Telephone response
   - Mail patient directions or give them over the telephone if able. There should be a map by the telephone with the office location marked so that all can give directions.
   - Ask who is calling and what you can do.
   - Do not give out information. Have patient send insurance form as you may not be talking to patient.
   - Ask patient to call you back as you also have calls waiting.
2. Supervisor will be monitoring you to help you use the telephone correctly. She will be listening to the accuracy of information given, tone of voice, diction, and terminology.
3. The standards are: the importance of the information, the urgency of the information, who gets the information, and the availability of that person.
4. Four advantages of an automated system are: decreases no-shows by making patient reminders; can request patients to call office; can give out normal test results in some limited cases; screen incoming calls; save practice money.

### F. Learning Level: Evaluation

1. Ten types of telephone calls are: New patient appointments; return appointments; inquiries about fees or bills; requests for insurance assistance; taking laboratory reports; satisfactory progress reports from patients; routine reports from hospitals; administration matters; requests for referrals; requests for prescription refills.
2. Referred calls include:
   a. calls from another physician—1. Buzz physician immediately
   b. patients who will not reveal symptoms—Message goes to physician desk
   c. unsatisfactory progress report—Message goes to physician desk
   d. request for test results—Message goes to physician desk
   e. third party information request—Message goes to physician desk
   f. complaints about care or fees—Message goes to physician desk
3. A preplanned telephone call is one made with notes concerning purpose, needs, and outcome desired. *Describe the process when making an outgoing telephone call.* Look up number for correct party; have the necessary information such as a chart; patient record, or invoice; note the time of day and call at an open or convenient time; physician should be waiting and ready to talk if the call is being placed for physician.

## PART 2 COMPETENCY CHALLENGE

Part 2 involves students applying the skills studied and reviewed in class. It is important that students hear their own voice on tape. Almost everyone has access to a tape deck to complete Activity A. Activity B involves using the CD-ROM ⊕ . Activity C allows the student to role-play calls. It is very effective when a barrier is placed between caller and receiver. Students may do this with the entire class listening. A barrier between the class allows for responses that are more natural. After all the calls are placed, students may then comment on themselves and each other. All students need to participate to build upon strengths and minimize fright and stumbling blocks.

## PART 3 CLINICAL APPLICATIONS

A. The calls that present opportunities for caller education are:

2. All information is given only by letter from physician.
3. If the medical assistant can find out why patient does not want to give information, the patient can be educated. Also, the M.D. can educate the patient.
4. Patients who want referrals should call the local medical society.
7. All bleeding from an orifice is important. Make appointment ASAP.
8. Patient needs to discuss with physician and probably should come into office.

The remainder of the activities in Part 3 help to develop critical thinking skills for the medical assistant, which will prepare him for practice. Offices need to have emergency numbers promptly posted. Students carry theirs with them. Ethical situations help students think about the application of principles and increase reasoning skills.

# 10

# Appointment Scheduling and Time Management

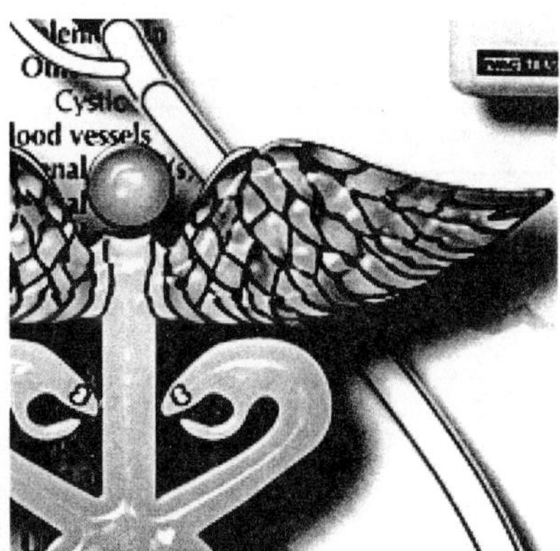

This chapter covers one of the most critical duties of the medical assistant. As instructors, it is important to provide adequate laboratory training and practice to ensure students the opportunity to further develop skills before the externship experience. A guest lecturer is very effective for this material. The chapter outline and use of the Mastery Manual is contained in the lesson plan to enable the instructor to complete all the content points. Assign students to read the chapter before discussion of the material. All of the Mastery Manual activities meet the objectives for content and performance. In addition, there are activities on the CD-ROM ⊕ that allow for completing competency objectives.

## USING THE LEARNING SYSTEM

### 1. MEDICAL ASSISTANT CONTENT AND COMPETENCIES

CONTENT

- Applications of medical terminology
- Medical ethics-related issues
- Risk management
- Basic principles
- Mental health and applied psychology
- Recognize and respond to verbal and nonverbal communications
- Adaptations for individual needs
- Applications of electronic technology
- Fundamental writing skills
- Professional components: Personal attributes
- Basic medical office functions

COMPETENCIES

- Schedule and maintain appointments
- Schedule inpatient and outpatient admissions and procedures
- Perform telephone and in-person screening
- Recognize and respond to verbal communications
- Demonstrate telephone techniques
- Perform within legal and ethical boundaries
- Document appropriately
- Perform risk management procedures

## 2. MEDICAL ASSISTANT ENTRY-LEVEL CURRICULUM INTERFACE

| TEXTBOOK OBJECTIVES | LEARNING SYSTEM LOCATION | MA CURRICULUM |
|---|---|---|
| Cognitive | | Content |
| 1. Define and spell the terms in the Vocabulary | • Text p. 121<br>• Manual 1-A | • Applications of medical terminology |
| 2. Describe four important features of an appointment book | • Text p. 122<br>• Lesson plan<br>• Manual Part 1-B<br>• CD-ROM Admin. duties | • Risk management<br>• Basic medical office functions |
| 3. List and explain three basic guidelines to follow in scheduling appointments | • Content & Text pp. 122,124,125<br>• Lesson plan<br>• Manual Part 1-B & 1-C<br>• Transparency Master 10-1 | • Basic principles and mental health<br>• Recognize and respond to verbal and nonverbal communications<br>• Adaptations for individual needs |
| 4. Identify and discuss advantages of wave scheduling | • Text p. 126<br>• Manual Part 1-A<br>• Lesson plan | • Basic medical office functions |
| 5. Cite three common situations requiring adjustment of appointment schedule | • Text p. 125<br>• Manual Parts 1-C and 2 | • Adaptations for individual needs<br>• Basic medical office functions |
| 6. Describe how to determine if a requested appointment is an emergency | • Lesson plan<br>• Manual Part 1-E | • Adaptations for individual needs<br>• Basic medical office functions |
| 7. State reasons for recording a failed appointment on chart | • Text p. 132<br>• Lesson plan<br>• Manual Parts 2 & 3 | • Risk management<br>• Basic psychology principles and mental health<br>• Basic medical office functions |
| 8. Discuss handling of cancellations and delays brought about by office situations | • Text p. 133<br>• Lecture opening<br>• Manual Part 2 | • Adaptations for individual needs<br>• Applications of electronic technology<br>• Personal attributes<br>• Basic medical office functions |
| 9. List seven points of information necessary in scheduling hospital surgery | • Text p. 134<br>• Manual Part 1-C<br>• Textbook memory jogger<br>• Lesson plan | • Recognize and respond to verbal and nonverbal communications<br>• Basic medical office functions |

| TEXTBOOK OBJECTIVES | LEARNING SYSTEM LOCATION | MA CURRICULUM |
|---|---|---|
| **Cognitive** | | **Content** |
| 10. State four items of information that must be available before arranging an outside laboratory appointment for a patient | • Lesson plan<br>• Manual Part 1-C<br>• Textbook memory jogger | • Recognize and respond to verbal and nonverbal communication<br>• Adaptations for individual needs |
| **Performance** | | **Competency** |
| 1. Select an appropriate appointment book to suit a given type of practice ⊕ | • Manual Part 2<br>• Procedure 10-1 | Perform clerical functions<br>• Schedule and maintain appointments:<br>• Schedule in and outpatient admissions and procedures |
| 2. Demonstrate advance preparation that must be done before using a new appointment book | • Manual Part 2<br>• Manual Competency Objective 10-1<br>• CD-ROM ⊕ | Perform clerical functions<br>• Schedule and maintain appointments<br>• Perform within legal boundaries |
| 3. Schedule patients according to urgency of complaints and anticipated treatment time | • Manual Part 2-E<br>• Manual Procedures 10-1 and 10-2<br>• CD-ROM ⊕ | • Perform telephone and in-person screening<br>• Perform within legal and ethical boundaries<br>• Document appropriately<br>• Perform risk management procedures |
| 4. Rearrange schedule in event that physician's arrival is delayed | • Manual Part 2-B | Perform clerical functions<br>• Schedule and maintain appointments<br>Communicate<br>• Recognize and respond to verbal communications<br>• Demonstrate telephone techniques<br>• Perform within legal and ethical boundaries<br>• Document appropriately<br>• Perform risk management procedures |
| 5. Explain physician's unavailability to patients in reception room | • Manual Part 2-B | • Recognize and respond to verbal communications<br>• Perform within legal and ethical boundaries<br>• Perform risk management procedures |

*Chart continues on following page*

| TEXTBOOK OBJECTIVES | LEARNING SYSTEM LOCATION | MA CURRICULUM |
|---|---|---|
| **Performance** | | **Competency** |
| 6. Arrange a referral appointment for a patient | • Manual Part 1-C<br>• CD-ROM ⊕ | • Schedule and maintain appointments<br>• Perform telephone and in-person screening<br>• Recognize and respond to verbal communications<br>• Demonstrate telephone techniques<br>• Document appropriately |
| 7. Demonstrate advance preparation that must be done before using a new appointment book | • Parts 1-C, 2 & 3<br>• Manual Procedure 10-3 | • Schedule outpatient procedures<br>• Recognize and respond to verbal communications |
| 8. Schedule a surgery with hospital, notifying all persons and departments concerned | • Manual Part 1-C<br>• CD-ROM ⊕ | • Schedule in- and outpatient admissions and procedures<br>• Recognize and respond to verbal communications<br>• Demonstrate telephone techniques<br>• Document appropriately |
| 9. Instruct a patient regarding pre-admission requirements, hospital stay, and insurance information needed | • Manual Part 2<br>• Externship | • Recognize and respond to verbal communications<br>• Perform within legal and ethical boundaries<br>• Document appropriately<br>• Perform risk management procedures |
| 10. Arrange for a patient's admission to a hospital as ordered by physician | • CD-ROM ⊕<br>• Manual Part 2<br>• Posttest<br>• Externship | • Schedule in- and outpatient admissions and procedures<br>• Recognize and respond to verbal communications<br>• Demonstrate telephone techniques<br>• Perform within legal and ethical boundaries<br>• Document appropriately<br>• Perform risk management procedures |

### 3. RESOURCES

Periodical: *PMA*, published by the AAMA. Free to all members.
Montane, D: *Power Building in Scheduling*, Philadelphia, W.B. Saunders Co., 1997. Exercises or medical office scheduling techniques.
Student software: allows students to practice scheduling

1. Medical Manager Versions from Southwest Publishers
2. Medi-soft, Mesa, AZ 1-800-334-4006 www.medisoft.com

http://search.yahoo.com/bin/search?p=management%2C+time **A site for articles and research on health care and time management concepts**

http://search.yahoo.com/bin/search?p=scheduling+appointments **A site with many links to appointment scheduling systems**

http://www.scheduling-medical.com/ **A scheduling system for small or large practices**

### 4. LESSON PLAN TIME 3 hours lecture, 9 hours lab

**Opening:** Plan to come to class 5 minutes late. Have a colleague come to class and ask students to wait 20 minutes quietly. After 3 or 4 minutes, come in and ask students how they felt about your being late. Then relate this to personal experience with late appointments.

**Pretest:** Identify feelings patients may have when they are kept waiting. Identify feelings the receptionist may experience when patients complain. Discuss psychology and ethics
Lesson 2: Identify the steps taken to arrange for a patient admission to a hospital.

**Objectives:** Write objectives on board or flip chart. Use grid to cover curriculum items with objectives in the lesson.

**Content outline:**
APPOINTMENT SCHEDULING—*Use medical terminology; follow lawful principles*
Open Office Hours, Scheduled Appointments, and Flexible Office Hours
THE APPOINTMENT BOOK—Selection, Advance Preparation
GUIDELINES FOR SCHEDULING—*Stress psychological principles to maintain good IPR*
Patient Need, Physician's Preferences and Habits, Available Facilities
PLANNING A TIME PATTERN—*Explain establishing the matrix and developing clerical skills*
TIME MANAGEMENT—*Develop principles of using time*
Wave Scheduling, Modified Wave Scheduling
Double Booking, Grouping Procedures
Advance Booking
DETAILS OF ARRANGING APPOINTMENTS—*Point out methods of meeting patient needs, office scheduling, and legal guidelines*
Telephone Triage, Arrangements by Telephone
Appointments for New Patients
Scheduling Return Appointments in Person or by Telephone
APPOINTMENT CARDS AND REMINDERS
EXCEPTIONS AND CHANGES—*Requires EMPHASIS of all curriculum content items*
Special Problems, Rescheduling Appointments
Emergency Calls, Acutely Ill Patients, Physician Referrals
Failed Appointments, No-Show Policy, Recording Failed Appointments, Charging for

*Chart continues on following page*

Failed Appointments
Cancellations and Delays by Patient, Physician Delayed, Called Out on Emergencies
Patients Without Appointments
Scheduling Outside Appointments—House Calls, Surgeries
Salesmen and Drug Reps
Preplanning for Next Day

**Assignment:** Student completes Part 1 in Mastery Manual before lab.
During lab, the instructor could use the time to have students complete Parts 2 and 3, leaving the scheduling for a week assignment until last. It is suggested that Part 2 activity E be completed as a laboratory class activity. Students will learn problem-solving skills as they make appointments for all classmates. Before the activity, have students write a diagnosis and preferred dates on a sheet of paper. This will allow some consistency. Have students rotate positions as appointment scheduler. Each student will build on the foundation.

**Posttest:** Use Examaster Chapter 10 questions. Students pass theory test before going on to practice of skills. Student passes competency objectives in Procedures 10-1; 10-2; and 10-3

## 5. MASTERY MANUAL ANSWERS

### PART 1 CONTENT MASTERY

#### A. Learning Level: Knowledge

1. j ; 2. i; 3. d; 4. h; 5. a; 6. b; 7. c; 8. f ; 9. e; 10. g

#### B. Learning Level: Comprehension

False statements are listed below according to the corresponding number in Mastery Manual:

2. With open office hours, the patients may come in anytime.

4. The success in the appointment system depends upon the guidelines for use and the keeping of the schedule by the physician.

6. Wave scheduling allows much flexibility in scheduling.

7. General practice is most adaptable to various procedures and patients scheduled throughout the day so as not to tie the physician up for too long.

11. The physician or written physician protocol decides when patient is to be seen.

#### C. Learning Level: Application

1. Basic guidelines in scheduling are: Patient need, physician preferences, available facilities
2. Information to schedule surgery is: Preferred date and time based on elective, urgent, or

emergent criteria; type of surgery; time required for surgery, gender, age, name, telephone number

3. Information needed for scheduling diagnostic tests: exact procedure or test, how soon, stat report, patient availability
4. Reasons to adjust appointment book are: physician illness, emergency, vacation; patient changes or cancels appointment; office unexpectedly closes; emergency causes excessive back-up

## D. Learning Level: Analysis

| Advantages | Disadvantages |
|---|---|
| **Wave or schedule** | |
| Patients can be seen at their convenience | Physician may be late |
| Booking can be made to fit physician time lines | Physician is not always realistic |
| **Open** | |
| Patients come at their convenience | Patient may have to wait |
| No running late or broken appointments | Physician may feel rushed if many waiting patients |

## E. Learning Level: Synthesis

A simple solution is to give mother the first available appointment in the morning. Child can have physical and be brought to school. If mother brings in the form early, some can be filled out. It is not an emergency as there is no illness involved. Physician is not responsible for mother's lack of planning.

## F. Learning Level: Evaluation

Three most important reasons for preparing calendar in advance:

1. Must be blocked off for as long in advance as appointments are booked
2. Medical assistant can plan use of office space when aware of physician availability
3. All schedulers, no matter what hours worked, are able to schedule appointments as the matrix is completed

## PART 2 COMPETENCY CHALLENGE

A. This requires the student to complete the matrix for a week. You will need to make a matrix for yourself. Set the *standards* for students. Each of the appointment forms at the end of the chapter covers only two days. Students will need to copy two more appointment forms and more for other exercises. Review each student's work in Laboratory as students indicate the activity is complete.

B. The first three appointments must be rescheduled. Make them all as late in the day as possible in case the physician is even later than expected. Cross off time until 3:30.

C. Students use the CD-ROM ⊕ and successfully complete Procedure 10-2. Evaluate students using the Procedure sheet in the Mastery Manual.

D. Students use the CD-ROM ⊕ and successfully complete Procedure 10-3. Evaluate students using the Competency Objective check in the Mastery Manual. Fill in Procedure competency evaluation forms for students. They are located in Appendix C of student Mastery Manual.

E. If students rotate their role as appointment scheduler they will truly get a feel of working out the complexities of appointment scheduling.

F. Preadmission steps and information needed are in the textbook, pp. 128 and 134.

## PART 3 CLINICAL APPLICATIONS

1. The purpose in recording missed appointments in patient chart is risk management protecting the physician and the medical assistant if problems arise. If appointments are removed from the book, another must be made at time of cancellation, or the cancelled appointment is then noted on the medical record. Some offices note cancelled appointments even when they are rebooked. Please note that the textbook uses the term "chart." Often medical offices call the same item a medical record or patient record.

**SELF-EVALUATIONS:** BE SURE STUDENTS HAVE COMPLETED SELF-EVALUATIONS BEFORE MOVING ON TO NEXT TOPIC.

# 11

# Correspondence and Mail Processing

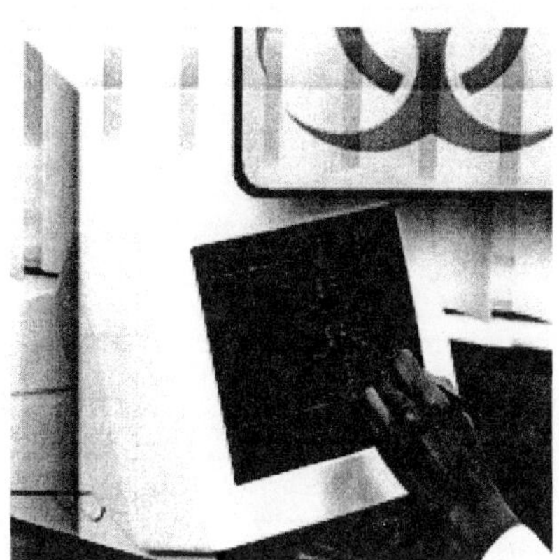

Developing basic secretarial skills is essential for the administrative medical assistant. It is therefore also essential that students have a basic grasp of parts of speech, grammar, punctuation, and spelling. Written correspondence will form lasting impressions, either positive or negative. The medical assistant needs expertise if letters are to be written for the physician or clinic. As an instructor it is beneficial to collect examples to use as a starting point in discussions. Instructors may find a variety of examples of poor grammar and English in written correspondence. Often students do not recognize these examples, and it is interesting to point them out.

## USING THE LEARNING SYSTEM

### 1. MEDICAL ASSISTANT CONTENT AND COMPETENCIES

CONTENT

- Principles of nonverbal communication
- Applications of electronic technology
- Fundamental writing skills
- Basic medical office functions
- Job readiness

COMPETENCIES

- Perform clerical functions
- Perform within legal and ethical boundaries
- Respond to written communications
- Document appropriately

## 2. MEDICAL ASSISTANT ENTRY-LEVEL CURRICULUM INTERFACE

| TEXTBOOK OBJECTIVES | LEARNING SYSTEM LOCATION | MA CURRICULUM |
|---|---|---|
| **Cognitive** | | **Content** |
| 1. Define and spell the terms in the Vocabulary | • Text p. 142<br>• Manual 1-A | • Principles of nonverbal communication |
| 2. Discuss the responsibility of the MA with respect to office equipment | • Text pp. 142-143<br>• Manual Part 1-F | • Fundamental writing skills<br>• Basic medical office functions |
| 3. Select stationery suitable for producing professional correspondence | • Text p. 143<br>• Manual Part 1-B & 1-C<br>• CD-ROM ⊕ | • Principles of nonverbal communication<br>• Fundamental writing skills<br>• Basic medical office functions<br>• Job readiness |
| 4. List the three basic sizes of letterhead stationery | • Text p. 143<br>• Manual Part 2 | • Basic medical office functions |
| 5. Name three types of essential references for the medical assistant's library | • Text p. 143<br>• Manual Part 1-E | • Basic medical office functions<br>• Job readiness |
| 6. Explain the five steps in getting ready to answer a letter | • Text p. 145<br>• Manual Part 1-D | • Basic medical office functions<br>• Job readiness<br>• Principles of nonverbal communication |
| 7. Discuss the process of developing a correspondence portfolio | • Text p. 146<br>• Manual Part 3 | • Basic medical office functions<br>• Job readiness |
| 8. Name four letter styles and discuss their differences | • Text pp. 146-149<br>• Manual Part 1-C | • Basic medical office functions<br>• Job readiness |
| 9. List the four main parts of any business letter | • Text pp. 149-151<br>• Manual Part 1-D | • Basic medical office functions<br>• Job readiness |
| 10. Explain how using ZIP Codes can save money for the mailer | • Text pp. 155-156 | • Basic medical office functions<br>• Job readiness<br>• Applications of electronic technology |

| TEXTBOOK OBJECTIVES | LEARNING SYSTEM LOCATION | MA CURRICULUM |
|---|---|---|
| **Performance** | | **Competency** |
| 1. Open, sort, and annotate incoming mail | • Text p. 161<br>• Manual Part 2<br>• Textbook Steps p. 162 | • Perform clerical functions<br>• Perform within legal and ethical boundaries<br>• Respond to written communications<br>• Document appropriately<br>• Principles of nonverbal communication |
| 2. Prepare a response to an inquiry letter | • Text p. 145<br>• Manual Part 2<br>• Procedure 11-2<br>• CD-ROM ⊕ | • Same as #1 competencies<br>• Applications of electronic technology |
| 3. Compose original letters | • Text p. 151<br>• Manual Part 2<br>• Procedure 11-1<br>• CD-ROM ⊕ | • Same as #1 competencies<br>• Applications of electronic technology |
| 4. Address envelopes for optical scanning | • Text p. 153<br>• Manual Part 2 | • Same as #1 competencies<br>• Applications of electronic technology |
| 5. Fold outgoing mail for insertion into three styles of envelopes | • Text p. 154<br>• Manual Part 2 | • Same as #1 competencies |

## 3. RESOURCES

www.mavisbeacon.com **A wonderful site for typists and instructors**

http://www.yahoo.com/Reference/ **A good source that will take you to postal ZIP codes, libraries, acronyms, abbreviations, English usage, and much more. This is one of the best reference sites around**

## 4. LESSON PLAN    TIME 3 hours lecture, 9 hours lab

**Opening:** An interesting opening might be to have a high school or college English teacher come in and give a quick test on the parts of speech and grammar. Have students keep their papers. Instructor reviews answers with group, has students mark their own papers, and then quietly tells students what level the test is aimed at. Tenth grade is usually the best for the Medical Assistant student.

**Pretest:** The above opening may be used as a pretest. Ask students how many need additional help based on the standard that it is best if all students are performing at 10th grade level. Students are usually surprised and may be motivated to get further education.

**Objectives:** See above and review with students.

**Content Outline:**
EQUIPMENT AND SUPPLIES: This chapter requires you to have a good supply of old mail that can be used to demonstrate sorting techniques. It may be collected as empty envelopes discarded by school or it may be made. Once established, it can be used yearly. Obtain post office regulations and procedures on current mail practice and duplicate. Get mail sorting supplies, date stamp, and ZIP code directory. Obtain a postage meter for demonstration. Obtain and discuss the state and federal regulations regarding mailing specimens.

In this chapter more of the activities require inductive and deductive reasoning. Whereas some of the previous chapter exercises could be taken directly from the 8th Edition Textbook, in this chapter students will have to use higher cognitive skills. Part 1-E-1 is an example of this. Some references are listed, others are acknowledged in other forms. The instructor is encouraged to add to the outline with personal notes for discussion. This becomes a complete lesson plan.

CORRESPONDENCE AND MAIL HANDLING:

1. Equipment and supplies
2. Personal tools—reference materials
3. Correspondence composing tips
    - Getting ready to write
    - Why a letter portfolio?
    - Letter styles
    - Punctuation
    - Spacing margins
    - Parts of letter
4. Mail
    - Preparing outgoing mail
    - Folding and inserting letters, sealing and stamping
    - Mailing procedures—Cost saving, speed, letter size, and classes

   Mail services and classifications—Postage meters, USPS, electronic mail, private services

    - Handling incoming mail: open, sort, and annotate
    - Special considerations and problems
5. Laboratory: Activities in Parts 2 and 3 will meet performance objectives. Composing letters and other procedures: time is used to complete all competencies. Have students spend a morning in the school office handling mail. Have students write a competence procedure for opening, sorting, and annotating mail.

**Assignment:** Students are to test each other on commonly misspelled words in Table 12-2. After the laboratory procedures are completed, have a team spelling contest. Team typing contests are another possibility with teams providing the letter to be typed to the opposing team. Teams may pick their own typist and proofreaders.

**Posttest:** Spelling test and another test on grammar and punctuation. It is good to repeat the test given as the pretest. Then discuss with students the need to learn their weaknesses so they may improve.

## 5. MASTERY MANUAL ANSWERS

### PART 1 CONTENT MASTERY

#### A. Learning Level: Knowledge

Misspelled words were:

1. inoculate
3. accommodate
6. hemorrhage
7. definitely
9. auxiliary
10. liquefy

#### B. Learning Level: Comprehension

TRUE or FALSE:
These statements now read correctly:

F 2. The first letter in the first word in the complimentary close is capitalized.

F 3. The attention line is placed on the second line below the inside address.

F 5. A letterhead is never used for the second page of a long letter.

F 7. In order to be forwarded, first class mail does not need to be placed in a new envelope. Cross out old address and put forwarding address.

F 10. Mail in the United States is delivered by a variety of public and private carriers.

#### C. Learning Level: Application

1. Basic knowledge necessary for composing a written document includes knowledge of:
   a. Sentence structure
   b. Spelling
   c. Punctuation
   d. Grammar

2. Types of letters described are:
   a. Block
   b. Modified block
   c. Modified block with indented paragraphs

#### D. Learning Level: Analysis

1. Main parts of a business letter are: a. heading, b. opening, c. body, d. closing
2. Preparatory steps to answering are: a. carefully read letter before answering; b. note questions asked or materials needed; c. formulate answer and verify information; d. draft a reply; e. proofread and rewrite for clarity if necessary

## E. Learning Level: Synthesis

1. Essential reference books are: standard dictionary, no more than 5 years old; medical dictionary, secretary's reference manual; English grammar guide; abbreviation book; telephone book
2. Mail is classified by a. type, b. weight, c. dimensions.
3. Largest standard 11 $^{1}/_{2}$ x 6 $^{1}/_{2}$ x $^{1}/_{4}$ inch thick
   Smallest is 3 $^{1}/_{2}$ x 5 x .0007 inches thick

## F. Learning Level: Evaluation

1. Matching 1. b; 2. a; 3. d; 4. e; 5. c
2. MA responsibilities with respect to office equipment include:
   Know how to use it to best advantage
   Keep it in good working order
   Keep equipment manual and have it handy to use
   Know how to perform or arrange for maintenance of equipment
3. Federal mail regulations prohibit opening mail marked personal.

## PART 2 COMPETENCY CHALLENGE

Hopefully the Medical Assistant program will require students to have typing proficiency before administrative tasks are begun. The purpose of all the activities in this Part is to have the students turn out letters that follow some firm guidelines. Physicians usually give guidelines to persons writing their correspondence. Students should work to be able to produce a perfect copy, folded and in an envelope, correctly addressed, within $^{1}/_{2}$ hour. Students might reasonably need many hours to complete Part 2 and work on the CD-ROM.

Suggested extra activity: Have students write a procedure for opening mail using p. 162 in the textbook as a guide. Obtain or make envelopes for Blackburn Medical Clinic and together review procedure, sorting and annotating mail.

## PART 3 CLINICAL APPLICATIONS

This Part contains a set of discussions and a calm way to end the lab after hours of difficult work. Students enjoy discussing ethical problems but do not always see that doing something the right way is an ethical decision. Many times circumstances are discussed when the application is simply right or wrong. Just because someone makes a mistake or makes a bad choice does not make him a bad person. These ideas seem incorrectly tied together very often in today's society. Students need this clarified and need encouragement to raise thinking to higher principled levels. This Part continues this thinking process.

# 12

# Dictation and Transcription

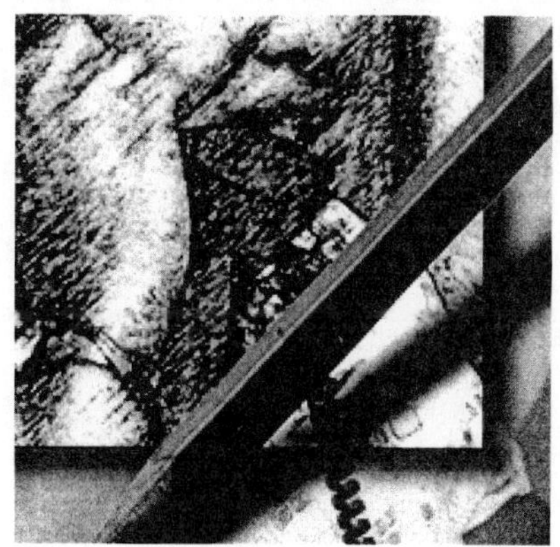

Some Medical Assistant students become extremely interested in medical transcription as a career. The average medical assistant does only a small amount of transcription. Therefore, practice transcribing progress notes and short reports will serve the student well. You may want to obtain the Saunders manual mentioned in the resource Part for this chapter. Have a few colleagues dictate some of the reports in the manual onto cassettes. Students may then practice some real transcribing skills. This will help students evaluate their skill and desires for this area of medical assisting. It is important to have a medical transcriptionist talk about professional preparation, skills, and the lifelong learning needed in this area. Sometimes a hospital can arrange for a tour of the facility and observation of the equipment used. Students often enjoy seeing these transcriptionists at work. MOST HOSPITAL TRANSCRIPTIONISTS TYPE OVER 100 WPM!

## USING THE LEARNING SYSTEM

### 1. MEDICAL ASSISTANT CONTENT AND COMPETENCIES

CONTENT

- Anatomy and physiology of all body systems
- Common pathology/disease
- Diagnostic/treatment modalities
- Applications of medical terminology
- Risk management
- Applications of electronic technology
- Fundamental writing skills

COMPETENCIES

- Perform medical transcription
- Respond to and initiate written communication
- Establish and maintain the medical record
- Document appropriately
- Utilize computer software to maintain office system

## 2. MEDICAL ASSISTANT ENTRY-LEVEL CURRICULUM INTERFACE

| TEXTBOOK OBJECTIVES | LEARNING SYSTEM LOCATION | MA CURRICULUM |
|---|---|---|
| **Cognitive** | | **Content** |
| 1. Define and spell the terms in the Vocabulary | • Text p. 166<br>• Manual Part 1 | • Applications of medical terminology |
| 2. List six basic educational requirements for the medical transcriptionist | • Text p. 166<br>• Manual Part 1-B | • Anatomy and physiology of all body systems<br>• Common pathology/disease<br>• Diagnostic/treatment modalities<br>• Applications of medical terminology<br>• Risk management<br>• Fundamental writing skill |
| 3. Name two primary requisites for the independently practicing transcriptionist | • Text p. 166<br>• Manual Part 3 | • Risk management<br>• Fundamental writing skill |
| 4. List the three stages of activity in the machine transcription process | • Text p. 167<br>• Manual Part 3-C | • Applications of electronic technology |
| 5. List five functional features of a typical transcribing unit | • Text p. 167<br>• Manual Part 1-C-1 | • Applications of electronic technology |
| 6. State the principal differences between a dedicated word processor and a computer | • Text pp. 165-166<br>• Manual Part 1-C-2 | • Applications of electronic technology |
| 7. Name three kinds of frequently dictated reports in the average physician's office | • Text p. 171<br>• Manual Part 2 | • Risk management<br>• Fundamental writing skill |
| **Performance** | | **Competency** |
| 1. Estimate the length of a finished document prior to transcribing it | • Text p. 175<br>• Manual Part 2 | • Respond to and initiate written communication |
| 2. Make any necessary corrections in keyboarding before removing the document from the machine | • Manual Part 1-D<br>• CD-ROM ⊕ | • Perform medical transcription<br>• Respond to and initiate written communication<br>• Establish and maintain the medical record<br>• Utilize computer software to maintain office system |

| TEXTBOOK OBJECTIVES | LEARNING SYSTEM LOCATION | MA CURRICULUM |
|---|---|---|
| **Performance** | | **Competency** |
| 3. Correctly utilize basic rules of capitalization | • Manual Part 2<br>• CD-ROM ⊕ | • Document appropriately<br>• Principles of nonverbal communication |
| 4. Follow the rules for word division | • Text p. 177<br>• Manual Part 2<br>• CD-ROM ⊕ | • Document appropriately |
| 5. Determine when to use figures for numbers | • Text p. 177<br>• Manual Part 2<br>• CD-ROM ⊕ | • Document appropriately |
| 6. Correctly format common medical reports | • Text pp. 174-177<br>• Manual Part 2<br>• CD-ROM ⊕ | • Perform medical transcription<br>• Respond to and initiate written communication<br>• Establish and maintain the medical record<br>• Document appropriately<br>• Utilize computer software to maintain office system |
| 7. Proofread and edit a transcribed document | • Text p. 177<br>• Manual Part 2<br>• CD-ROM ⊕ | • Perform medical transcription<br>• Respond to and initiate written communication<br>• Establish and maintain the medical record<br>• Document appropriately<br>• Utilize computer software to maintain office system |

## 3. RESOURCES

**Books**

American Association for Medical Transcription: *Code of Ethics of the American Association for Medical Transcription,* Modesto, California, 1987.

Diehl, M.O., Fordney, M.T.: *Medical Typing and Transcription Techniques and Procedures.* Philadelphia, W. B. Saunders, 1998.

Sloan, S., Fordney, M.T. (eds): *Saunders Manual of Medical Transcription,* Philadelphia, W. B. Saunders, 1994.

The above book is an excellent resource for the instructor. It contains principles of medical ethics, principles of transcription, the medical basis of transcription for all the specialties, and appendices of reference styles, terminology, and myriad items for which the transcriptionist may need quick reference.

See the Textbook, p. 180, for additional references.

Internet

www.NLM.nih.gov/pubs/factsheets/umls.html **This is the fact sheet for the unified Medical Language System information and connecting links**

**www.mavisbeacon.com** A wonderful site for typists and instructors

**http://www.mrc-group.com/** One of the largest private transcribing groups

## 4. LESSON PLAN **TIME 3 hours lecture, 9 hours lab**

**Opening:** Make a videotape of ER or another medical program. Show part of it, and have students write all the medical terms they can. Discuss the difficulty of hearing terms on tape. Discuss the process for trying to identify difficult words.

**Pretest:** Ask students to spell the medical words they wrote while watching the video. Review the correct spelling.

**Objectives:** Emphasize the performance objectives. Students may read, study and complete Mastery Manual Part 1 in class. Use time to review Part 1 in lab, then complete performance objectives in lab.

**Content:**

**Lesson**

1. Review cognitive objectives.
2. If there is time, review rules for spelling and punctuation. Give a basic English test for 12th grade. Sometimes a high school teacher will give you one.
3. Obtain a book on humorous transcription mistakes. Dictate some onto a tape or put on flip chart and let everyone figure out error and how to correct. These are usually excellent examples of grammar, spelling, and punctuation errors.
4. Explain and demonstrate the machine—transcription, dictation, and transcriber units.
5. Review content and format of history and physical, progress notes, consultation reports, operation reports, pathology reports, and discharge summary. Be sure to include format in Text page examples—Do not review content as students will be working on sample textbook report in Part 2 of manual. Bring sample formats of these reports from one hospital and one physician office. Students will see there is variety in formats. Use a transcribing Text page for samples also.
6. Have the department administrator of medical records come to the class and talk about standards and educational needs for transcriptionists in the hospital or a transcription business.

**Laboratory:**
1. It is recommended that all beginning students be able to type at 35 wpm
2. Set a typing meter for 35 wpm. Dictate one letter and one short patient report in the computer laboratory. Students may all type together. Help them to develop skills. Set a schedule for typing at completion of program.
3. Students complete all Part 2 activities in the Mastery Manual.
4. CD-ROM ⊕ Use the SOAP notes from Cases on the CD-ROM. Notes are also located in Appendix A ▲.

**Assignment:** Students complete Part 1 of Mastery Manual independently for review in last hour of class. If not enough, lab time assignments are to be taken home and finalized.

**Posttest:** Ask questions to objectives. Use Examaster testbank.

## 5. MASTERY MANUAL ANSWERS

### PART 1 CONTENT MASTERY

#### A. Learning Level: Knowledge

1. e; 2. h; 3. a; 4. i; 5. g; 6. j; 7. b; 8. c; 9. d; 10. f

#### B. Learning Level: Comprehension

The educational requirements for the medical transcriptionist:

1. Above average typing and word processing skills
2. Understanding of human anatomy and physiology and disease processes
3. Knowledge of medical terminology
4. Names and spellings of drugs, instruments, procedures, treatments
5. Superior command of grammar
6. Editing and proofreading skills

#### C. Learning Level: Application

1. Dials and indicators of a transcribing machine include: Start and stop controls, fast forward and back-up, speed control, volume control, tone control, indicator slips for special instructions.
2. Students may prefer either machine but should be able to list advantages of both.

#### D. Learning Level: Analysis

1. Errors to look for in a transcribed report include: Sentence structure, incomplete sentences, incorrect punctuation, unapproved hospital abbreviations, capitalization, style, format.
2. The transcriptionist may use only hospital-approved abbreviations.

## E. Learning Level: Synthesis

1. Change to two complete sentences.
2. Capitalize Professor. Add "and" after the word "times."
3. Spelling "appendices"
4. The sentence is correct. Students should begin to start making independent decisions. See Text p. 177.
5. Use complete word: Angiogram. Change "called" to small letters. This is one sentence.

## F. Learning Level: Evaluation

This activity is designed to be independent laboratory work. Student may use the Internet with this activity.

1. Proceed to page 171 in Textbook. Review progress notes and abbreviations with students
2. **The site where this information was obtained is** //www.rxlist.com/cgi/rxlist

Drugs underlined are:

Prednisone—prednisone—anti-inflammatory
Brethine—terbutaline sulfate—for bronchospasm
Theo-Dur—theophylline SR (slow release) —smooth muscle relaxant
Lanoxin—digoxin—cardiotonic
Coumadin—warfarin sodium—anticoagulant
Premarin— conjugated estrogens—hormone
Alupent—metaproterenol sulfate—sympathomimetic
Intal—cromolyn sodium—unclassified drug
Dyazide—Hydrochlorothiazide/triamterine—diuretic

## PART 2 COMPETENCY CHALLENGE

A. The transcription reports are in the Mastery Manual at the end.

Have students retype the reports in perfect form, no matter how many attempts are needed. Some instructors provide the final format and others do not. It is frustrating enough to type these correctly, and so it is suggested the correct and final copy be supplied. These are the reports taken from the 8th Edition Textbook Figures 12-7, 8, and 9. Refer the students to those pages if you want to provide correct formatting. You may want to copy these reports and place them in this resource.

B. Tape the TV show *ER* on NBC or T*rauma, Life in the ER* on TLC. Have the students listen to these tapes and write every medical word and diagnosis they can hear. This begins to develop listening skills for transcribing. These tapes can be used in later chapters.

## PART 3 CLINICAL APPLICATIONS

Discussion activities A and B are written to assist students in ethical decision making. Activity C will help students identify their skills and the reality of being medical transcriptionists. Students who do not have strong spelling, punctuation, and grammar skills or are not accurate and very speedy typists will have a difficult time succeeding as a medical transcriptionist.

Be sure to have students complete all self-evaluation forms when turning in work, or walk around the room and check Mastery Manual pages and assignments.

# 13

# The Computer in Medical Practice

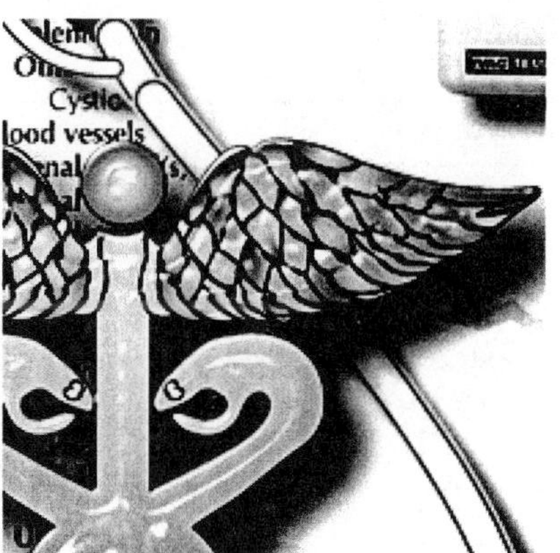

Today every medical assistant program needs to have a computer laboratory. It is imperative that the student be provided a good foundation in the use of a computer. Students learn these programs extremely well when working in pairs. It would be nice to have a minimum of one computer per two students. The student will have the opportunity to be competent in all the cognitive and performance objectives 1, 2, 3, 4, 9, and 10 at the completion of this chapter. The other objectives may be completed later in the program when skills in letter writing, billing, and insurance are learned. Instructors: Beg, borrow, or cajole, but do what it takes to obtain computers for students.

## USING THE LEARNING SYSTEM

### 1. MEDICAL ASSISTANT CONTENT AND COMPETENCIES

CONTENT

- Applications of electronic technology
- Basic medical office functions

COMPETENCIES

- Utilize computer software to maintain office systems
- Perform clerical functions
- Perform bookkeeping procedures
- Process insurance claims

## 2. MEDICAL ASSISTANT ENTRY-LEVEL CURRICULUM

| TEXTBOOK OBJECTIVES | LEARNING SYSTEM LOCATION | MA CURRICULUM |
|---|---|---|
| **Cognitive** | | **Content** |
| 1. Define and spell the terms in the Vocabulary | • Text p. 182<br>• Manual Part 1-A | • Applications of electronic technology |
| 2. Distinguish between the three types of computers | • Text p. 183<br>• Manual Part 1-C | • Applications of electronic technology<br>• Basic medical office functions |
| 3. List the four general categories of computer hardware devices | • Text pp. 183-184<br>• Manual Part 1-B | • Applications of electronic technology<br>• Basic medical office functions |
| 4. Name and state the functions of the most important computer hardware devices | • Text pp. 183-184<br>• Manual Part 1-B | • Applications of electronic technology<br>• Basic medical office functions |
| 5. Name the pointing device that controls the cursor | • Text p. 183<br>• Manual Part 1-A | • Applications of electronic technology<br>• Basic medical office functions |
| 6. Explain the function of the ENTER key | • Text p. 184<br>• Manual Part 1-A | • Applications of electronic technology<br>• Basic medical office functions |
| 7. Describe the cursor-control keys | • Text p. 184<br>• Manual Part 1-A | • Applications of electronic technology<br>• Basic medical office functions |
| 8. Name the output devices | • Text pp. 184-185<br>• Manual Part 1-A | • Applications of electronic technology<br>• Basic medical office functions |
| 9. Explain the purpose of diskettes | • Text p. 185<br>• Manual Part 1-E | • Applications of electronic technology<br>• Basic medical office functions |
| 10. List 10 administrative tasks that might utilize a computer | • Text pp. 187-191<br>• Manual Part 1-D | • Applications of electronic technology<br>• Basic medical office functions |
| **Performance** | **Locations** | **Competency** |
| 1. Start the computer | • Manual Part 2<br>• Procedure 13-1 | • Utilize computer software to maintain office systems<br>• Perform clerical functions |
| 2. Load a program | • Manual Part 2<br>• Procedure 13-1 | • Utilize computer software to maintain office systems<br>• Perform clerical functions |

| TEXTBOOK OBJECTIVES | LEARNING SYSTEM LOCATION | MA CURRICULUM |
|---|---|---|
| **Performance** | | **Competency** |
| 3. Format a disk | • Manual Part 2<br>• Procedure 13-1 | • Utilize computer software to maintain office systems<br>• Perform clerical functions |
| 4. Make a back-up copy of a document | • Manual Part 2<br>• Procedure 13-1 | • Utilize computer software to maintain office systems<br>• Perform clerical functions |
| 5. Generate a patient record | • Chapter 15<br>• CD-ROM ⊕ | • Utilize computer software to maintain office systems<br>• Perform clerical functions |
| 6. Prepare a billing statement | • Chapter 19<br>• CD-ROM ⊕ | • Perform bookkeeping procedures |
| 7. Complete a patient insurance form | • Chapter 21<br>• CD-ROM ⊕ | • Process insurance claims |
| 8. Personalize a computerized form letter | • Manual Part 2 | • Utilize computer software to maintain office systems<br>• Perform clerical functions |
| 9. Access, add, correct, and delete information on the computer | • Manual Part 2<br>• Procedure 13-1 | • Utilize computer software to maintain office systems<br>• Perform clerical functions |
| 10. Shut down the computer | • Manual Part 2 | • Utilize computer software to maintain office systems<br>• Perform clerical functions |

## 3. RESOURCES

Gylys, BA: *Computer Applications for the Medical Office.* Philadelphia, FA Davis, 1997.

www.ahima.org **For information about computerized medical records. American Health Information Management Association. 919 N. Michigan Ave. Suite 1400, Chicago, IL 60611-1683. There is also a state organization in every state.**

www.microsoft.com **This will give students links to learning about different PCs and usage.**

www.smithy.net/TMC/online.html **This site will give students access to information on Macintosh computers.**

## 4. LESSON PLAN Computers TIME 3 hours lecture, 9 hours lab

**Opening:** Meet in the computer lab if possible. Set up computerized overhead projector and screen.
It is important that every student obtain the theory in this chapter. So often computer frustration is relieved when theory is recalled. Students need to explain the problem and help to solve the problem. *Computers do not make input errors—people do.*

*True story for students:* A typist friend kept inadvertently deleting information on her word processor. When she was observed, it was noted that from years of keeping her fingers lightly on the keys, she was giving her computer all kinds of strange commands as the keypad was set to a very sensitive touch. When the keypad was adjusted and she was retrained to "get those fingers UP," the problem was cured.

**Equipment needed:** Make transparencies from the masters for this chapter located in Appendix D. Set up a classroom with a computer hooked up to a special projecting device, dry erase marker.

**Pretest:** Ask students how many are computer literate and who can name the parts of the computer shown on the projected image. Then let students name the parts while you put on labels.

**Objectives:**
**Lesson 1**—Discussion of content 8th Edition Textbook content objectives. Put them up and review in class with a computer for demonstration. Encourage questions and hands-on participation.
**Lesson 2**—Lab: Textbook performance objectives and Procedure 13-1 Competency Objective statement.

**Content:**

**Lesson 1**—Review objectives using the computer and follow outline.

- Computer design
  - CPU
  - Input devices
  - Output devices
- Hard disk management
- Software
- Common computer applications in the office
  - Appointments
  - Patient registration
  - Database management
  - Insurance
  - Bookkeeping entries
  - Billing and collections
  - Health information records
  - Word processing

*Legal and ethical considerations:*
You may want to discuss Part 3, CLINICAL APPLICATIONS, at this time
**Lesson 2**—In the lab: First demonstrate all the competencies in the textbook on the computer. This should be done in small groups of 4-5 while others work on Mastery Manual Part 1, CONTENT MASTERY. After all demonstrations, students may proceed with Mastery Manual Part 2 activities. Instructor needs to give individualized assistance. Students need reinforcement on ability to read and follow directions.

**Assignment:** Memorize all terms and parts of a computer.

**Posttest:** To the assignment above. Fill in the blanks are best for this material. There may be some applicable questions on Examaster Testbank.

## 5. MASTERY MANUAL ANSWERS

### PART 1 CONTENT MASTERY

#### A. Learning Level: Knowledge

1. d; 2. g; 3. j; 4. i; 5. b; 6. a; 7. f; 8. c; 9. h; 10. e
11. ROM is only erased when CPU battery dies or hard drive crashes.
12. Need a hard disk for every computer to store large amounts of programs and information.
13. Software applications are the most important, for they allow you to use information.
14. Modem connects via telephone lines.
15. The mouse or direction keys control the cursor.

#### B. Learning Level: Comprehension

1. Types of hardware devices are:
   Processing unit—CPU; input—keyboard or mouse, trackball, or pad; output—monitor, printer, modem; storage—ROM, RAM, floppy disks, back-up tapes

#### C. Learning Level: Application

Students draw a computer to use visual and tactile learning. Three types of computers are: Mainframes, PC's, and laptops or hand-carried machines. PC's are also called desktops and may be hooked up to a network.

#### D. Learning Level: Analysis

Students may need help understanding how each is accomplished. Review information applications for each of the following tasks: Complete insurance input, transmit claims, patient registration, patient scheduling, put in charges and insurance codes, insurance coverage information, compile billing information and print it, automatic calculating of accounts payable and receivable, bookkeeping entries, chart entries, operative reports, insurance and other letters, referrals, payroll, electronic signature. Students may get more tasks from 8th Edition Textbook.

#### E. Learning Level: Synthesis

This is an effective exercise to assist students in planning for their workspace and evaluating their needs. This can be related to learning styles.

#### F. Learning Level: Evaluation

This activity calls for self-evaluation and planning to obtain the information and skills needed.

### PART 2 COMPETENCY CHALLENGE

Writing directions for each phase of using the computer as listed in the Mastery Manual, p. 116, will give students ready access and also help tactile students. The directions then may be used to take each student through each competency. The second exercise will start the student applying a word processing program. One could have students type transcription reports and type a letter to begin familiarity with both processes on the word processing software application. Plan time to check-off students on Procedure 13-1, which is added as a tool for you to easily evaluate the performance objectives.

If students do not develop these basic skills at this point in the program, they will be spending too much time later catching up. With all the activities completed, they will have been through the learning process and basic computer skills should be theirs.

## PART 3 CLINICAL APPLICATIONS

This is a very important discussion. Some points follow.

- Security—Unauthorized persons should never have access to confidential information. Passwords should be given to each user with instructions not to share. Some persons have limited access, i.e., to appointments but not billing records.
- Sending e-mail—Those who do so again have access passwords and send over secure lines. No unauthorized or fun mail.
- None of these concerns are a problem if protection is taken. Usually care must be taken in large medical office complexes and hospitals due to hackers, disgruntled patients, and personnel with less than honest motives.
- There are many other points; these are but a few of the main ones.

# 14

# Filing Methods, Storage and Retention

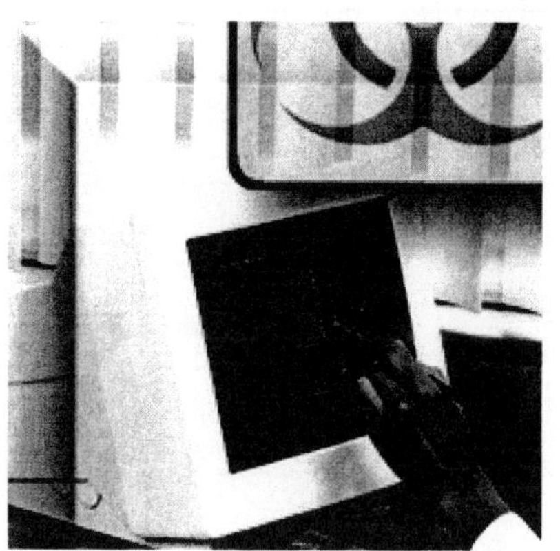

Filing is often one of the first tasks the medical assistant student is asked to perform in the externship experience. Students need the experience and once accomplished, they may advance to other duties. Every member of the health care team is needed to maintain patient charts in correct order, and students must learn the various systems and how to use them. Instructors will find this chapter comprehensive and easy to apply so the students will be interested. Instructors may accumulate all student files and have students make examples of all types of filing systems. New instructors will have students purchase files and then assign various filing sytem designs to different students. Students develop the systems and accomplish all the objectives. This contributes to the overall understanding of all types of filing and the efficiency of the medical assistant.

## USING THE LEARNING SYSTEM

### 1. MEDICAL ASSISTANT CONTENT AND COMPETENCIES

CONTENT

- Legal guidelines
- Risk management
- Basic medical office functions
- Workplace dynamics
- Recognition and response to verbal and nonverbal communication
- Fundamental writing skills

COMPETENCIES

- File medical records
- Organize a patient's medical record
- Identify and respond to issues of confidentiality
- Perform within legal and ethical boundaries
- Recognize and respond to verbal and nonverbal communication

## 2. MEDICAL ASSISTANT ENTRY-LEVEL CURRICULUM INTERFACE

| TEXTBOOK OBJECTIVES | LEARNING SYSTEM LOCATION | MA CURRICULUM |
|---|---|---|
| **Cognitive** | | **Content** |
| 1. List and discuss the basic equipment and supplies in a filing system | • Text pp. 195-199<br>• Manual Part 1-B | • File medical records<br>• Organize patient's medical record |
| 2. Describe the five sequential steps in filing a document | • Text pp. 199-200<br>• Manual Part 1 | • File medical records<br>• Organize patient's medical record<br>• Identify and respond to issues of confidentiality<br>• Perform within legal and ethical boundaries |
| 3. List and discuss application of the four basic filing systems | • Text pp. 202-204<br>• Manual Part 1-D, E, F | • File medical records<br>• Organize patient's medical record<br>• Recognize and respond to verbal and nonverbal communication |
| 4. Explain how color-coding of files can be advantageous in a health care facility | • Text pp. 204-205<br>• CD-ROM ⊕ | • File medical records<br>• Organize patient's medical record<br>• Perform within legal and ethical boundaries |
| **Performance** | **Locations** | **Competencies** |
| 1. Typewrite a list of names in indexing order and arrange them alphabetically for filing | • Manual Part 2<br>• CD-ROM ⊕ | • File medical records<br>• Organize patient's medical record<br>• Recognize and respond to verbal and nonverbal communication |
| 2. Arrange a group of patient numbers in filing sequence for a terminal digit filing system | • Manual Part 2<br>• CD-ROM ⊕ | • File medical records<br>• Organize patient's medical record |
| 3. Using the color key in this chapter, state the tab color to be used for a given list of names | • Manual Part 2<br>• CD-ROM ⊕ | • File medical records<br>• Organize patient's medical record<br>• Perform within legal and ethical boundaries<br>• Recognize and respond to verbal and nonverbal communication |

## 3. RESOURCES

See Lesson Plan opening to order VHS.
"The Eyes Have It In Color Filing," *Managing office technologies*, June 1994.

## 4. LESSON PLAN Filing TIME 3 hours lecture, 9 hours lab

**Opening:** AV VHS 14 minutes. "Set the Records Straight." Smead Manufacturing Company, 600 East Smead Boulevard, Hastings, MN 55033. Or have ten files on your desk that are labeled and in wrong order. Ask who can identify what is incorrect about the files as students come into class.

**Pretest:** You can use the opener as your pretest. Students may look at the files, write answers, and give them to you.

**Objectives:** Use the template in Appendix D and put the cognitive objectives up on an overhead projector. Use these objectives and fill the information in with a pen. Do not use permanent ink so that you can clean and use the transparency next year!

**Content:** Outline—Fill in with information you want to cover in short lecture.

FILING EQUIPMENT

Drawer Files — Shelf Files — Rotary Circular Files

Lateral File — Compactable Files — Automated Files

Card Files — Special Items

SUPPLIES

Divider Guides — OUTguides

Chart Covers or Folders — Labels

FILING PROCEDURES

Conditioning — Releasing — Indexing & Coding

Sorting — Storing & Filing

*Chart continues on following page*

SAFETY PRECAUTIONS
LOCATING MISPLACED FILES

INDEXING RULES

FILING SYSTEMS

Alphabetic
Numeric

Subject
Geographic

COLOR CODING

Alphabetic
Numeric
Other Applications

ORGANIZATION OF FILES

Patient health information

Health-related correspondence

General correspondence

Practice management file

Tickler files
Temporary files
Miscellaneous files

**Assignment:** Have students complete Part 2 and discuss the situation in Part 3. Students may be assigned a department in the school where for one hour or more they do the filing for the week. This takes a bit of time the first time it is arranged but usually proceeds smoothly. Often students are allowed to "give" an hour a week in a department to practice clerical skills such as filing, records management, telephone techniques, message taking, and computer skills. In return for this time, the instructor may grade students in a variety of methods or may consider it time in lab. Have students proceed to CD-ROM ⊕ and complete administrative exercise on filing. The procedures many be used with the activities. Look up topic in help file to find exact location.

**Posttest:** Take questions from testbank or objectives. Filing 10 folders may also be part of a "walk around" examination. Put out a filing cabinet with many files. Give each student a number of files and have them correctly file according to the system being used. Specify the time and accuracy. Ask students to write two things they learned in class and what they want clarified for next class or lab.

## 5. MASTERY MANUAL ANSWERS

### PART 1 CONTENT MASTERY

### A. Learning Level: Knowledge

1. e; 2. f; 3. d; 4. g; 5. c; 6. j; 7. b; 8. i; 9. a; 10. h

### B. Learning Level: Comprehension

1. List and describe five types of files.
   a. alphabetic—names in alphabetic order, they may also be indexed
   b. numeric—by numbers straight in order seen or by terminal digit
   c. geographic—according to demographics or location, not name or subject
   d. chronologic—according to date as in a tickler or A/P file
   e. subject—according to subject such as insurance received, EOB's, payroll

### C. Learning Level: Application

1. Give two examples of the use of the Librarians' Rule when filing.
   a. Lilley, A; Lilly, A., Lilly, ana, Lilly, Anne

   b. Mann, Carlotta, Mann-Wom; Carlotta
2. Code the following list of ten names, indicating Unit 1 with one underline, Unit 2 with two underlines, and Unit 3 with three underlines.

| One Underline | Double Underline | Triple Underline |
|---|---|---|
| Feldman | Ken | |
| MacLovell | John | Allen |
| Purcell | Agnes | M |
| Taylor | Adam | Q |
| Francis | Xavier | |
| Cicero | Sandy | Reed |
| Shirley | Cecil | A |
| Breck | W | A |
| Xavier | F | |
| Good | Arthur | Francis |

### D. Learning Level: Analysis

Describe the filing system being used.
1. alphanumeric
2. numeric
3. chronologic-tickler
4. geographic

### E. Learning Level: Synthesis

1. Name at least three methods for assigning numbers to patients for numeric filing.
   a. In order of appearance in office
   b. By Social Security number
   c. By terminal digit; also by birthday dates as terminal digits
2. Explain two reasons that medical offices use color coding with the main type of filing system.
   a. Color coding allows quicker retrieval; restricts the areas for storing and retrieving.
   b. Misfiled charts are easily spotted.

## F. Learning Level: Evaluation

1. Name two advantages of terminal digit filing.

   Allows unlimited expansion, saves time in retrieving

2. Write the type of filing system you would suggest for the following offices. List your rationale next to the system chosen. Answers reflect text guidelines.

   a. Alphanumeric with color coding

   b. Numeric with terminal digit—only system which can accurately handle that number of files

   c. Alphanumeric will handle the expected number over 10 years; color coding not needed. Could use alphabetic with color coding to make retrieving easier.

## PART 2 COMPETENCY CHALLENGE

Note: This activity will familiarize students with filing procedures. The reality is that many offices have an employee who sets up blank files for completion of records. One does not have to understand all the meanings of the records to put files in appropriate order and to label for filing.

These activities challenge the student to integrate and use the information. If the student does not know the material, the activities will be more difficult. The activities will help students meet all the objectives. They will take students through all the procedures. Students can use all the names in Part 2 and develop alphabetic, numeric, terminal digit, and subject files that may then be stored by the instructor for future use. Periodically take out the files, change the order, and have students refile the folders using different systems.

PROCEDURE 14-1: INITIATING A MEDICAL FILE FOR A NEW PATIENT
For alphabetic filing, provide the student with a file folder, label, and financial (ledger) card. For numeric filing, the student will also need an I .D. card and cross reference card. Students may be required to purchase these items.

A. Use Procedure 14-1: Initiating a Medical File for a New Patient. Establish charts for the four patients in the case studies in Appendix C▲. Decide the filing system and color coding you will use for medical record management. Use Appendix C▲ and copy all the chart forms for each of the patients and put them in the patients' files for future use. Save one copy of these forms, as they will need to be copied in future activities. As you encounter new patients, begin new medical files.

B. Establish charts for the following patients listed below in this activity: Abigail Anderson, Virginia Davies, Bertha Bogart, Connie Caldwell, Doris Dollar, Edith Edgewater, Rex Ingram, Mary Louise McCall, Claude Irvin, Thomas Ross, Johnnie Cramer, Jo McLinden, Rose Macdonald, Virginia Dement, Paul Leonard Alcorn, Leona Maxwell, Grace Schwartz, Karen Fox, Frances Schenk.

C. Disregarding the numbers next to the names, type each of the following 20 names in indexing order using the label page at the end of chapter or separate label paper, and then arrange the names in alphabetic order for filing. Place the labels on files and in alphabetic order. Place with above files from Part 2, activity 1 above. Establish a color coding system for the charts following Procedure 14-2.

PROCEDURE 14-2: COLOR CODING PATIENT CHARTS
You may be able to get practice kits from a supplier such as Safeguard or Bibbero Systems.

**Indexing order:**

| | | | |
|---|---|---|---|
| 90 73 00 | Ceccarini, Shirlee | 56 23 47 | John Murvall |
| 01 55 05 | Cecarini, Sibyl | 73 05 52 | Madam Shirlee |
| 03 43 17 | A & M Auto Supply | 51 98 54 | Arthur F. Goode |
| 18 43 17 | K. Felt | 65 77 73 | Kenneth Felt |
| 23 04 21 | Edw. Cecere | 15 00 77 | Dennis Mc Lain |
| 33 11 22 | Marian Fellows | 26 62 77 | The Fellows Medical Mfg. Co. |
| 36 93 27 | Wu See Po | 09 51 81 | Robert Murval |
| 29 87 32 | Dennis McLain | 21 78 83 | Wm. A. Breck, M.D. |
| 40 61 33 | Mrs. Robert Murval (Zelda) | 93 06 95 | AMA |
| 40 39 45 | Bill Fisher | 87 33 95 | Fisher & Bro. of Montana, Inc. |

D. Your instructor may have a filing activity for you in one of the school offices. Complete the activities and in the next laboratory explain the filing system used and your activities in the office. Have students put all files in alphabetical order.

Alcomb, Paul Leonard
AMA
A & M Auto Supply
Anderson, Abigail
Barnett, Joseph
Beck, William A.
Bogart, Bertha
Caldwell, Connie
Cecarini, Sibyl
Ceccarini, Shirlee
Cecere, Edw.
Cramer, Johnnie
Davies, Virginia
Dement, Virginia
Dollar, Doris
Edgewater, Edith
Fellows, Marian
Fellows Medical Mfg. Co. (The)
Felt, K.
Felt, Kenneth
Fisher, Bill
Fisher & Bro. of Montana, Inc.
Fischer, Cheryl
Fox, Karen
Goode, Arthur F. (attorney)
Ingram, Rex
Irvin, Claude
Lain, Dennis M.
Macdonald, Rose
Madame Shirlee
Maxwell, Leona
McCall, Mary Louise
McLain, Dennis
McLinden, Jo
Murval, Robert
Murval, Zelda (Mrs. Robert)
Murvall, John
Ross, Themes
Schenk, Frances
Schwartz, Grace
Po, Wu See

PART 3 CLINICAL APPLICATIONS
This discussion subject reinforces positive confidentiality behaviors. Keep files away from patients, keep names covered, do not ask another person for file locations in a loud voice, and do not let other patients hear names of patients who are not in the reception area.

# 15

# Health Information Management

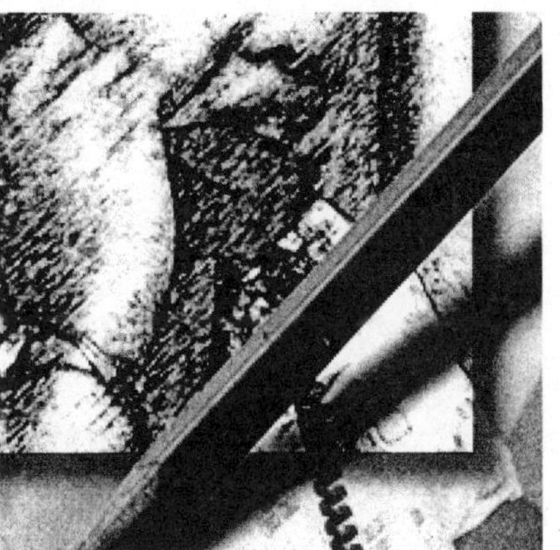

Government health insurance regulations, insurance company rules, and HMO contracts are requiring more accurate, timely, detailed, and legible documents. There are more audits of medical records than ever before. Many offices are being fined due to inadvertent errors. The topic of this chapter therefore takes on great importance in the medical office and clinic. Differentiate a file (blank) from a medical record, i.e., contains personal patient information. The medical assistant must be vigilant in protecting the physician by checking records for required information in greater depth and breadth than in the past. This chapter will begin to stress the importance of health information management (HIM) in today's medical office. This is another area where specialty certification and national credentials are available.

## USING THE LEARNING SYSTEM

### 1. MEDICAL ASSISTANT CONTENT AND COMPETENCIES

CONTENT

- Applications of medical terminology
- Legal guidelines
- Recognition and response to verbal and nonverbal communication
- Risk management

COMPETENCIES

- Establish and maintain the medical record
- Organize a patient's medical record
- Document accurately
- Inventory supplies and equipment

## 2. MEDICAL ASSISTANT ENTRY-LEVEL CURRICULUM INTERFACE

| TEXTBOOK OBJECTIVES | LEARNING SYSTEM LOCATION | MA CURRICULUM |
|---|---|---|
| **Cognitive** | | **Content** |
| 1. Define and spell the terms listed in the Vocabulary | • Text p. 209<br>• Manual Part 1-A | • Applications of medical terminology |
| 2. State five important reasons for keeping good medical records | • Text pp. 209-210<br>• Manual Part 1-B | • Legal guidelines<br>• Risk management |
| 3. Explain ownership of the medical record | • Text pp. 209 and 224<br>• Manual Part 3 | • Legal guidelines<br>• Risk management |
| 4. List three advantages of the POMR | • Text p. 214<br>• Manual Part 1-C | • Legal guidelines<br>• Risk management<br>• Recognition and response to verbal and nonverbal communication |
| 5. Explain the basic differences between the traditional and the problem-oriented medical record | • Text pp. 213-214<br>• Manual Part 1-A | • Legal guidelines<br>• Risk management<br>• Recognition and response to verbal and nonverbal communication |
| 6. Illustrate the meaning of subjective and objective information in a medical history | • Text p. 217<br>• Manual Part 1-D | • Recognition and response to verbal and nonverbal communication |
| 7. List four categories of subjective and objective information in a complete case history | • Text p. 214<br>• Manual Part 1-C | • Recognition and response to verbal and nonverbal communication |
| 8. List 15 items of personal data needed on a patient history | • Text p. 216<br>• Manual Part 2 | • Recognition and response to verbal and nonverbal communication<br>• Legal guidelines<br>• Risk management |
| 9. Discuss changing an entry in the medical record and the importance of following correct procedure | • Text p. 219<br>• Manual Part 1-E | • Recognition and response to verbal and nonverbal communication<br>• Legal guidelines<br>• Risk management |
| 10. List and describe the three classifications of patient files | • Text p. 223<br>• Manual Part 1-C | • Same as #5 |
| **Performance ⊕** | **Locations** | **Competencies** |
| 1. Assemble a medical record for a new patient | • Manual Part 2<br>• Procedure 14-1<br>• CD-ROM ⊕ | • Establish and maintain the medical record<br>• Inventory supplies and equipment |

## 2. MEDICAL ASSISTANT ENTRY-LEVEL CURRICULUM INTERFACE

| TEXTBOOK OBJECTIVES | LEARNING SYSTEM LOCATION | MA CURRICULUM |
|---|---|---|
| **Performance** | | **Competencies** |
| 2. Add reports and correspondence into the patient's file in the correct manner and sequence | • Manual Part 2<br>• Procedure 14-1<br>• CD-ROM ⊕ | • Organize a patient's medical record |
| 3. Make a correction in a patient's chart in a manner affording legal protection | • Text p. 219<br>• Manual Part 1-E<br>• CD-ROM ⊕ | • Document appropriately |

## 3. RESOURCES

**Internet Links Include**

http://www.ahima.org/ **American Health Information Management Association, specialists in medical records management**

www.mavisbeacon.com/edulink.htm **A nice link to many educational sites**

www.savetz.com/pd/ **A link to much public domain material. Not subject to any copyright laws**

**Books and Articles**

Goldwater S: *Electronic Patient Records.* PMA, September/October 1998.

Video: *The Medical Record, Clinical Skills for the medical assistant.* W. B. Saunders Co., The Curtis Center, Independence Square West, Philadelphia, PA 19106-3399.

Two good sources for Medical Office Management computer programs are:

Gylys, ME: *Computer Applications in the Medical Office.* Philadelphia, FA Davis Publisher, 1997.

Medical Office Management by Medisoft, Phoenix, AZ. This program is provided free to schools as a marketing tool.

There are other programs in regional areas that may be supplied to as marketing tools. For example, a California-based software program called Medical Manager has a student computer program available via Delmar Publishers.

## 4. LESSON PLAN Filing TIME 3 hours lecture, 9 hours lab

**Opening:** Discuss procrastination when not completing work or use an example that has affected students in the program. What is the problem with putting off work? How annoying is it when it is not done? How do others react? Relate to the workplace along with other negative behaviors, pejorative statements, etc.

**Pretest:** Have students spell five vocabulary words from chapter p. 209. Suggest they include some of the following: augment; chronologic; correlation; demographic, obliteration; parlance; pejorative; sequential.

**Objectives:** Post on a flip chart so that as content is covered it may be related to objectives.

**Content:** Have an RPT or MT come in and speak about the utilization of medical records and documentation problems for first hour.

Follow with a review of chapter and discussion of issues.

1. Review meanings of vocabulary words.
2. Talk about reasons for keeping medical records.
3. Clarify concept of ownership of the record.
4. Discuss source-oriented and POMR medical records.
5. List the advantages of POMR records.
6. Explain SOAP charting and differentiate subjective and objective information and facts!
7. Have students turn to patient registration form in Mastery Manual and review all the components for patient registration and then the 15 items on a patient history.
8. Legal documentation requires factual, timely, legible, dated, and signed records.
9. Discuss retention of files and records. Types are active, inactive, or closed.
10. Considerations for retention of records.
11. If time, students may complete Mastery Manual Part 1 activities.

**Lab:** Students complete Parts 2 and 3 in the laboratory. Take students on field trip to hospital or large clinic. Observe filing systems rationale, documentation requirements and data sets used.

**Assignment:** In preparation for this lesson, students should have read chapter. After lesson have students complete all Mastery Manual activities in the lab. Students may interview each other for patient registration activities.

**Posttest:** Use topic questions from Examaster testbank or subjective questions by turning objectives into questions.

## 5. MASTERY MANUAL ANSWERS

### PART 1 CONTENT MASTERY

### A. Learning Level: Knowledge

1. e; 2. i; 3. f; 4. j; 5. c; 6. b; 7. a; 8. d; 9. g; 10. h

### B. Learning Level: Comprehension

1. State the objectives of information management.
   a. saving space
   b. reducing unnecessary records
   c. faster information retrieval, legal compliance, saving physician and patient time
2. Explain five reasons for keeping health information records.
   a. provide best medical care
   b. provide statistical information
   c. provide legal protection
   d. to maintain financial and demographic information
   e. to meet health insurance and managed care participation requirements

### C. Learning Level: Application

1. Correct the following negative statements to neutral or positive.
   a. The patient *is not able to state* a specific complaint.
   b. *The patient states she is fearful* in giving insulin to son.
   c. Patient *states she is having a bad day.*
   d. *Patient is irritable, withdrawn, and states he wants pain medicine.*
   e. Fill in the answers. The meaning of POMR is problem-oriented medical record.
2. List five advantages of POMR over source-oriented medical records.
   a. Observations are together and chronological
   b. Problem list and resolution in the same area
   c. Treatment is numbered with problem
   d. SOAP notes are specific, concise, and accurate
   e. Logical relationship to chart entries

### D. Learning Level: Analysis

1. Research and obtain one type of medical record from one local hospital or long term care or rehabilitation facility. Where did you go? What type of record is kept? Answers will vary.
2. Is the following subjective or objective information?
   a. Patient has pain in lower leg. subjective
   b. Chest x-ray is normal. objective
   c. Hg. 14.2 objective
   d. Fatigue and malaise subjective
   e. Fell off the roof subjective
   f. Short of breath subjective
   g. Respirations 32 and labored objective
   h. The sky is azure blue. subjective
   i. The car was going at least 60. subjective
   j. This book is no good. subjective
3. List different methods of obtaining subjective or objective information.
   Subjective: interview, opinion, family history, recollection
   Objective: factual, scientific, may be proven, lab tests, observation, measurement, pictures

## E. Learning Level: Synthesis

Illustrate below the correct methods of making a correction to the medical record.

1. The chart states, "Mom says I think Robby has an ear date all ~~infection~~ obstruction."
   The physician says she told the medical assistant she thought he had an ear <u>obstruction</u>.
2. The chart states "Lab phoned. And reported Irma's FBS is 82." When the lab slip comes, it is 62. Correct by writing next to it, "Correction Lab slip indicated 62 and was verified by telephone with MA Woods, performing technician."
3. State **incorrect** practices in correcting a chart notation.
   <u>a. erase</u> <u>b. white out</u> <u>c. write in pencil</u>
4. Name four standards (qualities) for medical records to be documented correctly. Students should be able to write these from learning all the chapter information.
   a. factual documentation
   b. chart in a timely fashion, not late
   c. date and sign
   d. legible

## F. Learning Level: Evaluation

1. List as many storage forms for keeping records as you know.
   a. microfiche
   b. computer disk
   c. tape back-up
   d. micro film
2. The physician has told you to take three boxes of medical records and determine which, if any, need to be saved. What criteria should you use to make that determination?
   a. State law from last patient contact, or from when a child turns to age of majority
   b. Statute of limitations for business records—recommended 10 years
   c. Medicare and Medicaid charts—keep at least 5 years
   d. Forward to another physician if patient requires

## PART 2 COMPETENCY CHALLENGE

There are three student performance competencies. At completion of this activity, students will have assembled two patient files to add to patient charts assembled in previous chapters. Students again follow Procedure 14-1, 14-2, and 14-3 to complete this activity. There is one patient registration form at the end of the chapter for students to copy and use. There is another one in Appendix B▲. Students may use CD-ROM ⊕ activities to set up patient medical records also. Proceed to CD-ROM ⊕ administrative section, and find activities related to registering patients and using medical records.

Activities:

1. Use the Patient Registration form at the end of the chapter. Make two copies of the form. Interview any two adults and complete the forms. All the spaces must be filled in, or have N/A or a line in the space to indicate you have reviewed the entire form. If you have a medical computer program, you may be instructed to enter these patient's registration information. Your instructor will give you further directions for your Health Information Management activity.
2. Use the two completed patient registrations and establish a medical record (patient chart) for these patients. Use the filing system as directed by your instructor. When the file folder is labeled, place the registration and other chart forms in correct order and add these two records to those you made in Chapter 14, Filing. If you have not done so, make copies of the chart forms in Appendix B▲ and place a copy of each form in each patient folder.

## PART 3 CLINICAL APPLICATIONS

A. Why would a patient want to see his or her medical record? What would you say to the patient who asked to see his or her record?

Curiosity, concern about what is in it, understand the information and illness

One response might be "I will tell the physician of your request and he/she will probably review it with you."

B. When the court subpoenas an original case record, what should the medical assistant do? Consider all steps.

1. Notify the physician.
2. Copy entire chart x 2.
3. Put copied chart in medical record.
4. Place OUTguide in tickler file on date of promised return or status check.
5. Call subpoena service and have them pick up and sign for original.
6. Put in medical record.
7. Call if not returned.

C. The patient asks for a copy of the medical record. The physician does not want to provide the record because he does not feel the patient should see some psychiatric information.

What are the patient's rights in this matter?

What are the physician's rights?

How can the physician handle this?

How can the patient get a copy of the record even though the physician does not give it to the patient?

Who pays for the work and how much can legally be charged?

Do you have an opinion on this matter?

D. Your office procedure requires placing laboratory and other reports on the physician's desk. When the physician has seen the reports, they are checked and put in a central basket for placing on patient charts. If the physician wants a patient called, that is noted on the report. When the medical assistant and other personnel have time, they call up the charts, put the reports on them, and call the patients. Looking in the basket, you see reports that are over a month old. Think of a solution to update all charts in a timely manner and catch up on all the other calling and updating.

# 16

# Professional Fees and Credit Arrangements

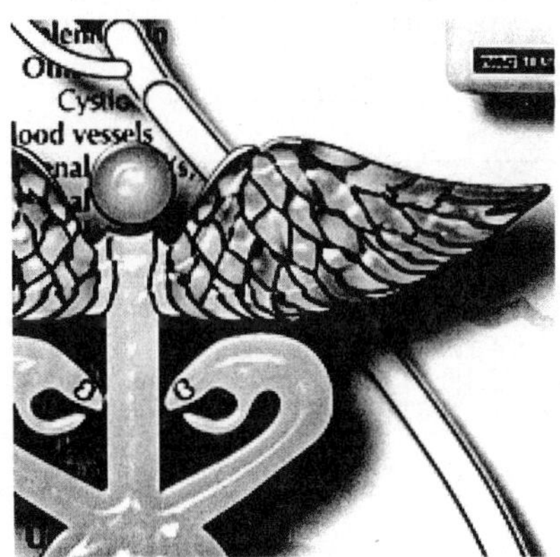

Most medical assistant students have little or no experience with asking for and collecting fees. It may be intimidating to most persons. Physicians, however, expect the medical assistant to keep monies owed to a minimum. It is important for students to learn that when done correctly, at the start of the professional relationship, late payments and collections rarely become a problem. Students need to learn these materials before completing the Mastery Manual. They must become comfortable and at ease with the procedures of explaining fees and making payment arrangements. These next four chapters should be given a total of 12 hours lecture/discussion and 48 hours laboratory/practice, field trips, and competency testing.

## USING THE LEARNING SYSTEM

### 1. MEDICAL ASSISTANT CONTENT AND COMPETENCIES

CONTENT

- Word building and definitions
- Legal guidelines/requirements for health care
- Medical ethics and related issues
- Hereditary, cultural, and environmental influences on behavior
- Principles of recognition and response to verbal and nonverbal communication
- Adaptations for individual needs
- Basic medical office functions
- Bookkeeping and basic accounting

COMPETENCIES

- Respond to and initiate written communications
- Recognize and respond to verbal communication
- Identify and respond to issues of confidentiality
- Document appropriately
- Explain general office policies
- Instruct individuals according to their needs
- Perform within legal and ethical boundaries
- Perform accounts receivable procedures
- Apply managed care policies and procedures
- Apply third-party guidelines
- Use a physician's fee schedule

## 2. MEDICAL ASSISTANT ENTRY-LEVEL CURRICULUM INTERFACE

| TEXTBOOK OBJECTIVES | LEARNING SYSTEM LOCATION | MA CURRICULUM |
|---|---|---|
| Cognitive | | Content |
| 1. Define and spell the terms listed in the Vocabulary | • Text p. 228<br>• Manual Part 1-A | • Word building and definitions |
| 2. Discuss how fees are determined | • Text p. 228<br>• Manual Part 1-D-3 | • Bookkeeping and basic accounting<br>• Adaptations for individual needs<br>• Legal guidelines/requirements for health care |
| 3. List three values that are considered in determining professional fees | • Text p. 228<br>• Manual Part 1-B | • Bookkeeping and basic accounting<br>• Adaptations for individual needs |
| 4. Give an example of a usual and customary fee | • Text p. 229<br>• Manual Part 1-D-3 | • Bookkeeping and basic accounting<br>• Legal guidelines/requirements for health care |
| 5. Explain how a physician's fee profile is determined | • Text p. 229<br>• Manual Part 1-D-3 | • Bookkeeping and basic accounting<br>• Legal guidelines/requirements for health care |
| 6. List three reasons for giving patients an estimate slip | • Text p. 231<br>• Manual Part 1-F | • Legal guidelines/requirements for health care<br>• Bookkeeping and basic accounting<br>• Hereditary, cultural, and environmental influences on behavior<br>• Adaptation to individual needs |
| 7. Discuss the concept of professional courtesy | • Text p. 232<br>• Manual Part 1-B | • Adaptation to individual needs<br>• Hereditary, cultural, and environmental influences on behavior<br>• Principles of recognition and response to verbal and nonverbal communication |
| 8. List four kinds of charges that should be avoided | • Text pp. 232-233<br>• Manual Part 1-D | • Legal guidelines/requirements for health care |
| 9. List the items to be included on a credit form | • Text pp. 234-235<br>• Manual Part 2-B | • Legal guidelines/requirements for health care |
| 10. Explain what is meant by third-party liability | • Text p. 235<br>• Manual Part 1-B | • Legal guidelines/requirements for health care |

## 2. MEDICAL ASSISTANT ENTRY-LEVEL CURRICULUM INTERFACE

| TEXTBOOK OBJECTIVES | LEARNING SYSTEM LOCATION | MA CURRICULUM |
|---|---|---|
| **Cognitive** | | **Content** |
| 11. Identify the three items of information that can be released in response to a request for credit information | • Text p. 236<br>• Manual Part 1-E | • Legal guidelines/requirements for health care<br>• Medical ethics and related issues<br>• Bookkeeping and basic accounting |
| 12. State three items that should be *excluded* in replying to a request for credit information | • Text p. 237<br>• Manual Part 3 | • Legal guidelines/requirements for health care |
| 13. Discuss the Truth in Lending Regulation | • Text pp. 236-237<br>• Manual Part 1-F | • Legal guidelines/requirements for health care |
| 14. Discuss how confidentiality relates to credit | • Text p. 237<br>• Manual Part 3<br>• CD-ROM ⊕ | • Legal guidelines/requirements for health care<br>• Medical ethics and related issues<br>• Hereditary, cultural, and environmental influences on behavior<br>• Principles of recognition and response to verbal and nonverbal communication<br>• Adaptations for individual needs |
| **Performance** | **Locations** | **Competencies** |
| 1. Respond to patient's request for explanation of the physician's fee | • Manual Part 2<br>• CD-ROM ⊕<br>• Procedure 16-1 | • Respond to and initiate written communications<br>• Recognize and respond to verbal communication<br>• Identify and respond to issues of confidentiality<br>• Document appropriately<br>• Explain general office policies<br>• Instruct individuals according to their needs<br>• Perform within legal and ethical boundaries<br>• Perform accounts receivable procedures<br>• Apply managed care policies and procedures<br>• Apply third-party guidelines<br>• Use a physician's fee schedule |

*chart continues on following page*

## 2. MEDICAL ASSISTIANT ENTRY-LEVEL CURRICULUM INTERFACE

| TEXTBOOK OBJECTIVES | LEARNING SYSTEM LOCATION | MA CURRICULUM |
|---|---|---|
| Performance | | Competency |
| 2. Make financial arrangements with a patient requesting credit | • Manual Part 2<br>• Procedure 16-2<br>• CD-ROM ⊕ | • Same as preceding #1 |
| 3. Prepare a Truth in Lending form | • Manual Part 2<br>• Sample on Text p. 236 | • Perform within legal and ethical boundaries<br>• Perform accounts receivable procedures |

## 3. RESOURCES

**http://www.law.cornell.edu/topics/consumer credit.html Cornell University consumer credit laws site including federal statutes and regulations**

http://search.yahoo.com/bin/search?p=credit+laws **This is a search engine for more credit information.**

## 4. LESSON PLAN Professional Fees TIME 3 hours lecture, 12 hours lab

**Opening:** Tell a story about the person who lost everything because she was responsible for a debt she wasn't aware of, and then tell the story of the person who never got his money back because he made a "gentleman's agreement," which the gentleman forgot about! The Purpose: Protect the patient and the physician.

**Pretest:** Ask if any one knows any consumer protection laws and have them explain. You may go to the Internet site and check on some laws before class.

**Objectives:** Ask students to write objectives. What do they think they will need to know? Write them on board, transparency, or easel. Teach to the objectives but get the essential materials in the outline below covered. The MA curriculum provides a total of 900 hours instruction. Medical offices require greater depth and breadth of understanding than ever before. As instructors, this requires increased time to master competencies. This and subsequent lessons reflect increased lab time.

**Content:** Chapter content has been rearranged into three topics below. This will help students organize concepts and emphasize the MA role in this area. Students learn the materials in the 8th Edition Textbook by relating the theory to personal experience and drawing analogies. Topics of the discussion of fees, adjusting fees, charges to avoid, and extending credit are all subjects that are familiar to most, although possibly not in relationship to the medical office. The two difficult concepts are first: the various ways fees are determined, which has little to do with the entry-level medical assistant, and secondly, extending credit, which may become a duty early on in the medical assistant career. Therefore cover these two areas first.

## LESSON PLAN *continued*

**Content continued:**

A. PROFESSIONAL FEES
- How Fees Are Determined
- The Effects of Managed Care
- Prevailing Rate in the Community
- Usual, Customary, and Reasonable Fee
- Fee Setting by Third-Party Payers
- Physician's Fee Profile
- Insurance Allowance

B. CREDIT ARRANGEMENTS
1. Extending Credit
   - Information from the patient
   - Health insurance information
   - Third-party liability
   - Assignment of benefits
2. Consent for Release of Information
3. Installment Buying of Medical Services
4. Credit Cards
   - Special Budget Plans
5. Truth in Lending Act
6. Confidentiality and Other Legal Issues
7. Obtaining Credit Information, Credit Bureaus

C. PROFESSIONAL FEES: medical assistant responsibilities
1. Advance Discussion of Fees
   - Responsibility to Discuss Fees
   - Explaining Additional Costs
2. Estimate Slips
3. Adjusting or Canceling Fees
   - Those Who Cannot Pay
   - Fee Adjustments
   - Fees in Hardship Cases
   - Professional Courtesy
4. Charges to Avoid
   - Telephone Calls
   - Missed Appointments
   - Late Payments
   - First Insurance Forms

**Lab:** Students all complete Part 2 in the Mastery Manual. Observe and evaluate explanations of Procedures 16-1 and 16 -2 for each student. Plan discussion time for the CLINICAL APPLICATIONS.

**Assignment:** Before lecture, students need to study this material. Give them the three major topics as outlined above and have them make index cards of three major topics to help organize their thoughts. Collecting the index cards will help you evaluate their ability to organize and recognize important concepts.

**Posttest:** The Examaster testbank has a wide variety of questions on this topic. Also, use some other ancillary testing materials. Students need to read multiple choice questions formatted by a variety of authors so they are preparing for certification as they progress in the program.

## 5. MASTERY MANUAL ANSWERS

### PART 1 CONTENT MASTERY

### A. Learning Level: Knowledge

**Short Answer**

1. Reduction or absence of fee to professional associates is **professional courtesy**.
2. A compilation of a physician's fees over a given time is **fee profile**.
3. A formula for determining medical benefits payable is **UCR**.
4. One who is able to take care of ordinary living expenses but who cannot afford medical care is **medically indigent**.
5. A statement authorizing the insurance company to pay the physician directly is **assignment of benefits**.
6. Someone who acts as a financial representative to insurance carriers is a **fiscal agent**.
7. Someone other than the patient, spouse, or parent who is responsible for paying all or part of patient's medical costs is **third-party payer**.
8. Payment system in which providers are paid a fixed fee for each enrolled patient whether seen by physician or not is termed **capitation**.
9. An organization that provides comprehensive health care to an enrolled group for a fixed period of time is **an HMO**.

### B. Learning Level: Comprehension

1. Explain why the statements are false on the lines provided.
   a. A third-party oral agreement is binding if it is made prior to treatment.
      Agreement must be written
   b. If a physician accepts a case and does not charge the patient, a record does not need to be made for the patient.
      Legally records must be kept for all medical care regardless of payment
   c. The extending of professional courtesy is made to all health care persons.
      May be made to any person, not obligated to any person
   d. An assignment of benefits authorizes medical payments for care to be made directly to the patient.
      Payment goes directly to physician
   e. The Truth in Lending Act applies to cases only when a finance charge is levied, applies any time credit is extended, and Regulation Z comes into effect when more than four payments.
2. Name the three commodities (values) the physician has to sell which helps to determine fees.
   Answer: a. time b. judgement c. services

### C. Learning Level: Application

1. Name two differences between payment in fee for service plans and managed care insurance plans

| Fee for Service | Managed Care |
|---|---|
| a. UCR basis of fee | Fee decided by managed care—basis not explained |
| b. Fee based on economic level of community alternative: Patients often pay 80% of allowed fee | Patient pays copay<br>Copay is the maximum payment |

2. State the knowledge needed when the medical assistant role is to explain fees.
   a. Know how fees are determined in office
   b. Know why charges may vary and how to determine
   c. Have knowledge of practice variables
   d. Know laws regarding credit
   e. Know any additional costs that are billable
   f. Know correct charges for each item
   g. Have knowledge of third-party regulations and payments

## D. Learning Level: Analysis

1. What types of service charges would the physician not want to make?
   - Telephone, late payment, missed appointment, filling insurance forms
2. Why would the physician want to avoid charges on the above services?
   - Most patients feel that physicians get paid enough
   - That this is not professional and it brings negative responses
3. Explain how physician fees are determined. How does that determination affect the physician fee profile?

   Physician fees are determined in a variety of ways
   - Prevailing rate in the community
   - UCR method
   - Settings by third-party payers for allowable amounts for procedures
   - Fee profile set by fiscal agents

   The fee profile is a compilation of individual physician charges over a number of years, so all the fees charged by that physician go into the profile and from which the customary fee for the physician is determined.

## E. Learning Level: Synthesis

As a medical assistant in the office, you have made an appointment with a new patient to see the physician. You ask if the patient has health insurance and patient states "Yes, I have insurance with Mutual Life through my job." What are the next steps you take?

1. Ask cash for first visit
2. Tell them whether credit cards and checks accepted
3. Ask patient to bring insurance card and employer information
4. Put note of conversation in patient chart

## F. Learning Level: Evaluation

1. Explain Regulation Z and give two examples of the types of medical offices where it might be used.

   Reg. Z requires that a written contract be made when debt is to be paid in more than four payments. The contract must disclose the terms of the payment including finance charges, meet specific information requirements, be drawn up and signed by physician and patient before the debt is incurred, and when payment will be in more than 4 payments.

   Types of offices could be

   1. Orthodontist
   2. Surgeon
   3. Physical therapist
2. Explain the difference between the application of Regulation Z to patient credit and the application of estimate slips. These are used to inform patients of surgical costs, explaining when patients may have to pay a substantial co-pay or % of insurance. Also, Medicare requires estimates at certain times. It is not an agreement for credit or more than four payments, although such an agreement may result from the estimate.

## PART 2 COMPETENCY CHALLENGE

A. The student will explain credit procedures to another student. When ready the student may complete the procedure to establish competency. Often students think they are ready and do not pass on the first attempt. The procedure is at the end of the chapter, and there is a fee schedule in Appendix C of Mastery Manual.

B. There are two situations for completion of Procedure 16-2. The items needed will be a patient ledger, a credit application, a surgical cost estimate sheet, and a federal Truth in Lending statement. You will need to provide these or the student will need to draw these up on the word processor and bring them to the lab. Credit applications may be obtained from your local credit bureau. Regulation Z may be obtained from the Internet. If the patient is a Medicare patient, more forms will be discussed in Chapter 20. Students need to be aware there will be more estimate requirements with Medicare.

## PART 3 CLINICAL APPLICATIONS

Have students sit in a circle and allow them at least 15 minutes discussion before moving on. Students might take turns leading discussion. Avoid personal input from years of experience until the discussion on each area has ended. These types of discussions raise levels of personal awareness and professionalism.

A. Discuss the ethical implications of reducing the physician fee after an insurance payment is made. Are there any legal restrictions to this practice? See text p. 237

B. List situations related to this chapter that you think may be appropriate education opportunities for patients. Extra charges for supplies, etc., federal rules, as soon as a new patient is booked

C. Discuss how is it that bankcards may avoid credit laws. Text p. 236

D. Discuss steps the medical assistant may take to avoid giving the appearance of extending credit to new or established patients. Text p. 236-237

E. Recall the questions which may not be asked on credit applications. Text p. 237

Have you ever seen those questions asked on applications? How do companies "get around" those questions yet still obtain the information? What is the applicant's recourse if those questions are asked?

F. List and discuss three applications of confidentiality around fee charges and credit.

Discuss balances, etc., in private areas, keep ledgers and statements away from patients and other employees (do not store on desk unless hidden from view), never discuss patients or their affairs with others, do not give information over the telephone. When requested to give information over the telephone, verify first with the patient and then initiate call to credit bureau. Do not give information because someone says they are from the credit bureau.

Remember to check assignments and self-evaluation forms. Update all procedural evaluation sheets.

# 17

# Managing Practice Finances

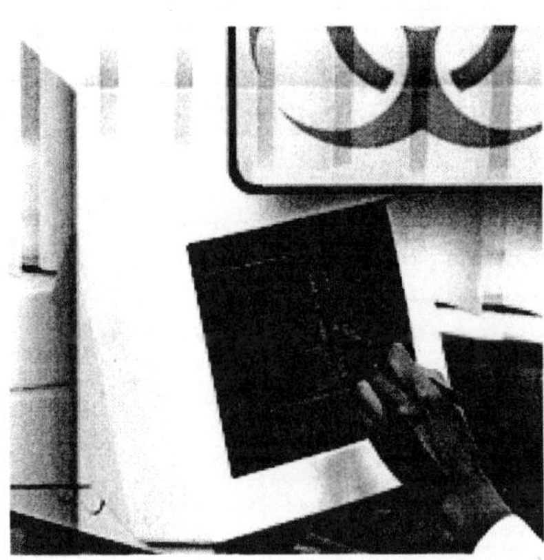

This topic on accounting services is a challenge for the students. Although a lot of the information in this chapter is basic, it is still confusing to the student. It takes ingenuity and patience to help students understand and become competent in the procedures in this chapter. Manual skills will require students to post charges and make adjustments to a pegboard system, account for petty cash, and make entries on a distribution journal.

## USING THE LEARNING SYSTEM

### 1. MEDICAL ASSISTANT CONTENT AND COMPETENCIES

CONTENT

- Word building and definitions
- Legal guidelines/requirements for health care
- Medical ethics and related issues
- Principles of recognition and response to verbal and nonverbal communication
- Adaptations for individual needs
- Basic medical office functions
- Bookkeeping and basic accounting

COMPETENCIES

- Post entries on a daysheet
- Perform accounts receivable procedures
- Perform accounts payable procedures
- Prepare a check
- Establish and maintain a petty cash fund
- Post adjustments, NSF checks

## 2. MEDICAL ASSISTANT ENTRY LEVEL-CURRICULUM INTERFACE

| TEXTBOOK OBJECTIVES | LEARNING SYSTEM LOCATION | MA CURRICULUM |
|---|---|---|
| **Cognitive** | | **Content** |
| 1. Define and spell the terms listed in the Vocabulary | • Text pp. 240-241<br>• Manual Part 1-A-1 | • Word building and definitions |
| 2. Name the two bases of accounting and explain their differences | • Textbook Table 17-2<br>• Manual Part 1-B | • Adaptations for individual needs<br>• Basic medical office functions<br>• Bookkeeping and basic accounting |
| 3. State the four kinds of information that the financial records of any business should show at all times | • Text p. 241<br>• Manual Part 1-B | • Basic medical office functions<br>• Bookkeeping and basic accounting |
| 4. Differentiate between a debit and a credit balance | • Text p. 242 | • Bookkeeping and basic accounting<br>• Legal guidelines/requirements for health care<br>• Principles of recognition and response to verbal and nonverbal communication |
| 5. Describe and demonstrate the entry for a credit balance | • Text p. 242, Table 17-2<br>• Manual Part 1-E | • Legal guidelines/requirements for health care<br>• Bookkeeping and basic accounting |
| 6. List six kinds of accounting records | • Text pp. 243-247<br>• Manual Part 1-C-1 | • Legal guidelines/requirements for health care<br>• Bookkeeping and basic accounting |
| 7. Compare the three most common systems used in the professional office | • Text pp. 247-249<br>• Manual Part 1-C | • Legal guidelines/requirements for health care<br>• Adaptations for individual needs<br>• Bookkeeping and basic accounting |
| 8. List four kinds of charges that should be avoided | • Text p. 248<br>• Manual Part 1-D | • Bookkeeping and basic accounting |
| 9. Discuss the importance of a trial balance | • Text p. 257<br>• Manual Part 1-D | • Bookkeeping and basic accounting |
| 10. Describe how to maintain a petty cash fund | • Text pp. 259-260<br>• Manual Part 2 | • Medical ethics and related issues<br>• Bookkeeping and basic accounting<br>• Adaptations for individual needs |
| 11. List and state the purpose of the five common periodic accounting summaries | • Text pp. 260-261 | • Bookkeeping and basic accounting |

## 2. MEDICAL ASSISTANT ENTRY-LEVEL CURRICULUM INTERFACE

| TEXTBOOK OBJECTIVES | LEARNING SYSTEM LOCATION | MA CURRICULUM |
|---|---|---|
| **Performance** | | **Competency** |
| 1. Prepare a ledger account for a new patient | • Manual Part 2<br>• Procedure 17-1<br>• CD-ROM ⊕ | • Perform accounts receivable procedures |
| 2. Prepare a patient charge slip | • Manual Part 2<br>• CD-ROM ⊕ | • Perform accounts receivable procedures |
| 3. Journalize service charges and payments using a single-entry system | • Manual Part 2<br>• CD-ROM ⊕ | • Post entries on a daysheet<br>• Perform accounts receivable procedures<br>• Perform accounts payable procedures<br>• Post adjustments, NSF checks |
| 4. Post the entries from the daily journal to patient ledger cards | • Manual Part 2<br>• CD-ROM ⊕ | • Perform accounts receivable procedures<br>• Perform accounts payable procedures<br>• Post adjustments, NSF checks |
| 5. Prepare a daily proof of posting | • Manual Part 2<br>• CD-ROM ⊕ | • Perform accounts receivable procedures<br>• Perform accounts payable procedures |
| 6. Prepare a daily proof of cash control | • Manual Part 2<br>• CD-ROM ⊕ | • Same as #5 above. |
| 7. Prepare a monthly trial balance | • Manual Part 2 | • Same as #5 above. |
| 8. Establish and maintain a petty cash fund | • Manual Part 2 | • Prepare a check<br>• Establish and maintain a petty cash fund |
| 9. Post service charges and payments using a pegboard | • Manual Part 2<br>• CD-ROM ⊕ | • Perform accounts receivable procedures<br>• Perform accounts payable procedures |

## 3. RESOURCES

www.gosafeguard.com/products **Nice on-line pictures of office files and bookkeeping pictures.**

Call toll free # 1-800-523-2422 for student packets. Sometimes they are available at a very reasonable price.

www.altavista.com/bookkeeping **Links to businesses throughout U.S. A good source for potential speakers.**

www.geocities.com/WallStreet/2924

www.yahoo.com/bin/search?p=bookeeping+ **Links to 250 sites about bookkeeping, businesses, and schools.**

## 4. LESSON PLAN Accounting Systems TIME 3 hours lecture, 12 hours lab

It often serves to have an accountant come to review the materials. Students should read the chapter first so they can write questions and ask them while the accountant is present. The accountant or you must distinguish the material that is essential to medical assistant practice and that which is background to provide understanding of bookkeeping procedures.

**Opening:** Bring in pegboard packets and hand them to students. Ask if anyone has done any bookkeeping. Opinions on student understanding of bookkeeping and degree of difficulty. Equipment needed: A complete pegboard set is preferable for each student. Sometimes local distributors will provide them to the students. One could also write the suppliers listed in resources above.

**Pretest:** Ask about personal budgets, how students track money, etc. Relate some terms to personal practices. A paycheck is a debit to our account and credit to bank account. Cash paid out is money spent and is recorded in the cash payment journal.

**Objectives:** Break lesson up into two or three discussions. Put up half of the objectives first lesson and half the second lesson.

**Content:** When discussing the content, you might want to use some of the Mastery Manual activities as a basis of discussion. The Part 2 activities may be completed using the ⊕ CD-ROM rather than using the Mastery Manual.

**Lesson 1** (2 hours): The vocabulary is complex. Often it is easier to show the parts to the pegboard and demonstrate its use, then go back to vocabulary and integrate it into pegboard use. Follow items below for the lesson.

1. Begin with using pegboard
2. What is accounting?
3. Cardinal rules of bookkeeping
4. Kinds of accounting records
5. A/R and A/P records
6. Short discussion of accounting systems
7. Review pegboard system and accounting adjustments in the system
   —Use # 7 as laboratory hour
8. Accounts receivable control
9. Trial Balance

**Lesson 2:** Have a guest speaker reinforce chapter materials and ensure students ask questions. Many local accountants are willing to speak to students—especially if they are serving physician offices at present.

**Lab:** Use laboratory hours for completing all items in Mastery Manual Part 2. Students must turn in 100% accurate activities. Make a copy of a daysheet. Enlarge it and make transparencies. Do the same with the distribution journal at the end of chapter in Mastery Manual. Complete Part 2 activities on these Transparency Masters once the students have completed theirs. Have students correct theirs using red pen as you proceed. Students may complete bookkeeping activities on the CD-ROM ⊕ . Look in the administrative menu.

**Assignment:**
**Lesson 1:** Study vocabulary—Make flash cards for vocabulary and come to class prepared to ask questions.
**Lesson 2:** Have students complete Mastery Manual Part 1.

**Posttest:** Give students short exercise to complete pegboard entries and take questions from the testbank.

## 5. MASTERY MANUAL ANSWERS

## PART 1 CONTENT MASTERY

### A. Learning Level: Knowledge

**Vocabulary**

1. adjustment column
2. balance column
3. balance sheet
4. cash flow statement
5. balance
6. credit
7. cash payment journal
8. packing slip
9. petty cash fund
10. statement
11. posting
12. receipts
13. superbill
14. bookkeeping
15. payables
16. transaction
17. trial balance
18. account
19. accounts payable
20. credit column
21. daily journal
22. cash basis of accounting
23. debit
24. disbursements
25. discount
26. general journal
27. credit balance
28. in balance
29. invoice
30. statement of income and expense
31. debit column
32. accounts receivable
33. accounts receivable control
34. accounting equation
35. receivables
36. accounts receivable ledger
37. account balance
38. accounts receivable trial balance
39. accrual basis of accounting
40. disbursement journal

### B. Learning Level: Comprehension

1. Of the common accounting systems, which do you think will be easier to use? Explain your answer. Students personal answer.
2. At all times, financial records should show the following information.
   a. earnings—income made or lost
   b. money charged or collected
   c. money owed to and by the practice
   d. distribution of expenses incurred

### C. Learning Level: Application

1. List the six kinds of accounting bookkeeping records.
   a. general journal
   b. ledger, patient ledger, or account
   c. checkbook
   d. disbursement journal
   e. petty cash record
   f. payroll record
2. Name the accounting records used for

   Accounts receivable procedures
   a. daysheet or general journal
   b. patient A/R ledger
   c. charge slips

   Accounts payable procedures
   a. checkbook
   b. distribution journal
   c. invoices
   d. payroll journal
3. Which type of bookkeeping system is used most commonly in your area? How will you obtain this information? Call medical society for information or survey some physician offices.

## D. Learning Level: Analysis

1. Explain the following about a trial balance:
   a. Purpose disclose discrepancies between journals and ledger
   b. When performed at the end of the month after all posting completed and before preparing monthly statements
   c. Procedure Pull all account cards with a balance, and total these cards. Total should equal A/R control.
   d. What to examine for locating errors:
      - Make sure all account cards are accounted for
      - Find the difference between the two
      - Look for an identical number
      - Check each balance for proper posting
      - Is it divisable by nine? Look for transposed number
      - Check for balance forward and previous balance amounts to be entered correctly
      - Check for sliding numbers
   e. Procedure when errors found correct error and redo trial balance
2. Explain the same for accounts receivable control:
   a. Purpose keep daily summary of what is owed to the practice—all unpaid money
   b. When performed every day
   c. Procedure total outstanding A/R from previous day plus today's charges minus today's payments minus today's adjustments equals balance A/R control to date.
   d. What to examine for locating errors Examine all ledgers for correct entries; make sure all checks and money received recorded. Bank deposit should equal today's payments.
   e. Procedure when errors found correct errorson record in question and correct A/R control

## E. Learning Level: Synthesis

1. Give examples of original source records (transactions) from which you would enter financial information into the records.
   a. charge slip
   b. superbill
   c. petty cash vouchers
   d. invoices

   Others? Payroll time cards, EOB's, checkbook
2. Write the A/R transactions that cause the following:
   a. a credit balance—overpayment, i.e., patient paid in advance, insurance payment causes overpayment
   b. a debit balance—charge to account and no payment, NSF check received
   c. a refund—overpayment

## F. Learning Level: Evaluation

1. Explain disbursement accounts.

   These moneys are paid out by the practice. In order to keep track of specific expenses, they are placed in different categories called accounts.
2. Give at least eight examples of different types of disbursements.
   a. Postage
   b. Office supplies
   c. Operating (clinical) supplies
   d. Utilities
   e. Rent
   f. Telephone
   g. Professional Fees
   h. Computer costs

   Other: surgical supplies, cleaning, stationary, and paper

## PART 2 COMPETENCY CHALLENGE

Students will use Procedures 17-1 and 17- 2 to complete posting for A/R and A/P activities for the pegboard. These are very simple activities that often cause much difficulty for students. There are forms at the back of the chapter in the Mastery Manual or you may obtain pegboard supplies from the local supplier. Using actual pegboard supplies helps the transition to the externship setting. Students may then correct their work if needed. The goal is to have the work completed with 100% accuracy, although the instructor may change the accuracy to whatever % desired. There is also a supplemental procedure for posting to a computerized accounts receivable system located at the end of this chapter.

## PART 3 CLINICAL APPLICATIONS

This part has one item each for discussion of ethical, legal, and educational application and evaluation.

**SUPPLEMENTAL PROCEDURE:** Accurately post patient charges and payments to the office computerized accounts receivable system.
Equipment: computer, software, patient charge slip, ledger cards if kept as hardcopy

1. Log onto or follow procedures for starting up the computer.
2. Select Accounts Receivable or Patient Billing option, depending on the system.
3. If making entries on a batch system (i.e., making multiple entries at one time, such as the end of the day), you will need to gather all documentary records of services rendered to patients since the last entries and all records of payments made or received since the last entries.
4. If making a single entry, such as upon patient checkout or departure, proceed to #5.
5. If **new patient,** you will need to first use a setup routine to record all patient personal, insurance, and billing information, prior to making any accounting entries. As a minimum, this usually requires name, address, phone number, responsible party, insurance plan name, member number, and physician of record. Most programs will guide you step by step through this procedure.
6. For an **existing patient,** you will need to call up the patient screen. This usually requires typing in the patient's last name or some portion of it. The transaction particulars must then be entered. Date usually defaults to the current date. The procedure (e.g., level 2 office visit) should be available
   a. Through a drop-down list from which a selection may be made or via entering a procedural code from the patient charge slip, superbill, or
   b. With item indicating procedures and charges provided by the physician or facility.
   c. The actual charge may be entered automatically by the system or you may be required to enter one from some other source. Depending on the system, you may also be required to enter other data such as diagnosis, referral, descriptive notes, medications prescribed, follow up appointments, etc.
7. Note whether patient has a balance, whether insurance has been billed, or whether patient owes the balance due. If patient owes balance, request amount due.
8. If the patient gives payment for services, or partial payment based on insurance company co-pay requirements, these must also be posted to the patient record.
9. Print out a record of service and or a receipt for the patient's records.
10. Manually enter charge and payment information on patient ledger card if medical facility keeps this information as backup.
11. Place payment with the deposit slip and enter the amount on the deposit slip.
12. When closing out the day, assure all payments received equal the total deposits on the deposit slip for the day.
13. Back-up computer when A/R day is closed out.

# 18

# Banking Services and Procedures

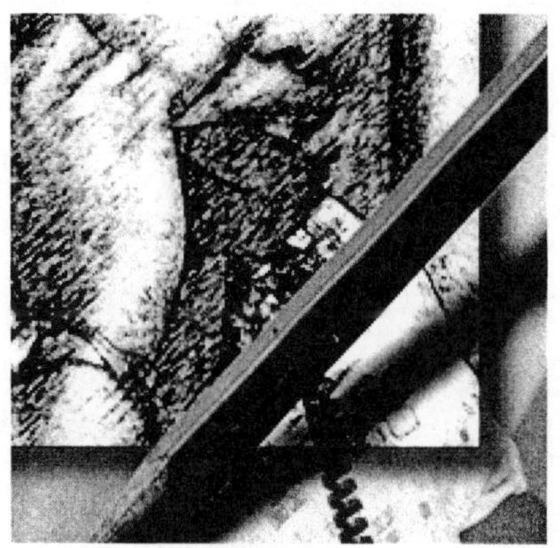

One of the challenges to the medical assistant instructor is to determine how students care for their personal accounts and then to sell them on the value and importance of handling office money. Students need to know the honor it is to be trusted with such responsibility and the inherent dangers in taking on responsibility with money. It is important to emphasize the correct way to write checks, to deposit all money received, and to reconcile the bank account monthly. One cannot treat the office money or accounts in any way but timely and according to financial management principles.

## USING THE LEARNING SYSTEM

### 1. MEDICAL ASSISTANT CONTENT AND COMPETENCIES

CONTENT

- Word building and definitions
- Legal guidelines/requirements for health care
- Principles of recognition and response to verbal and nonverbal communication
- Applications of electronic technology
- Basic medical office functions
- Bookkeeping and basic accounting
- Medical ethics and related issues

COMPETENCIES

- Prepare a bank deposit
- Reconcile a bank statement
- Process a credit balance
- Prepare a check
- Post adjustments, NSF checks
- Perform accounts payable procedures
- Process refunds

## 2. MEDICAL ASSISTANT ENTRY-LEVEL CURRICULUM INTERFACE

| TEXTBOOK OBJECTIVES | LEARNING SYSTEM LOCATION | MA CURRICULUM |
|---|---|---|
| **Cognitive** | | **Content** |
| 1. Define and spell the terms listed in the Vocabulary | • Text p. 264<br>• Manual Part 1-A | • Word building and definitions |
| 2. State the four requirements of a negotiable instrument | • Text p. 264<br>• Manual Part 1-B | • Legal guidelines/requirements for health care<br>• Applications of electronic technology<br>• Basic medical office functions<br>• Bookkeeping and basic accounting |
| 3. Discuss six advantages of using checks for the transfer of funds | • Text p. 264<br>• Manual Part 1-B | • Legal guidelines/requirements for health care<br>• Applications of electronic technology<br>• Basic medical office functions<br>• Bookkeeping and basic accounting |
| 4. State why it is important to complete the check stub before writing a check | • Text pp. 268-269 | • Same as #3 above and<br>• Principles of recognition and response to verbal and nonverbal communication |
| 5. Explain how you would handle mistakes made in preparing a check | • Text p. 271<br>• Manual Part 1-C | • Same as #4 above and<br>• Medical ethics and related issues |
| 6. List and discuss eight precautions to observe in accepting checks | • Text p. 273<br>• Manual Part 1-D | • Same as # 4 above and<br>• Medical ethics and related issues |
| 7. State the purpose of a check endorsement | • Text p. 273<br>• Manual Part 1-E | • Legal guidelines/requirements for health care<br>• Bookkeeping and basic accounting |
| 8. Name and compare four kinds of endorsements | • Text p. 274<br>• Manual Part 1-E | • Legal guidelines/requirements for health care<br>• Principles of recognition and response to verbal and nonverbal communication<br>• Bookkeeping and basic accounting |
| 9. Cite five reasons for depositing checks promptly | • Text p. 274<br>• Manual Part 1-F | • Same as #8 above |
| 10. Discuss the action necessary when a deposited check is returned | • Text p. 276<br>• Manual Part 1-F | • Same as #8 above |

## MEDICAL ASSISTANT ENTRY-LEVEL CURRICULUM INTERFACE

| TEXTBOOK OBJECTIVES | LEARNING SYSTEM LOCATION | MA CURRICULUM |
|---|---|---|
| **Performance** | | **Competencies** |
| 1. Prepare a bank deposit | • Manual Part 2<br>• Procedure 18-2<br>• CD-ROM ⊕ | • Prepare a bank deposit<br>• Post adjustments, NSF checks<br>• Perform accounts receivable and payable procedures |
| 2. Correctly write a check | • Manual Part 2<br>• Procedure 18-1<br>• CD-ROM ⊕ | • Prepare a check<br>• Perform accounts receivable and payable procedures |
| 3. Pay office bills by checks | • Manual Part 2<br>• Procedure 18-1<br>• CD-ROM ⊕ | • Prepare a check<br>• Post adjustments, NSF checks<br>• Perform accounts receivable and payable procedures |
| 4. Reconcile a bank statement with the checkbook balance | • Manual Part 2<br>• Procedure 18-3<br>• CD-ROM ⊕ | • Reconcile a bank statement<br>• Process a credit balance<br>• Post adjustments, NSF checks<br>• Perform accounts receivable and payable procedures<br>• Process refunds |

## 3. RESOURCES

http://search.yahoo.com/bin/search?p=banking+regulations **Banking regulations**

## 4. LESSON PLAN Banking TIME 3 hours lecture, 12 hours lab

**Opening:** This is an opening and a pretest in one activity. The day before class ask students to bring their checkbooks to class next time, but do not tell students why. Start off class having students write a check to themselves in their checkbook, write void where they sign it, rip out, and give to instructor. You immediately obtain feedback on students who need to learn how to write valid checks. If students do not have checks, hand a few out by copying checks at end of chapter in Mastery Manual.

**Equipment:** Try to have old cancelled checks available to critique with students. Go to banks and obtain brochures to discuss various account types for businesses. Samples of banking, reconciliation, and deposit forms.

**Pretest:** See opening

**Objectives:** Post on a flip chart and put MA curriculum next to them. Check them off as discussed or completed in lab.

**Content:** Use the content outline. Most students are not aware of the liability surrounding handling money and depositing checks. A good foundation is essential to competent performance and to reinforcing a strict moral code of honesty.

**Content outline:**

Checks

1. Types of Checks
    - Bank Draft
    - Cashier's Check
    - Certified Check
    - Limited Check
    - Money Orders
    - Traveler's Check
    - Voucher Check
    - Warrant
2. Advantages of Using Checks
3. ABA Number--Magnetic Ink Character Recognition (MICR)

Bank Accounts

1. Common Types of Accounts
    - Checking Account
    - Savings Accounts
    - Money Market Savings Account

Systemizing Bill Paying

1. The Business Checkbook
2. Computer Generated Checks
3. Checkbook Stubs
4. Lost and Stolen Checks
5. Writing Checks
6. Handling Corrections and Mistakes
7. Writing Cash Checks
8. One-Write Check Writing
9. Signing Checks
10. Mailing Checks

Special Problems with Checks

Account Overdrawn or Overdraft Stop-Payment Order

**Content Outline** *continued*

Payment from Patients
- Acknowledging Payment in Full
- Precautions in Accepting Checks

Endorsement of Checks
- Necessity for Endorsement
- Kinds of Endorsement
- Blank Endorsement
- Restrictive Endorsement
- Special Endorsement
- Qualified Endorsement
- Endorsement Procedures

Making Deposits
- Preparing the Deposit
- Depositing by Mail
- "Hold" on Account
- Returned Checks

Bank Statement
- Reconciling the Bank Statement

medical assistant's Position of Trust

**Lab:** The Mastery Manual Part 1 CONTENT MASTERY should be completed before proceeding to the competencies. Assure students complete all phases of banking from receiving payment to preparing deposits, writing checks for bills, and reconciling the account. Part 2 activities meet all performance objectives and MA curriculum competencies. CD-ROM ⊕ activities are listed in the index and encompass the performance skills listed as part of the 8th Edition Textbook objectives.

**Assignment:** Students go to lab and complete Part 2 work and begin to read Chapter 19.

**Posttest:** Take from testbank, develop a mini-bank to have students perform some of the competencies as part of the lab check-off.

## 5. MASTERY MANUAL ANSWERS

### PART 1 CONTENT MASTERY

#### A. Learning Level: Knowledge

1. f; 2. d; 3. g; 4. h; 5. b; 6. c; 7. j; 8. i; 9. e; 10 . a

#### B. Learning Level: Comprehension

1. Name the four qualities of a negotiable instrument.
   a. signed by maker
   b. promise or order to pay a sum of money
   c. payable on demand or specific date
   d. payable to order or bearer
2. Give examples of four types of negotiable instruments.
   a. bank draft
   b. cashier's check
   c. certified check
   d. limited check, money order, travelers check, voucher check, warrant

## C. Learning Level: Application

1. Write a check to city Medical Supplies for $ 321.76 with today's date and have physician sign the check. This is correct. To correct the incorrect check, cross out, initial, and write correct information above incorrect.

BLACKBURN PRIMARY CARE ASSOCIATES, PC  # 06228
1990 Turquoise Drive  78-31/5467
Blackburn, WI 54937

DATE Today's Date

Pay To the order of City Medical Supplies

Pay Three hundred twenty-one and 76/100 DOLLARS $ 321.76

FIRST BANK OF BLACKBURN—1231 SUN STREET, BLACKBURN, WI 54937

Memo: MEDICAL SUPPLIES  Dr. Chang MD

" 012345678 [12100101985] 00 010010 "

2. Demonstrate correcting the mistakes made in writing the check for the same amount. See check above for correct check.
3. How and when would you complete the check stub?

   Complete before writing check so you do not forget put in date, amount, payee, purpose, need to distribute expenses, and balance the accounts daily.

## D. Learning Level: Analysis

Describe the precautions the medical assistant must take when checks are received in the mail and before checks are prepared for deposit.
Precautions in accepting checks

- Scan the check carefully for the correct date, amount, and signature.
- Do not accept a check with corrections on it.
- If you do not know the person presenting a personal check, ask for identification and compare signatures.
- Accept an out-of-town check, government check, or payroll check only if you are well acquainted with the person presenting it and it does not exceed the amount of the payment.
- Acceptance of third-party checks is generally unwise. A third party check is one made out to your patient by a party unknown to you. A check from the patient's health insurance carrier is an exception.
- When accepting a postal money order for payment, make certain it has only one endorsement. Postal money orders with more than two endorsements will not be honored.
- Do not accept a check marked "Payment in Full" unless it does pay the account in full, up to and including the date on which it is received.
- Accepting checks written for more than the amount due is poor policy because, first, you will have to return cash for the difference between the amount of the check and the amount owed. Second, the canceled check could be used by the patient to indicate the amount paid on account.

## E. Learning Level: Synthesis

1. Name the types of endorsements and either describe or give an example of each type.
   Kinds of Endorsement
   a. Blank Endorsement—payee signs their name and makes payable to bearer. Only use for immediate cashing or deposit.
   b. Restrictive Endorsement—for deposit only this kind used in physician practice
   c. Special Endorsement—includes words specifying person to whom endorser makes check payable
   d. Qualified Endorsement—without recourse
2. Which is the most common type of endorsement used in the medical office?
   Restrictive endorsement

## F. Learning Level: Evaluation

1. Name three reasons that depositing checks once a week is poor financial practice.
   a. Patient may decide to stop payment
   b. Check may be stolen or lost
   c. Check may be good for limited time, it is a courtesy to the payer
2. What will the medical assistant do when a check is returned NSF?
   Add funds back into patient account. Call the patient and ask if it can be redeposited.

## PART 2 COMPETENCY CHALLENGE

Students will be processing checks for deposit, completing deposit slips, demonstrating proper check writing procedures, balancing the checkbook, recording disbursements, and balancing the disbursement journal. Procedures 18-1 and 18-2 are at the end of the chapter in the Mastery Manual along with the forms necessary. Students should also balance their personal checkbook and reconcile their account for one month.

1. Checks are written to the following companies
   The bills are:

| | |
|---|---|
| Shell Oil Company, auto expense | $87.54 |
| Physician's Management, subscription | $65.44 |
| W.B. Saunders Company, scientific books | $130.00 |
| Panel Laboratory, medical expense | $40.00 |
| Casey Stationers, office supplies | $32.89 |
| Professional Oxygen Service, medical expense | $57.50 |

2. The following payments from patients were received today and must be deposited in the bank at the end of the day. Using Procedure 18-2: Preparing a Bank Deposit, and the form provided at the end of the chapter, prepare a deposit slip for these receipts and enter the amount of the deposit in your checkbook.

| By check | Amount | Bank No. |
|---|---|---|
| Rexford Ingram | $30.00 | 15/355 |
| Mary Louise McCall | 425.00 | 10/401 |
| Claude Irvin | 25.00 | 12/298 |
| Thomas Ross | 100.00 | 12/296 |
| Johnnie Crammer | 65.00 | 1/15 |
| Total checks: | $645.00 | |
| By cash | | |
| Rose McDonnell | $15.50 | |
| Virginia DeMent | 25.00 | |
| Total cash | 40.50 | |
| Total deposit | $685.50 | |

3. Use Procedure 18-3: Reconciling a Bank Statement, and the simulated bank statement from the pages at the end of the chapter, to reconcile the checkbook balance with the bank statement balance. Show your calculations. If you have problems, refer to your 8th Edition Textbook for correcting errors in the checkbook balance.

For students who have trouble reconciling, put up Transparency Master and review the CHECKING for ERRORS in RECONCILIATION with them.

- Did you fail to correct your checkbook balance at the time of the previous statement?
- Is your arithmetic correct?
- Have you transposed a figure?
- Did you forget to include one of the outstanding checks?
- Did you fail to record a deposit or did you record it twice?
- Do all stubs and checks agree?
- Have you carried your figures forward correctly?
- Did someone write a check without your knowledge?

## PART 3 CLINICAL APPLICATIONS

Discuss topics A and B with students in lab.
There are many legal considerations around the situation presented to the students. It is very poor practice for any person to sign another's checks. If there are any missing funds or irregularities, one is assumed guilty because they have total access to an account. Students need to learn to protect their legal positions.

# 19

# Billing and Collecting Procedures

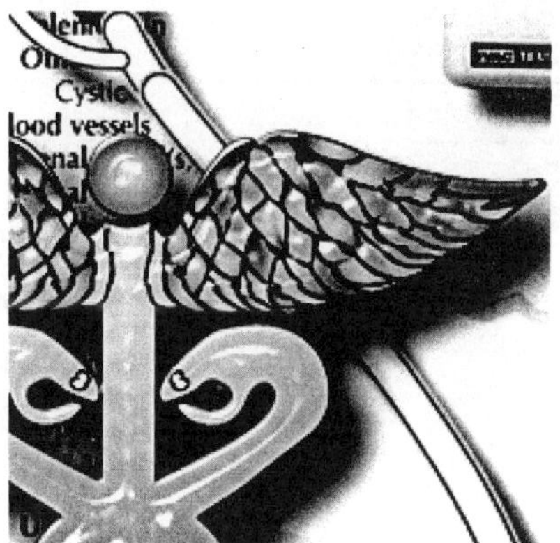


This is the last of four chapters in the unit on financial management. At this point it is important to specifically review the items in the objectives and MA curriculum topics for Medical Assisting administrative procedure content, and the competencies for performing bookkeeping procedures. As instructors, ensure that students have mastered the cognitive and performance objectives for all the finance chapters. When these objectives are mastered, the student will be able to perform basic entry finance skills. It is the instructor's responsibility to facilitate this process for the students. This chapter contains all the competencies for preparing billing statements and collecting delinquent accounts

## USING THE LEARNING SYSTEM

### 1. MEDICAL ASSISTANT CONTENT AND COMPETENCIES

CONTENT

- Word building and definitions
- Legal guidelines/requirements for health care
- Hereditary, cultural, and environmental influences on behavior
- Principles of recognition and response to verbal and nonverbal communication
- Applications of electronic technology
- Basic medical office functions
- Bookkeeping and basic accounting
- Medical ethics and related issues

COMPETENCIES

- Explain general office policies
- perform accounts receivable procedures
- Perform billing and collections procedures
- Prepare a check
- Post collection agency payment

## 2. MEDICAL ASSISTANT ENTRY-LEVEL CURRICULUM INTERFACE

| TEXTBOOK OBJECTIVES | LEARNING SYSTEM LOCATION | MA CURRICULUM |
|---|---|---|
| **Cognitive** | | **Content** |
| 1. Define and spell the terms listed in the Vocabulary | • Text p. 283<br>• Manual Part 1-A | • Word building and definitions |
| 2. Name three ways by which payment for medical services is accomplished | • Text p. 283<br>• Manual Part 1-B | • Legal guidelines/requirements for health care<br>• Principles of recognition and response to verbal and nonverbal communication<br>• Applications of electronic technology<br>• Basic medical office functions<br>• Bookkeeping and basic accounting |
| 3. List nine items to be addressed in developing a credit policy | • Text p. 284<br>• Manual Part 1-B | • Legal guidelines/requirements for health care<br>• Hereditary, cultural, and environmental influences on behavior<br>• Principles of recognition and response to verbal and nonverbal communication<br>• Applications of electronic technology<br>• Basic medical office functions<br>• Bookkeeping and basic accounting<br>• Medical ethics and related issues |
| 4. State three reasons for itemizing billing statements | • Text p. 287<br>• Manual Part 1-B | • Basic medical office functions<br>• Bookkeeping and basic accounting |
| 5. Describe cycle billing and its advantages | • Text p. 288<br>• Manual Part 1-B | • Basic medical office functions<br>• Bookkeeping and basic accounting |
| 6. Discuss the significance of determining the collection ratio and the accounts receivable ratio | • Text pp. 289-290<br>• Manual Part 2 | • Basic medical office functions<br>• Bookkeeping and basic accounting |
| 7. List the three most common reasons for patients' failure to pay accounts | • Text p. 290<br>• Manual Part 1-D | • Hereditary, cultural, and environmental influences on behavior<br>• Principles of recognition and response to verbal and nonverbal communication<br>• Medical ethics and related issues |

## MEDICAL ASSISTANT ENTRY-LEVEL CURRICULUM INTERFACE continued

| TEXTBOOK OBJECTIVES | LEARNING SYSTEM LOCATION | MA CURRICULUM |
|---|---|---|
| **Cognitive** | | **Content** |
| 8. Discuss the do's and don'ts of telephone collection procedures | • Text p. 293<br>• Manual Part 1-D | • Hereditary, cultural, and environmental influences on behavior<br>• Principles of recognition and response to verbal and nonverbal communication<br>• Legal guidelines/requirements for health care |
| 9. Name five sources of information in tracing skips | • Text p. 296<br>• Manual Part 1-E | • Principles of recognition and response to verbal and nonverbal communication<br>• Legal guidelines/requirements for health care |
| 10. State the procedure to follow upon receiving notice of a debtor's bankruptcy | • Text p. 297<br>• Manual Part 1-E | • Same as #9 above |
| 11. List three advantages of using small claims courts for collecting delinquent accounts | • Text p. 299<br>• Manual Part 1-F | • Same as #9 above |
| 12. Discuss five appropriate follow-up actions after assigning accounts to a collection agency | • Text pp. 299-300<br>• Manual Part 1-F | • Legal guidelines/requirements for health care<br>• Hereditary, cultural, and environmental influences on behavior<br>• Principles of recognition and response to verbal and nonverbal communication<br>• Medical ethics and related issues |
| **Performance** | **Locations** | **Competency** |
| 1. Prepare patient's monthly statements | • Manual Part 2<br>• Procedure 19-1<br>• CD-ROM ⊕ | • Explain general office policies<br>• Perform accounts receivable procedures |
| 2. Calculate a collection ratio and an accounts receivable ratio | • Manual Part 2<br>• CD-ROM ⊕ | • Perform accounts receivable procedures<br>• Perform billing and collections procedures<br>• Prepare a check<br>• Post collection agency payment |

*Chart continues on following page*

**MEDICAL ASSISTANT ENTRY-LEVEL CURRICULUM INTERFACE continued**

| TEXTBOOK OBJECTIVES | LEARNING SYSTEM LOCATION | MA CURRICULUM |
|---|---|---|
| **Performance** | | **Competency** |
| 3. Prepare an age analysis of accounts receivable | • Manual Part 2 | • Perform accounts receivable procedures<br>• Perform billing and collections procedures<br>• Prepare a check<br>• Post collection agency payment |
| 4. Initiate proceedings to collect delinquent accounts | • Manual Part 2<br>• Procedure 19-2 | • Same as #3 above |
| 5. Demonstrate telephone collection techniques | • Manual Part 2 | • Same as #3 above |

## 3. RESOURCES

www.conomikes.com **Conomikes Publications**

http://www.cftech.com/BrainBank/SPECIALREPORTS/NewRegsCrdtRptg.html **Links to credit regulations**

http://www.ftc.gov/ **The Federal Trade Commission**

http://www.ftc.gov/os/statutes/fcrajump.htm **Fair Credit Reporting Act**

http://www.ftc.gov/bcp/conline/edcams/fcra/index.html **A collection of educational materials related to the Fair Credit Reporting Act**

## 4. LESSON PLAN Billing and Collections TIME 3 hours lecture, 12 hours lab

**Opening:** Ask students to be detectives. Discuss locating a missing person. Relate to tracing skips. Remind students not to do anything illegal.

**Pretest:** How many federal laws relating to credit and collections?
Answer—at least four: Fair Credit Reporting Act, Truth in Lending Regulations, Fair Debt Collection Act, FCC regulations regarding telephone collections. Do you know others? Check Internet sites.

**Objectives:** Review the objectives as you discuss the materials. All the objectives are covered in the Intellectual Activities of the Mastery Manual and you could post objectives as responses are reviewed with students.

**Content:** Use this outline for major review and teaching points. It is important to relate these to medical assistant content and competencies listed in MA curriculum. Use time to review these materials and then tie the previous three chapters together to present a total financial picture.

**BILLING AND COLLECTIONS OUTLINE**

1. PAYMENT AT TIME OF SERVICE
2. BILLING AFTER EXTENSION OF CREDIT
    a. Credit Policy
    b. Outside Billing Methods
        Computerized
        Microfilm Billing
        Independent Billing Service
    c. Internal Billing by the medical assistant
        Encounter Form, Superbill, Charge Slip
        Typewritten Statement
        Photocopied Statement
        Computer-Generated Statement
    d. Procedure for Internal Billing
        Itemizing the First Statement
        Time and Frequency of Billing
        Once-a-Month Billing
        Cycle Billing
        Billing Third-Party Payers and Minors
3. PAYMENT COLLECTION
    a. Collection Goals
        Collection Ratio
        Accounts Receivable Ratio
    b. Importance of Collecting Delinquent Accounts
        Why Patients Do Not Pay
        When to Say No
    c. Aging Accounts Receivable
    d. Collection Techniques
        Telephone Collection Calls
        Collection Letters
        Observe Established Collection Policy
        Who Signs Collection Letters?
        Personal Interviews
    e. Special Collection Problems
        "Skip" Tracing
        Claims Against Estates
        Bankruptcy
    f. Statutes of Limitations
        Malpractice Statutes
        Collection Statutes
        Open Book Accounts Written Contracts Single-Entry Accounts
4. USING OUTSIDE COLLECTION ASSISTANCE
    a. Collecting Through the Court System
        Making the Decision to Sue
        Small Claims Court
    b. Using a Collection Agency
        Selecting the Agency Responsibilities to the Collection Agency

**Lab:** Use the time for students to complete all the CD-ROM ⊕ and COMPETENCY CHALLENGE from the Mastery Manual. Once students have finished the competencies, they should all be reviewed together in the lab. This helps students problem solve and helps instructor learn about common problems with these activities. Do not complete the activities—allow students to come to consensus on correct answers. This is an opportunity to allow a student to lead the class in this activity review.

**Assignment:** All procedures in these four chapters should be completed. Have students read Chapter 20, study vocabulary, and make flash cards. Ask them to pay attention to responding to the objectives.

**Posttest:** Use Examaster testbank questions. If students use CD-ROM ⊕ to gain competence, have students complete the Competency Challenge as test on this chapter.

## 5. MASTERY MANUAL ANSWERS

### PART 1 CONTENT MASTERY

### A. Learning Level: Knowledge

1. accounts receivable ratio A formula for measuring how fast outstanding accounts are being paid.
2. age analysis A procedure for classifying accounts receivable by age from the first date of billing.
3. collection ratio A formula for measuring the effectiveness of the billing system.
4. invasion of privacy Unauthorized disclosure of a person's private affairs.
5. statute of limitations The time limit within which an action may legally be brought upon a contract.
6. subsidize To aid or promote something (such as a private enterprise) with public money.
7. superbill A combination charge slip, statement, and insurance reporting form.

### B. Learning Level: Comprehension

1. Patients may pay for medical services
   a. at the time of service
   b. extension of credit
   c. outside collection assistance
2. Give three examples indicating why the medical office is advised to itemize bills.
   a. patient insurance requires itemization
   b. more than one service or procedure on the statement
   c. prevents misunderstandings; also a courtesy to patients
3. List three factors that would help the physician consider cycle billing over once-a-month billing.
   a. total number of billings so large it takes a large portion of a week for one person to complete
   b. allows equal sharing of billing over the weeks
   c. not as intensive; allows for less errors

### C. Learning Level: Application

1. Issues to be addressed in written credit policy
   - When payment is due from patients
   - When the practice requires payment at time of service
   - When or if assignment of insurance benefits is accepted
   - Whether insurance forms will be completed by the office staff
   - Billing procedures
   - Collection protocol
   - How long an account will be carried without payment
   - Telephone collection protocol
   - Sending accounts to a collection agency
2. What would you do if a patient asked you to extend credit and there was no credit policy in the office? You would offer to take a credit card or give the case to the office manager?

### D. Learning Level: Analysis

1. Mrs. Pepper has failed to pay any money on the account since the insurance payment 2 months ago. You are going to call her. What reasons might you expect her to give for not paying.
   a. "Oh, I forgot"—negligence
   b. "I am sorry, we are short of cash right now"—inability to pay
   c. "We think you charged too much"—unwilling to pay

2. You have to call her at work. What are the restrictions put on talking to her at work? How will you proceed with the call? You may want students to practice role-playing these types of calls to meet the performance objective.

   Do not call if employer does not allow. Do not make repeated messages. Do not state the call is from physician's office or about a bill. Ask patient if they are aware of an outstanding bill. Ask when you can expect payment.

## E. Learning Level: Synthesis

1. Actions you will take to attempt to find patient
   a. Reexamine registration card for address accuracy
   b. See if there is a call forwarding number
   c. Call employer on registration card or other contacts listed
   d. Call landlord
   e. Try them on the Internet 411 directory or another one
   f. Weigh the amount of the bill against the time and discuss turning over to collection or not pursuing.
2. You find out the patient is bankrupt because you have just received a note in the mail asking the physician to release debt to the bankruptcy court. As the medical assistant, what are your actions? Do not send statements or attempt to collect.
3. What will you do if you find out he is deceased? It is easiest to write off the debt for some persons due to a spouse with limited means, unless the insurance company will pay. Medicare will pay. If it is written off, the family should be told, it is a courtesy. If the patient is wealthy, the estate may be paying bills. If there is an estate, then the bill should be paid through the estate.

## F. Learning Level: Evaluation

| Small Claims Court | Collection Agency |
|---|---|
| **Advantages** | |
| 1. Saves time of suit or attorney | 1. Agency does all the work |
| 2. No commission charged | 2. Further delay lessens recovery chances |
| 3. Often defendant doesn't show and money is awarded | 3. Training often produces much better results |
| **Disadvantages** | |
| 1. Medical assistant must appear for physician | 1. Only 40-60% of amount to physician |
| 2. Still have to collect the money | 2. Often garnish wages |
| 3. Must serve subpoena or hire someone | 3. Make sure ledgers properly marked |

## PART 2 Competency Challenge

Use either the CD-ROM ⊕ or the Clinical Applications in the Mastery Manual to assist the student to gain competency in the two procedures Billing and Collections in the textbook and Mastery Manual.

A. Prepare a ledger card for Mr. Alcorn from the items below. You may have prepared the ledger card in Chapter 14 activities when you were preparing files and medical records. Type or write in all the information below on the ledger card monthly billing statement for Mr. Alcorn, dating it August 31. Also prepare statements for any other patients with account balances in your patient ledger files. Use Procedure 19-1: Preparing Monthly Billing Statements, and the ledger cards at the end of the chapter, to complete your work.

Patient: Paul Leonard Alcorn 244 Santa Inez Street

| Service | Charges | Paid | Balance |
|---|---|---|---|
| 1/31 Surgery | $450 | | $450 |
| 3/15 Paid on account | | $100 | $350 |
| 5/4 Paid on account | | $100 | $250 |
| 6/5 Office visit | $25 | | $275 |
| 6/5 Paid on account | | $100 | $175 |
| 8/1 Office visit $18 | $18 | | $193 |
| 8/4 Office visit | $25 | | $218 |
| 8/4 Laboratory | $33 | | $251 |
| 8/7 Office visit | $25 | | $276 |
| 8/7 Laboratory | $25 | | $301 |
| 8/10 Office visit | $18 | | $319 |
| 8/10 Paid on account | | $75 | $244 |
| 8/15 Office visit | $25 | | $269 |
| 8/22 Physical exam | $85 | | $354 |
| Paid on account | | $100 | $254 |
| 8/26 Hospital admission | | | |
| 8/27 Hospital visit | $45 | | $299 |
| 8/28 Hospital visit | $45 | | $354 |
| 8/29 Hospital visit and discharge | $65 | | $409 |

B. 1. On the chart below prepare an age analysis for Mr. Alcorn and any other patients having a balance due on August 31.

**AGE ANALYSIS for Aug 31 xxxx**

| NAME | Bal. TOTAL | 0-3 MO. | 3-6 MO. | 6-12 MO. | 1 YEAR+ |
|---|---|---|---|---|---|
| Alcorn | $409 | $409 | | | |
| | | | | | |
| | | | | | |
| | | | | | |

2. Using the following information, compute a collection ratio and an accounts receivable ratio.

| | |
|---|---|
| Gross charges for the year | $231,000 |
| Minus Courtesy discounts | $ 8,530 |
| Minus Insurance adjustments | $ 18,400 |
| Minus Other adjustments | $ 3,983 |
| Total collections | $182,332 |
| Accounts receivable balance | $ 38,230 |

Answer: Gross charges minus total adjustments = net charges of $204,070.00

Total collections of $182,332.00 divided by $204,070.00 = 89% collection ratio

Accounts receivable ratio

Annual gross charges divided by 12 = annual monthly gross charges = $19,252.00

$38,230 Current Acc/Rec Bal divided by $19,525 = 1.97 months = accounts receivable ratio

## PART 3 Clinical Applications

Three self-explanatory situations are presented for students to think about and discuss. Students who discuss these situations tend to practice better in the office. They understand their need for guidance and are more inclined to seek help rather than making errors.

# 20

# Health Insurance and Managed Care

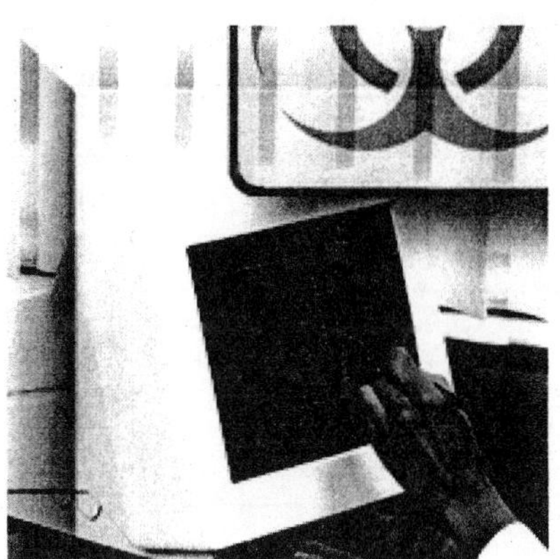

This chapter provides a foundation for understanding types of insurance policies, plans, benefits, and the impact of managed care on medical assistant responsibilities. Health insurance procedures begin with the first appointment by telephone and are completed when full payment is obtained. Whether practicing in the administrative or clinical area, the medical assistant must understand and apply guidelines to be an effective member of the team. The Internet resources and insurance specialists from a family practice office are essential contacts for assuring an accurate discussion of this topic.

## USING THE LEARNING SYSTEM

### 1. MEDICAL ASSISTANT CONTENT AND COMPETENCIES

CONTENT

- Word building and definitions
- Legal guidelines and requirements for health care
- Risk management
- Hereditary, cultural, and environmental influences on behavior
- Recognition and response to verbal and nonverbal behavior
- Insurance and coding administrative procedures
- Personal attributes
- Job readiness

## 2. MEDICAL ASSISTANT ENTRY-LEVEL CURRICULUM INTERFACE

| TEXTBOOK OBJECTIVES | LEARNING SYSTEM LOCATION | MA CURRICULUM |
|---|---|---|
| **Cognitive** | | **Content** |
| 1. Define and spell the terms listed in the Vocabulary | • Text p. 302<br>• Manual Part 1-A | • Word building and definitions |
| 2. Cite three advantages of group insurance policies over individual policies | • Text p. 304<br>• Manual Part 1-C | • Legal guidelines/requirements for health care<br>• Risk management<br>• Job readiness |
| 3. Name seven major types of health insurance benefits | • Text p. 305<br>• Manual Part 1-C | • Same as # 2 above and<br>• Insurance and coding administrative procedures |
| 4. State the meaning of the Birthday Law | • Text p. 303<br>• Manual Part 1-A | • Insurance and coding administrative procedures |
| 5. State the basic differences between indemnity and service benefit plans | • Text p. 306<br>• Manual Part 1-A | • Insurance and coding administrative procedures<br>• Legal guidelines and requirements for health care<br>• Risk management |
| 6. Describe the major government insurance plans | • Text pp. 307-310<br>• Manual Part 1-D | • Insurance and coding administrative procedures<br>• Legal guidelines and requirements for health care |
| 7. Discuss the implications of managed care for the medical assistant | • Text p. 310<br>• Manual Part 1-E | • Hereditary, cultural, and environmental influences on behavior<br>• Recognition and response to verbal and nonverbal behavior<br>• Insurance and coding administrative procedures<br>• Job readiness<br>• Legal guidelines and requirements for health care<br>• Risk management |
| 8. Explain the differences between health maintenance organizations (HMOs), independent practice associations (IPAs), and preferred provider organizations (PPOs) | • Text pp. 313-314<br>• Manual Part 1-E | • Insurance and coding administrative procedures |

## MEDICAL ASSISTANT ENTRY-LEVEL CURRICULUM INTERFACE *continued*

| TEXTBOOK OBJECTIVES | LEARNING SYSTEM LOCATION | MA CURRICULUM |
|---|---|---|
| **Cognitive** | | **Content** |
| 9. Describe the role of the medical assistant in obtaining referrals and authorizations for care | • Text pp. 315-317<br>• Manual Part 2 | • Hereditary, cultural and environmental influences on behavior<br>• Recognition and response to verbal and nonverbal behavior<br>• Insurance and coding administrative procedures<br>• Personal attributes |
| 10. Identify the legal implications of the medical records audit | • Text p. 319<br>• Manual Part 2 | • Insurance and coding administrative procedures<br>• Legal guidelines and requirements for health care |

## 3. RESOURCES


Fordney, M: *Insurance Handbook for the Medical Office,* 6th Edition. Philadelphia, W.B. Saunders Co., 1999.

Shapiro, JP: "There When You Need it," *US News and World Report,* October 5, 1998. A ranking and discussion of 271 of the nation's HMOs.

*Managed Care Week.* Atlantic Information Services, Inc. Publishers, 1100 17th Street NW., Suite 300, Washington, DC, 1-800-321-6388 **www.aispub.com**

www.bluecross.com
www.blueshield.com
www.aetnahealthcare.com

**4. LESSON PLAN Health Insurance** **TIME 3 hours lecture, 12 hours lab (some of this lab may carry over to the next chapter)**

**Opening:** It is not hard to learn information to successfully complete insurance claims and meet third-party regulations. It does require attention to detail, following directions, and lifelong learning: Completing information sheet and forms will make the process easier.

**Pretest:** Ask students how many insurance plans or carriers they can name. Write them on the board.

**Objectives:** Put objectives and content on flip chart. Have speaker cover this material. After speaker leaves, check-off all objectives as covered. Now students must learn information.

**Content:** Due to the rapidly changing insurance regulations and environment, it is important that the student understand all *current* concepts. When possible, ask an insurance specialist to review the chapter, present the material using the objectives as a guideline, and respond to student questions when possible. Then the instructor may review the chapter by completing Part 1 in the Mastery Manual and discussing each subject.

HEALTH INSURANCE AND MANAGED CARE—CHAPTER OUTLINE
Prepare for discussion by making copies if the insurance carrier information sheet. Students have one at the end of the chapter in the Mastery Manual. They will need between six and eight. More than eight is overwhelming to students.

1. BRIEF HISTORY OF HEALTH INSURANCE
2. PURPOSE OF HEALTH INSURANCE
   Cost of Coverage    Coordination of Benefits
3. AVAILABILITY OF HEALTH INSURANCE
   a. Group Policies
   b. Individual Policies
   c. Government Plans
4. TYPES OF INSURANCE BENEFITS
   a. Hospitalization
   b. Surgical
   c. Basic Medical
   d. Major Medical
   e. Disability (Loss of Income) Protection
   f. Dental Care
   g. Vision Care
   h. Medicare Supplement
   i. Special Class Insurance
   j. Special Risk Insurance
   k. Liability Insurance
   l. Life Insurance
5. HOW BENEFITS ARE DETERMINED
   a. Indemnity Schedules
   b. Service Benefit Plans
   c. Usual, Customary, and Reasonable Fee
6. KINDS OF PLANS
   a. Blue Cross/Blue Shield
   b. Blue Card

c. Foundations for Medical Care
d. Commercial Insurers
e. Government Plans
f. Medicare
    Part A: Hospital Insurance
    Part B: Medical Insurance
g. Medicaid
h. Medi/Medi
i. Military Medical Benefits
j. CHAMPUS
k. CHAMPVA
l. CHAMPVA/ TRICARE
m. Workers' Compensation
n. Managed Care Organizations
o. Health Maintenance Organization
p. Independent Practice Association
q. Preferred-Provider Organization
r. Life Insurance
s. Disability Insurance: State Mandated, Voluntary

7. KINDS OF MANAGED CARE ORGANIZATIONS
   a. Health Maintenance Organization
   b. Independent Practice Association
   c. Preferred-Provider Organization
8. WORKING WITH MANAGED CARE PLANS
   a. Precertification or Preauthorization
   b. New Patient Insurance Verification Procedure
   c. Provider Relations
   d. Member Services
   e. Claims Department
   f. Utilization Management
   g. Eligibility Services
   h. Medical Director
   i. Formulary
9. REFERRALS AND AUTHORIZATIONS
10. GUIDELINES FOR THE ASSISTANT IN SPECIALTY PRACTICE
11. MEDICAL RECORDS AUDIT
12. LEGAL AND ETHICAL RESPONSIBILITIES

**Lab:** Complete insurance carrier information forms. Arrange patient medical records in audit format as directed in Part 2.
Go to the main menu on the CD-ROM ⊕ and allow students to perform electronic and computer entries related to types of plans and assembly and audit of charts.

**Assignment:** Have students complete Part 1 of the Mastery Manual after first class. Have students complete in neat and easily readable form all the insurance carrier sheets for local and national plans you have assigned. These should be put into a binder for referral.

**Posttest:** Use the Examaster testbank. Grade the insurance carrier information sheets as part of a test. Ask objective questions related to the objectives. Do not let students proceed without 90% knowledge.

## 5. MASTERY MANUAL ANSWERS

### PART 1 CONTENT MASTERY

### A. Learning Level: Knowledge

VOCABULARY: Fill in the word or words which describe the meaning of the words below.

1. Individual policy—A policy usually held by a person who does not qualify for a group policy.
2. Beneficiary—The person receiving the benefits of an insurance policy.
3. Birthday law—The rule governing the hierarchy of coordination of benefits.
4. Claim—A demand to the insurer by the insured person for the payment of benefits under a policy.
5. Coinsurance/Copayment—A policy provision by which both the insured person and the insurer share in a specified ratio of the expenses resulting from an illness or injury.
6. Deductible—A statement in an insurance policy that the insuring company will pay the expenses incurred after the insured person has paid a specified amount.
7. Assignment of insurance benefits—A statement authorizing the insurance company to pay benefits directly to the physician.
8. Fee schedule—A list of services or procedures indemnified by the insurance company and the specific dollar amounts that will be paid for each service.
9. Fringe benefit—A benefit granted by an employer that involves a money cost but does not affect the basic wage rates of employees.
10. Coordination of benefits (COB)—The provision in an insurance contract that limits benefits to 100% of the cost.
11. Member physician—A physician who has agreed to accept the contracts of an insurer; this usually includes accepting the insurance benefits as payment in full.
12. Subscriber—A person named as principal in an insurance contract.
13. Prepaid plan—A plan that provides all covered services to a policyholder for payment of a monthly fee.
14. Professional standards review organization (PSRO)—A group of physicians working with the government to review cases for hospital admission and discharge under government guidelines; sometimes referred to as Peer Review.
15. Service benefit plan—A plan that agrees to pay for certain surgical and medical services and that is not restricted to a fee schedule.
16. Capitation—Reimbursement to a health care provider based on a fixed amount per member for a given period.
17. Co-payment—A fixed dollar amount that the insured must pay each time service is rendered.
18. Utilization review—Approval for health care by an outside group.

### B. Learning Level: Comprehension

1. Give the meaning of the following abbreviations

| | |
|---|---|
| a. Benefits ID card | BIC |
| b. Utilization Review Dept | URD |
| c. Explanation of benefits | EOB |
| d. Independent provider assoc | IPA |
| e. Prospective payment system | PPS |
| f. Member services | MS |
| g. Primary care physician | PCP |
| h. Preferred provider org. | PPO |
| i. Supplemental Security Income | SSI |
| j. Utilization management | UM |

2. Name the responsibilities involved in processing an insurance claim.
   a. Obtain authorization and referrals
   b. Prepare insurance claims forms
   c. Maintain an insurance claims register
   d. Trace unpaid claims
   e. Evaluate claims rejection
   f. Report procedures to prepaid care plans
   g. Translate medical terminology into procedural and diagnostic codes

## C. Learning Level: Application

1. Insurance plan evaluation

| | Group Plan | Individual Plan | No Health Insurance |
|---|---|---|---|
| a. Cost | Paid by employer | About $110/month | Nothing until needed |
| b. Deductibles | $5/visit | 20% or $15/visit<br>Average HMO | Nothing |
| c. Covered services | Most everything | No preventative | Nothing |
| d. Physical required | No | Yes | |
| e. Maximum paid | $5/visit or hosp | Depends upon plan | 100% of everything |
| f. Coverage for whom | Employee and family | Employee alone | |
| g. Exclusions (Riders) | None | Exclude husband on heart<br>Child would need physical | |

2. Premium, deductibles or non-covered expenses

## D. Learning Level: Analysis

1. What types of health insurance benefits would the patient have for the situations below?
   a. AARP pays the person $70 for every day in the hospital but nothing for physician bills. Hospitalization
   b. Baby Ann has run out of medical coverage for sleep apnea due to prematurity. Fortunately her parents have a supplement to the basic coverage. Major medical
   c. Blue Cross paid Mr. Dement $2000 for the laparoscopic inguinal hernia repair, but Mr. Dement had to pay for the one-day hospital stay. Surgery
   d. Mr. Acorn is 74 years old. After his bypass surgery, the medical office sent the bill to the Medicare carrier and told him that Medicare would forward the claim on to his Medicare supplement policy.
   e. Mr. Kieffer was in getting a broken tooth capped. The dentist wanted the hygienist to clean his teeth before putting the cap on. Mr. Kieffer said as long as he had dental insurance it would be OK.
2. List seven kinds of plans and describe each so that looking at the patient's card, one could identify the kind of plan and what the benefits might be.
   a. Blue Cross/Blue Shield—May have one or both symbols on card-cross or shield or both. Need to call company for specifics
   b. Foundation for Medical Care is an intermediary for an insurance company. The card has the company name on it—not the foundation name
   c. Commercial plans—Private insurance companies such as Aetna, Columbia Care, or Healthnet insure persons and unless HMO may even send payment to patient
   d. Medicare card indicates Medicare and Part A or Part B or both.
   e. Medicaid—Plastic BIC cards indicate name and coverage status when used with authorization machine
   f. Military—CHAMPUS or CHAMPVA indicated on card
   g. Workers' Compensation—Only insurance for on-the-job injuries and must be verified by employer as to insurance carrier coverage

   Other types of insurance include disability, life, medi/medi, and managed care plans.

## E. Learning Level: Synthesis

Managed care questions

1. What do you see as the major differences in an HMO and a PPO?

   Two major differences—

   a. how fees are paid

   b. types of care that may be given without referral

2. Give four examples of HMO plans and state which type they are. You may list local plans or federal or state.

   a. Medicare HMO network

   b. Kaiser—staff model

   c. Blue Cross/BlueShield—Network

   d. TRICARE—IPA

   e. Suggest instructor use local plans for other examples.

3. An AARP plan or any similar plan that just pays the insured for days in the hospital is not a health care plan, it is just an insurance plan and not subject to health care guidelines.

## F. Learning Level: Evaluation

1. Managed care contracts require procedures common to all in order to insure the physician is complying and will be paid.

   What are the procedures for which the medical assistant is responsible?

   a. Verify insurance

   b. Obtain precertification and preauthorization for surgeries, labs, tests

   c. Obtain referrals

   d. Provide chart for medical records audit

2. Which department in the managed care organization would you refer the patient or yourself to in the following situations?

   a. The physician wants you to appeal a claim—provider relations

   b. Submit a copy of authorization when requesting payment to—claims dept

   c. You are verifying membership in HMO—eligibility services

   d. The list of covered drugs and prescriptions—formulary

   e. Patient needs to question coverage—member services

3. The Birthday Law applies in HMOs when both parents are covered by insurance unless the decree provides for only one party to be responsible. Even then the other spouse may be subject to it if both belong to the same HMO.

## PART 2 COMPETENCY CHALLENGE

All the activities in this part may be completed in lab and prepare the student to understand information regarding national and local carriers so they may apply the knowledge in the next chapter when coding and preparing claims. The main menu on the CD-ROM ⊕ also allows compiling files correctly for audit.

1. Use the Insurance Carrier Information sheet at the end of the chapter and begin to fill it out for the major insurance carriers and HMOs that serve your local area. Have students copy the sheet and fill it out for all the major carriers in your area. Use Transparency Master 21-6 with an eraseable pen and use lab time to complete each form for each carrier.
2. Design an insurance claims register form that allows you to track the following: claims sent, claims paid, amount paid, denials, partial payments, downcoding, adjustments to charges, and patient balances.
3. Take all the patient medical records you have put together to date. Organize them in the order necessary to comply with a medical records audit. Assure that the materials in all charts are consistent in content and organization. Complete the audit by using the forms for chart organization and audit checklist at the end of the chapter for all patient charts.

## PART 3 CLINICAL APPLICATIONS

This activity should produce a lively discussion for objective 10. A written answer may also be required. This question may be discussed in a separate law and ethics course. The medical assistant should verify insurance for all patients. No matter what patient's think, the person who contracts with the office to give care is the responsible party and must pay the bill. This is especially true when one parent lives out of state.

Discuss the following situation.
Mrs. Solce brought her son Robby in to see the physician in November. When you go to collect from her insurance, they tell you that she is no longer covered under the policy. What did you forget to do? You call Mrs. Solce and tell her the situation. She tells you to bill Robby's father, who is the responsible party according to the divorce decree. He resides in the adjacent state. How do you proceed? Consider the legal, ethical, and patient education points and opportunities.

## Insurance Carrier Information Form

**Insurance Carrier/HMO** ________________________ Date Prepared ____________

**Name of Program** ________________________

**Claims Filing Address** ________________________

________________________

**PRD Contact Name:** ________________________ Telephone ____________

**MS Contact Name:** ________________________ Telephone ____________

**Pre-authorization requirements??** Circle one: **YES** (List below) **NO**

For ________________________

________________________

**Second opinion** required for surgery?? Circle one **YES** **NO**

**Claim Form used:** ____________ Code Books: Dx: ____________ Procedure: ____________

**Filing deadline** ________________________

**Card verification markings:** ________________________

**Circle one:** Co-pay / Fee for service / Cost of share / Not collectible from patient

**What is the deductible/co-pay/COS/amount?** For: OV ________, ER ________

HOSP ________, ASC ________, PT ________, Other ________________

**Does deductible apply to all services?** Circle one **YES** **NO**

**Non-covered services:** ________________________

________________________

**Appeals:** Name & Address: ________________________

________________________

Form #________ or Letter ______ Timelines : ________________

**Claims tips for filing:**

________________________

________________________

****On insurance forms put specific information required if different than field description (i.e.: Medicare and Medicaid regulations).**

# 21

# Coding and Claims Processing

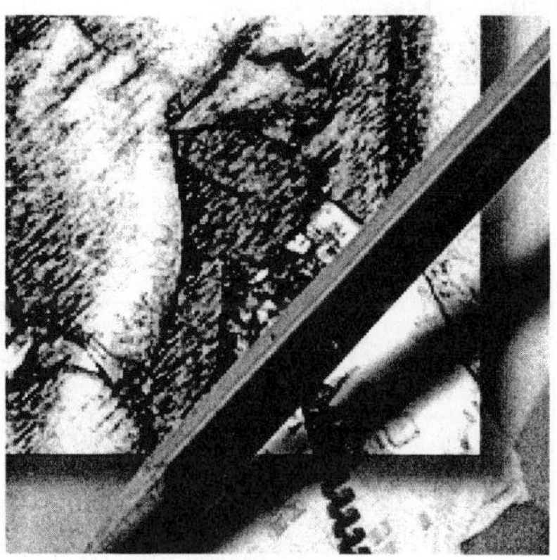

This chapter continues the insurance process. Because the process begins when the patient first makes an appointment, the medical assistant is involved and must learn all the requirements in order to process forms and claims correctly. The physician's office cannot be waiting for money because of the medical assistant, lack of performance. It is important to stress the need for attention to detail but also the relative ease of the process when one reads carefully and follows established procedures. The rules change, but if the necessary reading is done, there is not a problem.

## USING THE LEARNING SYSTEM

### 1. MEDICAL ASSISTANT CONTENT AND COMPETENCIES

CONTENT

- Word building and definitions
- Legal guidelines and requirements for health care
- Risk management
- Recognition and response to verbal and nonverbal communication
- Insurance and coding administrative procedures
- Job readiness

COMPETENCIES

- Apply managed care policies and procedures
- Apply third-party guidelines
- Obtain managed care referrals and precertifications
- Perform procedural coding
- Perform diagnostic coding
- Complete insurance claim forms
- Use a physician's fee schedule
- Respond to and initiate written communications
- Perform within legal and ethical boundaries
- Instruct individuals according to their needs
- Utilize computer software to maintain office systems

## 2. MEDICAL ASSISTANT ENTRY-LEVEL CURRICULUM INTERFACE

| TEXTBOOK OBJECTIVES | LEARNING SYSTEM LOCATION | MA CURRICULUM |
|---|---|---|
| **Cognitive** | | **Content** |
| 1. Define and spell the terms listed in the Vocabulary | • Text p. 322<br>• Manual Part 1-A | • Word building and definitions<br>• Recognition and response to verbal and nonverbal communication |
| 2. Identify four purposes of numeric diagnostic and procedural coding | • Text p. 323<br>• Manual Part 1-B | • Legal guidelines and requirements for health care<br>• Risk management<br>• Insurance and coding administrative procedures<br>• Job readiness |
| 3. Name the principal coding systems that link the medical profession and insurance system | • Text pp. 323-324<br>• Manual Part 1-B | • Same as #2 above<br>• Recognition and response to verbal and nonverbal communications |
| 4. List 10 reasons for possible rejection of insurance claims | • Text pp. 325, 330 | • Same as #3 above |
| 5. State the maximum billing period for Medicare claims | • Text p. 330 | • Same as #2 above |
| 6. Explain why a patient's care under workers' compensation should be recorded separately from the patient's private care chart | • Text p. 332<br>• Manual Part 3 | • Same as #2 above |
| 7. List and briefly describe three types of managed care organizations | • Text pp. 335-336 | • Same as #2 above |
| **Performance** | **Locations** | **Competency** |
| 1. Identify and complete the appropriate insurance forms for patients covered by:<br>a. Medicare<br>b. CHAMPUS<br>c. Workers' Compensation<br>d. Blue Cross and Blue Shield | • Manual Part 2<br>• CD-ROM ⊕ | • Apply managed care policies and procedures<br>• Apply third-party guidelines<br>• Perform procedural coding<br>• Perform diagnostic coding<br>• Complete insurance claim forms<br>• Use a physician's fee schedule<br>• Initiate written communications<br>• Perform within legal and ethical boundaries<br>• Utilize computer software to maintain office systems |

## MEDICAL ASSISTANT ENTRY-LEVEL CURRICULUM INTERFACE *continued*

| TEXTBOOK OBJECTIVES | LEARNING SYSTEM LOCATION | MA CURRICULUM |
|---|---|---|
| Performance | | Competency |
| 2. Calculate the billing for patients whose insurance includes deductibles and copayments or coinsurance | • Manual Part 2<br>• CD-ROM ⊕ | • Apply managed care policies and procedures<br>• Apply third-party guidelines<br>• Use a physician's fee schedule<br>• Perform within legal and ethical boundaries |

## 3. RESOURCES

Fordney, M: *Insurance Handbook for the Medical Office,* 6th Edition. Philadelphia, W.B. Saunders Co., 1999.

www.hcfa.gov **This site gives the latest regulations and correct instructions for completing HCFA 1500.**

www.medicarerights.org

## 4. LESSON PLAN Health Insurance TIME 3 hours lecture, 12 hours lab

**Opening:** Usually it is good to posttest and refresh using some concept from previous chapter. Whether students have read the chapter or not, students may be quite confused and intimidated by insurance processing. Discuss coding and its history. The ICD 10 is in use in Europe and may be used in the U.S. by 2001, although HCFA is denying the possibility.

**Pretest:** Differentiate a procedure from a diagnosis. Give examples. Discuss.

**Objectives:** You probably want to add a few specific ones of your own. Be prepared to teach to the objectives and use them in post-testing to see if they "got it."

**Content:** Use the activities in the Mastery Manual to discuss all the important points in an orderly fashion. After students have mastered vocabulary and had preliminary chapter discussion, it may be advisable to complete the Mastery Manual as a group and complete a lot of problem solving. Students will then be able to function independently with the CD-ROM activities. Fill in important concepts as necessary.

*chart continues on following page*

## LESSON PLAN Health Insurance *continued*

1. VOCABULARY
2. FEE SCHEDULES
   Relative Value Scales (RVS)
   Resource-Based Relative Value Scale (RBRVS)
3. PROCEDURAL CODING
   CPT organization
   HCPCS coding system
4. DIAGNOSTIC CODING
   International Classification of Diseases, Ninth Revision, Clinical Modification (ICD-9-CM)
5. CODING GUIDELINES REVIEW IN TEXT
6. GUIDELINES FOR CLAIMS PROCESSING
   Verifying insurance
   Claim forms used
   Superbill
   Assignment of benefits
   Tracking claims
   Electronic claims submission
   Claim rejection
   Procedure 21-1: Completing Paper HCFA 1500
   Procedure 21-2: Electronic Medicare Submission
7. BILLING REQUIREMENTS
   Medicare—par & non-par, timelines, preauthorizations
   Medicaid—physician responsibilities, billing limits, BIC card
   Medi-Medi—send to Medicare and crossover will occur if both boxes checked
   Blue Plans—follow directions in carrier provider books
   CHAMPUS and CHAMPVA—HCFA 1500 for physician fee
   Workers' Compensation—keep separate records, bill insurance carrier, never bill patient
8. HEALTH CARE AND COST CONTAINMENT
   Health care Reform
   HMO PRO PPS DRGs
9. LEGAL AND ETHICAL ISSUES
   HCFA regulations
   Workers' Compensation laws
   Physician must provide codes—must be accurate or fraud

**Lab:** Complete all Part 2 and 3 activities in lab. This would include the CD-ROM ⊕ activities for insurance billing of the patient case studies. The billing and claims processing activities are contained in the CD-ROM main menu under administrative skills. Students may complete the insurance billing separately from other administrative activities. Also, if an activity was done incorrectly due to limited foundation, this is a good time to repeat insurance skills.

**Assignment:** Most assignments will be directed toward applying vocabulary, understanding the use of the coding books, and evaluating HCFA 1500 forms for accurate completion. Use the Examaster testbank for objective style questions. Fill out a couple of HCFA 1500 forms incorrectly and have students identify inaccurate information. Use medical management computer program (Medisoft, Medical Manager, or Gylys book, *Computer Applications in the Medical Office,* by FA Davis publishers, 1995) and complete insurance forms for the program.

**Posttest:** Test to class objectives for each class.

## 6. MASTERY MANUAL ANSWERS

### PART 1 CONTENT MASTERY

#### A. Learning Level: Knowledge

Students need to master terminology to correctly process claims

1. comorbidity—A pre-existing condition that will, because of its presence with a specific principal diagnosis, cause an increase in length of stay by at least one day in approximately 75% of the cases.
2. DRG creep—The process of inflating diagnoses to obtain a higher payment rate.
3. site—A designated place or point.
4. TEFRA—Federal Law in 1982. Contains provisions for major changes in Medicare reimbursement.
5. pre-existing condition—A physical condition of an insured person that existed prior to the insurance policy.
6. peer review organization—An entity that is composed of a substantial number of licensed doctors of medicine and osteopathy engaged in the practice of medicine or surgery in the area, or an entity that has available to it the services of a sufficient number of physicians engaged in the practice of medicine or surgery, to assure the adequate peer review of the services provided by the various medical specialties and subspecialties.
7. mandated—Required by an authority or law.
8. grouper—Computer software program that is used by the fiscal intermediary in all cases to assign discharges to the appropriate DRGs.
9. crossover claim—A claim for benefits under both Medicare and Medicaid.
10. discharge face sheet—A summary of the hospital stay prepared at time of patient's discharge from the hospital.
11. etiology—Classifying a claim according to the cause of the disorder.
12. established patient—A patient who has received care from the physician within the last 3 years.
13. non-participating provider—A physician who does not accept assignment under Medicare or the Blue Plans (i.e., non-par).
14. principal procedure—One that was performed for definitive treatment rather than for diagnostic or exploratory purposes, or one necessary to take care of a complication. It is that procedure most related to the principal diagnosis.
15. uniform hospital discharge data sheet—A minimum data set required to be collected for each Medicare patient on discharge.
16. preauthorization—Permission by insurance carrier obtained prior to giving certain treatment to a patient.
17. ancillary diagnostic services—Services that support patient diagnoses, e.g., laboratory or x-ray.
18. ICD-9-CM—A system for classifying diseases to facilitate collection of uniform and comparable health information.
19. new patient—A patient who has not received any professional services from the physician in the past 3 years.
20. coding—Converting verbal descriptions of diseases, injuries, and procedures into numeric and alphanumeric designations.
21. complication—A condition that arises during the hospital stay that prolongs the length.
22. electronic billing—The submission of a claim via computer to computer.
23. fiscal intermediary—An organization that handles claims from hospitals, nursing facilities, intermediate and long-term care facilities, and home health agencies.
24. participating provider, i.e., par—A physician who accepts assignment under Medicare or the Blue Plans.
25. principal diagnosis—That condition that after study is determined to be chiefly responsible for occasioning the admission of the patient to the hospital.

## B. Learning Level: Comprehension

1. Name three coding systems and indicate whether they are procedural or diagnostic codes.
   a. CPT procedural
   b. HCPCS procedural
   c. ICD-9 diagnostic
2. Summarize what the RBRVS is to health claims processing today.

   A fee for service schedule to provide uniform national payments after being adjusted to reflect for different practice costs in different geographic areas. It contains a single conversion factor for different areas, i.e., medical, surgical, or laboratory services.
3. What is the procedural coding system used by Medicare? HCPCS
   Explain its use.

## C. Learning Level: Application

1. Name all the CPT sections from which the codes are obtained and explain usage.

2. A 25-year-old new patient came into the office and had an examination so he could play football with a local team. The physician also took off a mole. When you went to code the excision of the mole, there was a star next to the procedure. Can you bill for the office visit and the procedure? yes

   Explain. In this case the procedure was not the main reason the patient came to the office. It may then be added to the bill for the sports physical. Bill for level under preventative medicine, i.e., 99385 and mole removal—needs more description

## D. Learning Level: Analysis

1. Describe how you would use a diagnostic code to its highest level of specificity. If you need an example, refer to the diagnosis of diabetes in the ICD-9 book.
2. Why can't a diagnosis code be used when there is the word probable, suspected, or rule out in the diagnosis statement?

   Because these terms indicate the diagnosis has not been finalized so it must be billed by the symptom stated.
3. Look at the coding guidelines in Chapter 21 in the textbook and analyze the items that need to be listed on the claim for the situation below. What sections of the code books will you look in? If you have the code books available, code the items you chose.

   A 48-year-old woman with a history of breast cancer, bilateral mastectomy, and breast reconstruction was seen by her primary care physician for a complaint of shortness of breath. A chest x-ray was taken, and it demonstrated a small pleural effusion in the left. The physician performed an aspiration thoracentesis, drew off the fluid, and sent it for cytology and chemistry.

| Diagnosis items—ICD | Section and # codes | Procedural items from CPT | Section and # codes |
|---|---|---|---|
| Left pleural effusion<br>Personal Hx of breast cancer | Respiratory 511.9<br>Persons with potential health hazards related to personal Hx V10.3 | Office visit | 99213 - 25 Explain modifier use |
| | | Thoracentesis | 32000 ★ Explain star |
| | | Chest x-ray AP and Lat. 2 views | Radiology 71020 |
| | | Thoracentesis tray<br><br>Specimen to lab | Special services<br>99070<br>99000 |

## E. Learning Level: Synthesis

A. Complete the CPT coding exercises: Point out need-to-know terminology in different format, i.e., an excision is an "ectomy" and need to interpret when reading descriptors.

1. First visit, multiple complaints, medications for arthritis, depression, and hypertension reviewed and medications changed. 99205
2. Eight-year-old seen second time in a week for severe sore throat and fatigue. 99212
3. Initial hospital consult for diabetic male with incisional infection following back surgery. 99223
4. Dermatology office consult for teenager with severe acne. 99244
5. Debridement of skin and subcutaneous tissue for infection of right arm. 11000
6. Second-stage Mohs procedure, 4 specimens. 17305
7. Partial acromionectomy. 23130 left
8. MMR injection. 90707
9. Initial hospital newborn screen. 99431
10. Four-year-old preschool physical with vision screen and hearing tests. 99393
11. Parietal pleurectomy. 32310
12. ERCP with biopsy. 43261

B. Complete the diagnostic coding exercises.

| | |
|---|---|
| Acute anterior wall MI | 410.10 |
| Acute cholecystitis | 575.0 |
| Alcohol abuse, continuous | 305.01 |
| Alzheimer's disease | 330.0 |
| Ataxia | 781.3 |
| Carbuncle, neck | 680.1 |
| Chronic sinusitis, maxillary | 473.0 |
| Corneal foreign body | 930.0 |
| Diaphragmatic hernia | 553.3 |
| Endometriosis | 617.9 |
| Fracture distal end of radius closed | 813.41 |
| Hemangioma | 228.00 |
| Hematuria | 599.7 |
| Hemorrhoids | 558.8 |
| Hodgkin's disease, unspecified | 201.9 |
| Impacted cerumen | 380.4 |
| Multiple sclerosis | 340 |
| Nosebleed | 784.7 |
| Open angle glaucoma | 365.10 |
| Osteoarthritis, left hip | 715.5 |
| Post-menopausal hormone replacement therapy | V07.4 |
| Recurrent shoulder dislocation | 718.31 |
| Routine infant check | V20.2 |
| Threatened abortion | 640.00 |

## F. Learning Level: Evaluation

Read the comprehensive evaluation below and assess for each item whether the item needs to be put on a claims reimbursement form. Give your reasons.

RE: Patient Mrs. X

COMPREHENSIVE EVALUATION

DATE: 2-4-99

The patient comes in today to establish care for complete evaluation. A comprehensive history and physical was performed and will not be repeated here.

In summary, the patient is a 48-year-old with the following problems:

1. Chest pressure syndrome—is not clearly exertional, seems to be relieved with rest, has some radiation to her left shoulder, no associated shortness of breath or diaphoresis, suggestive of angina in somebody who has multiple risk factors.

   Yes, this is a specific diagnosis
2. Family history of premature coronary disease in both her father and mother.

   No, not related to a dx for patient
3. Morbid obesity—has been a lifelong dieter and believes that she has gained an excessive amount of weight, despite eating normally. Most people who eat what she eats weigh a lot more.

   Yes, relates to diagnosis established from exam
4. Polyuria and nocturia—rule out diabetes.

   Yes, symptoms are diagnostic; do not include R/O
5. Suspected syndrome X—needs lipid status and uric acid checked.

   No, suspected may not be coded
6. Dysphagia with frequent regurgitation after eating. Treated empirically for reflux and has had some help with an upper GI

   Yes, part of current problem
7. Essential hypertension—her blood pressure today was 160/94 in both arms.

   Yes, part of current evaluation
8. Moderately strong suspicion of sleep apnea—she wakes up frequently and awakens in the morning feeling sleepy. She also has some orthopnea and the body habitus consistent with sleep apnea.

   No, see #5
9. History of asthma, followed by an allergist.

   No, not part of this evaluation
10. Status post-pneumonia.

    No, see #9
11. Family history of colon cancer.

    No, see #9

PLAN: Today I have done a 12 lead ECG and given her Pneumovax. Tested occult blood, feces and negative. Obtained blood for full screen lab studies for # 3, 4, and 5. Will arrange a stress test and had a long discussion of all her problems. Will follow with all test results in 1 week.

**Coding answers for Mrs. X**

| Diagnosis | Service |
|---|---|
| Chest pressure syndrome 786.50 or 786.59 | Established patient comprehensive examination 99215 |
| Obesity 278 | ECG 93000 |
| Polyuria 788.42 | Pneumovax 90--- |
| Nocturia 788.43 | Stool occult blood 82270 |
| Dysphagia 787.2 or 536.8 | |
| Essential hypertension 401.9 | |

## PART 2 COMPETENCY CHALLENGE

1. Use the CD-ROM and complete the HCFA 1500 for all the case studies presented in the Administrative Skills section from the main menu. If the CD-ROM is not available, copy the HCFA × 8 and use the Appendix to obtain the patient information to complete the claims process. Procedure 15-1 is the instructions for completing the paper HCFA 1500, and Procedure 15-2 is the instructions for electronic claims billing—**For Medicare patients only.**

**CD-ROM case study coding answers**

*Case 1 Mr. Ivan Shapiro*

Diagnosis:
Chest pain on exertion 786.59 probably the closest
Coronary artery disease 414.00
Hypertension 402.90
Service:
New patient comprehensive examination 99205
ECG 93000
Urinalysis complete, dipstick 81000

*Case 2 Mr. Raymond Johnson*

Diagnosis:
Chronic obstructive asthma 493.21 or 493211 or 493.91
Acute URI 465.9
Service:
Established patient limited examination 99213
Subcutaneous injection of Susphrine 90782
Spirometry 94010
IPPB 94650
OV on emergency basis 99058
Venipuncture 36415

*Case 3 Robby Soto, 4 1/2-month-old child*

Diagnosis:
Well child care V20.2
Service:
Estab patient preventative service 99391
Immunizations DtaP 90720
Hib 90721
Oral polio 90712

*Case 4 Lucy Ferguson*

Diagnosis:
UTI 599.0
Arteriosclerosis not treated
Osteoporosis 733.0 dietetic counselling
Dyspnea 786.09
Degenerative arthritis 715.90
Service:
New patient comprehensive examination 99205
Vaginal examination—part of NP examination
Dipstick urinalysis 81000
Pap smear
X-rays and lab referred to outside facilities

2. Using the HCFA 1500 at the end of the chapter, complete a claims reimbursement for Mrs. X in Part 1-F, the comprehensive evaluation report.

## PART 3 CLINICAL APPLICATIONS

1. Mr. Souci, a postal worker, was bitten on his route by a dog. Dr. Healer has treated him twice for the wound, which appears to be infected. When you bring the patient to the physician, you notice that all of this patient's records are in one chart. What are the dangers with this situation? How could this impact your employer and you?

   Worker's Comp. records must be separated from patient medical record.

2. When you see patient for B/P checks, you write the actual service on the charge slip. As a medical assistant, what codes may the insurance billing person use for medical assistant services such as B/P check, removal of stitches, or diet education? Why did you give the answer you did? If other codes are used, what is the problem?

   Use 99211—lowest code available—minimal service with MD supervision

# 22

# Assisting with Library, Research, Travel, and Meetings

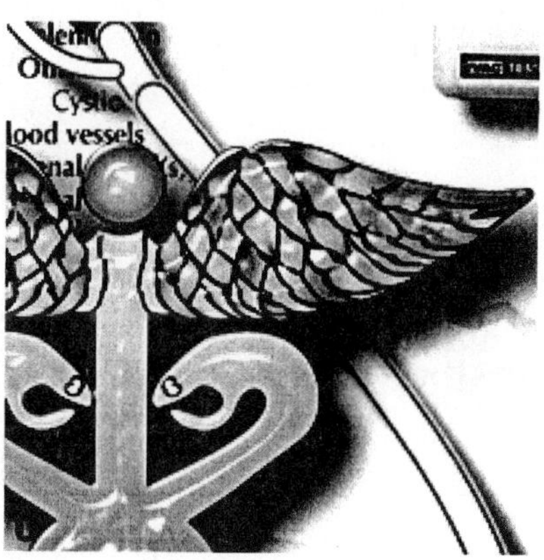

It is not the responsibility of the support staff of medical assistants to correct speeches or complete other editorial duties or make physician travel arrangements, but often the medical assistant is requested to assist in these matters. The medical assistant who becomes active in a professional association may hold office or write for a journal, and the knowledge for procedures for arranging meetings and scheduling travel plus preparing manuscripts will help with these functions. Chapters 22, 23, and 24 may be offered as continuing education for the professional medical assistant. If they are so offered, the activities and competencies must be increased in the depth of knowledge and performance for the practicing medical assistant.

## USING THE LEARNING SYSTEM

### 1. MEDICAL ASSISTANT CONTENT AND COMPETENCIES

CONTENT

- Respond to and initiate written communications
- Receive, organize, and prioritize information
- Identify community resources
- Fundamental writing skills
- Personal attributes
- Workplace dynamics

COMPETENCIES

- Identify community resources
- Demonstrate telephone techniques
- Document appropriately
- Recognize and respond to verbal communications for travel arrangements and group meetings

## 2. MEDICAL ASSISTANT ENTRY-LEVEL CURRICULUM INTERFACE

| TEXTBOOK OBJECTIVES | LEARNING SYSTEM INTERFACE | MA CURRICULUM |
|---|---|---|
| **Cognitive** | **Locations** | **Content** |
| 1. Define and spell the terms listed in the Vocabulary | • Text p. 340<br>• Manual Part 1-B | • Word building and definitions |
| 2. Originate and maintain a card catalog for a personal library | • Text pp. 343-344 | • Respond to and initiate written communications<br>• Receive, organize and prioritize information<br>• Identify community resources<br>• Fundamental writing skills<br>• Personal attributes<br>• Workplace dynamics |
| 3. Discuss the nature and importance of an abstract | • Text p. 341<br>• Manual Part 1-F | • Same as #2 above |
| 4. List the four items to include on a cross reference card for a general reference file | • Text p. 343<br>• Manual Part 1-C | • Same as #3 above |
| 5. Name five items of information to include on a diagnostic file card | • Text p. 342<br>• Manual Part 1-C | • Respond to and initiate written communications<br>• Receive, organize, and prioritize information |
| 6. Name two of the largest medical databases for electronic retrieval of information | • Text p. 343 | • Respond to and initiate written communications<br>• Receive, organize, and prioritize information |
| 7. List the seven items of information needed for each reference in a bibliography | • Text p. 344<br>• Manual Part 1-C | • Same as #6 above |
| 8. Briefly outline the general procedure for preparing a manuscript for publication in a periodical | • Text pp. 345-347 | • Same as #6 above |
| 9. List five items that should be included in the first paragraph of the minutes of a meeting | • Text p. 350 | • Same as #6 above |
| **Performance** | **Locations** | **Competency** |
| 1. Prepare cards for an abstract file | • Text p. 341<br>• Manual Part 1-E | • Identify community resources<br>• Document appropriately<br>• Recognize and respond to verbal communications |

**MEDICAL ASSISTANT ENTRY-LEVEL CURRICULUM INTERFACE *continued***

| TEXTBOOK OBJECTIVES | LEARNING SYSTEM INTERFACE | MA CURRICULUM |
|---|---|---|
| **Performance** | **Locations** | **Competency** |
| 2. Set up a diagnostic file, including subject cards and the necessary subheadings to accommodate the patient charts | • Text p. 342<br>• Manual Part 2 | • Identify community resources<br>• Document appropriately<br>• Recognize and respond to verbal communications |
| 3. Retype a manuscript that has been edited using proofreader's marks | • Manual Part 2 | • Identify community resources<br>• Document appropriately<br>• Recognize and respond to verbal communications |
| 4. Make travel arrangements for a proposed trip | • Manual Part 3 | • Recognize and respond to verbal communications for travel arrangements and group meetings |
| 5. Prepare a typewritten itinerary | • Manual Part 3 | • Recognize and respond to verbal communications for travel arrangements and group meetings<br>• Document appropriately |
| 6. Make arrangements for a group meeting | • Manual Part 2 | • Recognize and respond to verbal communications for travel arrangements and group meetings |
| 7. From a rough draft, type the minutes of a meeting in correct form, including the secretary's signature | • Manual Part 2 | • Document appropriately<br>• Recognize and respond to verbal communications |

## 3. RESOURCES

Plotnik, A: *The Elements of Editing,* Collier Books, Macmillan Publishing Co., 1982. Still the definitive short book for editing.

*The Oxford Companion to the English Language,* Edited by Tom McArthur, Oxford University Press, New York, 1992.

*Roberts Rules of Order.* Parliamentary procedure for chairing a meeting.

www.travelocity.com
www.1travelcom.crs.htm/
**For maps go to** www.yahoo.com

## 4. LESSON PLAN Editorial Duties TIME 3 hours lecture, 3 hours lab

**Opening:** An interesting opening might be to have a manager who is involved in these activities come in and talk to students.

**Pretest:** Bring students to library and give them a library orientation test. Those who need to will then go through the library orientation.

**Objectives:** Review with students. Write on flip chart.

**Content:** Have librarian discuss all cognitive objectives with students and the discussion items in Mastery Manual Part 3.
Instructor is encouraged to add to the outline with notes for discussion. This becomes a complete lesson plan.

EDITORIAL DUTIES

1. Physician's library
   a. Organizing the library
   b. Card catalog
   c. Periodical files, reprints, other reference files, diagnostic files
2. Patient library
3. Gathering information
   Resources, public library, Internet searches
4. Manuscript preparation—*Hint: bring an English teacher in to cover this in an hour*
   a. Library will have proper footnote and bibliography formats
   b. Assign students to write a two-page paper on a disease
5. Mailing manuscript—refer to Chapter 11
6. Travel and meeting arrangements

Procedure 22-1 Making travel arrangements
Procedure 22-2 Arranging group meetings

Students may complete these Competency Objectives as they go to class meetings or even arrange field trips to a travel agency. Compare modes of travel and schedules. Use the Internet for travel sites.

**Assignment:** Students prepare two-page paper, give it to another to proofread, correct, and turn in with proofed copy (using proofreader's marks), signed by student who proofread it, teams providing the letter to be typed to the opposing team. Teams may pick their own typist and proofreaders.

**Posttest:** Talk with travel agent. Bring back a short report.

## 5. MASTERY MANUAL ANSWERS

### PART 1 CONTENT MASTERY

#### A. Learning Level: Knowledge

Answers: 1. T; 2. T; 3. T; 4. F; 5. F; 6. T; 7. T; 8. F; 9. T; 10. F

#### B. Learning Level: Comprehension

Answers: 1. c; 2. k; 3. i; 4. a; 5. h; 6. d; 7. j; 8. f; 9. b; 10. e

#### C. Learning Level: Application

1. Name four items of information that should be included when organizing a card index for a reference file of articles that have been clipped or photocopied:
   a. Title of article or book chapter
   b. Author
   c. Periodical or book in which item appeared
   d. Date of publication

2. List four headings to be included on each patient card in organizing a diagnostic file:
   a. Patient Name
   b. Diagnosis
   c. Treatment
   d. Prognosis
3. List four items of information to be included in a footnote reference:
   a. Author's name
   b. Title of work cited
   c. Publication information
   d. Page of citation

#### D. Learning Level: Analysis

List the seven items of information that should be recorded for each reference in a bibliography:

Subject

Author

Title of book or author

Volume and number

Page number(s)

Publisher or periodical name

Date of publication

## E. Learning Level: Synthesis

**Multiple Choice**
Mark the one best answer to each question by circling the letter preceding it.
* = correct answer

1. In abstract of a paper is a/an:
   * A. Summary of its main points.
   B. Quotation from the article.
   C. Introduction to the paper.
   D. Critical evaluation of a paper.

2. In systematically organizing the doctor's personal library, books should be classified:
   A. Alphabetically
   * B. By subject groupings
   C. Chronologically by publication date
   D. By name of author

3. The typeset proof returned by an editor to the author is called what kind of proof?
   A. Editor's
   B. Final
   * C. Galley
   D. Author's

4. How many cards should be prepared for each book in cataloging a library?
   A. One
   B. Two
   * C. Three
   D. Four

5. The system that uses decimal numbers to indicate specific subjects and arranges the book collection in numeric sequence is called the:
   A. Library of Congress System
   B. Boston Medical Library System
   C. Barnard Classification
   * D. Dewey System

6. In the following number combinations representing minutes/words per page, indicate which would correspond to the average number of minutes required to read one page of double-spaced copy:
   A. five/500 to 550
   B. four/400 to 450
   C. three/300 to 350
   * D. two/200 to 250

7. The parliamentary authority for most organizations is:
   A. Their bylaws
   B. The society's parliamentarian
   C. The members
   * D. Robert's Rules of Order

## F. Learning Level: Evaluation

1. Answers will vary.

## PART 2 COMPETENCY CHALLENGE

Students are instructed to complete the following:

1. Prepare a paper in manuscript form, including a bibliography. Choose a disease and follow your instructor's directions.
2. Proofread another student's manuscript using appropriate proofreader's marks.
3. Retype the paper you wrote, which was proofread by a classmate.
4. Make arrangements for a class meeting as a group. Hold the meeting from a prepared agenda, and take notes of the meeting. As a class, each student should read the minutes they took and compare and critique the minutes.
5. Type the minutes from rough draft and sign your name as secretary.
6. Set up a diagnostic file, including subject cards and necessary information to accommodate the patient charts.
7. As instructed, complete the other Competency Objectives for Procedure 22-1 located at the end of the chapter.

## PART 3 CLINICAL APPLICATIONS

Students benefit greatly if they are taken to either the school library of public library and the librarian spends an hour with them discussing the following topics and orientating them to setting up a simple reference system.

Suggested applications include discussing the following topics.

1. How to set up a general reference file. If you have a special library in your classroom, students can participate in cataloging the books.
2. Describe ways in which a diagnostic file might be used by a physician.
3. The impact of electronic transmission and information retrieval on modern reference libraries.
4. How to use a reference library.

# 23

# Facility Environment

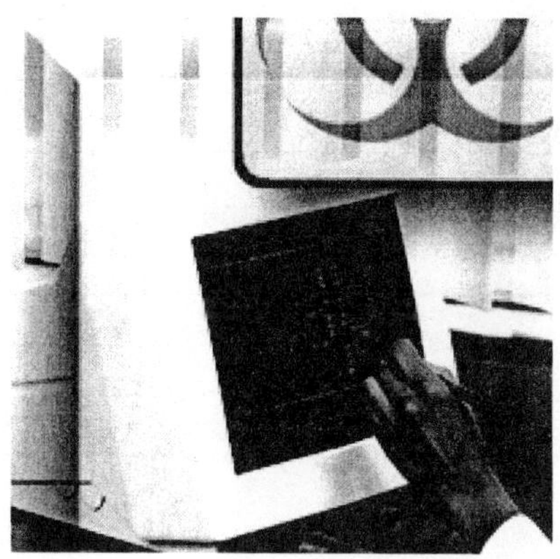

This chapter discusses the requirements to manage the physical plant, supplies, and office environment. It is therapeutic for patients to have a comfortable environment, one that is clean, safe, and has appropriate supplies and equipment to accomplish the tasks to keep the office functioning smoothly. Usually these responsibilities are those of the office manager, but the entire team helps in accomplishing the above goals. When the medical assistant is aware of the office requirements, he becomes a more effective team member because he performs some of these tasks.

## USING THE LEARNING SYSTEM

### 1. MEDICAL ASSISTANT CONTENT AND COMPETENCIES

CONTENT

- Risk management
- Respond to and initiate written communications
- Receive, organize, and prioritize information
- Fundamental writing skills
- Workplace dynamics
- Facility management

COMPETENCIES

- Perform all clerical functions
- Perform an inventory of supplies and equipment
- Perform routine maintenance of all equipment
- Identify community resources

## 2. MEDICAL ASSISTANT ENTRY-LEVEL CURRICULUM INTERFACE

| TEXTBOOK OBJECTIVES | LEARNING SYSTEM LOCATION | MA CURRICULUM |
|---|---|---|
| **Cognitive** | | **Content** |
| 1. Define and spell the terms listed in the Vocabulary | • Text p. 354<br>• Manual Part 1-B | • Fundamental writing skills |
| 2. List seven items of concern in controlling the general environment of the medical facility | • Text p. 354<br>• Manual Part 1-D | • Risk management<br>• Respond to and initiate written communications<br>• Receive, organize, and prioritize information<br>• Workplace dynamics<br>• Facility management |
| 3. Discuss the utilization of various areas of the medical facility | • Text pp. 354-356<br>• Manual Part 1-A | • Same as #2 above |
| 4. Describe how the medical assistant would arrange for and supervise a maintenance service | • Text pp. 356-357<br>• Manual Part 1-C | • Same as #2 above |
| 5. Explain the inventory process | • Text p. 360<br>• Manual Part 1-2<br>• Procedure 23-1 | • Fundamental writing skills |
| 6. Explain the importance of the instructions and warranties accompanying new equipment purchases | • Text p. 359 | • Fundamental writing skills<br>• Risk management<br>• Respond to and initiate written communications<br>• Receive, organize, and prioritize information<br>• Workplace dynamics<br>• Facility management |
| 7. Cite precautions to be observed in storing poisons, narcotics, acids and caustics, and flammable items | • Text p. 356<br>• Manual Part 1-C | • Same as #6 above |
| 8. Discuss the procedure for storing supplies and drug samples | • Text p. 360<br>• Transparency Master 23-3 | • Risk management<br>• Workplace dynamics<br>• Facility management |
| 9. List six possible safety hazards in a medical facility | • Text pp. 361-362<br>• Manual Part 1-D | • Risk management<br>• Workplace dynamics<br>• Facility management<br>• Receive, organize, and prioritize information |

## MEDICAL ASSISTANT ENTRY-LEVEL CURRICULUM INTERFACE *continued*

| TEXTBOOK OBJECTIVES | LEARNING SYSTEM LOCATION | MA CURRICULUM |
|---|---|---|
| **Cognitive** | | **Content** |
| 10. Discuss the importance of and procedures in routine office security | • Text p. 362 | • Fundamental writing skills<br>• Receive, organize, and prioritize information<br>• Risk management<br>• Workplace dynamics |
| **Performance** | | **Competencies** |
| 1. Write instructions for a maintenance service | • Manual Part 1-F | • Perform all clerical functions<br>• Fundamental writing skills |
| 2. Set up an equipment inventory | • Manual Part 2<br>• Procedure 23-1 | • Perform all clerical functions<br>• Perform an inventory of supplies and equipment<br>• Perform routine maintenance of all equipment<br>• Fundamental writing skills |
| 3. Organize and dispose of drug samples | • Manual Part 2 | • Perform an inventory of supplies and equipment<br>• Identify community resources |
| 4. Establish and maintain a supply inventory and ordering system | • Manual Part 2<br>• Procedure 23-1 | • Fundamental writing skills<br>• Perform all clerical functions<br>• Perform an inventory of supplies and equipment |

## 3. RESOURCES

a. Catalogs from medical suppliers and surgical suppliers. Call a local hospital and request old catalogs. Local medical representatives may come and demonstrate common equipment or specialized equipment.

b. Obtain warranties for medical assistant equipment in the lab and show to students

**4. LESSON PLAN Facility Environment** **TIME 3 hours lecture, 3 hours lab**

**Opening:** An interesting opening might be to have a manager who is involved in these activities come in and talk to students. Bring a card file and inventory to demonstrate.

**Pretest:** Have students describe the areas involved in facilities environment in a medical office and in the school building.

**Objectives:** Put on flip chart along with content and competencies and discuss a manager's functions and how the medical assistant assists in this area.

**Content:** Instructor is encouraged to add to the outline with notes for discussion to complete the lesson plan. Content discussion may be drawn from personal experience.

**Outline:**

PLANNING AND ORGANIZING FACILITIES

1. General environment includes:
   temperature lighting walls traffic and sound controls
   privacy efficiency
2. Area utilization and care.
3. Maintenance.
4. Furniture and equipment considerations include:
   acquisition warranties service inventory
5. Supply considerations
   selecting suppliers ordering preventing waste
   receiving and storing drug samples inventory
6. Physician bag
7. Safety and security.
   DEA smoke alarms and extinguishers fire exits
   security systems routine office precautions and security
8. Legal and ethical considerations

**Lab:** Because these are advanced skills, the activities have been simplified for the medical assistant student, not the manager student. The activities do meet the objectives and students have the opportunity to help establish or maintain inventory control in the medical assistant class, laboratory, and with office supplies. Rotating responsibility gives all students the opportunity for experience. Emphasize the legal responsibilities with drugs, safety, and OSHA regulations

**Assignment:** Students may inventory class, lab, and any other assigned areas.

**Posttest:** Take questions from Examaster testbank. Part of grade may be completion of class and lab inventory.

## 5. MASTERY MANUAL ANSWERS

### PART 1 CONTENT MASTERY

#### A. Learning Level: Knowledge

Answers: 1. F; 2. T; 3. F; 4. T; 5. F; 6. F; 7. T; 8. F; 9. T; 10. F

#### B. Learning Level: Comprehension

Answers: 1. d; 2. j; 3. g; 4. f; 5. h; 6. a; 7. i; 8. c; 9. e; 10. b

#### C. Learning Level: Application

1. List six steps in supervising the office maintenance service and prioritize from 1, low to 6, high:
   a. communicate with person in charge
   b. prepare written list of expectations
   c. review list with person in charge
   d. be specific about limitations and boundaries
   e. set up regular schedule
   f. evaluate regularly

2. Apply the precautions to be observed in the storage of:
   a. Drugs and solutions—cool dark locked cupboard
   b. Poisons—locked cupboard away from other supplies
   c. Narcotics—locked cupboard and inventory daily
   d. Acids and caustics—resistant lids, stored below and in cleaning area
   e. Inflammables—away from heat, usually in lab

#### D. Learning Level: Analysis

1. Describe six possible safety hazards in a medical facility:
   a. Unsafe chairs
   b. Exposed wires or electric cords
   c. Unsteady lamps
   d. Reachable sharps, hazardous liquids, any medications
   e. Spills, wet floors, slippery floors
   f. Poor lighting

2. List seven items of concern in controlling the general environment of a medical facility:
   a. temperature
   b. lighting
   c. walls and floor coverings
   d. traffic control
   e. sound control
   f. privacy
   g. efficiency

#### E. Learning Level: Synthesis

If you were to assign cleaning tasks according to working areas, what locations would you make those assignments to?

Reception, administration, clinical, lavatories and laboratories, storage and utility

## F. Learning Level: Evaluation

The maintenance crew has quit and there will be no outside service providing services for the next week. You are going to assign all the medical assistants to do essential cleaning. Write a list of the tasks and decide when and how often they must be done over the next five days.

Student answers will vary here . It is important to discuss all the possible solutions. The examination rooms and reception areas are the primary importance as they are patient areas

## PART 2 COMPETENCY CHALLENGE

1. Students may be directed to do the following: According to Procedure 23-1, establish an inventory of the equipment in your facility.
2. Establish and maintain a supply inventory and ordering system throughout the semester.
3. Obtain supply requisitions for your facility and complete them for missing supplies.

## PART 3 CLINICAL APPLICATIONS

As time allows, discuss the following situations, considering legal and ethical ramifications. Also consider the possible message being sent to patients when 1 , 2, and 3 are not followed.

1. The essentials of a comfortable, attractive, and clean environment, and how patients are influenced by surroundings.
2. Precautions to be observed in storing poisons, narcotics, acids and caustics, and flammable items.
3. Safety hazards and office security. Are there any safety hazards in the classroom?
4. The importance of preserving instructions and warranties that accompany new equipment purchases.

# 24

# Management Responsibilities

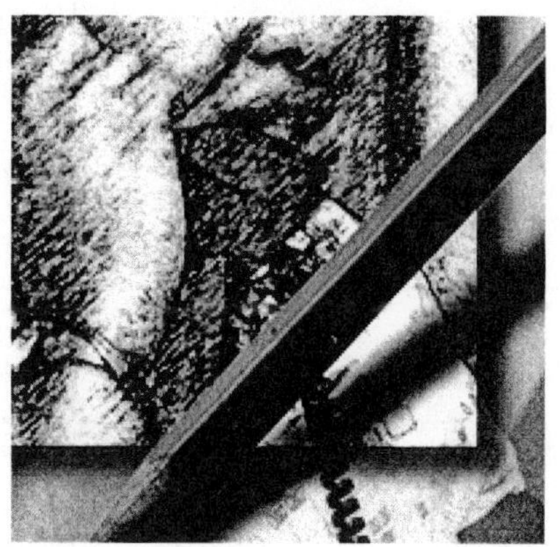

This chapter is for students who wish to become acquainted with management functions as a first step toward professional growth. There are many activities that may help the student prepare for employment. Students who are aware of the many facets of a well-run office are better able to evaluate an office position for which they are interviewing, such as the presence of job descriptions and regular evaluations. Advanced administrative procedures include orienting and training personnel, maintaining liability coverage, monitoring legislation related to health care and third party payers, maintaining licenses and accreditation, and performing advanced payroll and financial report functions.

## USING THE LEARNING SYSTEM

### 1. MEDICAL ASSISTANT CONTENT AND COMPETENCIES

CONTENT

- Respond to and initiate written communications
- Receive, organize, and prioritize information
- Identify community resources
- Fundamental writing skills
- Personal attributes
- Workplace dynamics
- Facility management

COMPETENCIES

- Perform within legal and ethical boundaries
- Identify and respond to issues of confidentiality
- Document appropriately
- Perform risk management procedures
- Identify community resources
- Perform accounts payable procedures
- Explain general office policies
- Instruct individuals according to their need
- Identify community resources

## 2. MEDICAL ASSISTANT ENTRY-LEVEL CURRICULUM INTERFACE

| TEXTBOOK OBJECTIVES | LEARNING SYSTEM LOCATION | MA CURRICULUM |
|---|---|---|
| Cognitive | | Content |
| 1. Define and spell the terms listed in the Vocabulary | • Text p. 364<br>• Manual Part 1-A | • Receive, organize, and prioritize information |
| 2. State the purpose and goals of medical office management | • Text p. 364<br>• Manual Part 1-B | • Receive, organize, and prioritize information |
| 3. Discuss the desirable qualities of an office manager and their importance in the selection of a supervisor | • Text p. 365<br>• Manual Part 1-C | • Respond to and initiate written communications<br>• Receive, organize, and prioritize information<br>• Identify community resources<br>• Fundamental writing skills<br>• Personal attributes<br>• Workplace dynamics<br>• Facility management |
| 4. Identify goals of an office policy manual and how they may be achieved | • Text p. 365<br>• Manual Part 1-B | • Facility management<br>• Respond to and initiate written communications<br>• Receive, organize, and prioritize information |
| 5. Explain the inventory process | • Text pp. 364-365<br>• Manual Part 1-B | • Same as #4 above |
| 6. Discuss the steps in the hiring and dismissal of employees | • Text pp. 368-372<br>• Manual Part 1-F | • Facility management<br>• Respond to and initiate written communications<br>• Receive, organize, and prioritize information<br>• Workplace dynamics |
| 7. List five kinds of staff meetings | • Text p. 379<br>• Manual Part 1-B | • Facility management |
| 8. Discuss the concept of practice development and its importance | • Text pp. 379-380<br>• Manual Part 1-F | • Facility management<br>• Receive, organize, and prioritize information |
| 9. List at least 10 features of a patient information folder | • Manual Part 3 | • Same as #8 above |
| 10. State two advantages of patient instruction sheets | • Text p. 380<br>• Manual Part 3 | • Same as #8 above |

**MEDICAL ASSISTANT ENTRY-LEVEL CURRICULUM INTERFACE *continued***

| TEXTBOOK OBJECTIVES | LEARNING SYSTEM LOCATION | MA CURRICULUM |
|---|---|---|
| **Cognitive** | | **Content** |
| 11. Discuss the supervisor's role in financial management | • Text p. 382<br>• Manual Part 1-D | • Facility management<br>• Workplace dynamics |
| 12. Identify the source of reference for information on employer taxes and deposit requirements | • Text p. 382<br>• Manual Part 1-F | • Facility management<br>• Identify community resources |
| **Performance** | | **Competencies** |
| 1. Interview an applicant for a position, utilizing the guidelines in this chapter | • Manual Part 2 | • Perform within legal and ethical boundaries<br>• Identify and respond to issues of confidentiality<br>• Document appropriately<br>• Perform risk management procedures<br>• Identify community resources<br>• Explain general office policies<br>• Instruct individuals according to their need<br>• Identify community resources |
| 2. Prepare an outline of contents for a basic office policy manual | • Manual Part 2 | • Same as # 1 above |
| 3. Write a procedure sheet for a specific task | • Manual Part 2 | • Same as # 1 above |
| 4. Outline a patient information folder | • Manual Part 2 | • Same as # 1 above |
| 5. Outline a financial policies folder | • Manual Part 2 | • Perform accounts payable procedures |
| 6. Write a patient instruction sheet | • Manual Part 3<br>• Procedure 11-2 | • Same as # 1 above |

## 3. RESOURCES

Sample tests

Lane, K: *medical assistant Examination Guide,* Philadelphia, FA Davis, Publisher.

Palko, Palko, : *Review for the medical assistant,* Norwalk, CT, Appleton, Lange Publishers, 1995

1-800-TAX-FORM for forms such as W-4, SS-4 and Federal Employers' Tax Guide, i.e., Circular E

## 4. LESSON PLAN

**TIME 3 hours lecture, 3 hours lab**

**Opening:** Ask students why you are covering this topic in a basic preparation program. Explain the value of this knowledge as discussed in the opening paragraph.

**Pretest:** Ask students the need for this information in a manager. Ask same question as part of posttest.

**Objectives:** Discuss objectives.

**Content:** There are many interesting concepts that will help prepare the student to look for an ideal rather than a haphazard office. Policy and procedure manuals, job descriptions, leadership qualities, and use of patient information sheets make the job of the medical assistant easier to carry out. Students need this information to make informed choices about a potential work environments.

1. PURPOSE OF MANAGEMENT: Who's in Charge, Avoiding Management Problems
2. QUALITIES OF A SUPERVISOR
3. MANAGEMENT DUTIES
   a. Personnel Management
      Office Policy Manual: Preparation; Expectations; Using the Policy Manual: Development
      Office Procedures Manual; Job Description; Procedure Sheets Benefits and Recruitment.
         Preliminary Steps
         Arranging the Personal Interview
         The Interview
         Follow-Up Activities
         Checking References
         Hiring
      Orientation and Training
      Performance and Salary Review
      Dismissal
4. BUSINESS MANAGEMENT: See Mastery Manual Activity Part 1-F
   Staff Meetings
   Practice Development
   Patient Education
   Patient Information Folder
   Financial Policy Folder
   Patient Instruction Sheets
5. FINANCIAL MANAGEMENT: See Mastery Manual Activity Part 1-F
   Payroll Records
   Payroll Reporting Forms
   Income Tax Withholding
   Employer's Income Tax
   Social Security, Medicare, and Income Tax Withholding
   Quarterly Returns
   Annual Returns
   How to Deposit
   Federal Unemployment Tax Deposits
   Annual Return
   State Unemployment Taxes
   State Disability Insurance

6. SPECIAL DUTIES
   a. Moving a Practice and Planning the New Quarters
      Establishing a Moving Date and Notifying Utilities and Mailers
      Packing and Moving Day Strategy
      Follow-Up
   b. Closing a Practice
      Advance Notice to Patients and Avoiding Abandonment Charge
      Public Announcement and Other Notices
      Patient Transfer and Patient Records
      Financial Concerns
      Disposition of Controlled Substances
      Professional Liability Insurance
      Furnishings and Equipment

Legal/Ethical Issues—Probationary Employee and Long-term Employee

**Lab activities:** The manual meets the objectives but uses a bit of a different format to cover the objectives in a simple style. Part 3 activities are not related to procedures, but could be done in small groups and then present to the class in a short lab. Use lab time to complete all Mastery Manual activities. Advanced classes for CEUs will need longer times and increased depth of management functions. See the end of the chapter for advanced activity ideas.

**Assignment:** Students will complete this chapter and probably the course unless they continue with clinical, in which case they begin on Chapter 25, reading learning terms and picking the most important concept.

**Posttest:** Complete administrative test from the Examaster testbank or sample tests from FA Davis, *medical assistant Examination Guide* by Karen Lane, or Appleton, Lange *Review for the medical assistant*, by Palko and Palko.

## 5. MASTERY MANUAL ANSWERS

## PART 1 CONTENT MASTERY

### A. Learning Level: Knowledge

Answers: 1. d; 2. f; 3. a; 4. g; 5. c; 6. i; 7. b; 8. j; 9. e; 10. h

Answers: 11. D; 12. C; 13. A; 14. A

### B. Learning Level: Comprehension

Answers: 1. F; 2. F; 3. F; 4. T; 5. T; 6. F; 7. F; 8. F

Complete the following statements:

9. The policy manual is an office manager's best friend when it
   a. Gives information to new employees
   b. Is a ready and complete reference for temporary employees
   c. Contains policies for all employees
   d. Serves as back-up for disagreements and conflict
10. A policy manual tells *what to do* and the procedure manual tells *how to do it.*

## C. Learning Level: Application

1. The qualities a supervisor will need are:
   a. Leadership ability
   b. Good judgment
   c. Good health
   d. Ability to organize
   e. Ability to learn and improve
   f. Original ideas
   g. A sense of fairness
   h. Strength to stand firm on policy, but enough flexibility to recognize when an exception should be made
2. List at least 10 items included in patient information folders.

   Practice name, location, telephone, philosophy, policies regarding appointments, cancellations, telephone calls, any extra or ancillary services, office hours, emergency procedures, financial policy folder, andnames of personnel.
3. Why would a practice give out patient information folders to patients? Because it reduces confusion and informational calls by 20–30%. Would you mail these to new patients? Why or why not? Hand it to patients and if possible review it with them.

## D. Learning Level: Analysis

Differentiate practice management business responsibilities from financial responsibilities and give examples.

**Business: includes all the running of the office not associated with money**

- Prepare and update policy and procedure manuals and job descriptions
- Recruitment
- Orientation and training
- Performance and salary review
- Dismissal
- Plan staff meetings
- Maintain staff harmony
- Establish work flow guidelines
- Improve office efficiency
- Supervise purchase and care of equipment
- Patient education
- Eliminate time-wasting tasks for the physician
- Practice marketing
- Making provisions for:

  Practice insurance
  Workers' compensation
  Disability insurance
  Professional liability
  Employee's health benefits
  Unemployment insurance

**Financial Management**

- Supervise cash transactions
- Maintain payroll records
- Manage employee benefits
- Advanced responsibilities
- Supervising cash receipts
- Banking, billing, and collections
- Preparing periodic profit and loss statements
- Computing collection ratios

- Writing payroll checks
- Paying bills
- Preparing reports for government agencies
- Serving as liaison with the accountant

## E. Learning Level: Synthesis

1. Now that you have read and worked with the information, would you like to be an office manager? Explain why or why not related to your personality and the job requirements.

   Student answers vary

2. You are in charge of payroll and filing the necessary reports and deposits. Where do you go to obtain the requirements?

   IRS circular E, also known as Federal Employers Tax Guide

3. How do you make the deposits?

   With a deposit form at your local bank

## F. Learning Level: Evaluation

You are going to interview three candidates for a medical assistant administrative position. The person will be scheduling appointments and greeting patients when they arrive. The medical assistant will be training with the present appointment person with the intent that the office is getting very busy, and in a month or two, two persons will be needed in the position. What are the five most important things for you to do during the interview so that you can get the best person for the job?

1. Ask all persons the same questions
2. Ask all persons what they think the job entails
3. Ask all why they want to work in your office
4. Ask them what their goals are and what types of projects they like to be involved in
5. Give them a situation to decide how to handle

## PART 2 COMPETENCY CHALLENGE

Students should complete the following activities.

1. Use the form at the back of Mastery Manual Chapter 24, interview someone for a position, and fill out the applicant rating form
2. Prepare an outline of the contents for a basic office policy manual
3. Write a procedure sheet for a specific task
4. Outline the contents of a financial policy folder

## PART 3 CLINICAL APPLICATIONS

1. Give two advantages of patient instruction sheets. Write a patient instruction sheet for the patients to obtain insurance referral to a specialist or a topic assigned by your instructor. You will need to give these instructions with a sheet when you are in practice. Use Procedure 11-2 at the end of Chapter 11 as a guide.
2. If a person applies for a job and her credit and personal references are not satisfactory, what are you obliged to tell her in your state?

**Advanced activity ideas**

1. Compute payroll for five persons on different salaries and for differing number of hours in the work period. Calculate deductions from W-4 information. Compute the federal and state payroll taxes due.
2. Collect samples of policy manuals from offices and have students develop one manual for the lab.
3. Have a guest speaker to discuss personnel and work laws.

4. Have students write a critique of their positive points relating to management qualities. Then define their weaknesses and prescribe strategies for overcoming them.
5. Have students make a schedule for one week, including home and school activities. Prioritize them. Return in one week with tasks accomplished and reasons for not finishing other tasks.
6. Go to the library and find a book or magazine on time management. List the most important ideas you found in the book. Write the bibliography for the book using correct format as recommended by the reference librarian.

# 25

# Patient Assessment

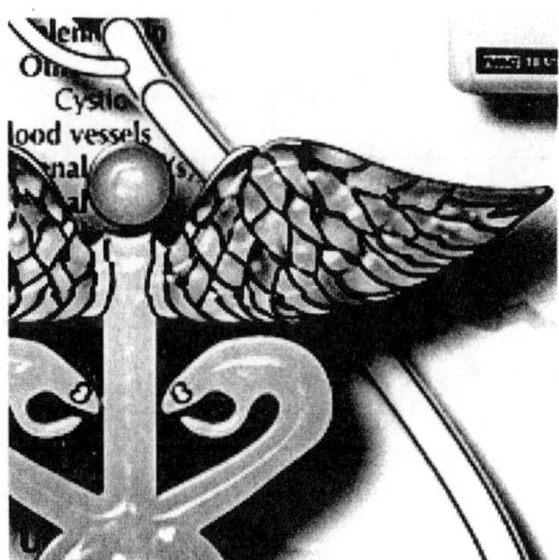

The clinical experience for the medical assistant student begins with this chapter. The material includes information on interview techniques, including collection of medical histories, and documenting on the medical record. The medical assistant must understand interviewing techniques in order to interview patients appropriately. Interviewing skills are used to establish baseline observable assessments for the physician. These assessments are recorded in the patient history and progress notes. The interview often provides an opportunity to reinforce physician teachings regarding health promotion and disease prevention. It takes a good deal of practice to develop the skills to interview and record accurately, with empathy, and in a confidential comfortable environment. There is opportunity for practice in obtaining histories and developing a short teaching plan in Parts 2 and 3.

## USING THE LEARNING SYSTEM

### 1. MEDICAL ASSISTING CONTENT AND COMPETENCIES

CONTENT

- Application of medical terminology
- Legal guidelines and requirements for medical care
- Medical ethics and related issues
- Developmental stages of the life cycle
- Recognize and respond to verbal and nonverbal communications
- Basic medical office functions

COMPETENCIES

- Organize medical record
- Document appropriately
- Obtain and record patient history
- Respond to and initiate written communications
- Recognize and respond to verbal communications
- Explain general office policies
- Instruct individuals according to their needs
- Document appropriately

Each of the above items is important for medical assistant students to understand as they prepare to enter the externship portion of the program. As instructors, it is important to mention the competencies related to each skill. For instance, the medical assistant adheres to ethical standards by providing patients privacy and not discussing patient problems with others.

## 2. MEDICAL ASSISTING ENTRY-LEVEL CURRICULUM INTERFACE

| TEXTBOOK OBJECTIVES | LEARNING SYSTEM LOCATION | MA CURRICULUM |
|---|---|---|
| Cognitive | | Content |
| 1. Define and spell the terms listed in the Vocabulary | • Text p. 398<br>• Manual Part 1-A | • Application of medical terminology |
| 2. State the purpose of the medical history and how personal anxieties can affect the process | • Text p. 399<br>• Manual Part 1-B | • Legal guidelines and requirements for medical care<br>• Medical ethics and related issues<br>• Developmental stages of the life cycle<br>• Recognize and respond to verbal and nonverbal communications<br>• Basic medical office functions |
| 3. List the three types of body language that can indicate your interest in the patient | • Text p. 400<br>• Manual Part 1-C | • Recognize and respond to verbal and nonverbal communications |
| 4. List the components of the medical history and explain the importance of each one | • Text pp. 399–400<br>• Manual Part 1-A | • Application of medical terminology<br>• Legal guidelines and requirements for medical care<br>• Basic medical office functions<br>• Medical ethics and related issues<br>• Developmental stages of the life cycle |
| 5. Identify and explain the internal factors of communicating | • Text p. 400<br>• Manual Part 1-C | • Recognize and respond to verbal and nonverbal communications |
| 6. List and give an example of the external factors of communicating | • Text p. 401<br>• Manual Part 1-D | • Recognize and respond to verbal and nonverbal communications |
| 7. State when you should use open-ended questions | • Text p. 401<br>• Manual Part 1-D | • Recognize and respond to verbal and nonverbal communications<br>• Legal guidelines and requirements for medical care<br>• Medical ethics and related issues |
| 8. Describe the purpose and usage of direct questions | • Text p. 402<br>• Manual Part 1-D | • Recognize and respond to verbal and nonverbal communications |

| TEXTBOOK OBJECTIVES | LEARNING SYSTEM LOCATION | MA CURRICULUM |
|---|---|---|
| **Cognitive** | | **Content** |
| 9. State the meaning of interviewing restraints | • Text p. 403<br>• Manual Part 1-F | • Recognize and respond to verbal and nonverbal communications<br>• Legal guidelines and requirements for medical care<br>• Medical ethics and related issues |
| 10. Describe the medical assistant's role during the system review | • Manual Part 1-F | • All MA Content requirements listed above |
| 11. Differentiate between a sign and a symptom | • Text pp. 406–407<br>• Manual Part 1-D | • Application of medical terminology<br>• Basic medical office functions |
| 12. List the three medical record systems used in physician's offices | • Text pp. 408–409<br>• Lab | • Legal guidelines and requirements for medical care<br>• Basic medical office functions |
| **Performance** | | **Competencies** |
| 1. Distinguish between verbal and nonverbal communication | • Text p. 400<br>• Manual Part 1-B | • Respond to and initiate written communications<br>• Recognize and respond to verbal communications<br>• Explain general office policies |
| 2. Provide examples of interviewing restraints | • Text p. 403<br>• Manual Parts 2 and 3<br>• ⊕ CD-ROM | • Respond to and initiate written communications<br>• Recognize and respond to verbal communications |
| 3. Discuss the terminology used in the assessment process | • Text p. 406<br>• Manual Part 2 | • Application of medical terminology<br>• Organize medical record<br>• Document appropriately<br>• Obtain and record patient history |
| 4. State your legal responsibilities in handling the patient's medical record | • Manual Part 3<br>• ⊕ CD-ROM | • Organize medical record<br>• Document appropriately<br>• Obtain and record patient history<br>• Respond to and initiate written communications<br>• Recognize and respond to verbal communications<br>• Explain general office policies<br>• Instruct individuals according to their needs<br>• Document appropriately |

## 3. RESOURCES

http://search.yahoo.com/bin/search?p=interview+techniques

http://www.yahoo.com/Social_Science/Communications/ **A general site with many links to specific communication topics**

Books and publications on communication techniques: See resource list in Chapter 7.

## 4. LESSON PLAN Patient Assessment TIME 3 hours lecture, 12 hours lab

Students need to read, review, and grasp the six main concepts discussed in the 8th Edition Textbook items A-H in the lesson plan before you attempt a review of the materials. This chapter begins the study of clinical information, and it is presented with understanding and simplicity.

**Opening:** Role-model a short taking of patient history. Obtain the volunteer beforehand. When finished, ask students to critique. The critique becomes the pretest to see if they have completed the assignment of reading and studying the chapter.

**Pretest:** Ask students to discuss and evaluate your collecting of the history, interviewing strategies and skills, and your use of interviewing restraints and assessment questions.

**Objectives:** Review the textbook objectives and apply them to MA content requirements above. Write two performance objectives adapted from the procedures in Parts 2 and 3.
Suggested:
1. Complete two patient medical histories.

2. Teach a classmate to complete a medical history.

**Content:**

A. THE MEDICAL HISTORY
   Collecting the History Information
   Components of the Medical History
   Database
   Past History
   Family History
   Social History
   Systems Review

B. INTERVIEWING STRATEGIES
   The Process of Communication
   Internal Factors
   Empathy
   Observation
   Ensure Privacy
   Comfortable Surroundings
   Liking Others
   The Ability to Listen
   External Factors
   Refuse Interruptions
   Note-Taking

C. INTERVIEWING THE PATIENT
- Introductions
- Open-Ended Questions
- Direct Questions

D. INTERVIEWING RESTRAINTS
- Providing Assurance
- Giving Advice
- Using Professional Terms
- Leading Questions
- Talking Too Much

E. ASSESSING THE PATIENT
- Signs and Symptoms
- Subjective Findings
- Objective Findings

F. CHARTING
- Terminology
- Methods
- Problem-Oriented Medical Record (POMR)
- Source-Oriented Medical Record (SOMR)
- Computerized Medical Record (CMR)

G. LEGAL AND ETHICAL RESPONSIBILITIES

**Lab activities:** Discuss with students specific aspects of the chapter, such as when to use and when to avoid medical terminology. Have students make a 3x5 card with notes on correct charting. Differentiate the three major methods of charting. List advantages and disadvantages of different types of charting for MA, physician, or other caregivers. Demonstrate history taking to students using the form in Appendix B.

**Assignment:** After first discussion and history-taking demonstration, have student take a history on a family member. Students should have mastered this chapter and be ready to move to the next one, which is Aseptic Concepts and Infection Control. Students will read, outline, and make terminology cards for Chapter 26. Have students use medical terminology and begin to break words into component parts. This helps them understand the terminology in an easier format.

**Posttest:** Repeat earlier pretest and have students complete written critique or use testbank.

## 5. MASTERY MANUAL ANSWERS

### PART 1 CONTENT MASTERY

### A. Learning Level: Knowledge

1. Define and spell the following terms. Study them first and define in simple, accurate words.
   a. **biophysical**—pertaining to the science dealing with the application of physical methods and theories; technological problems
   b. **cognitive**—pertaining to the operation of the mind process by which we become aware of perceiving, thinking, and remembering.
   c. **diagnosis**—a concise technical description of the cause, nature, or manifestations of a condition or problem.
   d. **familial**—occurring in or affecting members of a family more than would be expected by chance.
   e. **hereditary**—transmitted from parent to offspring; genetically determined.
   f. **psychosocial**—pertaining to or involving psychic (behavior) and communal activity.
   g. **rapport**—a relationship of harmony and accord between patient and physician.

2. From the communication technique state the value or benefit given.

| **Technique** | **Value—from Table 25-2, text p. 402** |
|---|---|
| a. Open-ended Question | Encourages patients to respond in manner comfortable to them. |
| b. Direct Questions | Ask for specific information. Usually reply is a yes or no answer. |
| c. Listening | Nonverbally communicates your interest in the patient. |
| d. Silence | Nonverbally communicates your acceptance of the patient. |
| e. Establish Guidelines | Helps the patient to know what is expected of him/her. |
| f. Acknowledgment | Shows the importance of the patient's role. |
| g. Restating | Checks your interpretation of the message for validation. |
| h. Reflecting | Shows the patient the importance of his/her feelings. |
| i. Summarizing | Helps patient to separate relevant from irrelevant material. |

### B. Learning Level: Comprehension

1. Explain the purpose of the medical history.
   To provide consistent medical care, and for the evaluation, diagnosis, and treatment of patient status.
2. How would a patient's anxieties affect your taking of the medical history? List three effects and explain what you do to decrease each anxiety.
   Patient's anxieties will make the history less accurate.
   a. will be forgetful and not remember—can mail history to home
   b. may not speak freely—provide very private area, i.e., examination room
   c. may not be attentive—medical assistant needs to sit and give full attention to patient and refocus
3. Give an example of nonverbal communication observation regarding each area listed below.

| **Area** | **Hearing** | **Visual Observation** |
|---|---|---|
| Breathing | Prolonging respirations<br>Sighing | Shallow fast respirations<br>Thoracic breathing |
| Arm and leg placement | Short impersonal response<br>Tapping feet | Arms folded across chest<br>Continuous movement |
| Eye movement | N/A | Looking side to side<br>Looking down<br>Avoiding eye contact |

## C. Learning Level: Application

1. Choose three types of body language personally known to you that would indicate your interest in the patient and what the patient is saying.
   a. smiling face, bending toward patient to listen
   b. sit facing with arms on lap, do not engage in other activities
   c. asking questions and waiting for answers, clarifying questions
   d. Others?

2. What specific communication technique do the above answers in C-1 communicate to the patient?
   Listening

3. What other factors would you choose to develop to be an effective listener for your patients and friends?
   a. relax
   b. be patient and nonjudgmental
   c. do not interupt
   d. do not intimidate

## D. Learning Level: Analysis

In the following brief examples, state whether one should use open-ended or direct questions. Place a 1 if open-ended is the best type of question to use and a 2 if a direct question is appropriate. Then write a question for the type chosen. The questions are subjective and must be evaluated by instructor.

1. Mrs. Woods states she has terrible pain in her abdomen. 1
2. You need to know the patient's cardiac history. 2
3. You have to ask the adolescent about sexual practices. 2
4. You want to know about the patient's nutritional status 1

## E. Learning Level: Synthesis

You have learned about signs and symptoms in previous chapters. Define each term and make a list of at least ten signs and symptoms that a patient may discuss with you.

1. A sign is observable; may be measured or is seen or heard; an objective finding. Signs include diagnostic test results, skin lesions, heart murmurs, blood pressure, temperature, respirations, pulse, anything that can be percussed, auscultated, or elicit sounds (tamponade).
2. A symptom is subjective and may be perceived only by the person. Feelings, some smells, vision difficulties, pain, ringing in the ears, headache, numbness, tingling are symptoms.
3. Ten examples of each: See items 1 and 2 above with definitions.

## F. Learning Level: Evaluation

1. What does the acronym RATATQ mean?
   restraining, assurance, advice, terminology, talking and questions

2. After reading and learning the chapter materials, what do you conclude to be the medical assistant's role in systems review? Name five in order of priority.
   a. Put the patient at ease as much as possible
   b. Obtain a beginning accurate history
   c. Obtain patient's vital signs
   d. Document in patient chart
   e. Teach the patient

## PART 2 COMPETENCY CHALLENGE

Demonstrate history taking on a volunteer student. This role models professional communication and skills. Students may then proceed to complete Part 2 activities in their Mastery Manual. It is important to review their self-evaluation of their history-taking skills located in items C and D below. There is also a medical history form at the end of the chapter in the Mastery Manual.

A. Use Procedure 25-1, Obtaining a Medical History, at the very end of the chapter and the Patient History form in Appendix C ▲. You may use the CD-ROM ⊕ for Cases 1–4 and obtain a history on these patients and answer the interactive questions.

B. If you use the activities in this part, follow the procedure and obtain two medical histories, first on a family member, then on a classmate. There is also a medical history form at the end of the chapter before the procedure. When you are finished, ask the family member if you asked any questions that made him or her anxious or did anything to cause discomfort. As the classmate being interviewed for the medical history, try to be difficult in the interview. Identify the interviewing restraints that you avoided using with the difficult interview.

C. I restrained myself from the following—check applicable.

Unwarranted assurance ________

Professional terms ________

Leading questions ________

Talking too much ________

Giving advice ________

D. Complete a short self-evaluation of your performance.

1. What area was easiest for you to complete?
2. What area caused you the most difficulty?
3. Why do you think it was a problem?
4. What steps can you take to decrease the problem?
5. Is the form easy to use?
6. What changes would you make to the form?

## PART 3 CLINICAL APPLICATIONS

A. Practice teaching a classmate how to take a history. This will help you become proficient in history taking before you proceed to the externship experience. Use the short Practice Activity Guideline, Developing a Teaching Plan, at the end of the chapter. This plan may also be used for patient teaching. Fill in the teaching plan and then teach a classmate to take a history. Turn the plan in to your instructor.

B. State two medical assistant responsibilities in handling the patient's medical record.

C. Discuss interviewing restraints. How easy is it to give a patient advice or unwarranted assurance? What responses can you make to patients who need assurance or advice?

# 26

# Aseptic Concepts and Infection Control

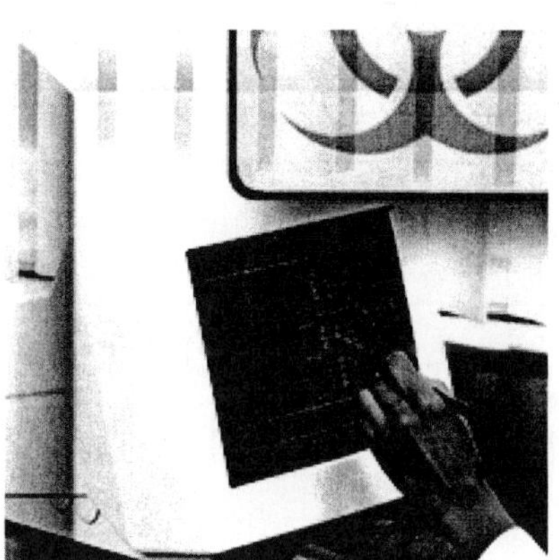

The concept that the greatest danger to a sick person is the introduction of microorganisms that will further weaken resistance to disease is extremely important for students to understand. The second concept, that something is either sterile or it is not, is also essential. This chapter conveys knowledge on how to prevent introducing or spreading disease-causing microorganisms. Students will then have the opportunity to practice four procedures to develop competency in applying principles of aseptic technique. Students will differentiate medical and surgical principles and practices. Preparing students to use this information correctly in the medical office is the first and most important protection we can offer students and the patient. Aseptic technique and medical asepsis is the patients' and students' most valuable protector. Students need to develop a conscious and positive attitude about the practices in this chapter. The lesson plan contains an extensive outline of the textbook materials.

## USING THE LEARNING SYSTEM

### 1. MEDICAL ASSISTING CONTENT AND COMPETENCIES

CONTENT

- Asepsis and infection control
- Patient care
- Job readiness
- Hereditary, cultural, and environmental influences on behavior
- Legal guidelines/requirements for health care
- Risk management

COMPETENCIES

- Fundamental principles
- Perform handwashing
- Wrap items for autoclaving
- Perform sterilization techniques
- Dispose of biohazard materials
- Practice standard precautions

## 2. MEDICAL ASSISTING ENTRY-LEVEL CURRICULUM INTERFACE

| TEXTBOOK OBJECTIVES | LEARNING SYSTEM LOCATION | MA CURRICULUM |
|---|---|---|
| **Cognitive** | | **Content** |
| 1. Define and spell all terms in the Vocabulary | • Text p. 413<br>• Manual Part 1-A | • Applications of medical terminology |
| 2. Explain the five links in the chain of infection | • Text pp. 415–417<br>• Manual Part 1-B | • Asepsis and infection control<br>• Job readiness<br>• Hereditary, cultural, and environmental influences on behavior<br>• Risk management |
| 3. Identify the specific reactions the body initiates as the inflammatory response | • Text pp. 417–418<br>• Manual Part 1-CA | • Asepsis and infection control<br>• Hereditary, cultural, and environmental influences on behavior |
| 4. Differentiate among the four types of infections | • Text p. 418<br>• Manual Part 1-D | • Asepsis and infection control |
| 5. Compare virus and bacteria cell invasion | • Text pp. 418–419<br>• Manual Part 1-D | • Asepsis and infection control |
| 6. List the infectious materials covered in the Standard Precautions | • Text p. 419<br>• Manual Part 1-E | • Asepsis and infection control<br>• Legal guidelines/requirements for health care |
| 7. Identify the four major areas included in the OSHA Compliance Guidelines | • Text pp. 420–424<br>• Manual Part 1-B | • Asepsis and infection control<br>• Job readiness<br>• Legal guidelines/requirements for health care<br>• Risk management |
| 8. Differentiate medical and surgical asepsis | • Text p. 424 | • Asepsis and infection control<br>• Risk management |
| 9. Differentiate between sanitization, disinfection, and sterilization | • Text pp. 425–430<br>• Manual Part 1-A | • Asepsis and infection control<br>• Risk management |
| 10. Explain the types and uses of indicators | • Text pp. 431–432<br>• Manual Part 1-E | • Asepsis and infection control<br>• Risk management |
| 11. Discuss legal and ethical concerns for medical asepsis and infection control | • Text p. 438<br>• Manual Part 3 | • Asepsis and infection control<br>• Legal guidelines/requirements for health care<br>• Job readiness<br>• Hereditary, cultural, and environmental influences on behavior<br>• Risk management |

| TEXTBOOK OBJECTIVES | LEARNING SYSTEM LOCATION | MA CURRICULUM |
|---|---|---|
| **Cognitive** | | **Content** |
| 12. List possible methods of patient education | • Text p. 438<br>• Manual Part 3 | • Job readiness<br>• Hereditary, cultural, and environmental influences on behavior<br>• Risk management |
| **Performance** | | **Competencies** |
| 1. Demonstrate proper handwashing technique for medical asepsis | • Manual Part 2<br>• Procedure 26-1, p. 426 | • Fundamental principles<br>• Perform handwashing<br>• Practice standard precautions |
| 2. Clean and wrap instruments and equipment for autoclaving | • Manual Part 2<br>• Procedures 26-2 and 26-3, pp. 428 and 432 | • Wrap items for autoclaving<br>• Dispose of biohazard materials<br>• Practice standard precautions |
| 3. Load and run autoclave with accuracy | • Manual Part 2<br>• Procedure 26-4, p. 437 | • Perform sterilization techniques |

## 3. RESOURCES

http://www.yahoo.com/Health/Medicine/Infectious_Diseases/ **Infectious disease information**

http://www.yahoo.com/Health/Medicine/Immunology/ **Information on vaccines and research**

http://wwwindex.nlm.nih.gov/pubs/factsheets/dirlinfs.html **Site to direct health and bioscientific information**

http://wwwindex.nlm.nih.gov/index/medindex.html **Consumer health information resources**

Saunders CLINICAL SKILLS FOR THE MEDICAL ASSISTANT, 1995, W.B. Saunders Co. ISBN 0-7216-9750-X—for entire set

3M Films and Tapes Medical Products Division/3M, 3M Center, St. Paul, MN 55144:

*Introduction to Sterilization Monitoring*

*Chemical Monitoring*

*Biological Monitoring*

## 4. LESSON PLAN Asepsis and Infection Control TIME 3 hours lecture, 12 hours lab

**Opening:** Begin with a personal situation, such as a simple procedure where the physician does not wash hands or where there is an examination and the physician does not wash hands—you know the previous patient had hepatitis. How do you, as patient, feel? Is this ethical behavior? Another interesting opening is to have a sterile field with some equipment on it. Although not used until much later in the teaching cycle, this gets the students' attention. Next to this have the equipment used for protective barriers. Do not immediately tell students that one represents surgical asepsis and the other medical.

**Pretest:** Discuss or have students write something on the ethics of medical asepsis and "shortcuts." While this is not a pretest, one does get an idea of student values. Ask students if they can differentiate the use of this equipment. This is a good lead-in to determining if some people read the chapter. Others may even be able to synthesize the information and answer the question. In either case, this will lead to a discussion of the objectives.

**Objectives:** Review objectives and compare to MA curriculum requirements.

**Content:**
A complete chapter outline is included to help present this material. Use the 3-hour lecture time to review the entire outline. The lab time includes demonstration, practice, and check-off for competency of all four procedures.

**INFECTIOUS DISEASES**
- The Chain of Infection
- The Inflammatory Response

TYPES OF INFECTION
- Acute Infection
- Chronic Infection
- Latent Infection
- Slow Infection

TYPES OF ORGANISMS
- Viruses
- Bacteria
- Spirochetes
- Fungus

PREVENTION OF DISEASE TRANSMISSION
- Staying Healthy with Lifestyle Choices

OSHA BLOODBORNE PATHOGEN STANDARDS
- Compliance Guidelines
- Barrier Protection
- Environment Protection
- Housekeeping Controls
- Exposure Control Plan

**ASEPSIS—Medical and Surgical**
- Handwashing
- Sanitization and Ultrasonics
- Disinfection
  - Alcohol
  - Alkalies
  - Disinfection by Boiling

Sterilization
- Moist Heat Sterilization
- Wrapping Materials
- Wrapping Instruments
- Indicators
  - Autoclave Tape
  - Sterilization Indicator Strips
  - Culture Tube Test
- Sterilization Indicator Bags
- The Steam Autoclave
- Loading the Autoclave
- Unloading the Autoclave
  - Storage of Wrapped Supplies

Gas Sterilization
- Sterilization of Containers
- Jars, Bottles, and Trays

THE MEDICAL ASSISTANT'S ROLE IN ASEPSIS
LEGAL AND ETHICAL RESPONSIBILITIES
PATIENT EDUCATION

**Assignment:** Have students study 8th Edition Textbook and complete Part 1 in the Mastery Manual in preparation for posttest and lab lesson.

**Posttest:** Students need a posttest and must pass before proceeding to lab, where the procedures and discussions will be held. Take questions from Examaster testbank. Make them specific to textbook objectives and MA content requirements.

## 5. MASTERY MANUAL ANSWERS

### PART 1 CONTENT MASTERY

### A. Learning Level: Knowledge

1. v; 2. u; 3. t; 4. s; 5. p; 6. r; 7. q; 8. o; 9. n; 10. m; 11. l; 12. k; 13. j; 14. i; 15. h; 16. g; 17. f; 18. e; 19. d; 20. c; 21. b; 22. a

### B. Learning Level: Comprehension

1. Explain the five links in the chain of infection and give an example of each.

   This chart may be copied and enlarged for a Transparency Master.

| Link | Example |
|---|---|
| 1. Reservoir host | Insect, animal, human |
| 2. Means of exit | All body orifices |
| 3. Means of transmission | Direct—discharge<br>Indirect—droplets, vectors, fomites |
| 4. Means of entry | All body orifices and broken skin |
| 5. Susceptible host | Virulence, location, health of individual, dose |

2. State the purpose of standard precautions.

   To reduce the risk of cross-infection of any person from any infective agent; this includes the patient and the caregiver.

3. Recall as many infectious materials included in standard precautions as possible.

   All body fluids from external openings of body, fluids from serous and mucous membranes, all body cavity fluids, amniotic fluids, any blood-contaminated fluid, blood, unknown body fluids, human tissues, cells, or exudates

*Sterilization Record Keeping*

4. What four major areas are included in the OSHA guidelines?
   a. barrier protection
   b. environment protection
   c. housekeeping controls
   d. exposure controls plan

## C. Learning Level: Application

1. Sketch the inflammatory response described in your 8th Edition Textbook and label each stage.

2. Describe what you have sketched if you have not labeled the sketch. Try to keep it simple. The description should read:
   1. Wound, blood vessels dilate; 2. white cells increase and cause redness; 3. phagocytosis; 4. fluids increase to area causing edema; 5. pressure from edema on nerves causes pain; 6. increased blood supply causes heat; if not treated, there will be 7. supporation; 8. swollen glands; and finally, 9. septicemia

3. Name the methods, means, and advantages of the two types of sterilization.

| Types | Methods | Means | Advantages |
|---|---|---|---|
| Dry heat | Gas under pressure | Gas autoclave | Can sterilize glass, rubber, tubes |
| Moist heat | Steam under pressure | Steam autoclave | Kills all pathogens and spores, small office size |

## D. Learning Level: Analysis

1. Describe characteristics of bacterium and virus in the following areas.

| Characteristics | Bacterium | Virus |
|---|---|---|
| Enter body | Open wounds, orifices | Open wounds, orifices |
| Secrete or produce | Toxins | Interferon |
| Resistant forms | Spores, drugs | HIV antibiotics |
| Treatment | Antibiotics | Interferon, antivirals |

2. Name the type of infection described.
   A. This infection is sometimes called "mad cow disease" and caused the ban on exporting cows from another country to the U.S. **Slow infection**
   B. The infection is present but the symptoms come and go. **Latent**
   C. Has a rapid onset, severe symptoms, and quick resolution. **Acute**
   D. Can be detected and transmitted, but no sign in the host. **Chronic**

## E. Learning Level: Synthesis

1. Of all the breaks in medical asepsis, which do you think is the most common and why?
   The most common break is in handwashing, and it is because people do not train themselves to wash before and after all patient contact.

2. Of all the common breaks in disinfection and sanitization of instruments, which do you think is the most common and why?

   The most common error is the failure to remove all organisms with mechanical scrubbing. Usually not enough time is spent on surfaces and in cracks and grooves.

3. Indicate the cleaning process you would choose for each item listed below.

| | Sanitation | Disinfection | Chemical Sterilization | Steam Sterilization |
|---|---|---|---|---|
| Suture removal instruments | | | | X |
| Vaginal speculum | | X | | |
| Surgical scissors | | | | X |
| Mercury thermometer | | X | | |
| Cystoscope that cannot be autoclaved | | | X | |

## F. Learning Level: Evaluation

1. Write a daily and weekly housekeeping plan for a medical office that will conform to OSHA guidelines.

   Plan must include:

   a. Decontaminate surfaces after spills, procedures, first thing in A.M. and at close of day.
   b. Cleaning reusable containers with bleach weekly.
   c. Empty lined containers daily.
   d. Check sharps containers daily and dispose of when 3/4 full.
   e. Provide double bags for all linens. Remove from examining area in single bag and place into double bag daily.
   f. All dressings and potentially infected waste must go into biohazard bag. Remove bags and replace daily.
   g. Soak, wash, scrub soak and sterilize instruments daily.

## PART 2: COMPETENCY CHALLENGE

Mastery Manual activities are listed below.

Suggested instructor lab activities:

1. Have the students gown, glove, mask and goggle for a procedure with potential for body fluid splashing.
2. Students may see procedures demonstrated and become involved with the CD-ROM ⊕. This is the first preference for performing competencies. The procedures are included at the end of the chapter in the Mastery Manual. The instructor should identify that all four procedure competencies (handwashing, sanitizing, wrapping instruments, and using the autoclave) will need to be practiced for mastery. If CD-ROM is not available, all skills may be demonstrated in the lab. It would be beneficial to have the tapes CLINICAL SKILLS FOR THE MEDICAL ASSISTANT, 1995, available from W.B. Saunders, for viewing before instructor demonstration.
3. Due to student fears it is best to demonstrate the loading and use of the autoclave whenever possible. Run it through a full cycle and allow as many students as possible to participate.

ACTIVITIES IN MASTERY MANUAL:

A. See the main menu and click on clinical skills on the CD-ROM ⊕ to find the procedures in this chapter. If instructed, you may follow the activities below.
   1. Proceed to APPENDIX C ⚠ and read the case study for each patient. Determine the competencies needed for each patient as listed in Chapter 26 procedures. List each patient and the competencies learned in Chapter 26 that you will need to perform for each patient.

Competencies needed: See first page of chapter and grid.

   2. After identifying these skills, students are to turn to the end of this chapter and practice these skills until they are ready to have their instructor check their competency.

B. Use the telephone yellow pages or the Internet and find all the agencies that have to do with immune and infectious diseases. Bring the list to class.

## PART 3: CLINICAL APPLICATIONS

These topics will bring students into awareness of personal feelings, which are important in guiding patient care. Personal attitudes must be recognized and acknowledged.
Students may discuss the activity in small groups. Then hold a class discussion. Time the entire activity so it doesn't get out of control.

1. Discuss implications to you, personally, in taking care of the patients below.
   - Consider how you feel about the condition.
   - Do you feel threatened by the diagnosis or lack of diagnosis?
   - Do you feel you can refuse to care for a patient with that diagnosis?
   - How will you handle these feelings in the workplace?
   - Is it legal to refuse care to these patients?
   - Is it ethical?

   The patients are:

   a. No diagnosis, cough, weight loss, night sweats
   b. A child with possible meningitis
   c. A child with chickenpox
   d. A 35-year-old man with hepatitis B
   e. A 42-year-old HIV-positive woman
2. Your patient has an infected leg ulcer. The physician wants you to explain medical aseptic technique for home use, after which the physician will show the patient how to care for the covering put on the ulcer. Write all the teaching points you want to explain to the patient. Bring the list to class for discussion. Have students use the Patient Activity "Developing a Teaching Plan" from Chapter 25 and fill it in together.
3. What do you think are five legal or ethical responsibilities of the medical assistant regarding medical asepsis and infection control? Be specific.

   Wash hands between patients every time.

   Do not go to work when ill.

   Do not compromise technique.

   Use quality controls.

   Follow federal and OSHA guidelines.

# 27

# Vital Signs and Anthropometric Measurements

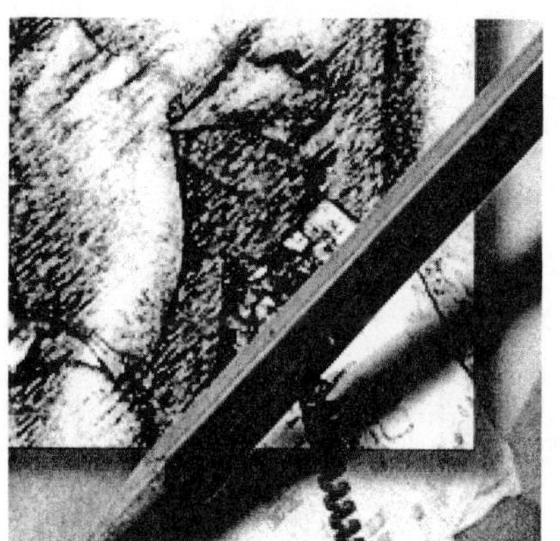

Vital signs are the primary clinical evaluation tools from which the physician proceeds to more specific diagnostic procedures and physical examination. Since the medical assistant is chiefly responsible for obtaining these measurements, it is essential to have theoretical knowledge in anatomy, physiology, normal and abnormal values, factors affecting values, conditions causing abnormal values, and the principles and procedures for measuring vital signs. The physician needs to count on students' mastery of these skills.

## USING THE LEARNING SYSTEM

### 1. MEDICAL ASSISTING CONTENT AND COMPETENCIES

CONTENT

- Anatomy and physiology of all the body systems
- Applications of medical terminology
- Legal requirements for health care
- Developmental stages of the life cycle
- Recognition of and response to verbal and nonverbal communication
- Asepsis and infection control
- Patient care
- Adaptations for individual needs
- Job readiness

COMPETENCIES

- Practice standard precautions
- Obtain vital signs
- Prepare and maintain examination and treatment areas
- Instruct and demonstrate use and care of patient equipment
- Recognize and respond to verbal and nonverbal communication
- Perform within legal and ethical boundaries
- Perform routine maintenance of clinical equipment
- Instruct individuals according to their needs

## 2. MEDICAL ASSISTING ENTRY-LEVEL CURRICULUM INTERFACE

| TEXTBOOK OBJECTIVES | LEARNING SYSTEM LOCATION | MA CURRICULUM |
|---|---|---|
| Cognitive | | Content |
| 1. Define and spell the terms in the Vocabulary | • Text p. 441<br>• Manual Part 1-A | • Anatomy and physiology of all the body systems<br>• Applications of medical terminology |
| 2. Cite the average values of body temperatures, pulse rates, respiratory rates, and blood pressure | • Text pp. 442, 460, 463, 466, and 467<br>• Manual Part 1-B | • Developmental stages of the life cycle<br>• Recognition of and response to verbal and nonverbal communication<br>• Adaptations for individual needs<br>• Patient care<br>• Job readiness |
| 3. Describe how emotional and physical factors cause body temperature to increase or decrease | • Text p. 442 | • Same as 2. above |
| 4. Identify the 24-hour patterns for three types of fevers | • Text p. 443<br>• Textbook memory jogger #3 | • Anatomy and physiology of all the body systems<br>• Patient care |
| 5. List six methods for obtaining a patient's temperature | • Text pp. 444–457<br>• Manual Part 1-C | • Patient care<br>• Developmental stages of the life cycle<br>• Recognition of and response to verbal and nonverbal communication<br>• Adaptations for individual needs<br>• Legal requirements for health care |
| 6. Describe pulse rate, volume, and rhythm | • Text pp. 460–461<br>• Manual Part 1-C | • Anatomy and physiology of body systems<br>• Developmental stages of the life cycle<br>• Recognition and response to verbal and nonverbal communication<br>• Adaptations for individual needs |
| 7. List four important characteristics to note when taking a pulse | • Text p. 460<br>• Manual Part 1-E | • Anatomy and physiology of body systems<br>• Patient care<br>• Adaptations for individual needs<br>• Legal requirements for health care |

| TEXTBOOK OBJECTIVES | LEARNING SYSTEM LOCATION | MA CURRICULUM |
|---|---|---|
| **Cognitive** | | **Content** |
| 8. List six respiratory rate variations | • Text p. 463<br>• Manual Parts 1-C and 1-E | • Anatomy and physiology of body systems<br>• Adaptations for individual needs<br>• Patient care |
| 9. Describe the best way to obtain accurate respiration counts | • Text p. 464<br>• Manual Part 2<br>• Textbook memory jogger #9 | • Patient care<br>• Adaptations for individual needs<br>• Legal requirements for health care |
| 10. List four physiological factors affecting blood pressure | • Text p. 465<br>• Manual Parts 1-D and 1-F<br>• Memory jogger #10 | • Anatomy and physiology of all the body systems<br>• Adaptations for individual needs |
| 11. Differentiate between essential and secondary hypertension | • Text p. 463<br>• Manual Part 1-B | • Anatomy and physiology of all the body systems |
| 12. Describe the methods for obtaining weight and height of a patient | • Text pp. 471–474<br>• Manual Part 2 | • Anatomy and physiology of all the body systems<br>• Adaptations for individual needs |
| 13. Identify patient education possibilities | • Text p. 474<br>• Manual Part 3 | • Patient care<br>• Anatomy and physiology of body systems<br>• Adaptations for individual needs |
| 14. Describe ethical and legal responsibilities in obtaining vital signs | • Text p. 474<br>• Manual Part 3 | • Patient care<br>• Legal requirements for health care<br>• Adaptations for individual needs |
| **Performance** | | **Competencies** |
| 1. Locate eight pulse sites | • Manual Part 1-B<br>• Procedure 27-7 | • Practice standard precautions<br>• Obtain vital signs<br>• Recognize and respond to verbal and nonverbal communication<br>• Instruct individuals according to their needs |
| 2. Identify the different Korotkoff phases | • Procedure 27-9 | • Same as 1. above |
| 3. Convert kilograms to pounds and pounds to kg | • Textbook memory jogger #13 | • Practice standard precautions<br>• Obtain vital signs |

*chart continues on following page*

## MEDICAL ASSISTING ENTRY-LEVEL CURRICULUM INTERFACE continued

| TEXTBOOK OBJECTIVES | LEARNING SYSTEM LOCATION | MA CURRICULUM |
|---|---|---|
| **Performance** | | **Competencies** |
| 4. Complete all assigned chapter procedures at the satisfactory level determined by your instructor | • ⊕ CD-ROM<br>• Manual Part 2 | • Practice standard precautions<br>• Obtain vital signs<br>• Prepare and maintain examination and treatment areas<br>• Instruct and demonstrate use and care of patient equipment<br>• Recognize and respond to verbal and nonverbal communication<br>• Perform within legal and ethical boundaries<br>• Perform routine maintenance of clinical equipment<br>• Instruct individuals according to their needs |

## 3. RESOURCES

www.mayoclinic.com **A site for all types of health information**

http://dingo.vut.edu.au/~michaelb/welcome.htm **This leads to a site to obtain a CD-ROM specifically for teaching B/P; comes from Victoria University of Technology**

http://www.dinamap.com **Shows different types of monitoring equipment**

## 4. LESSON PLAN Vital Signs TIME 3 hours lecture, 12 hours lab

**Opening:** Bring in B/P cuff and stethoscope. Be taking B/P as students arrive. Watch responses. Obtain comments on students' personal experience with this procedure. Does everyone complete the procedure the same way?

**Pretest:** Ask students to define vital signs, what specific signs they are and how they came to be called that. Students who know medical history will realize that for years they were the easiest way to verify life. With pulse oximeters and other monitors clinics are able to use other techniques, but vital signs are still the mainstay in the physician office.

**Objectives:** There are many objectives associated with this material. It is helpful to put objectives up for each hour of class or lab; then students are not overwhelmed. Use Part 1 in the manual to meet all cognitive objectives. Use the CD-ROM and lab to meet all performance objectives. Review the CD-ROM activities before assigning to students. ⊕ All the skills essential to vital signs are located here. Check the main menu and choose clinical skills for exact location. Students should have a demonstration of techniques and complete the CD-ROM before they are allowed to practice to achieve competence.

**Content:** Use the outline below to cover important points. Use the textbook to present information and answer questions. Reinforce the importance of paying attention to accuracy. Discuss common errors.

VITAL SIGNS AND ANTHROPOMETRIC MEASUREMENTS

Factors That May Influence Vital Signs
TEMPERATURE
- Physiology
- Fever
- Temperature Readings

TYPES OF THERMOMETERS, USAGE, and SANITIZING
- Glass
- Electronic
- Rectal
- Tympanic
- Axillary
- Disposable

PULSE SITES
- Temporal
- Apical
- Radial
- Popliteal
- Carotid
- Brachial
- Femoral
- Dorsalis Pedis (Pedal)

CHARACTERISTICS OF PULSE
- Rate
- Volume
- Average Pulse Rates
- Vessel Elasticity
- Rhythm

DETERMINING PULSE

RESPIRATION

*lesson plan continues on following page*

**LESSON PLAN** ***continued***

CHARACTERISTICS OF RESPIRATIONS Rate Rhythm Depth

COUNTING RESPIRATIONS

BLOOD PRESSURE

FACTORS AFFECTING BLOOD PRESSURE

Volume Peripheral Resistance

Vessel Elasticity Heart Muscle

Pulse Pressure

EVALUATING BLOOD PRESSURE

MEASURING BLOOD PRESSURE

HEART SOUNDS

Korotkoff Sounds

Phase I Phase III

Phase II Phase IV

Phase V

Palpatory Method

TIPS FOR TAKING VITAL SIGNS

ANTHROPOMETRIC MEASUREMENT

MEASURING HEIGHT AND WEIGHT

To Convert Kilograms to Pounds—To Convert Pounds to Kilograms

LEGAL AND ETHICAL RESPONSIBILITIES PATIENT EDUCATION

**Assignment:** Complete the Mastery Manual Part 1 activities. View videos on vital signs. Complete the CD-ROM ⊕ in preparation for the demonstration in lab and subsequent practice. Study all material and techniques. Be prepared to observe demonstration and begin lab practice.

**Posttest:** Use the Examaster testbank to ask as many multiple choices on this material as possible. Be sure that normal values are in agreement with national testing standards.

## 5. MASTERY MANUAL ANSWERS

### PART 1 CONTENT MASTERY

### A. Learning Level: Knowledge

1. Write in the term for each definition given below.

cerumen A waxy secretion in the ear canal.
elastic pulse Pulse with regular alterations of weak and strong beats without cycle changes.
essential hypertension Elevated blood pressure that develops for no apparent reason.
intermittent pulse A pulse in which occasional beats are skipped.
orthostatic blood pressure Inflammation of the middle ear.
otitis media Blood pressure taken at standing and erect positions.
pulse deficit Difference between the apical pulse and the radial pulse.
pulse pressure Difference between the systolic and the diastolic blood pressures.
rales Abnormal or crackling chest sounds during breathing.
remittent fever Fever in which temperature fluctuates greatly but never falls to normal.

| | |
|---|---|
| rhonchi | Rattling noises in the throat that may resemble snoring. |
| stertorous | Describing a deep snoring sound that occurs with each inspiration. |
| thready pulse | A pulse that is scarcely perceptible. |
| unequal pulses | Difference felt between right and left radial and/or femoral pulse points. |

2. Define all the medical terminology listed below. Attempt to break it into parts with slash (/) marks and define each prefix, root, or suffix.

   A/pnea—no/breathing The absence or cessation of breathing.

   Ar/rhythm/ia—-without/rhythm Irregular heart rhythm.

   Brady/cardia—-slow/heart Slow heartbeat; a pulse below 60 beats per minute.

   Brady/pnea—Respirations that are regular in rhythm but slower than normal in rate.

   Dys/pnea—Difficult breathing.

   Homeo/stasis—same/balance or stability Internal adaptation and Hughese in response to environmental factors.

   Hyper/pnea—excessive/respiration Increased rate of respiration.

   Hyper/tension—High blood pressure (systolic pressure consistently above 160 mm Hg, and diastolic pressure above 90 mm Hg)

   Hyper/ventila/tion—excessive /breathing Abnormally prolonged and deep breathing usually associated with acute anxiety or emotional tension.

   Hypo/tension—Blood pressure that is below normal (systolic pressure below 90 mm Hg, and diastolic pressure below 50 mm Hg)

   Ortho/pnea—straight/breathing Breathing in an upright position.

   Tachy/pnea—fast/breathing Respirations that are regular in rhythm but faster than normal in rate.

## B. Learning Level: Comprehension

1. The pulses with markers from top to bottom are: temporal, carotid, apical, brachial, radial, femoral, popliteal and pedal
2. Answers to multiple choice are: 1-A; 2- C; 3 - C; 4 - D; 5 - B; 6 - B; 7 - A; 8 D; 9 - C; 10 -B

## C. Learning Level: Application

1. Choose the patient vital signs you would report to the physician before the physician sees the patient. Mark the choices with an X.
   a. T 99°F (A) at 9 A.M. X
   b. T 99°F (R) at 4 P.M.
   c. P 120 in a 4-year-old
   d. P 120 in an adult X
   e. R 30 in an asthmatic 12-year-old X
   f. R 30 in a 1-year-old
2. Fill in the chart with five tips for taking each of the vital signs.

   Review the material with the students.

## D. Learning Level: Analysis

Name some possible causes for the following.

1. 16-year-old shows up for sports physical. He is sweaty, with pulse and respirations elevated.

Ans: He probably ran to get to office on time. Ask him if he has been exercising.

2. Mom brings 2-year-old in and says baby has a temp of 105°F. Baby is not flushed, red, or irritable. Pulse and respirations are normal. When you take tympanic temperature it is 98.6°F.

Ans: What type thermometer was used? Did she insert it correctly? Did she read it wrong?

3. What might a 60-year-old patient with an irregular pulse have?

Ans: Heart disease, arrhythmia

4. ⚠ Mrs. Ferguson, a patient from the case studies, has been in before and comes back for her revisit with the physician. The first time she was seen, her B/P was within normal limits. Today it is 150/94.

Ans: Anxious, sleepless, rushing to appointment, or medical assistant may have taken reading incorrectly.

## E. Learning Level: Synthesis

Using the above situations, describe your actions in caring for these patients.

1. 16-year-old shows up for sports physical. He is sweaty, with pulse and respirations elevated.

Ans: Have patient rest for 5 minutes, then retake. If symptoms still present, notify the physician.

2. Mom brings 2-year-old in and says baby has a temp of 105°F. Baby is not flushed, red, or irritable. Pulse and respirations are normal. When you take tympanic temperature, it is 98.6°F.

Ans: Ask Mom about how she took the temp. What kind of thermometer did she use? Where did she insert it and how long did she leave it in? Also, about hot drinks. Educate Mom about correct use of thermometer in a nonthreatening manner; appeal to her need not to worry when using correct technique.

3. What might a 60-year-old patient with an irregular pulse have?

Ans: A heart condition. Take apical and radial pulse and have patient rest. Make sure patient has no pulse deficit or pain. Report to physician and prepare to take EKG.

4. ⚠ Mrs. Ferguson, a patient from the case studies, has been in before and comes back for her revisit with the physician. The first time she was seen, her B/P was within normal limits. Today it is 150/94.

Ans: Take cuff off and recheck, paying attention to correct technique. If still high, ask her if she is anxious, uncomfortable, restless. Ask her to rest some more before taking it again. If it remains high, notify physician.

## F. Learning Level: Evaluation

1. Why would you tell a patient with high blood pressure not to take any medication that increases heart rate?

Ans: Because these medications will increase the B/P and make the heart less efficient in pumping blood to essential body areas.

2. Do you know of any common OTC medications that increase heart rate?

Ans: Antihistamines, allergy medicines, some cold medicines.

3. Why do we tell patients not to hyperventilate before holding breath under water?

Ans: It may cause them to stop breathing or lose consciousness from oxygen and carbon dioxide imbalance.

4. Why do we tell moms not to let babies sleep on their sides or stomachs?

Ans: Because it causes a higher incidence of sleep apnea and death, i.e. sudden infant death syndrome.

5. Name four situations in which you would avoid taking a B/P in an upper extremity.

Ans: 1. IV in the arm, 2. Injured or diseased arm, 3. Removal of radial artery, 4. Renal shunt or fistula; 5, Same side as recent mastectomy

6. In what situations would you avoid taking an oral temperature?

Ans: 1. Unconscious, 2. Uncooperative, 3. Infant or very young, 4. Disoriented, 5. Respiratory difficulties, 6. Oral surgery

## PART 2 STUDENT ACTIVITIES COMPETENCY CHALLENGE

1. Before proceeding to the CD-ROM, be sure to see at least one demonstration of the procedures. ⊕ Use the CD-ROM to perform and gain competence in measuring all the vital signs, height, and weight. The procedure evaluation sheets are located at the end of this chapter for you to use with the CD-ROM and for practice and mastery testing. Go to the main menu and choose clinical skills to find the interactive scenarios for you to use to gain competence. When you are ready for evaluation, notify your instructor. Your instructor will use a stethoscope with two sets of earpieces and tubing so that your readings may be accurately determined.

2. For more complete demonstrations, watch the videos *Recording Temperature, Pulse and Respirations and Vital Signs: Blood Pressure.*
3. If the CD-ROM is not available, obtain graphic vital signs forms from a hospital or clinic and take and record vital signs on at least 10 of your classmates. When you complete this practice, take three blood pressures on three persons and complete the chart below. Use Procedure 27-10 and also take height and weight on the same three persons and record it next to their numbers in the chart. Some volunteers may want to remain anonymous.

Instructors: The following are some hints for preparing for demonstration or student practice.

PROCEDURES 27-1 AND 27-2 OBTAINING AN ORAL TEMPERATURE USING GLASS/MERCURY OR ELECTRONIC THERMOMETER

Have oral and electronic thermometers available. Demonstrate the technique, stressing patient identification, sanitization, and disinfection procedures. Have students practice reading both Fahrenheit and Centigrade glass thermometers and electronic thermometers if available. Observe for accuracy in the recording of the results. Students should practice until proficient before attempting the performance test in the Student Mastery Manual.

PROCEDURE 27-3 OBTAINING AN AURAL TEMPERATURE USING TYMPANIC SYSTEM

Have the processing unit with disposable probe covers available. Demonstrate the techniques, following the manufacturer's directions. Remind students to put thermometer in TYMPANIC mode.

PROCEDURE 27-6 OBTAINING AN AXILLARY TEMPERATURE

Gloves, warm water, soap, and a towel should be available. Students may take each other's axillary temperatures.

PROCEDURE 27-7 DETERMINING RATE AND ASSESSING PULSE

Students will need a watch with a second hand. Students should have patient in a comfortable position with the palm downward. Observe the students for proper finger placement; be sure that the thumb is not being used. Identify any irregularities.

PROCEDURE 27-8 DETERMINING RESPIRATIONS

A watch with a second hand is needed. Some students may have difficulty counting respirations. Advise students that respirations may be counted before or after the pulse and should be done without the patient's knowledge.

PROCEDURE 27-9 DETERMINING A PATIENT'S BLOOD PRESSURE

Students should not use the digital readout blood pressure equipment until they have mastered the mercury and/or aneroid technique.

Students will need a sphygmomanometer and a stethoscope. Mercury and aneroid types should be used. The LED readout may be demonstrated, but it is best that students learn on the aneroid and mercury types. Be sure to demonstrate the procedure, EVEN IF THE VIDEOS OR THE INTERACTIVE CD-ROM are used. It is best to have a teaching stethoscope. You can demonstrate on students and they can listen to their own blood pressure. Some students have difficulty hearing the sounds at first; some also have difficulty reading the scale. They should repeat the full procedure on as many different students as possible and a variety of age groups. The performance test should be attempted once the student feels confident and competent.

PROCEDURE 27-10 MEASURING A PATIENT'S HEIGHT AND WEIGHT

A balance scale with a measuring bar should be available. It may be borrowed from the school clinic. Students should weigh at least three other persons after balancing the scale.

## PART 3 CLINICAL APPLICATIONS

This is an important area for patients. The medical assistant should, with the physician's permission, teach all patients about their vital signs and their normal values. Older patients are encouraged to take and record vital signs biweekly. Some offices give patients booklets; others just let patients keep their own written record, which they are asked to bring when they come in at least yearly when over 50. (Females will need Pap smears taken and males will need a prostate check.)

Student activities for discussion

1. Each student is to make a list for teaching patients about their vital signs. If necessary, go to Chapter 25 and use the patient teaching plan form. The list will consist of just important teaching points, not a complete patient teaching plan.
2. You take Mrs. Ferguson's B/P and TPR. You are pretty sure you heard her B/P reading at 140/90. When you check her last visit, it was 150/94. These seem consistent. What do you do now?
3. Mr. Pepper comes in for his 1-year follow-up after quadruple bypass. All his vital signs are normal; however, you think his pulse is a little weak and it is 74. How do you proceed and why?

# 28

# Assisting with the Primary Physical Examination

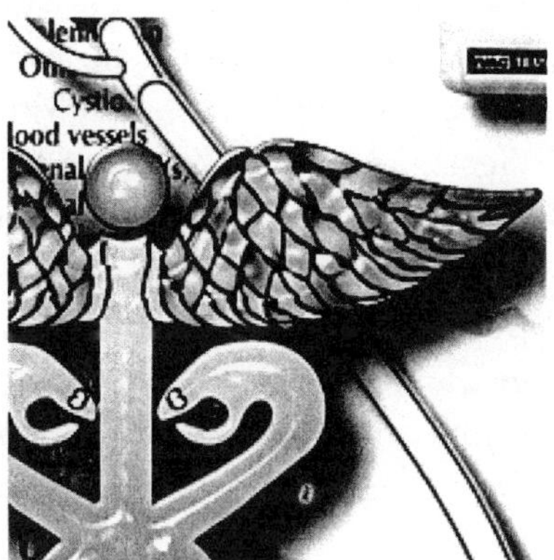

Assisting with the primary physical examination is a major responsibility of the clinical medical assistant. As the instructor, you will want to emphasize the importance of preparing the patient, preparing and maintaining the treatment areas, and assisting the physician. Often it is necessary to get close to patients and make contact with them. Students who are aware of cultural diversity within the community will be able to position patients with more comfort. Some students and some patients may be reluctant to have this type of personal contact. Medical assistants should allow patients to do what they can for themselves and stand by to assist as necessary. The instructor may serve as a role model when demonstrating positioning and moving patients. Review discussions of diverse cultural preferences and aseptic techniques. Review circumstances that require standard precautions.

## USING THE LEARNING SYSTEM

### 1. MEDICAL ASSISTING CONTENT AND COMPETENCIES

The list below applies to Chapters 28 through 39, primary and specialty assisting chapters. All these assisting chapters cover MA curriculum content and competencies applicable to textbook objectives. As instructors, it is important to discuss and apply the curriculum requirements within the total learning system. This will be provided to you in the interface grids for each chapter.

CONTENT

Review areas

- Anatomy and physiology for all body systems
- Common pathology and disease
- Applications of medical terminology
- Basic principles of psychology
- Job readiness
- Personal attributes
- Asepsis and infection control

New content

- Diagnostic/treatment modalities
- Diagnostic testing
- Legal guidelines and requirements for health care
- Medical ethics and related issues
- Risk management
- Recognition and response to verbal and nonverbal communication
- Adaptations for individual needs
- Specimen collection and processing
- Patient care

COMPETENCIES

- All fundamental principles of handwashing, autoclaving, sterilizing, standard precautions
- Prepare and maintain examination and treatment areas
- Prepare patient for and assist with routine and specialty examinations
- Prepare patient and assist with specialty procedures and treatments
- Recognize and respond to verbal and nonverbal communication
- Identify and respond to issues of confidentiality
- Document appropriately
- Instruct patients according to needs
- Identify community resources
- Provide instruction for health maintenance and disease prevention
- Instruct patients in collection of specimens
- Perform specialty noninvasive diagnostic tests
- Use methods of quality control
- Screen and follow up test results
- Demonstrate use and care of patient equipment
- Perform an inventory of supplies and equipment

## 2. MEDICAL ASSISTING ENTRY-LEVEL CURRICULUM INTERFACE

| TEXTBOOK OBJECTIVES | LEARNING SYSTEM LOCATION | MA CURRICULUM |
|---|---|---|
| **Cognitive** | | **Content** |
| 1. Define and spell the words in the Vocabulary | • Text p. 478<br>• Manual Part 1-A | • Applications of medical terminology |
| 2. Describe the structural development of the human body | • Text p. 479<br>• Manual Part 1-B | • Anatomy and physiology for all body systems |
| 3. Identify the eleven body systems and the major organs or units in each | • Text p. 479<br>• Manual Part 1-F | • Anatomy and physiology<br>• Common pathology and disease |
| 4. List ten instruments used during a physical examination | • Text pp. 480–484<br>• Manual Part 1-B | • Asepsis and infection control |
| 5. Describe the six methods of examination and give an example for each | • Text pp. 485–486<br>• Manual Part 1-C | • Adaptations for individual needs |
| 6. Outline basic principles of properly draping a patient for examination | • Text p. 486<br>• Manual Part 2 | • Diagnostic/treatment modalities<br>• Basic principles of psychology<br>• Patient care<br>• Recognition of and response to verbal and nonverbal communication |

| TEXTBOOK OBJECTIVES | LEARNING SYSTEM LOCATION | MA CURRICULUM |
|---|---|---|
| **Cognitive** | | **Content** |
| 7. List eight positions that may be used in examinations | • Text pp. 486–489<br>• Manual Part 1-B | • Diagnostic/treatment modalities<br>• Basic principles of psychology<br>• Patient care |
| 8. Outline the sequence of a routine physical examination | • Text pp. 489–490<br>• Manual Part 2 | • Job readiness<br>• Personal attributes<br>• Specimen collection and processing<br>• Diagnostic testing<br>• Patient care |
| 9. Identify medical specialty for each body system | • Text pp. 490–492<br>• Manual Part 1-F | • Common pathology and disease |
| 10. Discuss the legal and ethical implications of the physical examination | • Text pp. 494–495<br>• Manual Part 3 | • Legal guidelines and requirements for health care<br>• Medical ethics and related issues<br>• Risk management |
| **Performance** | | **Competencies** |
| 1. Prepare the examination room and instruments for a physical examination | • Manual Part 2<br>• ⊕ CD-ROM | • All fundamental principles of handwashing, autoclaving, sterilizing, standard precautions<br>• Prepare and maintain examination and treatment areas<br>• Prepare patient for and assist with routine and specialty examinations<br>• Perform an inventory of supplies and equipment<br>• Demonstrate use and care of patient equipment |
| 2. Position and drape a patient in six different examining positions with ease while being mindful of patient modesty | • Manual Part 2<br>• ⊕ CD-ROM | • Prepare patient and assist with specialty procedures and treatments<br>• Recognize and respond to verbal and nonverbal communication |

*chart continues on following page*

## MEDICAL ASSISTING ENTRY-LEVEL CURRICULUM INTERFACE continued

| TEXTBOOK OBJECTIVES | LEARNING SYSTEM LOCATION | MA CURRICULUM |
|---|---|---|
| **Performance** | | **Competencies** |
| 3. Assist in the physical examination of a patient, correctly completing each step of the procedure in the proper sequence | • Procedure 28-2<br>• Manual Part 2<br>• ⊕ CD-ROM | • Identify and respond to issues of confidentiality<br>• Document appropriately<br>• Instruct patients according to needs<br>• Identify community resources<br>• Provide instruction for health maintenance and disease prevention<br>• Instruct patients in collection of specimens<br>• Perform specialty noninvasive diagnostic tests<br>• Use methods of quality control<br>• Screen and follow up test results |

## 3. RESOURCES

1. *The Physical Examination Explained* Film—16 min.
   Madison General Hospital, 202 South Park Street, Madison, WI 53715
   PMA/AAMA-1998-3.
2. Medcom/Trainex, PO Box 6003, 6060 Phyllis Drive, Cypress, California, 90630
   1-800-877-1443 Bates Physical Examination Series
3. Obtain surgical instrument catalogues—old ones available from hospitals.

**4. LESSON PLAN Primary Physical Exam** **TIME 3 hours lecture, 12 hours lab**

**Opening:** Set up a patient so that students walk into class with a patient lying on bed or table in a supine position and covered with a blanket.

**Pretest:** Ask students to identify patient's position in medical terminology. Require use of medical terminology in all clinical classes. Ask questions from the textbook and establish the level of student preparation. Give a written quiz and count it!

**Objectives:** Review textbook objectives. Place the objectives into the four major topic headings included in the lesson plan chapter outline below.

**Content:** Use the outline below to cover important points. Use the textbook to present information and answer questions. Reinforce the importance of paying attention to accuracy. Discuss common errors.

**CHAPTER OUTLINE**

1. Anatomy and Physiology
   Structural Development
   A. Cells
   B. Tissues
   D. Organs
   D. Systems, p. 479, Table 28-1
2. Medical Specialties and Family Care Physician, Text, p. 479, Table 28-2
3. Physical Examination
   A. Preparing for the Physical Examination
   B. Medical Assisting Duties—Preparing room and equipment, preparing patient, assisting physician
   C. Instruments and Equipment Needed— See list in text, p. 493, Procedure 28-1. Have students make 3x5 card with list and memorize list

| | |
|---|---|
| Nasal Speculum | Gloves |
| Ophthalmoscope | Tape Measure |
| Otoscope | Headlight or Penlight |
| Tongue Depressor | Additional Supplies |
| Stethoscope | Assisting with the Examination |

   D. Methods of Examination

| | |
|---|---|
| Inspection | Auscultation |
| Palpation | Mensuration |
| Percussion | Manipulation |

   E. Positioning and Draping, Text pp. 479 and 480

| | |
|---|---|
| Supine | Dorsal Recumbent |
| Lithotomy | Trendelenburg |
| Fowler | Prone |
| Sims | Knee-Chest |

   F. Examination Sequence

| | |
|---|---|
| Presenting Appearance | Neck |
| Nutrition and Stature | Eyes |
| Speech | Ears |
| Breath Odors | Mouth and Throat |
| Skin | Nose and Sinuses |
| Reflexes | Chest and Abdomen |
| Head | Rectum |

*lesson plan continues on following page*

**LESSON PLAN** ***continued***

4. Legal and Ethical Responsibilities, Patient Education. Discuss international and local cultures in the immediate area of the school. Have students explain their personal culture's attitudes regarding illness, examination, bodily exposure. What are MA responsibilites in this area?
5. Lab: The Mastery Manual covers the entire chapter in great depth, as the information is so important to the students. Activity in Part 1-F-2 is a good tool for summarizing much of the material and it makes the students use all the accumulated clinical information to date. Have students practice assisting two times with peer evaluation before you set up scenarios and evaluate each student.

**Assignment:** Assign students to read and study this chapter beforehand. After this lesson and lab, proceed to Chapter 29 and have students review anatomy of the heart and all the chapter materials. Tell them the pretest will be to name the structures of the heart—this is if they have studied anatomy separately. If not, say nothing.

**Posttest:** Use Examaster testbank questions. Put out a "wander around" test where students go to different test areas and identify instruments and pictures of positions.

## 5. MASTERY MANUAL ANSWERS

### PART 1 CONTENT MASTERY

### A. Learning Level: Knowledge

Across Answers
1. PAP
3. dorsal
6. supine
9. POMR
10. UCD
13. hydrocele
15. prone
16. PI
17. PH
18. palpation
19. nevi
21. acidosis
23. bilirubin
24. gait
26. tinnitus
28. oral
29. cyanosis

Down Answers
2. apnea
4. ROM
5. stridor
6. Sims
7. percussion
8. jaundice
9. pallor
10. uremia
11. FH
12. inspection
14. emphysema
20. vertigo
21. atrophy
22. SR
23. bruit
25. thrush
27. SOAP
29. CC
30. PH

## B. Learning Level: Comprehension

1. Name the positions illustrated below.

   a. supine  d.Trendelenburg
   b. dorsal recumbent  e. Fowler
   c. lithotomy  f. jackknife

2. Name the instruments used in physical examination that are illustrated below from page 490, figure 28-20. Students may name in different order.

   a. Stethoscope  e. Penlight
   b. Tuning fork  f. Nasal speculum
   c. Otoscope  g. Tongue blade
   d. Ophthalmoscope

## C. Learning Level: Application

1. Demonstrate in a drawing or on the examining table the missing position above from B-1.
   Ans.wer: Have students demonstrate prone position.
2. Name at least one examination or specific body part examined with each of the instruments pictured above. Place the body system examined next to the body part name.
   a. Stethoscope: chest, abdomen—cardiac, GI
   b. Tuning fork: bone conduction, reflexes—senses, ears; nervous system
   c. Otoscope: ears—senses
   d. Ophthalmoscope: eyes—senses
   e. Penlight: orifices of head—senses; GI
   f. Tongue blade: mouth—GI
   g. Nasal speculum: nose—respiratory

3. Name the four standard methods of physical examination and list at least two body parts and two systems examined using each method.

| Methods | Body Parts Examined | Systems Examined |
|---|---|---|
| 1. Inspection | General, posture, mannerisms, color, injuries, deformities, rashes, gait | Overall view of all systems through observation of talking, walking, and general health |
| 2. Palpation—touch | Abdomen, rectum, vagina | GI, skin, reproductive |
| 3. Percussion—tapping | Chest, abdomen | Respiratory, GI |
| 4. Auscultation—listening | Lungs, heart, abdomen | Respiratory, cardiac, GI |

## D. Learning Level: Analysis

1. Name the two other types of examination not discussed above.
   Answer: mensuration and manipulation
2. In what types of patient examinations would you use the missing position from the picture in item in Part 1 A.1? Name at least two.
   Answer: This position is used most commonly for spinal manipulation.
   a. spinal  b. rectal and neuromuscular
3. Explain why this position is used in these types of examinations.
   spinal—to examine entire area in resting position; also for manipulation
   rectal—to examine anal area, more comfortable for patient and physician

## E. Learning Level: Synthesis

Direct and assist a "patient" to assume this position. Write patient directions below.

Answer: When the student can position a patient through oral directions, the skill is mastered.

"Mrs. Jones, I am going to help you lie on your abdomen. Sit all the way back on the examining table. Now take your left arm, cross it in front of your chest, and lean it on the table. I will help you bring your legs up as you lower yourself on your side to the pillow. Now come to the back of the table near me and we will roll you forward on your tummy while I come around and help you get comfy from the side you are facing. I do not want you to feel as though you are going to fall off the table." You may now place patient in true prone or a Sims position.

## F. Learning Level: Evaluation

1. In what instance would you not use this position although it is normally indicated in the type of examination the patient is prepared to have?

   Any difficulty breathing, any chest pain

2. On a separate sheet of paper, make a chart for your use when you arrive on your externship site. Make five columns. On the left side of the paper, write in the first column the 11 body systems. Head the other columns: 1. Instruments Needed; 2. Methods of Examination; 3. Positions, and 4. Special Assisting Needs. Fill in the chart as best you can. Continue to fill in and turn in to your instructor for grading when requested.

   Complete this activity in class or lab. Put students in small groups, assign each group two or three body systems. When complete, review and fill in as a class. Use a flip chart for visualization, and students may complete one for themselves. Example below.

| Body Systems | Instruments Needed | Method of Examination | Positions | Special Assisting Needs |
|---|---|---|---|---|
| | | | | |
| | | | | |

## PART 2 COMPETENCY CHALLENGE

Instructors: Direct students to all expected activities. Have students use the CD-ROM ⊕ and procedure "Assisting with a Physical Examination" in the student Mastery Manual at the end of the chapter. It incorporates all the components including: (1) prepare for and assist with examination of a patient, (2) care for the exam room, specimens, and the patient's medical record, and (3) conduct an exit interview. When demonstrating, please demonstrate all possible positions needed and review the types of examinations performed for each position as shown in the text on page 479 or 480. Stress the importance of both assisting the physician and helping the patient.

1. Supplies needed for Procedure 28-1 include:

   Stethoscope, ophthalmoscope, scale, tongue depressors, cotton balls, examination light, percussion hammer, lubricating gel, examination gloves, sphygmomanometer, otoscope, tape measure, head mirror, penlight, nasal speculum, tuning fork, biohazard container, laboratory request form, specimen bottle, glass slides, patient gown, drape, thermometer, finger cots, and cotton-tipped applicators.

   If possible, ask a physician in the area to come in and perform a mock examination on a volunteer or on you, the instructor. Have students ask questions and critique the procedure.

2. Have students complete a teaching plan for assisting patients into different positions. Students must realize that every contact with a patient is a teaching opportunity. Relate this to the medical assisting Content and Competencies Topic 4.0, titled "Instruction," which includes the items. Explain procedures and policies, instruct individuals according to their needs, and teach methods of health promotion and disease prevention.

3. Have students interchange the role of the medical assistant and the patient while practicing positioning and draping. Be sure the students learn to position the patient under the drape. Adjust the drape after positioning is completed.

## PART 3 CLINICAL APPLICATIONS

There are many assessments of situations in this Part. Students may be aware of cultural differences and potential problems from their own experience. This may be a good place from which to start a discussion. Considering that most patients sue because of poor communication and attention, it is important to treat each patient within both legal and ethical boundaries.

1. Students complete a simple teaching plan for positioning patients using the practice activity at the end of the chapter. Pick the type of examination and position, and complete the teaching plan for the patient.
2. Discuss the ethical or legal implications of the following:
   a. Miss Amir from Saudi Arabia is 36. After the physician completes a physical examination and leaves the room, she tells you she is engaged and her fiancé has brought her in for examination. Miss Amir tells you that she has to bring her fiancé in to the physician now to assure him she is a virgin.
   b. What are the laws in your state regarding the treatment of teenagers, parent's rights, and legal responsibility?
   c. Discuss and make a list to establish what people want from physician's office staff. What are the expectations of men, women, teenagers, and children? Before you complete the list in class, talk with some friends of all age groups. What are the similarities and differences in the needs of these four groups? Explain them.

# 29

# Assisting in Cardiovascular Medicine

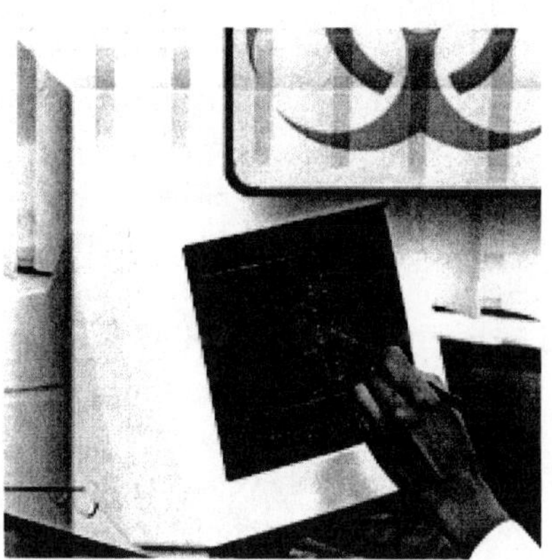

The instructor may also use the CD-ROM here also to reassign vital sign skills before moving on to obtaining the ECG. Because the electrocardiographs are often multichannel and automated, the skill development is simplified. The knowledge base is large, and students will need to spend a good amount of time reviewing cardiac and respiratory functions and structure. If the program has a 12-lead ECG, expand the steps in the procedure and have students learn on these machines. Applying the Holter monitor can be simulated with electrodes, monofilament line, and cutouts. The activities in the Mastery Manual become more demanding and require students to give more input to the levels of knowledge designated. For example, most matching is gone and students must know terms by definition or define terms. Analysis and application levels require putting information together in chart form. Synthesis and evaluation levels have situations for examination and problem solving. The Mastery Manual should be completed after the lecture and before the demonstration and practice of the skills. Most programs may simulate the ECG, but it is difficult to obtain the Holter monitor as offices rarely have extras. Students may practice placing electrodes and counting pulse beats. Rhythms may be identified if the instructor can obtain sample strips from physician offices or hospitals. The CCU is a wonderful source for tracings. Be sure all patient identifiers are removed.

## USING THE LEARNING SYSTEM

### 1. MEDICAL ASSISTING CONTENT AND COMPETENCIES

CONTENT

Review areas

- Anatomy and physiology for all body systems
- Common pathology and disease
- Applications of medical terminology
- Basic principles of psychology
- Job readiness
- Personal attributes
- Asepsis and infection control

New content

- Diagnostic/treatment modalities
- Diagnostic testing
- Legal guidelines and requirements for health care
- Medical ethics and related issues
- Risk management
- Recognition of and response to verbal and nonverbal communication
- Adaptations for individual needs
- Specimen collection and processing
- Patient care

COMPETENCIES

- All fundamental principles of handwashing, autoclaving, sterilizing, standard precautions
- Prepare and maintain examination and treatment areas
- Prepare patient for and assist with routine and specialty examinations
- Prepare patient and assist with specialty procedures and treatments
- Recognize and respond to verbal and nonverbal communication
- Identify and respond to issues of confidentiality
- Document appropriately
- Instruct patients according to needs
- Identify community resources
- Provide instruction for health maintenance and disease prevention
- Instruct patients in collection of specimens
- Perform specialty noninvasive diagnostic tests
- Use methods of quality control
- Screen and follow up test results
- Demonstrate use and care of patient equipment
- Perform an inventory of supplies and equipment

## 2. MEDICAL ASSISTING ENTRY LEVEL-CURRICULUM INTERFACE

| TEXTBOOK OBJECTIVES | LEARNING SYSTEM LOCATION | MA CURRICULUM |
|---|---|---|
| **Cognitive** | | **Content** |
| 1. Define and spell the terms in the Vocabulary | • Text p. 497<br>• Manual Part 1-A | • Applications of medical terminology |
| 2. Anatomically and physiologically describe the heart and its significant structures | • Text p. 499<br>• Manual Part 1-B | • Anatomy and physiology for all body systems<br>• Common pathology and disease |
| 3. Identify the important presenting symptoms of cardiovascular disease | • Text p. 501<br>• Manual Part 1-F | • Same as # 2 |
| 4. List the signs, symptoms, diagnostic and therapeutic procedures employed with coronary artery disease and hypertension | • Text pp. 501–505<br>• Manual Part 1-F | • Anatomy and physiology for all body systems<br>• Common pathology and disease<br>• Diagnostic/treatment modalities<br>• Diagnostic testing<br>• Specimen collection and processing |
| 5. Anatomically and physiologically describe the circulatory vessels | • Text p. 505<br>• Manual Part 1-D | • Same as # 2 |
| 6. List the most frequently diagnosed vascular conditions | • Text p. 505<br>• Manual Part 1-C-1 | • Same as # 4 |

| TEXTBOOK OBJECTIVES | LEARNING SYSTEM LOCATION | MA CURRICULUM |
|---|---|---|
| **Cognitive** | | **Content** |
| 7. Trace the electric conduction system through the heart | • Textbook | • Same as # 2 |
| 8. State the meaning of the horizontal and vertical lines on the ECG paper | • Text p. 510<br>• Manual Part 1-D<br>• Table 29-1 | • Same as # 4 |
| 9. List four types of artifacts commonly seen and explain the probable cause for each | • Text pp. 515–517<br>• Manual Part 1-D | • Same as # 4 |
| 10. Discuss the process of obtaining the ECG | • Text pp. 517–522<br>• Manual Part 2<br>• Procedure 29-1 | • Recognition of and response to verbal and nonverbal communication |
| 11. Recognize the differences between patient preparation of the basic ECG and the stress test | • Text pp. 521–525<br>• Manual Part 1-F | • Basic principles of psychology<br>• Job readiness<br>• Personal attributes<br>• Diagnostic/treatment modalities<br>• Diagnostic testing<br>• Legal guidelines and requirements for health care<br>• Medical ethics and related issues<br>• Risk management<br>• Adaptations for individual needs<br>• Patient care |
| **Performance** | | **Competencies** |
| 1. Match the contractions of the heart with the deflections on the ECG tracing | • Manual Part 2 | • Provide instruction for health maintenance and disease prevention<br>• Perform specialty noninvasive diagnostic tests<br>• Use methods of quality control<br>• Screen and follow up test results |
| 2. Point out the 12 leads recorded on an ECG; state the electrical activity of each; and identify the coding used for each | • Text p. 510<br>• Manual Part 2<br>• Table 29-1<br>• ⊕ CD-ROM | • Provide instruction for health maintenance and disease prevention<br>• Use methods of quality control<br>• Screen and follow up test results |

*chart continues on following page*

## MEDICAL ASSISTING ENTRY-LEVEL CURRICULUM INTERFACE continued

| TEXTBOOK OBJECTIVES | LEARNING SYSTEM LOCATION | MA CURRICULUM |
|---|---|---|
| **Performance** | | **Competencies** |
| 3. Obtain a 12-lead ECG tracing | • Procedure 29-1<br>• Manual Part 2<br>• ⊕ CD-ROM | • All fundamental principles of handwashing, autoclaving, sterilizing, standard precautions<br>• Prepare and maintain examination and treatment areas<br>• Prepare patient for and assist with routine and specialty examinations.<br>• Prepare patient and assist with specialty procedures and treatments<br>• Recognize and respond to verbal and nonverbal communication<br>• Identify and respond to issues of confidentiality<br>• Document appropriately<br>• Instruct patients according to needs<br>• Identify community resources<br>• Provide instruction for health maintenance and disease prevention<br>• Instruct patients in collection of specimens<br>• Perform specialty noninvasive diagnostic tests<br>• Use methods of quality control<br>• Screen and follow up test results<br>• Demonstrate use and care of patient equipment<br>• Perform an inventory of supplies and equipment |
| 4. Obtain a multichannel ECG | • Same as 2. | • Same as # 3 above—Be sure to emphasize competencies as they apply to each step |
| 5. Apply and connect the Holter monitor | • Procedure 29-1<br>• Manual Part 2 | • Same as # 3 above—Be sure to emphasize competencies as they apply to each step |

## 3. RESOURCES

1. THE BODY HUMAN CD-ROM is available for purchase. It is excellent for student illustrations.
2. Models of specific body parts and wall charts of human anatomy are available from Denoyer-Geppert. Call for catalogue 1-753-561-9200.
3. Obtain a heart from the butcher, clean it and cut in half to show students. Some students cannot handle this without preparation!!
4. Some Internet Heart sites are not copyright-protected. They have pictures that can be printed and turned into color or black-and-white transparencies.

http://www.heartinfo.org/hinf_hp.html **This is THE HEART SITE. Check it for all sorts of new information, education, research pictures, etc.**

http://www.medicinenet.com/hp.asp?li=MNI **This site will take students to one of the best resources for education of patients and students. The disclaimer must be agreed to before access is granted. Choosing C in the alphabet for congestive heart failure will take students to information on heart attacks and high blood pressure, both major topics in the textbook.**

http://www.healthgate.com/HealthGate/free/dph/static/index.html **A site for diagnostic procedures. Choose C from the alphabet, and a world of cardiac procedures and descriptions opens up to patient and student.**

## 4. LESSON PLAN Cardiovascular Assisting TIME 3 hours lecture, 12 hours lab

**Opening:** Point out that the chapter discusses roles as applied to family practice or cardiology office. Explain a cardiology tech to students. This chapter stops short of preparing students for the tech role, but with physician training or another 6 months of school, the medical assistant could proceed up that multidisciplinary ladder and eventually be trained in echocardiography and assisting with cardiac catheterization.

**Pretest:** Use vocabulary list as a pretest. Go around the room asking each student to define a word, breaking it into its component parts. You might also have the equipment out to complete the procedures and see what students can identify. As you discuss the lesson, use the equipment, including heart models, the ECG machine, stethoscope, B/P equipment, a Holter monitor, and some ECG tracings.

**Objectives:** Put on flip chart and point to each as covered. Objectives are covered in all areas of the learning system, and students will need to use all information.

**Content**

**CHAPTER OUTLINE**

A. Vocabulary: Assign students to make flash cards for all cardiac terms.

B. Circulatory System

1. Heart: Keeping with the following analogy, it is easy to teach the anatomy and then name all the parts, especially when it is also related to medical terminology.
The heart is like a two-story house: atria above and ventricles below. Many homes are constructed on hillsides, where we enter through the top and go down to the bedrooms, as in the heart where the blood enters through the top structure and passes to the bottom ventricles. Homes are built with three layers, as is the heart. The house has external siding, the insulation and interior walls.
2. Layers of the Heart
3. Heart Chambers and Valves
4. Heart Conduction
5. Heart Diseases; Symptoms
   a. Coronary Artery Disease—Risks; S and S; Diagnosis; Treatment
   b. Hypertensive Heart Disease—Risks; S and S; Diagnosis; Treatment
6. Blood Vessels—Similarities and Differences
   a. Arteries Veins Capillaries
7. Vascular Disorders
   a. Emboli and Thrombi—Risks; S and S; Diagnosis; Treatment
   b. Atherosclerosis and Arteriosclerosis—Risks; S and S; Diagnosis; Treatment
   c. Aneurysms—Risks; S and S; Diagnosis; Treatment
   d. Phlebitis and Varicose Veins—Risks; S and S; Diagnosis; Treatment

C. MEDICAL ASSISTANT'S ROLE

1. Obtain VITAL SIGNS sitting and lying and in both arms
2. Obtain medication list, including OTC's
3. List presence or lack of symptoms
4. Assist with procedures, including ECG and applying Holter monitor
5. Assist with treadmill
6. Prepare patient for radiological procedures

## LESSON PLAN *continued*

D. Electrocardiography and the Cardiac Cycle
Electrocardiogram
ECG Paper — Electrodes and Electrolytes
Leads
Standard
Augmented Leads
Chest or Precordial Leads Standardization
Tracing an Error in Limb Lead Placement
Artifacts
Wandering Baseline — Somatic Tremor
Alternating Current — Baseline Interruption
Pathological Tracings
Obtaining the ECG
Preparing the Room and Patient
Applying the Electrolyte and Leads
Recording the ECG
Caring for the Equipment
Mounting the ECG
Interpretation of the ECG
Multichannel Automatic ECG
Automatic Lead Control Switch
Telephone Transmissions
Interpretive Electrocardiographs
E. Cardiac Stress Testing
Differences in Stress Testing and Obtaining ECG
F. Echocardiography
G. Holter Monitor Cardiograph
H. Heart Catheterization and Angioplasty
I. Legal, ethical, and patient education responsibilities: create a community resource list of agencies that help patients with heart conditions or promote heart health. Do this for every chapter from 29–39.

**Lab:** Obtain radiographs of angiography and show vessels to students. Have students name vessels.

Students should complete CD-ROM activities for Mr. Shapiro, then practice and complete two ECGs before evaluation.

If a Holter monitor is available, the same should be done. Sometimes an internist will come and demonstrate application to you. Larger facilities may arrange to have students observe procedures with a physician or a trained cardiology technician.

**Assignment:** Complete the Mastery Manual and know all steps in procedures. After students demonstrate procedure, ask questions that indicate knowledge of purpose behind procedural steps. Students should know the purpose of each step.

**Posttest:** Use Examaster testbank questions. Be sure to include A&P, diseases, treatments and ECG information.

## 5. MASTERY MANUAL ANSWERS

### PART 1 CONTENT MASTERY

#### A. Learning Level: Knowledge

Matching: 1. i; 2. j; 3. h; 4. d; 5. f; 6. g; 7. e; 8. b; 9. a; 10. c

#### B. Learning Level: Comprehension

1. See illustration in textbook figures 29-2, -3, -4.
2. 1. d; 2. c; 3. f; 4. b; 5. e; 6. a
3. 1 = Lead 2; 2 = AVL; 3 = Lead 1; 4 = AVR; 5 = Lead 3; 6 = AVF

#### C. Learning Level: Application

Fill in the chart below with information on vascular disorders.

| Common Disorders | Symptoms | Diagnostic Tests | Treatment |
|---|---|---|---|
| Embolus and thrombus | Lower leg pain, chest pain with dyspnea, cyanosis, decreased B/P | Doppler, angiogram | Streptokinase, heparin, Coumadin, angioplasty |
| Atherosclerosis | Those of MI | Stress ECG, cardiac catheterization | Cholesterol-lowering drugs, angioplasty, diet modification, decrease stress and stop smoking |
| Aneurysm | Bruit, severe headache, abdominal palpitations | Ultrasound, angiography | Surgery, watch and wait |
| Phlebitis | Leg pain, usually swollen, knotty veins<br>May have small ruptures and spider hemangiomas | Pain, especially with knee and ankle flexed | Support stockings, rest, laser Rx, saline injection or surgical ligation and stripping |

#### D. Learning Level: Analysis

Differentiate the structure and function of arteries, veins, and capillaries in the chart below.

| Vessel | Structure | Function |
|---|---|---|
| Arteries | Carry blood from the heart, three layers, thick muscle wall, very elastic outer layer | Contract and relax |
| Veins | Thinner, less muscle layer, valves help prevent back flow | Return blood to heart |
| Capillaries | One cell thick | Allow nutrients and WBCs to pass to other organs and tissues |

## E. Learning Level: Synthesis

Students will need to think about the chapter information presented and then decide how to prevent artifacts before the ECG is attempted. When everything is set up correctly, artifacts may be kept to a minimum.

1. What do the horizontal lines indicate on the ECG paper? **Time 04 second**
2. What do the vertical lines indicate? **Time and force (electrical force)**
3. Pictured below are four different types of artifact. **Label the types, and below each type write the steps to prevent this type.**

   a. wandering baseline

   See Fig 29.19, p 515, from 8th Edition Textbook:

   Steps to prevent —**Unnoticed patient movement, electrode interference caused by pulling, poor application or quality of paste, pulling on electrodes or corroded electrodes—check electrodes, date of paste, etc. before applying.**

   b. somatic tremor

   See Fig 29.20, p. 516 from 8th Edition Textbook:

   Steps to prevent—**Ask patients to be totally still and not talk, ask them if they feel relaxed, give a pillow, instruct them to take slow deep breaths, do not allow chilling.**

   c. AC interference

   See Fig 29.21, p. 516 from 8th Edition Textbook:

   Steps to prevent—**Usual causes are new pieces of equipment, patient holding onto metal, wires touching and crossed, improper grounding.**

   d. baseline interruption

   See Fig 29.22, p. 517 from 8th Edition Textbook:

   Steps to prevent—**Check for broken wires, interruption in current before starting, and watch for patient movement and pulled electrodes.**

## F. Learning Level: Evaluation

1. Mr. Shapiro comes to see Dr. Hughes. He is being seen for a cholesterol check and annual examination. As you take the history, he says he has been feeling great except for a bit of indigestion after eating. He also gets a bit sweaty at night. When you ask him to describe the indigestion, he states it is just below his nipples and is just uncomfortable although he has been taking Pepcid AC and his belching has decreased some.

   So far, what do your suspicions lead you to think?

   Answer: Either GI or cardiac symptoms

   What other symptoms would you ask the patient about which might help the physician's assessment?

   Answer: Ask him about dyspnea, tachypnea, palpitations, cyanosis, edema, syncope, fatigue. He has mentioned chest pain and diaphoresis.

2. The physician has told Mr. Shapiro he is going to have a test at another office. Mr. Shapiro cannot remember the name but it is where he will be wearing the EKG equipment and doing some exercising. He wants to know what it is called and why the physician is ordering it. He was so nervous he cannot remember what he was told. The name and purpose of this test is:

   Answer: A stress test is done to evaluate the condition of blood supply to the heart and ability to tolerate a normal workload.

## PART 2 COMPETENCY CHALLENGE

1. Have students complete Procedure 29-1, Performing a Multichannel ECG. Patient position and clearance of the wires needs to be stressed. Use fresh electrode paste if leads are not prepasted. Most offices now have multichannel machines except in rural areas. Students must check standardization and coding on older machines. Be sure to mark strips as the leads are taken if the machine is not automated. Be sure to stress the need for precise, accurate, sufficient tracings.
2. Students develop a plan to teach patient

   A. how to prevent or minimize varicosities.

   B. nutrition and diet plan for coronary artery disease.

   Use the teaching plan at the end of Chapter 28. For varicose and phlebitis prevention include rest, support hose that are full length, lose weight, avoid standing in one position. Exercise with raising and lowering heels off the ground while standing at job, walk one mile daily.
3. When you are taking Mr. Shapiro's ECG, you note that the distance between the QRS waves does not seem to be even. In some cases it looks like there are two beats where in other areas there is one beat. What should you do and why? Write your response below.

   Answer: Any time the medical assistant sees what appears to be an abnormal tracing, the tracing should be quietly and efficiently completed and taken directly to the physician. Do not wait for the physician to return to the examination room.

## PART 3 CLINICAL APPLICATIONS

Items 1, 2, and 3 are stimulating for small group discussion, especially if students need a "pick-up" time. Sometimes it is interesting to have groups come to consensus on the best way to handle the situation. See if each group independently came up with the same "best" solution.

1. You are preparing Mr. Shapiro for an ECG test. While placing the electrodes on his forearms, you notice that his fists are clenched and he is extremely talkative. He tells you repeatedly that this is his first ECG. You observe that he is perspiring, and as he blinks you see what looks like a tear run down his cheek.
2. Mrs. Mullin, an extremely obese 50-year-old female, is to have an ECG as part of her physical examination. You give her a gown and disrobing instructions. When you return, you find she has not removed her bra. You offer to help her in removing it, but she says she does not want to remove her bra and will not have the ECG if you insist. The bra is made of cotton and does not have an underwire.
3. Johnny is a ten-year-old who has experienced many contrast media x-rays that involved an injectable dye prior to the test. You are to perform an ECG. He is very frightened and does not believe you when you tell him that this test will not hurt and that there are no needles. He clings very tightly to his mother for security. How can you gain Johnny's confidence?

# 30

# Assisting in Pulmonary Medicine

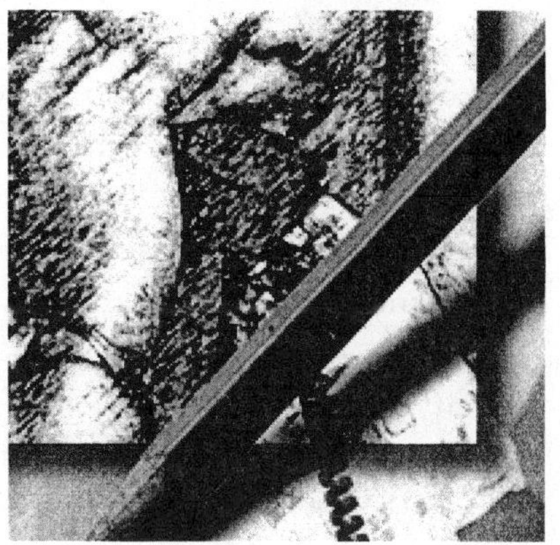

The medical assistant is involved in pulmonary medicine daily. From pediatrics to the elderly, the most common diseases involve the respiratory system. Activities will reinforce MA curriculum content for knowledge of anatomy, diseases, symptoms, treatments, use of standards of infection control, communication, and practice providing patient reassurance and education. The competencies and procedures included in this chapter require applying previous competencies such as medical asepsis and standard precautions. New content will allow you to present principles for administering or performing diagnostic tests and collecting specimens, all of which require barrier protection, exacting detail, and quality control. The students need to perform skills while providing for adequate patient ventilation and reassurance to those with difficult or obstructed breathing. All the competencies may be actually performed or simulated.

## USING THE LEARNING SYSTEM

### 1. MEDICAL ASSISTING CONTENT AND COMPETENCIES

CONTENT

- Anatomy and physiology for all body systems
- Applications of medical terminology
- Common pathology and disease
- Diagnostic/treatment modalities
- Asepsis and infection control
- Specimen collection and processing
- Diagnostic testing
- Legal guidelines and requirements for health care
- Medical ethics and related issues
- Risk management
- Basic principles of psychology
- Recognition and response to verbal and nonverbal communication
- Adaptations for individual needs
- Patient care
- Job readiness
- Personal attributes

COMPETENCIES

- All fundamental principles of handwashing, autoclaving, sterilizing, standard precautions
- Prepare and maintain examination and treatment areas
- Prepare patient for and assist with routine and specialty examinations
- Prepare patient and assist with specialty procedures and treatments
- Recognize and respond to verbal and nonverbal communication
- Identify and respond to issues of confidentiality
- Document appropriately
- Instruct patients according to needs
- Identify community resources
- Provide instruction for health maintenance and disease prevention
- Instruct patients in collection of specimens
- Perform specialty noninvasive diagnostic tests
- Use methods of quality control
- Screen and follow up test results
- Demonstrate use and care of patient equipment

## 2. MEDICAL ASSISTING ENTRY-LEVEL CURRICULUM INTERFACE

| TEXTBOOK OBJECTIVES | LEARNING SYSTEM LOCATION | MA CURRICULUM |
|---|---|---|
| **Cognitive** | | **Content** |
| 1. Name and locate the structures of the respiratory system | • Text pp. 535–537<br>• Manual Part 1-A | • Anatomy and physiology for all body systems<br>• Applications of medical terminology |
| 2. Describe the functioning purpose of each respiratory structure | • Text pp. 535–537<br>• Manual Part 1-B | • Anatomy and physiology for all body systems<br>• Applications of medical terminology |
| 3. Demonstrate understanding of ventilation | • Text p. 537<br>• Manual Part 1-C | • Anatomy and physiology for all body systems |
| 4. Identify the major categories of respiratory diseases | • Text pp. 538–542<br>• Manual Part 1-C | • Common pathology and disease<br>• Diagnostic/treatment modalities<br>• Asepsis and infection control<br>• Specimen collection and processing<br>• Diagnostic testing |
| 5. Differentiate the signs and symptoms and the diagnosis and treatment for the diseases discussed in this chapter | • Text pp. 538–542<br>• Manual Part 1-D | • Common pathology and disease<br>• Diagnostic/treatment modalities<br>• Asepsis and infection control<br>• Specimen collection and processing<br>• Diagnostic testing |

| TEXTBOOK OBJECTIVES | LEARNING SYSTEM LOCATION | MA CURRICULUM |
|---|---|---|
| **Cognitive** | | **Content** |
| 6. Be able to assist the pulmonary care physician in the examination of the chest and lungs | • Text pp. 543–546; 550–554<br>• Manual Part 1-E | • Legal guidelines and requirements for health care<br>• Medical ethics and related issues<br>• Risk management<br>• Basic principles of psychology<br>• Recognition of and response to verbal and nonverbal communication<br>• Adaptations for individual needs<br>• Patient care<br>• Job readiness<br>• Personal attributes |
| **Performance** | | **Competencies** |
| 1. Accurately administer a Mantoux tuberculin skin test | • Chapter 49<br>• Procedure 30-1 | • All fundamental principles of handwashing, autoclaving, sterilizing, standard precautions<br>• Instruct patients in collection of specimens<br>• Identify community resources<br>• Document appropriately |
| 2. Prepare a patient for pulmonary function testing | • Manual Part 1-F<br>• Procedure 30-2 | • Prepare patient and assist with specialty procedures and treatments<br>• Recognize and respond to verbal and nonverbal communication<br>• Identify and respond to issues of confidentiality<br>• Instruct patients according to needs<br>• Provide instruction for health maintenance and disease prevention<br>• Document appropriately |

*chart continues on following page*

## MEDICAL ASSISTING ENTRY-LEVEL CURRICULUM INTERFACE continued

| TEXTBOOK OBJECTIVES | LEARNING SYSTEM LOCATION | MA CURRICULUM |
|---|---|---|
| **Performance** | | **Competencies** |
| 3. Obtain an accurate volume capacity spirometric test | • Manual Part 2<br>• Procedure 30-2 | • Prepare and maintain examination and treatment areas<br>• Perform specialty noninvasive diagnostic tests<br>• Use methods of quality control<br>• Screen and follow up test results<br>• Demonstrate use and care of patient equipment |
| 4. Prepare a patient for throat culture | • Manual Part 2<br>• Procedure 30-3 | • Prepare patient for and assist with routine and specialty examinations<br>• Perform specialty noninvasive diagnostic tests<br>• Demonstrate use and care of patient equipment |
| 5. Collect a specimen by swab for throat culture | • Manual Part 2<br>• Procedure 30-3 | • Perform specialty noninvasive diagnostic tests<br>• Use methods of quality control<br>• Screen and follow up test results<br>• Demonstrate use and care of patient equipment |
| 6. Demonstrate the standard safety precautions used when handling a sputum sample | • Manual Part 2 | • Use methods of quality control<br>• Demonstrate use and care of patient equipment<br>• Risk management |
| 7. Prepare the patient and obtain a sputum specimen for culture | • Procedure 30-3 | • All of the above |

## 3. RESOURCES

www.ahhh-allegra.com/pollen **For pollen forecasts throughout the U.S.**

American Lung Assoc. 1740 Broadway, NY, NY 10019 1-800-586-4872

National Institute of Allergy and Infectious Diseases (NIAID)
9000 Rockville Pike, Bethesda, MD 20892 1-301-496-5717
www.niaia.nih.gov/

National Foundation for Asthma, PO Box 5034, Tucson, AZ 85703

Black Lung Association, 2 Hale St, Charleston, WV 25301
304-347-7100

National Institutes of Health Publication #93-3511

## 4. LESSON PLAN Pulmonary Assisting — TIME 3 hours lecture, 12 hours lab

**Opening:** Have a torso or transparency available to show the chest. Bring in some grapes on the stems and a picture of an upside-down tree. Use the grapes and the tree to make an analogy to the trachea, mainstem bronchi, bronchioles and alveoli.

**Pretest:** Can any student show where lungs are located and what the boundaries are? For example, diaphragm, ribs, mediastinum.

**Objectives:** Refer students to objectives. Write them on a large flip chart. Cross them off as you have students meet the objectives.

**Content:** Follow the outline below. Use the Mastery Manual to involve students. The textbook has some new pictures, which can be copied and enlarged for anatomy transparencies when there is class discussion. It is important to confirm that students have read the chapter before beginning discussions or activities. The memory jogger questions cover the main ideas and some of the objectives. They are a good basis for discussion.

RESPIRATORY SYSTEM OUTLINE

A. Review objectives and vocabulary. Break terms into component parts for meaning Bring in model and **explain anatomy**—external and internal

B. **Describe** how the lungs work in both stages of ventilation

C. **Respiratory system diseases:** include names, S and S, Diagnosis and Rx.

1. Infectious—URI, pneumonia, TB
2. Immune—Asthma, allergic rhinitis
3. Environmental—COPD results from most
4. Tumors—Lung cancer, laryngeal cancer

D. **Procedures:**

1. Administering the Mantoux test
2. Performing volume capacity spirometry
3. Collecting a specimen by swab for throat culture
4. Obtain a sputum specimen sample for culture

E. **Medical Assistant role** in examination

F. **Issues** in law, ethics and education: Have students complete Part 3 before discussion.

**Lab:** All of the areas in Parts 1 and 2 should be reviewed in the lab. It is beneficial to see if students have completed the manual and then complete a review and discussion of the items. Allow students to make corrections to their work.

CD-ROM ⊕ Check the clinical skills area on the CD-ROM for respiratory skills related to Raymond Johnson, the patient with asthma. If spirometry equipment is available, students may learn to perform this test.

**Assignment:** Have students design equipment at home that could be used to simulate spirometry testing. Bring it to class and explain usage. Complete Mastery Manual, Demonstrate provide time for student practice, followed by evaluation.

**Posttest:** Vocabulary matching from Mastery Manual if not completed earlier or questions from textbook. Examaster testbank.

## 5. MASTERY MANUAL ANSWERS

### PART 1 CONTENT MASTERY

#### A. Learning Level: Knowledge

Matching: 1. f; 2. s; 3. c; 4. q; 5. j; 6. t; 7. n; 8. o; 9. b; 10. p
11. d; 12. r; 13. h; 14. a; 15. k; 16. l; 17. m; 18. i; 19. g; 20. e

#### B. Learning Level: Comprehension

Name the respiratory structures described below.

1. Allows exchange of gases at cellular level. alveoli
2. Defends body from pathogens in air as brought into respiratory system. pharynx
3. Cartilaginous rings hold passage open. trachea
4. Cleans, warms and moistens air. nasal cavity/nose
5. Collects dust and foreign particles and initiates coughing. cilia
6. Turbulence makes it difficult for invading organisms to remain in. bronchi
7. Soft, spongy tissues with air sacs. lungs
8. Draw a picture of the respiratory system including all structures mentioned in items 1–7.

See Text pp. 535–537. You may want a student to draw structures on the board.

#### C. Learning Level: Application

1. Which of the major categories of respiratory diseases are missing?
   a. environmental, b. tumors, c. infections, and d. immune diseases
2. Fill in the chart below for the common diseases of the above missing categories.

| Major Category | Name of Diseases | Signs and Symptoms | Diagnosis | Treatment |
|---|---|---|---|---|
| 1. Infectious | 1. URI | Rhinorrhea, sneezing, watery eyes, pharyngitis, coughing, hoarseness | Observation, culture of sputum, CBC | Palliative |
| | 2. Pneumonia | Fever, chills, malaise, dyspnea, tachypnea, pain on inspiration, rusty sputum | Auscultation, rales, rhonchi, chest x-ray, sputum culture, CBC | Destroy organism, antibiotic, antifungals, rest |
| | 3. TB | Intermittent fever, night sweats, weight loss, malaise, productive cough | Sputum culture, bronchoscopy, chest x-ray | Isoniazid, Ethambutol, Rifampin, usually 2 in combination for 6–9 mos |
| 2. | 1. Asthma | Expiratory wheeze, rapid shallow breathing, increased pulse and respirations, dyspnea, rhonchi | Decreased breath sounds, pulmonary function tests, chest x-ray, IgG and eosinophils elevated | Inhalation therapy, bronchodilators, cortisone inhalers, allergy shots |
| | 2. Allergic rhinitis | Sneezing, watery red eyes, rhinorrhea | History, increased eosinophils | Antihistamines, orally and inhalers, beclamethasone inhaler |

## D. Learning Level: Analysis

Compare ventilation by filling in the following chart.

| Stage | Inspiration | Expiration |
|---|---|---|
| Initiated by | Signal from medulla in brain to diaphragm | Relax of diaphragm and intercostal muscle |
| Physiological Processes | Diaphragm flattens and pulls down; intercostals contract and pull ribs out, chest cavity enlarges as air is forced in by pressure changes | Chest moves inward as pressure equalizes and then air is lost to atmosphere and lungs decrease in volume. When pressure in chest is higher than outside, the process begins again |
| Effect on Gas Exchange | Air brings in oxygen, which crosses into bloodstream | Blood gives up carbon dioxide to air and it is exhaled |

## E. Learning Level: Synthesis

Describe in order the steps the medical assistant takes in assisting the physician with a respiratory examination. List at least seven steps.

1. Patient disrobes to waist
2. Put on gown closing in front or back as physician or patient prefers
3. Sit on end of table
4. Take V/S and record
5. Ask patient about chief complaint
6. Explain examination to patient
7. Help move gown during examination to maintain patient's dignity

## F. Learning level: Evaluation

1. Often you will be taught new skills while in the specialist's office, and you must be prepared to gather the information needed to perform the skill accurately. If the physician were to teach you to accurately read a PPD, what information would you need? List at least six items.
   a. Site and date of injection
   b. Ruler or test cards scaled in mm
   c. Practice inspecting and reading five tests with physician
   d. Know standards for positive and negative readings
   e. Recognize adverse reactions to test
   f. Record as physician prefers

2. What signs would indicate that your patient was short of breath, aside from counting respirations?
   a. Doesn't want to lie down
   b. Has to sleep on more than two pillows i.e., upright
   c. Holds self upright with arms at sides
   d. Cyanotic around lips and nail beds
   e. Talks about sudden lack of energy and tiredness

## PART 2 COMPETENCY CHALLENGE

1. Before students complete the CD-ROM activity and Mastery Manual activities demonstrate all the procedures.
2. Demonstrate and explain the proper steps for teaching the patient the correct maneuvers for accurate spirometry testing. These are covered in Procedure 30-1 at the end of the chapter. When students can demonstrate and get a patient to return demonstration with 100% accuracy, they are competent.
3. Students will need a demonstration and practice before testing for competence using Procedure 30-3.

   Students should complete this activity and demonstrate to the instructor. Often sputum specimens turn out to be saliva specimens, as patients are not instructed accurately.
4. Instruct a patient (one of your classmates) on the proper collection of a sputum specimen. The next morning collect the specimen from your classmate using Procedure 30-4.
5. Have the students make the equipment needed to simulate performing a volume capacity test on a peer in the school health laboratory (TP and paper towel rolls, etc.) so it may be disposed of after demonstration of Procedure 30-1.

## PART 3 CLINICAL APPLICATIONS

1. When you are learning new procedures in the medical office, is it necessary to tell the patient you are practicing on them? What are the legal or ethical ramifications of not informing the patient?

   Answer: This situation has legal points—are students experimenting? Do patients have a right to know? To refuse? Ethically, what is the morally correct action?

2. Go to the resources in Appendix B and find places to obtain educational materials. Have the class split assignments as designated by your instructor and bring all available literature to class for posting.

   Use this for discussion in small groups.
3. When you develop administering intradermal medication competency techniques, return to Procedure 30-1 and demonstrate administration of the Mantoux skin test. This competency will be developed with Chapter 49 activities, so it may be postponed, but not forgotten.

# 31

# Assisting with Ophthalmology and Otorhinolaryngology Procedures

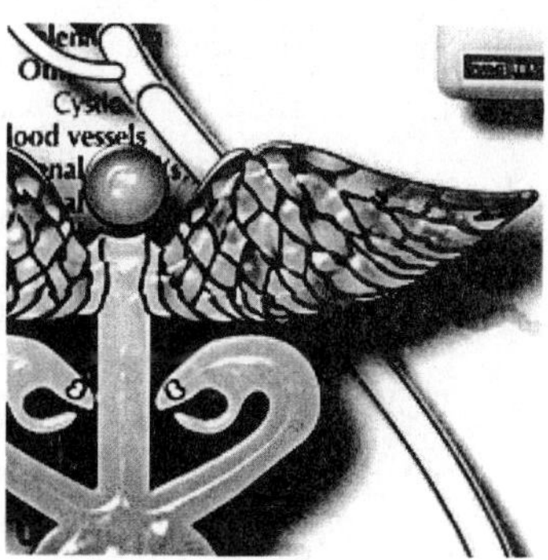

The eye and ear are sense organs that often are initially examined and treated in the primary practitioner's office. The medical assistant prepares the patient and then assists the physician. This includes anticipating physician needs, having the potentially needed equipment, and performing the procedures included in the chapter. The medical assistant also obtains the patient's vital signs and chief complaint. The equipment needed for demonstration and practice are included in the procedures. Usually one can use commercial eye drops for instilling medication. Also, sterile saline drops are available for eye procedures. For ear procedures, students might use a wax loosener such as Debrox for practice. Ensure that students have no allergies to the products. It is advisable to have students review Chapter 49 on preparing and administering medications before attempting Procedures 31-3, 31-5, and 31-6.

## USING THE LEARNING SYSTEM

### 1. MEDICAL ASSISTING ENTRY-LEVEL CONTENT AND COMPETENCIES

CONTENT

- Applications of medical terminology
- Anatomy and physiology for all body systems
- Common pathology and disease
- Diagnostic/treatment modalities
- Asepsis and infection control
- Specimen collection and processing
- Diagnostic testing
- Patient care
- Legal guidelines and requirements for health care
- Medical ethics and related issues
- Risk management
- Basic principles of psychology
- Recognition and response to verbal and nonverbal communication
- Adaptations for individual needs
- Job readiness
- Personal attributes

COMPETENCIES

- All fundamental principles of handwashing, autoclaving, sterilizing, standard precautions
- Prepare and maintain examination and treatment areas
- Prepare patient for and assist with routine and specialty examinations
- Prepare patient for and assist with specialty procedures and treatments
- Recognize and respond to verbal and nonverbal communication
- Identify and respond to issues of confidentiality
- Document appropriately
- Instruct patients according to needs
- Identify community resources
- Provide instruction for health maintenance and disease prevention
- Instruct patients in collection of specimens
- Perform specialty noninvasive diagnostic tests
- Use methods of quality control
- Screen and follow up test results
- Demonstrate use and care of patient equipment

## 2. MEDICAL ASSISTING ENTRY-LEVEL CURRICULUM INTERFACE

| TEXTBOOK OBJECTIVES | LEARNING SYSTEM LOCATION | MA CURRICULUM |
|---|---|---|
| **Cognitive** | | **Content** |
| 1. Explain differences between an ophthalmologist, an optometrist, and an optician | • Text p. 558<br>• Manual Part 1-A | • Applications of medical terminology<br>• Anatomy and physiology for all body systems |
| 2. Identify the anatomical structures that form the eye | • Text p. 560<br>• Manual Part 1-B | • Same as #1 above<br>• Job readiness |
| 3. Describe how vision occurs | • Text p. 560<br>• Manual Part 1-B | • Same as #1 above |
| 4. Differentiate between the four major types of refractive errors | • Text pp. 560–561<br>• Manual Part 1-CA | • Common pathology and disease<br>• Job readiness |
| 5. Be able to give the three reasons for eye irrigation and eye instillation | • Text pp. 572–573<br>• Manual Part 1-CA | • Diagnostic/treatment modalities<br>• Asepsis and infection control<br>• Specimen collection and processing<br>• Diagnostic testing<br>• Patient care<br>• Adaptations for individual needs |
| 6. Identify the structures and explain external, middle, and internal ear functions | • Text p. 577<br>• Manual Part 1-B | • Same as #1 above |
| 7. List disorders that can cause hearing losses | • Text pp. 576–577 | • Common pathology and disease<br>• Job readiness |

| TEXTBOOK OBJECTIVES | LEARNING SYSTEM LOCATION | MA CURRICULUM |
|---|---|---|
| **Cognitive** | | **Content** |
| 8. Differentiate between conductive and sensory losses | • Text p. 578 | • Common pathology and disease<br>• Job readiness |
| 9. Describe four methods used to assess hearing acuity | • Text pp. 581–582<br>• Manual Part 1-C | • Same as #5 above |
| 10. State three reasons for ear irrigation and/or ear instillation | • Text p. 583<br>• Manual Part 1-D | • Same as #5 above |
| 11. State reasons for ensuring aseptic technique in both eye and ear procedures | • Manual Part 1-D | • Diagnostic/treatment modalities<br>• Asepsis and infection control<br>• Patient care<br>• Legal guidelines and requirements for health care<br>• Medical ethics and related issues<br>• Risk management<br>• Basic principles of psychology<br>• Recognition and response to verbal and nonverbal communication<br>• Personal attributes |
| **Performance** | | **Competencies** |
| 1. Correctly label the results of a Snellen vision test | • Manual Part 1-F<br>• Procedure 31-1 | • Document appropriately |
| 2. Accurately measure distance visual acuity | • Manual Part 1-F<br>• Procedure 31-1 | • Perform specialty noninvasive diagnostic tests<br>• Use methods of quality control<br>• Screen and follow up test results<br>• Demonstrate use and care of patient equipment |
| 3. Assess color acuity | • Manual Part 2<br>• Procedure 31-2 | • Same as #2 above |
| 4. Properly irrigate a patient's eyes | • Manual Part 2<br>• Procedure 31-3 | • All fundamental principles of handwashing, autoclaving, sterilizing, standard precautions<br>• Prepare and maintain examination and treatment areas<br>• Prepare patient for and assist with routine and specialty examinations. |

*chart continues on following page*

**MEDICAL ASSISTING ENTRY LEVEL CURRICULUM INTERFACE continued**

| TEXTBOOK OBJECTIVES | LEARNING SYSTEM LOCATION | MA CURRICULUM |
|---|---|---|
| Performance | | Competencies |
| 4. Properly irrigate a patient's eyes *(continued)* | | • Prepare patient and assist with specialty procedures and treatments<br>• Recognize and respond to verbal and nonverbal communication<br>• Identify and respond to issues of confidentiality<br>• Document appropriately<br>• Instruct patients according to needs<br>• Identify community resources<br>• Provide instruction for health maintenance and disease prevention<br>• Instruct patients in collection of specimens |
| 5. Accurately instill eye medication | • Manual Part 2<br>• Procedure 31-4 | • Same as #4 above |
| 6. Assist with removal of a foreign object from an eye | • Text p. 572<br>• Procedure 31-3 | • Same as #4 above |
| 7. Properly irrigate a patient's ears | • Manual Part 2<br>• Procedure 31-5 | • Same as #4 above |
| 8. Accurately instill otic drops | • Manual Part 2<br>• Procedure 31-6 | • Same as #4 above |

## 3. RESOURCES

A. Krames Communications, 312 90th Street, Daly City, CA 94015. Publications for a variety of specialties and conditions—excellent pictures and information

B. American Academy of Ophthalmology, PO Box 7424, San Francisco, CA 94120. Publications on refractive errors, vision and disorders

C. *Nursing* magazine January 1995, Glaucoma, excellent illustrations and patient care

D. See Part 3 answers for Internet sites

E. National Association for Hearing and Speech Action, 1-800-638-8255, 10801 Rockville Pike, Rockville, MD 20852

F. National Eye Care Project, 1-800-222-EYES. Free exams for the elderly. PO Box 9688, San Francisco 94101-9688

G. National Federation of the Blind, 1-301-659-9314, Baltimore, MD

## 4. LESSON PLAN Ophthalmology and Otorhinolaryngology

### TIME 3 hours lecture, 12 hours lab

**Opening:** When everyone is seated, put up Snellen chart. Ask TWO students who are sitting 20 feet away to assist you. Demonstrate the correct way to give and record the test. Talk about advanced training in both areas. Find an ophthalmology OR tech or an audiologist to come and have a short discussion on the specialty training available.

**Pretest:** Ask about student experience with disorders and symptoms of eye and ear; often much will be known about children and the frequency of ear disorders. Discuss new treatments for ear infections, i.e., withholding antibiotics unless infection is obvious or cultured from specimen. There are too many drug-resistant bacteria. Also may use Part 1 activity C-2 for a pretest.

**Objectives:** There is a transparency master to review objectives. Students may be asked to check objectives when they are met. Review objectives with MA curriculum content and competencies and discuss applicability to the "real world."

**Content:** This outline may be filled in to contain the materials in the depth desired.

**Ophthalmology Overview**

1. Anatomy and Physiology of the Eye, Eyeball, Vision
2. Common Disorders of the Eye
   Refractive Errors—Signs, Symptoms, Diagnosis, Treatment, Associated Procedure
   Hyperopia Myopia Presbyopia Astigmatism
   Strabismus
3. Disorders of the Orbit—Signs, Symptoms, Diagnosis, Treatment, Associated Procedure
4. Disorders of the Eyeball—Signs, Symptoms, Diagnosis, Treatment, Associated Procedure
   Cataract and Glaucoma
5. Medical Assistant's Role in Ophthalmology
   A. Examination
   B. Diagnostic Procedures
   C. Laboratory Tests
   D. Special Needs Patients—Blind, Hearing or Mobility Impaired, ESL
6. Theory and Demonstration of Procedures
   Measuring Visual Acuity—Procedure 31-1: Measuring Distance Visual Acuity
   The Ishihara Test—Procedure 31-2: Assessment of Color Acuity
   Eye Irrigation—Procedure 31-3: Irrigating a Patient's Eye
   Eye Instillation—Procedure 31-4: Instilling Eye Medication
   Foreign Bodies

**Otology**

1. Anatomy and Physiology of the Ear
   Outer or External Ear
   Middle Ear
   Inner Ear
2. Disorders of the Ear—Signs, Symptoms, Diagnosis, Treatment, Associated Procedure
   Deafness
   Otitis

*lesson plan continues on following page*

## 5. LESSON PLAN Ophthalmology and Otorhinolaryngology *continued*

Cerumen Impaction

3. Medical Assistant Role in Otology Procedures
   The Examination
   Tests—Weber, Rinne, Audiometric
   Aseptic Procedures
      Procedure 31-5: Irrigating the patient's ear
      Procedure 31-6: Instillation of otic drops

**Patient Education/Legal and Ethical Implications:** Use this content to reinforce patient preparation, confidentiality, risk management, and community resources, especially for the blind and deaf or hard of hearing. Have students research local resources.

**Lab:** Students will need every hour for demonstration, practice, and return demonstration.

**Assignment:** Students prepare for laboratory with home practice of procedures and completing the Mastery Manual.

**Posttest:** Use the Examaster testbank and blank Transparency Master illustrations to test students' knowledge. Begin to use current examination guides for Medical Assistant to ask questions in the style and type of those used on national and state certificate examinations.

## 5. MASTERY MANUAL ANSWERS

### PART 1 CONTENT MASTERY

### A. Learning Level: Knowledge

Terminology Review: Break the following words associated with the chapter into component parts and give the meanings of each part. Example: Optic = opt = eye; ic = pertaining to

| | |
|---|---|
| 1. Ambly/opia | dull/vision |
| 2. An/alges/ic | no/sensation/pertaining to |
| 3. Audio/logist | hearing/one who studies |
| 4. Blepharopt/itis | eyelid/ inflammation of |
| 5. Cerumin/ous | Wax/substance |
| 6. Conjunctiv/a | To join together/membrane, lining, eyelid and eyeball |
| 7. Di/plopia | double/vision |
| 8. Ex/ophthalmia | out/eye/condition |
| 9. Hordeolum | stye |
| 10. Kera/titis | cornea/inflammation |
| 11. Ophthalmo/logist | eye/one who specializes in the study of |
| 12. Op/tic/ian | vision/pertaining to/one who |
| 13. Opto/metr/ist | vision/measure/one who |
| 14. Ot/algia | ear/pain |
| 15. Oto/sclerosis | ear/hardening |
| 16. Ptosis | drooping |
| 17. Re/fract/ion | again/bend/condition |
| 18. Sebo/rrhea | sebum/flowing |
| 19. Tinni/tus | ringing/a |
| 20. Vitre/ous | glassy/chemical or substance |

## B. Learning Level: Comprehension

1. Label the parts of the eye on the figure. Illustrate how light enters and where vision occurs.

   Note to Instructors: The figure is on page 560 in text. Review anatomy with students.

2. Illustrate the parts of the ear on the figure below. Next to it, draw the organ of Corti.

   Note to Instructors: The figure is on page 577 in text. Review anatomy with students.

## C. Learning Level: Application

1. Choose the description that best describes the test or procedure given. Put the description next to the correct letter for the test.

| | | | | |
|---|---|---|---|---|
| a. | 3 | Most routine test | 1. | Views fine details of anterior eye |
| b. | 6 | Ophthalmoscope | 2. | Differentiates hearing variances in each ear |
| c. | 1 | Slit-lamp | 3. | Visual acuity |
| d. | 5 | Snellen | 4. | Used in persons over 40 |
| e. | 7 | Ishihara | 5. | Distance visual acuity |
| f. | 2 | Weber | 6. | Examines retina and optic nerve |
| g. | 8 | Rinne | 7. | Color vision test |
| h. | 4 | Near vision acuity | 8. | Compares air and bone conduction |

2. Give the medical name for the following layperson terms and conditions. State the cause of the disorder.

| | | |
|---|---|---|
| a. | Pinkeye | conjunctivitis—bacteria or virus |
| b. | Nearsighted | myopia—light focuses in front of retina |
| c. | Farsighted | hyperopia—eyeball too short and light cannot focus on retina |
| d. | Cross-eyed | strabismus—weak muscles pull eye inward or outward |
| e. | Droopy-eyed | blepharoptosis—eyelid muscle or tissue weakens |
| f. | Increased eye pressure | glaucoma—obstruction of the canal of Sclem prevents fluid from being reabsorbed |
| g. | Ear infection | otis externa or otis media—bacteria or fungus |
| h. | Ruptured eardrum | myringorrhexis—ruptured tympanic membrane |

## D. Learning Level: Analysis

1. Contrast and distinguish the use of the following visual acuity tests.

| | | |
|---|---|---|
| a. | Snellen | distance visual acuity screening for over 4 to 5 years to adult |
| b. | Picture chart with animals | for children and nonreaders |
| c. | E chart | generally for nonreaders and children |

2. Choose the procedures the physician could be expected to perform for the following conditions.

| | | |
|---|---|---|
| a. | Eye infection | medication instillation |
| b. | Ear drainage | examination, not irrigation or medication if tympanic rupture |
| c. | Eye drainage | possible irrigation, medication, cleaning of debris or hordeolum before medication |
| d. | Eye foreign body | examination, gentle irrigation by physician |
| e. | Impacted cerumen | examination, irrigation by qualified medical assistant |

3. Which of the above procedures require aseptic technique? All of them

## E. Learning Level: Synthesis

What would you expect to do when assisting the physician and patient in the following examinations? What, if any, barrier protection would you use?

1. The patient is called to the clinical area and you note a patch over the right eye. He states he has something in his eye.

   Answer: sterile setup for examination for foreign body and eye irrigation

2. Your patient comes into the examining room with red, watery, itching eyes and states, "This has been going on for 4 days and this morning some dried drainage made them hard to open." There are crusts around the eyelids. Patient has no fever and states he has no allergies or hay fever.

   Answer: setup for examination and possible eye irrigation, soaks and medication, i.e., sterile equipment

3. Mother brings in Robby, who is rubbing his ear and saying "In dere, in dere." What do you think Robby is saying and what does it possibly mean? What equipment will you get ready for the physician?

   Answer: Robby is saying, "In there, in there." Could mean it hurts or he put something in his ear. Get otoscope, equipment to remove foreign body, ear forceps, and equipment to irrigate ear

## F. Learning Level: Evaluation

Before assigning this exercise, demonstrate the proper technique for testing distance visual acuity as in Procedure 31-1. Instructors may use this exercise to check students' accuracy and identify problems in using the Snellen test.

## PART 2 COMPETENCY CHALLENGE

There are six procedures in this chapter. There are no procedures on the CD-ROM. All of the procedures must be practiced to develop competence. The procedure instructions are very specific, and the illustrations in the 8th Edition Textbook very clear. First, demonstrate the procedures to the students. Give suggestions and methods for practice at home. Students may use dolls or practice with another student. Practice must be accomplished using sterile technique. Do this for Procedure 31-3, Irrigating the Patient's Eye; Procedure 31-4, Instilling Eye Medication; Procedure 31-5, Irrigating the Patient's Ear; and Procedure 31-6, Instilling Ear Medication. All procedures are located at the end of the chapter in the Mastery Manual.

## PART 3 CLINICAL APPLICATIONS

1. Case 3 on the CD-ROM concerns Robbie Soto, a 4 ½-month-old child whose mother thinks her child may have an ear infection. Babies often have narrow ear canals, and cerumen accumulates. Describe how you would irrigate this child's ear if ordered to do so. What is the anatomic difference in a child's and adult's ear which affects the method of irrigation?

   Answer: Ear would be irrigated with small 1 cc syringe. In adult ear canal, pull pinna up and back; in child, pull pinna straight down. MA should not atempt procedure unless trained in pediatrics.

2. In the office in which you are working, there are medical assistants who did not go to any school. The physician tells "one of you" to irrigate the patient's ear to remove cerumen. The "untrained medical assistant" has been caring for the patient and says she will do it. Later on you see the patient leaving and you say goodbye. She says, "Goodbye forever. I am never letting anyone here touch me again." What do you do?

   Answer: Allow students to come up with as many actions as possible. Some questions to ask include:

   Does student get patient to explain?

   Does medical assistant try to correct problem?

   Was other medical assistant qualified according to your state laws?

   Is this relevant?

   Does medical assistant ask co-worker what happened?

   Is this reported at all and, if so, to whom—manager or physician?

3. The textbook indicates there are opportunities for Medical Assistant multiskilled advancement in the fields of ophthalmology and otology. Some resource sites are:

   http://www.yahoo.com/Health/Medicine/Organizations/Professional Medical_Associations_and_Societies/ **This is an area for research.**

   http://www.yahoo.com/Health/Employment/ **For jobs associated with these specialties, search Yahoo for Ophthalmic + technician.**

   Also direct students to the Dictionary of Occupational Titles.

# 32

# Assisting in Gastroenterology and Proctology

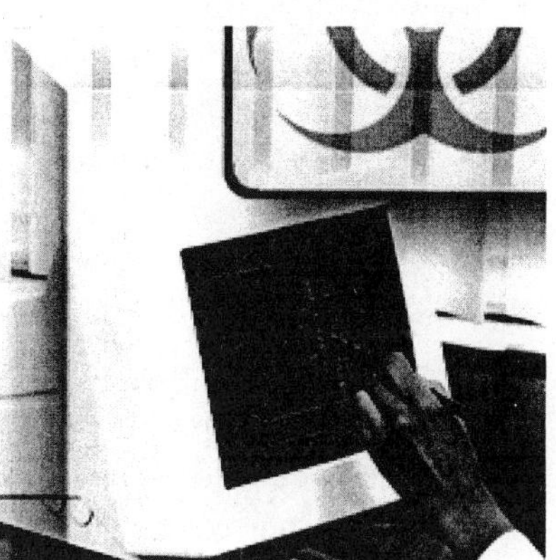

This chapter contains information and procedures of a very personal nature. Examination of and procedures on the lower GI tract are potentially frightening, upsetting, and represent loss of dignity and control to many patients. Most of the procedures will have to be simulated, or in the case of Procedure 32-3, students may perform the testing using their own samples. It is suggested that students do this, as it greatly increases their awareness of patient feelings, allowing the medical assistant to become more supportive and empathetic.

## USING THE LEARNING SYSTEM

### 1. MEDICAL ASSISTING ENTRY-LEVEL CONTENT AND COMPETENCIES

CONTENT

- Applications of medical terminology
- Anatomy and physiology for all body systems
- Common pathology and disease
- Diagnostic/treatment modalities
- Asepsis and infection control
- Specimen collection and processing
- Diagnostic testing
- Patient care
- Legal guidelines and requirements for health care
- Medical ethics and related issues
- Risk management
- Basic principles of psychology
- Recognition and response to verbal and nonverbal communication
- Adaptations for individual needs
- Job readiness
- Personal attributes

COMPETENCIES

- All fundamental principles of handwashing, autoclaving, sterilizing, standard precautions
- Prepare and maintain examination and treatment areas
- Prepare patient for and assist with routine and specialty examinations
- Prepare patient for and assist with specialty procedures and treatments
- Recognize and respond to verbal and nonverbal communication
- Identify and respond to issues of confidentiality
- Document appropriately
- Instruct patients according to needs
- Identify community resources
- Provide instruction for health maintenance and disease prevention
- Instruct patients in collection of specimens
- Perform specialty noninvasive diagnostic tests
- Use methods of quality control
- Screen and follow up test results
- Demonstrate use and care of patient equipment

## 2. MEDICAL ASSISTING ENTRY-LEVEL CURRICULUM INTERFACE

| TEXTBOOK OBJECTIVES | LEARNING SYSTEM LOCATION | MA CURRICULUM |
|---|---|---|
| **Cognitive** | | **Content** |
| 1. Describe the three primary functions of the GI system | • Text p. 592<br>• Manual Part 1-A | • Applications of medical terminology<br>• Anatomy and physiology for all body systems |
| 2. Identify major functions of the system and describe physiology of each phase | • Text pp. 592–594<br>• Manual Part 1-A | • Same as #1 |
| 3. Name the six fundamental aspects of the gastrointestinal system | • Text p. 592<br>• Manual Part 1-A | • Same as #1 |
| 4. List eight diseases or disorders of the gastrointestinal system and the signs, symptoms, methods of diagnosis, and treatment for each | • Text pp. 594–602<br>• Manual Part 1-B | • Common pathology and disease<br>• Diagnostic/treatment modalities<br>• Asepsis and infection control<br>• Specimen collection and processing<br>• Diagnostic testing<br>• Patient care<br>• Legal guidelines and requirements for health care |
| 5. Describe the significance of the gastrointestinal system and its relationship with other body systems | • Text p. 603<br>• Manual Part 1-B | • Anatomy and physiology for all body systems<br>• Patient care<br>• Common pathology and disease<br>• Basic principles of psychology |

| TEXTBOOK OBJECTIVES | LEARNING SYSTEM LOCATION | MA CURRICULUM |
|---|---|---|
| **Cognitive** | | **Content** |
| 6. Define hepatitis and describe the similarities and differences of the five types | • Text pp. 602–603<br>• Manual Part 1-C | • Common pathology and disease<br>• Diagnostic testing<br>• Patient care<br>• Legal guidelines and requirements for health care |
| 7. Identify the methods used to diagnose gallstones | • Text p. 605<br>• Manual Part 1-E<br>• Operative report | • Diagnostic/treatment modalities<br>• Asepsis and infection control<br>• Specimen collection and processing<br>• Diagnostic testing |
| 8. Identify the types of disorders that might be referred to a proctologist | • Text p. 607<br>• Manual Part 1-E | • Common pathology and disease<br>• Risk management<br>• Adaptations for individual needs |
| 9. List 10 possible laboratory procedures that could be ordered to assist the physician in obtaining a diagnosis | • Text pp. 610–615<br>• Manual Part 1-C | • Job readiness<br>• Personal attributes<br>• Medical ethics and related issues<br>• Diagnostic testing |
| 10. Explain the indication of a positive occult blood screening | • Text p. 612<br>• Manual Part 2 | • Diagnostic testing<br>• Risk management<br>• Basic principles of psychology |
| 11. List types of laboratory samples that can be obtained during endoscopic procedures | • Text p. 613<br>• Manual Part 1-E | • Diagnostic testing<br>• Adaptations for individual needs<br>• Risk management |
| **Performance** | | **Competencies** |
| 1. Demonstrate the medical assistant's role during the physical examination of the gastrointestinal area | • Text pp. 605–609<br>• Procedure 32-1<br>• Manual Part 2 | • All fundamental principles of handwashing, autoclaving, sterilizing, standard precautions<br>• Prepare and maintain examination and treatment areas<br>• Prepare patient for and assist with routine and specialty examinations |

*chart continues on following page*

**MEDICAL ASSISTING ENTRY-LEVEL CURRICULUM INTERFACE continued**

| TEXTBOOK OBJECTIVES | LEARNING SYSTEM LOCATION | MA CURRICULUM |
|---|---|---|
| Performance | | Competencies |
| 2. Demonstrate the preparation of a patient for a colorectal procedure | • Procedure 32-1<br>• Manual Part 2 | • Prepare patient and assist with specialty procedures and treatments<br>• Recognize and respond to verbal and nonverbal communication<br>• Instruct patients according to needs |
| 3. Assist with a colon examination | • Procedure 32-1<br>• Manual Part 2 | • Prepare patient and assist with specialty procedures and treatments<br>• Identify and respond to issues of confidentiality<br>• Document appropriately<br>• Instruct patients according to needs |
| 4. Accurately obtain a stool specimen collection | • Procedure 32-2<br>• Manual Part 2 | • Perform specialty noninvasive diagnostic tests<br>• Use methods of quality control<br>• Screen and follow up test results<br>• Demonstrate use and care of patient equipment<br>• Identify community resources |
| 5. Demonstrate the points that need to be explained to the patient who will be receiving a suppository or rectal ointment | • Procedure 32-3<br>• Manual Part 2 | • Instruct patients in collection of specimens<br>• Provide instruction for health maintenance and disease prevention |
| 6. Properly insert a rectal suppository | • Procedure 32-3<br>• Manual Part 2 | • Same as #3 |

## 3. RESOURCES

www.yahoo.com/health **Then proceed to gastrointestinal topics**

www.liverfoundation.org am **Liver Foundation. 1-800-465-4837**


1. Tierney, McPhee and Papadakis, Editors. Current Medical Diagnosis and Treatment 1998. Appleton and Lange, Norwalk, CT 1995
2. United Ostomy Association, Inc., 19772 MacArthur Blvd, Suite 200, Irvine CA 92612-2405
3. Juvenile Diabetes Foundation, 432 Park Ave, NY, NY 10010 1-212-889-7575
4. Alcoholics Anonymous, www.aa.org
5. National Foundation for Ileitis and Colitis, 1-800-343-3637
6. National Health Information, 1-800-336-4797—Patient education materials, information, and referrals
7. *PMA* March/April 1999, Viral Hepatitis.

## 4. LESSON PLAN Assisting in Gastrointestinal TIME 3 hours lecture, 12 hours lab

**Opening:** When possible, obtain a flexible sigmoidoscope. It is helpful to have a gastroenterologist come and talk about assisting and equipment for about an hour. Also, show some OTC medications and preparations such as Fleet enemas, laxatives, etc. Relate meds to the number of people who self-medicate before seeing a professional.

**Pretest:** Pretest with medical terminology word parts by building words from vocabulary list, text p. 591. This helps students to realize they know much of the vocabulary if it is kept simple. Put up the words *masticate, absorb, biopsy, digest,* and *eliminate* and have students define them. These are all English words with common applications.

**Objectives:** The objectives are in the textbook. Review them before beginning discussion. Encourage student questions.

**Content:** The topic of gastrointestinal specialty is so large that only the most common disorders are presented here. Using the Mastery Manual after lecture and before evaluation on procedures will allow students to meet the chapter objectives easily. The information presented is basic, and students should learn it well enough to be able to sit in lab and complete the manual Part 1 as a posttest.

1. Overview
2. Anatomy and Physiology—Use Procedure #32-1.
3. Major Diseases of the GI System
   Food Poisoning; Oral Tumors and Cancer; Herpes Simplex (Cold Sores)
   Gastric and Duodenal Ulcers, Gastric Cancer; Hernias (Hiatal, Abdominal, Inguinal)
   Ulcerative Colitis; Hemorrhoids (Piles)
4. Diseases of the Accessory Organs—Discuss Signs and Symptoms; Diagnosis and Treatment; Viral Hepatitis; Cirrhosis of the Liver; Cholelithiasis
5. Medical Assistant's Role
   A. Assisting with the Examination
      1. Proctologic Examination
         a. Patient Preparation
         b. Patient Positioning on a Proctologic Table
      2. Sigmoidoscopy and Colonoscopy Procedure 32-1: Assisting with a Colon Exam
   B. Laboratory Tests
      1. Occult Blood Screening Procedure 32-2: Stool Collection
      2. Endoscopic Observations
         a. Rectal Suppository Medication Procedure 32-3
         b. Instilling of Ointment

**Lab:** Have one student take role of physician and have another simulate assisting with the colon examination. Other procedures may be practiced and simulated on a mannequin. Students need reinforcement and discussions of privacy, dignity, confidentiality. This is another place to discuss personal attitudes about sensitive topics such as rectal functions.

**Assignment:** Prepare to be evaluated for procedure competency. Be able to state purpose of steps.

**Posttest:** Name as many signs and symptoms of GI disease as possible or have students write the medical assistant's role in examination of abdomen and colon. Use the Examaster testbank questions from the chapter.

## 5. MASTERY MANUAL ANSWERS

### PART 1 CONTENT MASTERY

### A. Learning Level: Knowledge

1. Place the name of the primary function of the GI system next to its description. Then number the order of the phases.
   - a. Food is mechanically and chemically changed. digestion #1
   - b. Feces are product of last phase. elimination #3
   - c. Food products pass through small intestine walls. absorption #2
2. Which of the above functions is further divided into other separate functions?
   Answer: digestion
3. What are the names of those other functions? Ingestion, mastication, peristalsis

### B. Learning Level: Comprehension

1. Without referring to your 8th Edition Textbook, fill in the chart below.

| Disease | Signs and Symptoms | Method of Diagnosis | Treatment |
|---|---|---|---|
| 1. Food poisoning | Severe abdominal cramping, N and V, malaise, fever | Pt. hx, stool and blood cultures | Maintain electrolyte balance; medication to control nausea |
| 2. Oral cancers | Small lumps; ulcers; sore or slit lip that will not heal | Biopsy | Surgical resection or excision |
| 3. Herpes simplex | Blisters around mouth and lips | Small, fluid-filled blisters, itch, pain, ulcer, may spread | Antiviral drugs, rest, analgesics |
| 4. Gastric ulcer | Intense pain in abdominal region about 2 hours after food, N and V, blood in vomit or feces | UGI series, endoscopy, biopsy, stool test, Hg and Hct | Histamine $H_2$ blockers, antibiotic; diet modification |
| 5. Gastric cancer | Usually silent or complication of ulcer; weight loss, malaise, anemia | Upper GI series; endoscopy; gastric analysis; biopsy | Gastrectomy; radiation; chemotherapy |
| 6. Hernias—Abnormal protrusion of a body part through structure holding it in place | Abdominal, inguinal may be reducible; hiatal causes indigestion due to regurgitation, pain on lying down, and relief on sitting | Palpation, Valsalva's maneuver, x-ray, upper GI series, CT | Herniorrhaphy, herniplasty; antacids; anticholinergics; histamine $H_2$ antagonists; diet modification |
| 7. Ulcerative colitis—Chronic inflammatory disease of colon lining | Bloody diarrhea, abdominal cramping, urge to defecate, loose stools or mucus in BM | Stool analysis, patient hx.; Hg, CBC, colonoscopy, biopsy | Dietary modification, antiemetics, surgical resection |
| 8. Hemorrhoids—Varicose veins of anus and rectum | Pain, itching, burning, discomfort straining, bleeding | Palpation, proctoscopy, Hg, RBC | Stool softeners, high-fiber diet, ointments, hemorrhoidectomy |

2. Hepatitis is the most common disease of health care workers. National law requires that the employer immunize persons employed in health care. It is essential to know the information below. Fill in this chart.

| **Disease Transmission** | **Signs and Symptoms** | **Method of Diagnosis** | **Treatment** | **Prevention** |
|---|---|---|---|---|
| Hepatitis A HAV-contaminated water/food | Usually asymptomatic. Fever, malaise, low WBC, abnormal liver tests | Anti-HAV antibody | Bed rest—immune globulin to all close contacts | Vaccination; wash and scrub hands after toilet; household bleach to disinfect food surfaces |
| Hepatitis B Infected blood or blood products, maternal barrier, infected needles, tattoos | Insidious onset. Fever, malaise, arthralgia, anorexia, skin rash, URQ pain | HBsAG marker positive, low WBC, abnormal liver tests, jaundice | Antivirals; bed rest, pain medication, no alchohol; liver tests indicate severity and recovery; most severe form. May be chronic or fatal. | HBV immune globulin to contacts; vaccination |
| Hepatitis C 4% due to posttransfusion, 50% to IV drug use, body piercings | Usually asymptomatic, then malaise, fever, N and V, 50% become chronic | Immunoassay RIBA tests specific antigens | 50% become chronic; Interferon | Do not share razors, toothbrushes, needles |
| Hepatitis D | With Hepatitis B only | Same as B | Interferon, delta agent occurs with Hepatitis B. $HB_SAG$ marker | Clears when $HB_SAG$ marker clears |
| Hepatitis E Non-a non-b; waterborne | Mexico, India, Burma, Algeria | Same as B | No vaccine; boil water; Hepatitis B vaccine | High mortality rate; 10–20% in women |

## C. Learning Level: Application

1. Seven diagnostic and laboratory tests are listed. Write the GI function or disorder for which the physician may be looking.
   a. AST and ALT — liver damage
   b. Barium swallow — gastric ulcer
   c. Endoscopy — gastric, colon disorder
   d. Barium enema — cancer, polyps
   e. Occult blood — cancer, ulcerative colitis
   f. Sigmoidoscopy — any colon or sigmoid abnormalities
   g. Proctoscopy — cancer, hemorrhoids

2. Name three other tests, not listed above, that diagnose GI system disorder.
   Gastric analysis, biopsy, upper GI series, lower GI series

## D. Learning Level: Analysis

1. Examine the importance of the GI system to the rest of the body. How does it interact with other systems? What would happen if there were no GI system?
   Nutrients supplied through GI system, materials for growth, and repair must be synthesized. Cannot supplement completely without. Person would eventually expire.

2. List as many procedures for GI disorders that you can.

   See the charts in Part 1-C above and also the exercise in E-2 following. Have students write them on the board.

## E. Learning Level: Synthesis

1. After you have gowned the patient and taken the vital signs, you might ask the patient to point to an area that he says is painful. While inspecting the area, what skin markings or changes might you see?

   Scars, lesions, moles, petechiae, jaundice, bulges

   If the pain is under the right ribs, how would you describe it in your notes?

   RUQ or right hypochondriac region

2. Look up all the unknown terms in the operative report below. With your instructor, review the procedures performed on the patient and identify anatomic landmarks.

   Review all the terms with the students. Explain procedures using Figure 32-3 in text.

**PREOPERATIVE DIAGNOSIS:** Painless, obstructive jaundice (probable carcinoma head of pancreas).
**POSTOPERATIVE DIAGNOSIS:** Cancer, common duct distal to cystic duct, with complete obstruction (tentative, pending histology).
**PROCEDURES PERFORMED:**

1. Exploratory laparotomy.
2. Multiple punch biopsies of tumor.
3. Duodenotomy with pancreaticocholangiogram using the C-Arm, and cholangiogram using overhead x-ray.
4. Resection of:
   A) Distal common duct
   B) Head and uncinate process of the pancreas
   C) Antrum
   D) First and second part of the duodenum
5. Truncal vagotomy.
6. Pancreaticocholecystogastrojejunostomy and jejunojejunostomy.
7. Jejunal feeding tube (#12 Foley catheter).
8. Jackson-Pratt drainage of right subhepatic space.

**FINDINGS:** On entering this patient's abdomen, it was deeply stained with bilirubin. The liver was free of evidence of metastases. The gallbladder was tense. The common duct was dilated to greater than 1 cm. A firm area, distal to the cystic duct and confluent with the duodenum and head of pancreas, was noted after tedious dissection. Multiple punch biopsies were taken of the hardest areas in this tumorous process, but though the specimens were all suspicious for carcinoma, on frozen section they were not conclusive. The duodenum was not grossly involved in the process and there was no evidence of obstruction of the duodenum. The stomach was normal. The small and large bowel and omentum were normal and free of evidence of disease, and there was only one lymph node encountered adjacent to the specimen which was submitted in continuity with the specimen. The common duct was totally obstructed, approximately 2 cm distal to the entrance of the cystic duct. There was no evidence of cholelithiasis or choledocholithiasis, and the bile was thick and dark, greenish-black. The ampulla of Vater appeared normal. When cannulated and pancreaticocholangio-gram obtained, the pancreatic duct of Santorini was noted, but no dye progressed up the common duct. A cholangiogram was obtained using an angiocath, and the common duct was found totally obstructed, as mentioned above, greatly dilated, as were the gallbladder and intrahepatic radicals.

3. Name the medical specialty that would treat the following conditions.

| | |
|---|---|
| a. Coronary artery disease | CV |
| b. Tinnitus | Otology |
| c. Hordeolum | Ophthalmology |
| d. Influenza | Respiratory |
| e. Cirrhosis | GI |
| f. Aortic stenosis | CV |
| g. Hemorrhoids | GI |
| h. Ulcerative colitis | GI |
| i. Otitis media | Otology |
| j. Glaucoma | Ophthalmology |

## F. Learning Level: Evaluation

BH, a 50-year-old architect and new patient, comes to the gastroenterologist for treatment of recurrent cramping, mucus stool, and recently some blood streaking in the stool. The patient has 1/2 hour with the physician and in order to facilitate the time given the patient, the physician asks you to complete the history as much as possible. Mr. BH is 5′10″ and weighs 200 pounds. His Vital Signs are 162/100, P 110, R 24, and T 100. Patient is sweating excessively ("diaphoretic"). Patient says he has no real medical history. He gave up a pack a day for 30 years and quit 5 years ago, drinks at least one drink a night, and doesn't exercise as he is too busy building his business. No immediate family or siblings with a history of heart, lung, or cancer problems. Father died 15 years ago, but "we weren't close." Patient uses the bathroom and provides specimen for Hematest. There is a blue color around the smear.

1. Name three health risks in this patient's history.
   a. Hx smoking and drinking
   b. Overweight
   c No exercise

2. What abnormal findings did you note?

   Weight, blood pressure, pulse, respirations, temperature, and blood in stool

## PART 2 COMPETENCY CHALLENGE

There are three procedures in this chapter in which the student will develop mastery. Use the supplies list from the procedures in the textbook to ensure that all necessary supplies are ready for demonstration and practice. Have students purchase glycerin suppositories and a box of nonsterile gloves for these and subsequent procedures.

1. You are expected to be able to demonstrate the medical assistant's role in a gastrointestinal examination. This includes the entire GI tract from mouth to anus. On a separate paper write a procedure for assisting with the gastrointestinal examination, including all the necessary procedural steps. This is not the same procedure as assisting with the colon examination, although many steps may be extracted from this procedure.
2. Demonstrate your procedure, then proceed directly to practice and demonstrate Procedure 31-1, Assisting with the Colon Examination.
3. While this may be difficult, you will need to complete Procedure 32-2 in the following manner. Obtain three personal samples from home, observing dietary restrictions. Bring the samples to the lab and test them following the procedure. Record the results.

Answer the following questions.

a. When do patients routinely have this test performed?

   With every adult physical examination and about every 5 years for patients over 50

b. How do you think they feel about doing the test?

   Uncomfortable and squeamish

c. What do you think the percentage of home compliance is?

   Less than 50%

d. What is the significance of a positive test?

   Slow bleeding from some spot in intestinal wall

4. Follow Procedure 32-3 located at the end of the chapter, and using a lab mannequin, insert a glycerin rectal suppository. When ready, demonstrate the procedure to your instructor. Be sure to include the pertinent points of explanation before starting the procedure—even though you are talking to a dummy!

## PART 3 CLINICAL APPLICATIONS

It is important to review the legal implications and medical assistant's responsibilities for giving medications, especially if the unit on this topic has not been completed. Students may not give medications until the units on administering medications and competencies have been successfully evaluated. How does one prevent errors?

1. Review the legal implications of giving suppositories in the medical office.

   How often would you imagine suppositories are given in the medical office? Which specialties use them the most? What are the bookkeeping requirements when giving scheduled drugs? Are all suppositories considered medication? How quickly would you expect a suppository to be absorbed and begin acting?

2. Develop a teaching plan to accompany stool specimen collection, Procedure 32-2. Use the activity from Chapter 28. Plan some tools to help the patient remember the diet and the rules.

# 33

# Assisting in Gynecology and Obstetrics

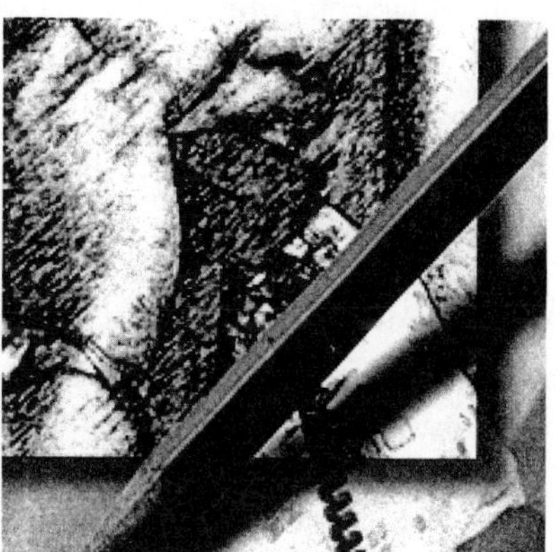

It is important to explain to students that an increased number of basic specialty examinations are being performed in the primary care office. Many such offices have an OB/GYN nurse practitioner, who may perform gynecological examination, culdoscopy, and colposcopy. Students therefore need to have a wide range of skills in this area. They need to understand conception choices, recognize symptoms of complications related to pregnancy, and prepare and assist with procedures testing for STDs. This is a very good time to clear up misconceptions in these areas. State and federal laws related to sterilization and care of minors should be reviewed.

## USING THE LEARNING SYSTEM

### 1. MEDICAL ASSISTING ENTRY-LEVEL CONTENT AND COMPETENCIES

CONTENT

- Applications of medical terminology
- Anatomy and physiology for all body systems
- Common pathology and disease
- Diagnostic/treatment modalities
- Asepsis and infection control
- Specimen collection and processing
- Diagnostic testing
- Patient care
- Legal guidelines and requirements for health care
- Medical ethics and related issues
- Risk management
- Basic principles of psychology
- Recognition of and response to verbal and nonverbal communication
- Adaptations for individual needs
- Job readiness
- Personal attributes

COMPETENCIES

- All fundamental principles of handwashing, autoclaving, sterilizing, standard precautions
- Prepare and maintain examination and treatment areas
- Prepare patient for and assist with routine and specialty examinations
- Prepare patient and assist with specialty procedures and treatments
- Recognize and respond to verbal and nonverbal communication
- Identify and respond to issues of confidentiality
- Document appropriately
- Instruct patients according to needs
- Identify community resources
- Provide instruction for health maintenance and disease prevention
- Instruct patients in collection of specimens
- Perform specialty noninvasive diagnostic tests
- Use methods of quality control
- Screen and follow up test results
- Demonstrate use and care of patient equipment

## 2. MEDICAL ASSISTING ENTRY-LEVEL CURRICULUM INTERFACE

| TEXTBOOK OBJECTIVES | LEARNING SYSTEM LOCATION | MA CURRICULUM |
|---|---|---|
| **Cognitive** | | **Content** |
| 1. Identify the major organs of the female reproductive system and explain the primary function of each | • Text pp. 619–620<br>• Manual Part 1-A<br>• Memory jogger #1 | • Applications of medical terminology<br>• Anatomy and physiology for all body systems |
| 2. Trace the ova through the three phases of menstruation | • Text pp. 620–621<br>• Manual Part 1-B | • Same as #1 |
| 3. Explain the physiology of pregnancy from conception through the three trimesters and parturition | • Text pp. 621–623<br>• Manual Part 1-C | • Same as #1 |
| 4. Identify the three types of pregnancy complications | • Text p. 623<br>• Memory jogger #5 | • Common pathology and disease |
| 5. List and explain the diseases and disorders that may affect the female | • Text pp. 625–628<br>• Manual Part 1-D | • Same as #4 |
| 6. Name and describe the seven sexually transmitted diseases | • Text pp. 628–630<br>• Manual Part 1-D | • Same as #4 |
| 7. Outline the medical assistant's role in the reproductive examination | • Text pp. 631–634<br>• Manual Part 1-D | • Diagnostic/treatment modalities<br>• Asepsis and infection control<br>• Specimen collection and processing<br>• Diagnostic testing<br>• Patient care |

| TEXTBOOK OBJECTIVES | LEARNING SYSTEM LOCATION | MA CURRICULUM |
|---|---|---|
| **Cognitive** | | **Content** |
| 7. Outline the medical assistant's role in the reproductive examination (continued) | | • Legal guidelines and requirements for health care<br>• Medical ethics and related issues<br>• Risk management<br>• Basic principles of psychology<br>• Recognition and response to verbal and nonverbal communication<br>• Adaptations for individual needs<br>• Job readiness<br>• Personal attributes |
| 8. Compare and contrast a yearly physical exam with an initial pregnancy examination | • Text p. 631<br>• Manual Part 1-D | • Diagnostic/treatment modalities<br>• Legal guidelines and requirements for health care |
| 9. Name and describe the medical assistant's role in seven diagnostic tests that may be done in evaluating the female reproductive system | • Text pp. 638–642<br>• Manual Part 1-F<br>• ⊕ CD-ROM | • Asepsis and infection control<br>• Specimen collection and processing<br>• Diagnostic testing<br>• Patient care<br>• Recognition and response to verbal and nonverbal communication<br>• Adaptations for individual needs<br>• Job readiness |
| 10. Define family planning and the three classifications of birth control that are used | • Text pp. 642–643<br>• Manual Part 1-D | • Diagnostic testing<br>• Patient care<br>• Legal guidelines and requirements for health care<br>• Medical ethics and related issues<br>• Risk management<br>• Basic principles of psychology<br>• Recognition of and response to verbal and nonverbal communication<br>• Adaptations for individual needs<br>• Job readiness<br>• Personal attributes |

*chart continues on following page*

## MEDICAL ASSISTING ENTRY-LEVEL CURRICULUM INTERFACE *continued*

| TEXTBOOK OBJECTIVES | LEARNING SYSTEM LOCATION | MA CURRICULUM |
|---|---|---|
| **Performance** | | **Competencies** |
| 1. Prepare the instruments and equipment for a female examination, including a Pap test | • Procedure 33-1<br>• Manual Part 2<br>• ⊕ CD-ROM | • All fundamental principles of handwashing, autoclaving, sterilizing, standard precautions<br>• Prepare and maintain examination and treatment areas<br>• Prepare patient for and assist with routine and specialty examinations.<br>• Instruct patients in collection of specimens<br>• Perform specialty noninvasive diagnostic tests<br>• Demonstrate use and care of patient equipment |
| 2. Teach a person how to perform a self-breast examination | • Procedure 33-2<br>• Manual Part 2<br>• ⊕ CD-ROM | • Instruct patients according to needs<br>• Identify community resources<br>• Provide instruction for health maintenance and disease prevention<br>• Identify and respond to issues of confidentiality<br>• Document appropriately |
| 3. Describe cryosurgery preparation to a patient | • Procedure 33-3<br>• Manual Part 2<br>• ⊕ CD-ROM | • Prepare patient and assist with specialty procedures and treatments<br>• Recognize and respond to verbal and nonverbal communication<br>• Use methods of quality control<br>• Screen and follow up test results<br>• Document appropriately |
| 4. Determine the estimated day of confinement when given the date of last menstrual period | • Procedure 33-3<br>• Manual Part 2<br>• ⊕ CD-ROM | • Same as #2 above |

## 3. RESOURCES

www.yahoo.com/health **There are many sites for reproductive health, diseases, treatments, etc.**

www.ahn.com **Anatomy and diseases**

www.cdc.gov

American Social Health Resource, PO Box 13827, Triangle Park, NC 27709 1-800-227-8922 is the STD hotline

Upjohn and GlaxoWellcome pharmaceutical companies have women's health issues on the Internet.

March of Dimes Birth Defects Foundation 1-914-428-7100
1275 Mamaroneck Ave., White Plains, NY 10605

## 4. LESSON PLAN OB/GYN

**TIME 3 hours lecture, 12 hours lab**

**Opening:** Ask how many students have had a gyn examination, Pap smear, or prenatal examination. Relate to feelings about dignity and how each responds. How does a person want to be treated during these exams? What are the barriers to people going and having these types of examinations?

**Pretest:** There is much new vocabulary in this chapter. Choose 10 words from the vocabulary list and ask students to define them. Most students will know the common words, and this will give them a feeling of success.

**Objectives:** Review with students and explain those that will be covered in class and in lab.

**Content:** Overview of the Female System

1. Anatomy and Physiology—Internal Organs, External and Mammary Glands; Functions
2. Menstruation—Follicular Phase Luteal Phase Menstrual Phase
3. Pregnancy
   First Trimester Second Trimester Third Trimester Parturition
4. Pregnancy Complications
   Abnormal Fertilization Improper Implantation Interruption of Pregnancy
   Abortion Spontaneous, Complete, Incomplete, Missed, Threatened, Induced
5. Diseases and Disorders
   Cervicitis Cervical Polyps Cystocele Endometriosis
   Fibrocystic Breast Fibroid Tumors Ovarian Cysts
   Pelvic Inflammatory Disease
   Rectocele Breast Cancer STDs Herpes Simplex Virus
   Gonorrhea Syphilis Trichomoniasis Candidiasis
   Chlamydia Acquired Immunodeficiency Syndrome
6. Medical Assistant's Role
   Examination Preparation
   Assisting with the Examination
   Breast Examination
   Abdominal Examination
   Pelvic Examination
   Post-Exam Duties
7. Diagnostic Testing
   Ultrasonogram Mammogram Papanicolaou Test Schiller's Test
   Colposcopy Cryosurgery Pregnancy Testing Lunar Method
8. Family Planning

*lesson plan continued on following page*

**LESSON PLAN continued**

9. Sterilization Procedures
10. Patient education opportunities
11. Legal and ethical considerations. This topic alone could use 12 hours! Major points revolve around fertility drugs, abortion, clones, proper preparation for procedures, medicating for procedural pain.

**Lab:** Students may set patients up and simulate assisting with the gynecological examination. Students should be able to identify the equipment needed for examination and testing for STDs. Students should actually complete the teaching of another student for breast self-examination. This may be done on a teaching mannequin. Have students calculate EDD by giving days of LMP. Cryosurgery is painful and may be very painful; most offices pre-medicate patients before the procedure. The CD-ROM ⊕ has one case, which requires assisting with the female examination and Pap smear. This is the case for Mrs. Ferguson. Proceed to this case and complete all activities. Then have students practice and be evaluated on.

Procedure 33-1: Assisting with Gynecologic Examination
Procedure 33-2: Teaching the Patient Breast Self-Examination
Procedure 33-3: Preparing the Patient for Cryosurgery
Procedure 33-4: Establishing the EDD Using Nagel's Rule and Lunar Method

**Assignment:** Independently practice procedures and complete Mastery Manual activities. Study pediatric chapter after last class on Chapter 33.

**Posttest:** Choose test questions from Examaster testbank to meet objectives and MA curriculum.

## 5. MASTERY MANUAL ANSWERS

### PART 1 CONTENT MASTERY

### A. Learning Level: Knowledge

1. Label the parts in the figures below.
   Instructors: see 8th Edition Textbook pp. 619–620
   Ingestion, mastication, peristalsis

### B. Learning Level: Comprehension

Complete the chart to trace the menstrual cycle. This chart may be enlarged and used for teaching purposes.

| Phase | Ovary Action | Hormone Produced | Endometrial Change |
|---|---|---|---|
| Follicular | Produce mature graafian follicle | Estrogen | Grows and thickens, increased blood supply |
| Luteal | Follicle bursts from ovary | Progesterone | Extensive growth of potential implantation layer |
| Menstrual | Follicle (egg) not fertilized | None | Endometrial tissue sloughs |

## C. Learning Level: Application

1. How are STDs transmitted? **through transmission of bodily fluids**

2. Fill in the chart for the following examinations

| STD | Supplies Needed | DiagnosisTest and Lesions | Treatment |
|---|---|---|---|
| Trichomoniasis | Microscope and slide | Protozoa—discharge foul, profuse, yellow, frothy | Must treat both partners with antibiotic |
| Candidiasis | Microscope, slide, 10% KOH on slide | Yeast-like fungus | OTC Vagisil, Monistat—antifungals |
| Gonorrhea | Microscope. Gram stain, obtain culture | Greenish yellow | Antibiotic |
| Herpes Simplex; Lesions highly contagious | Culture tube and swabs | HSV-2; Observation of vesicles, tissue cultures | Antiviral meds and sulfa creams |
| Chlamydia | Lab—serologic tests and observation | Chlamydia trachomatis: urethritis, burning, PID, epididymitis | Antibiotics for both partners |

3. Name the essential information that is contained in the gyn history.
   a. age at menarche
   b. regularity of cycle
   c. amount and duration of flow
   d. menstrual problems, difficulties
   e. intermenstrual or postmenopausal bleeding
   f. vaginal discharge
   g. LMP

## D. Learning Level: Analysis

1. Mrs. Nuygen calls the office. She has missed her period. She took a pregnancy test 2 weeks ago and it was positive. She was to see Dr. Lawler in 2 weeks, but yesterday she started having pain in her LLQ and today it is getting worse.
   a. What actions do you take?
   Notify doctor, who may send for immediate ultrasound or have her come in.
   b. Why? **Could be ectopic pregnancy or mild infection**
   **c. Do you have any idea what the problem might be?**
   **MA not to dx but UQ pain may indicate many things, including ectopic pregnancy.**

2. Name common female diseases for each category.

| Infectious | Growth disorders | Inflammatory |
|---|---|---|
| STDs | Cysts | Cystocele |
| Cervicitis | Cancer | Endometriosis |
| Urethritis | Polyps | |

3. List seven STDs according to the common name and causative organism.

| Bacteria | Virus | Fungus | Protozoa |
|---|---|---|---|
| Gonorrhea | HSV | Candida | Trichomoniasis |
| Syphilis | HIV | | |
| Chlamydia | | | |

## E. Learning Level: Synthesis

1. Consider the situation and answer the question. A patient comes to the physician office. She was referred by a friend and is visiting from out of town. Patient is complaining of numbness in legs and feet which just started in past week. She states she is on AZT and acyclovir for a "viral infection."What diseases do you know to be treated with more than one antiviral drug at a time?

   HIV infection There are now others, but not STDs

2. Describe the extra components added to a physical examination when it is the first prenatal visit. List the supplies will you need.

   Extra parts: obtain pelvic measurements—ultrasound, serologic tests, lab tests

   Preparation and supplies: empty bladder, slides, urinalysis

## F. Learning Level: Evaluation

1. Measure the Estimated Date of Confinement using both Nagel's rule and the lunar method.

| LMP | EDD—Nagel's Rule | EDD—Lunar method |
|---|---|---|
| July 16, 1999 | LMP - 3 mos + 1 year + 7 days = April 23, 2000 | LMP + 9 mos + 7 days =4/23/2000 |
| August 31, 1999 | June 8, 2000 | same |
| December 13, 1999 | Sept. 20, 2000 | same |

2. Think about the differences in the medical assistant's role in the diagnostic tests listed below. Give your opinion. Which tests are more difficult on the patient? Which are more difficult on the medical assistant? Fill in below. What supplies are needed, and what does the patient need to be taught?

| Test | Description | Location/Supplies | Teaching |
|---|---|---|---|
| Ultrasound | Transducer on abdomen. No pain, may be image alone or image and sound Doppler | If in office—jelly and machine | Nonpainful, visual picture, no x-ray |
| Mammogram | X-ray compression of each breast | Diagnostic imaging office | May cause severe pressure, especially in large or very small breasts |
| Pap test | Sampling of cells at head of cervix | Microscopic slides, fixative for smear, slide tops, vaginal spatula, lab slips | Should not be painful, keep patient covered, maintain dignity |
| Schiller test | Iodine painted on mucous membrane | Iodine, speculum, flashlight | Maintain dignity |
| Colposcopy | Visual examination of vagina and cervix with microscope and camera | Colposcope, speculum | Discomfort or bleeding only when biopsy done |
| Cryosurgery | Placing probe against problem area with liquid nitrogen for 3–4 minutes to freeze and kill cells | | Premedicate; painful and may have slight bleeding or watery discharge |

## PART 2 COMPETENCY CHALLENGE

1. The CD-ROM ⊕ has one case, which requires assisting with the female examination and Pap smear. This is the case for Mrs. Ferguson. Proceed to this case and complete all activities.
2. Students should be able to practice the procedures with video demonstration. You might want to review placing the patient into lithotomy position when students are ready to practice.

   33-1 Assisting with the Female Examination

   33-2 Teaching the Patient Self-Breast Examination

   33-3 Preparing the Patient for Cryosurgery

   33-4 Establish the EDD Using Nagels and the Lunar Method

## PART 3 CLINICAL APPLICATIONS

1. Describe the methods and list advantages and disadvantages.

   The methods are: oral contraceptives; RU486; diaphragm; spermicides; IUD; condom; rhythm method; Norplant; Depo-Provera
2. Patient comes in for her yearly gyn examination and Pap smear. She is on oral contraceptives and uses foam also "because 5% of the people get pregnant anyway." She tells you she douched last night so the foam would not affect her test. In addition, she did not wear perfume. Do you have any thoughts on this conversation?

   Physician needs to be notified because the douche may interfere with the Pap smear.

3. SBE Procedure 33-2.
4. Discuss legal and ethical implications of this situation. Mother is upset because she got a bill for services and daughter will not discuss it with her.

   Mother has to pay as child is dependent. Physician office may not give out information—neither can physician if treatment is contraception-related in some states. In other states, this information may be given to parents. Check your state law.

# 34

# Assisting in Pediatrics

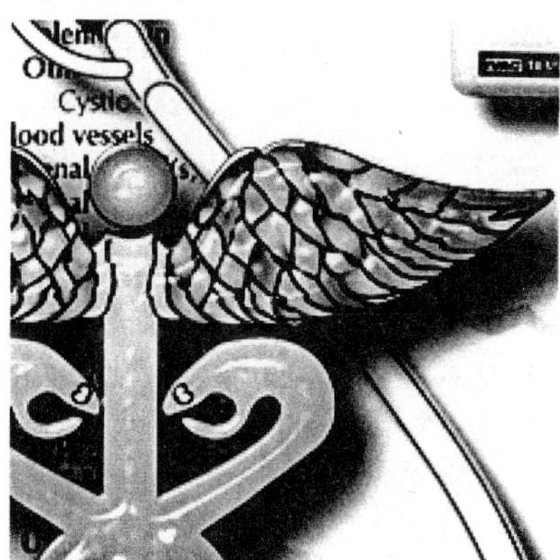

The biggest challenges to working with children are eliciting cooperation and compensating our procedures to their small sizes. Children require special procedures and medication dosages. They have different reactions than adults. In the chapter the Medical Assistant student will begin to learn about childhood disease, vaccinations, and other procedures, which will help the student deal with children in an effective and competent manner. The performance objective for pediatric medications will be covered in Chapter 49. If real children can be used for the attainment of competency, students will have much better job readiness to serve their externship and be employed in a pediatric office.

## USING THE LEARNING SYSTEM

### 1. MEDICAL ASSISTING ENTRY-LEVEL CONTENT AND COMPETENCIES

CONTENT

- Applications of medical terminology
- Anatomy and physiology for all body systems
- Common pathology and disease
- Diagnostic/treatment modalities
- Asepsis and infection control
- Specimen collection and processing
- Diagnostic testing
- Patient care
- Legal guidelines and requirements for health care
- Medical ethics and related issues
- Risk management
- Basic principles of psychology
- Recognition and response to verbal and nonverbal communication
- Adaptations for individual needs
- Job readiness
- Personal attributes
- Developmental stages of the life cycle
- Heredity, cultural, and environmental influences on behavior

COMPETENCIES

- All fundamental principles of handwashing, autoclaving, sterilizing, standard precautions
- Prepare and maintain examination and treatment areas
- Prepare patient for and assist with routine and specialty examinations
- Prepare patient for and assist with specialty procedures and treatments
- Recognize and respond to verbal and nonverbal communication
- Identify and respond to issues of confidentiality
- Document appropriately
- Instruct patients according to needs
- Identify community resources
- Provide instruction for health maintenance and disease prevention
- Instruct patients in collection of specimens
- Perform specialty noninvasive diagnostic tests
- Use methods of quality control
- Screen and follow up test results
- Demonstrate use and care of patient equipment

## 2. MEDICAL ASSISTING ENTRY-LEVEL CURRICULUM INTERFACE

| TEXTBOOK OBJECTIVES | LEARNING SYSTEM LOCATION | MA CURRICULUM |
|---|---|---|
| **Cognitive** | | **Content** |
| 1. Compare the different growth and development patterns | • Text pp. 646–648<br>• Manual Part 1-A | • Developmental stages of the life cycle<br>• Heredity, cultural, and environmental influences on behavior |
| 2. Name and briefly explain the major diseases explained in the chapter | • Text pp. 650–653<br>• Manual Part 1-B | • Common pathology and disease<br>• Diagnostic/treatment modalities<br>• Basic principles of psychology<br>• Recognition and response to verbal and nonverbal communication<br>• Adaptations for individual needs<br>• Job readiness<br>• Personal attributes |
| 3. Understand how vaccines are made | • Text p. 653<br>• Manual Part 1 | • Diagnostic/treatment modalities<br>• Risk management |
| 4. List the AAP-approved immunizations and appropriate age at which each is given | • Text p. 654<br>• Manual Part 1<br>• Internet site | • Asepsis and infection control<br>• Adaptations for individual needs<br>• Job readiness |

| TEXTBOOK OBJECTIVES | LEARNING SYSTEM LOCATION | MA CURRICULUM |
|---|---|---|
| **Cognitive** | | **Content** |
| 5. Compare and contrast the well-child and the sick-child examinations | • Text pp. 655–656<br>• Manual Part 1 | • Developmental stages of the life cycle<br>• Heredity, cultural, and environmental influences on behavior |
| 6. Understand the medical assistant's role in the pediatric examination | • Text p. 657<br>• Manual Part 2 | • Specimen collection and processing<br>• Diagnostic testing<br>• Patient care<br>• Legal guidelines and requirements for health care<br>• Medical ethics and related issues |
| 7. Be able to obtain accurate pediatric measurements | • Text p. 658<br>• Manual Part 2 | • Obtain vital signs<br>• Legal guidelines and requirements for health care |
| 8. Accurately obtain pediatric vital signs | • Text pp. 664–665<br>• Manual Part 2<br>• Procedure 34-2 | • Obtain vital signs<br>• Legal guidelines and requirements for health care |
| 9. Understand when and how to apply restraints | • Text p. 667<br>• Manual Part 2<br>• Procedure 34-3 | • Adaptations for individual needs<br>• Job readiness |
| 10. Show knowledge in handling child abuse | • Text p. 671<br>• Manual Part 3 | • Adaptations for individual needs<br>• Job readiness |
| 11. Spell and define the terms in the vocabulary | • Manual Part 1-E | • Applications of medical terminology<br>• Anatomy and physiology for all body systems |
| **Performance** | | **Competencies** |
| 1. Properly obtain head measurement | • Manual Part 2 | • Prepare patient for and assist with routine and specialty examinations<br>• Document appropriately<br>• Instruct patients according to needs |
| 2. Accurately obtain pediatric vital signs | • Manual Part 2 | • Prepare patient for and assist with routine and specialty examinations<br>• Obtain vital signs<br>• Document appropriately<br>• Instruct patients according to needs |

*chart continues on following page*

## MEDICAL ASSISTING ENTRY-LEVEL CURRICULUM INTERFACE continued

| TEXTBOOK OBJECTIVES | LEARNING SYSTEM LOCATION | MA CURRICULUM |
|---|---|---|
| **Performance** | | **Competencies** |
| 3. Apply pediatric restraints–Large sheet | • Manual Part 2 | • Prepare patient for and assist with routine and specialty examinations |
| 4. Correctly obtain a pediatric urine sample | • Manual Part 2 | • All fundamental principles of handwashing, autoclaving, sterilizing, standard precautions<br>• Prepare and maintain examination and treatment areas<br>• Prepare patient and assist with specialty procedures and treatments<br>• Recognize and respond to verbal and nonverbal communication<br>• Document appropriately<br>• Instruct patients according to needs<br>• Instruct patients in collection of specimens<br>• Perform specialty noninvasive diagnostic tests<br>• Use methods of quality control<br>• Screen and follow up test results<br>• Demonstrate use and care of patient equipment |
| 5. Correctly obtain a pediatric urine sample | • Chapter 49<br>• All procedures | • See Chapter 49 |

## 3. RESOURCES

www.vaccines.com **Site for parents giving updated vaccines**

www.aap.org **American Academy of Pediatrics**

www.cdc.gov **Centers for Disease Control will have recommended vaccination schedule**

www.yahoo.com/health **Proceed to immunology and vaccine choices**

## 4. LESSON PLAN Pediatrics

**TIME 3 hours lecture, 6 hours lab**

**Opening:** If one of the students has a baby and would like to bring baby in, this is a good way to start class. Ask student to show class what helps baby relax and how to change diapers. Find out how many have never held a baby. Use the opportunity to demonstrate Procedures 34-1, 34-2, 34-3 and 34-4 if mother will allow.

**Pretest:** Ask students to define the words and have papers handed to you.
anomaly—a marked deviation from normal, congenital deformity
attenuated—weakened or change in the virulence of a pathogenic microorganism
congenital—Present at and existing from birth.
electrolyte —a chemical substance when dissolved, dissociates into electrically charged particles and is capable of conducting an electric current; essential to normal cell function.
excoriation—a scratch or similar abrasion to the skin.
hydrocephaly—An enlargement of the cranium caused by abnormal accumulation of cerebrospinal fluid within the cerebral system.

**Objectives:** The objectives should be reviewed after putting on a flip chart. Pay particular attention to information on growth, diseases, vaccinations, and handy patients

**Content:** Use the outline in the lesson plan to have a lively discussion about pediatrics. Emphasize the need for knowledge of growth, development, diseases, and vaccinations. All the charts for completion are finished in the Mastery Manual answer section.

**Overview**

1. Normal Growth and Development
2. Growth Patterns
3. Denver Developmental Screening Test
4. Developmental Patterns
5. Diseases and Disorders
6. The Pediatric Patient
   Well-Child Visits     Sick-Child Visits
   Children with Special Needs
7. The Medical Assistant's Role
8. Adapting to Physical and Chronologic Changes
9. Measurements
10. Child Abuse
11. Patient Education
12. Legal and Ethical Issues

**Lab:** Time to have a children's day in the lab. Get permission if needed. Ask parents to bring their children in and then demonstrate all the procedures on the children. Use an older child and obtain cooperation before attempting preventive wrapping. Supervise taking rectal temperatures for each child.

**Assignment:** Students need to practice skills and have them evaluated. They must know the purpose of the procedural steps.

**Posttest:** Use the Examaster testbank. Obtain growth and development charts and have students graph them. Have students volunteer to demonstrate a procedure as part of the grade. Have students teach others the procedures and grade them with the average their students obtain when they attempt evaluation.

## 5. MASTERY MANUAL ANSWERS

### PART 1 CONTENT MASTERY

### A. Learning Level: Knowledge

1. Complete the chart below to summarize pediatric growth and development patterns.

| Age | Weight Gain | Height Growth | Developmental Patterns |
|---|---|---|---|
| 6 mos. | Doubled from birth | Sitting | Reflex and grasping |
| 1 year | Tripled from birth | Grown 10–12 inches since birth | Manipulate objects/cooing and crying; pulling self up, may walk |
| 1–2 years | Gain about 1/2 pound per month | Grow 3 1/2 to 5 inches | Talking in words, running |
| 2–3 years | 3–5 pounds in year | Grow about 2–2 1/2 inches | Increased independence—temper tantrums, more social |
| 3–6 years | 3–5 pounds in year | Growth slows to 1 1/2 to 2 1/2 inches | Initiates activities, good gross motor skill. Full simple and some complex sentences; literal, doesn't get "sayings" |
| 6–12 years | Same as above | Same as above until puberty growth rate | Perfected fine motor skills; self-esteem developing, tests rules |
| 12–18 years | Gains almost half adult weight: girls 20–25 pounds; boys 15–20 pounds | Girls grow 5–6 inches; boys grow 4–5 inches | Attempting to establish identity, adult role experimenting, testing |
| Over 18 years | | Girls' skeletal maturation at 15–16; Boys' skeletal maturation at 17–18 | |

### B. Learning Level: Comprehension

1. List the four major testing areas in the Denver Developmental Test. Text p. 647
   a. gross motor skills
   b. fine motor skills
   c. language
   d. personal skills; socialization

2. Give examples of four signs of child abuse. Text p. 671
   malnutrion, frequent injuries, trauma, previous filed reports, shoulder dislocations, bruising to buttocks and back

3. The common childhood diseases are listed below. Fill in the missing information.

| Disease | Usual Age | Symptoms | Cause | Treatment |
|---|---|---|---|---|
| Croup | 1–4 years | At night, high-pitched, raspy cough | Virus, edema and spasm of vocal cords—stridor | Cold, moist vapor Upright position |
| Colic | Newborn to 6 | Draws up legs, clenches fist, painful cry | Unknown, air swallow or milk allergy | Find cause, help parents via counseling |
| Asthma | 1–adulthood | Nonproductive cough, expiratory wheeze, shallow respirations | Allergy, broncho-spasm, stress, infection, exercise, noxious fumes, shallow breathing, increased pulse, rhonchi | Pulmonary function tests, bronchodilators, antibiotics, prednisone |
| Diarrhea | 2 mos.–4 years | two or more watery stools in 24 hours | Viral or bacterial | Stool evaluation, restrict foods, antibiotics, electrolyte in balance |
| Chicken pox | School age if not vaccinated | slight fever, lesions small vesicles, very itchy | Varicella virus | Palliative—cool baths, anti-itch cream |
| Influenza | Infants, toddlers | High fever, restless, aches, respiratory complications | Haemophilus Influenza B virus | Bed rest, fluids, analgesics, antibiotic if opportunistic infection |
| Otitis media | Infants, toddlers | Fever, rubbing ears, purulent drainage | Cold, allergy, infection | Analgesics, decongestants, antibiotics |
| Tonsillitis | 1–10 years | Sore throat, red, painful, fever | Bacteria—often beta hemolytic streptococcus | Bed rest, liquid diet, gargling, antibiotics |
| Reye's syndrome | Children | 5 stages, from restless; N&V; liver dysfunction; coma & death | Aspirin during fever or illness but unknown | |

## C. Learning level: Application

1. Check the conditions for which childhood immunizations are recommended. Call public health department or go to AAP Web site and obtain CURRENT recommendations as the textbook may not be current. Recommendations are changing at least yearly.

| | | | |
|---|---|---|---|
| ✓ | Pertussis | ✓ | Diphtheria |
| ✓ | Rubella | ___ | Rabies |
| ✓ | Varicella | ✓ | Hepatitis B |
| ___ | Hepatitis A | ✓ | Haemophilus B |
| ___ | Asthma | ___ | Influenza |
| ___ | Tuberculosis | ___ | Pneumonia |

2. Explain well-child and sick-child areas in your physician's office and explain to patients the reasons for separate areas and when you use each area.

   Students need to explain the communicability of sick children and importance of using techniques to prevent spread. Refer to Chapter 50 on spread of microorganisms.

3. Name four pediatric screening tests.

   Vision, U/A, HG, hearing

4. After giving a vaccine, for what untoward effects will you tell the parent to observe?

   high fever, swelling at site or neck, breathing difficulties, severe headache, convulsions

## D. Learning Level: Analysis

1. Under what conditions would a physician decide not to give a vaccine?

   High fever, acute illness, patient has had disease, allergy to vaccine components—eggs or yeast; cardiovascular disease for Hepatitis B vaccine

2. Go to the following Internet site and print the most recent schedule for vaccines as recommended by CDC. www.cdc.gov

## E. Learning Level: Synthesis

When little Robby came in, the medical assistant noticed he had (a) purulent drainage from his ear. He also had (b) excoriations on his arm. When the medical assistant took measurements, the head circumference seemed very large for his size. The medical assistant reports her findings of possible enlarged head or (c)__________ and (d)__________ from the ear to the physician. The physician states that Robby had a natural rupture of the ear drum. When a surgical procedure, this is termed a (e)__________.

a. pus-forming

b. scratches

c. hydrocephaly

d. supporation

e. myringotomy

## F. Learning Level: Evaluation

Write at least four methods that you personally can use to gain the trust and cooperation of a pediatric patient.

This personal answer includes: letting mother help; offering patient a distracting toy; telling child not to move but allowing them to cry—encourage it!! Give them a reward before starting.

## PART 2 COMPETENCY CHALLENGE

1. Use the information on Case Study for Robbie Soto in the CD-ROM to develop techniques for dealing with children.
2. First demonstrate correct procedures; then have students use other students, children, or a life-size doll. Students should practice and be evaluated for the five procedures at the end of the chapter in the Mastery Manual. Evaluate students using procedure sheets when they indicate readiness or according to your timetable.

## PART 3 CLINICAL APPLICATIONS

1. Discuss result with students. Have them hand in results of survey.

   Interview a family with preschool children. Ask questions to determine what they want from the administrative and clinical staff. Obtain viewpoints from the child and parent or guardian. Why do you think the needs are different?

2. The situation described is in the Mastery Manual.

   Review the signs of child abuse and point out what the physician saw. Medical assistant went over to hospital to ensure that child got care and child protective services would arrive in time to investigate.

# 35

# Assisting in Neurology

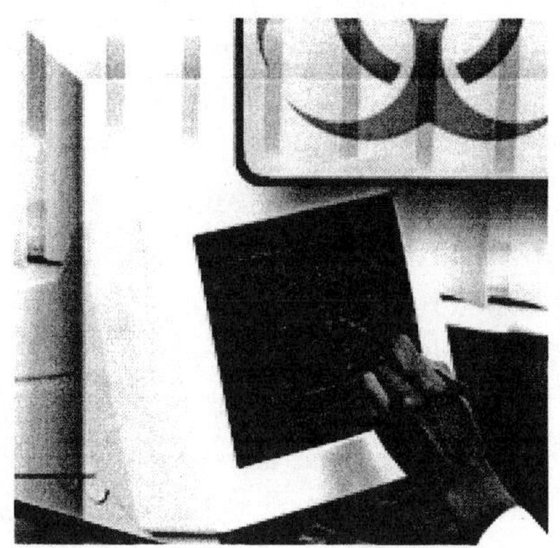

Neurology and neuroscience are one of the more complex areas of medical practice. Neurological examination is done in the primary care office as part of the overall examination. The medical assistant usually is involved with the neurology examination as with the physical examination procedure in Chapter 28. It is important for the medical assistant to recognize the mental, sensory and motor components of the physical examination and some normal responses in these areas. The medical assistant often picks up changes in these areas because of the close contact and interaction with patients. The specialty requires advance training if the medical assistant is going to perform procedures. Often the neurologist will give the training.

## USING THE LEARNING SYSTEM

### 1. MEDICAL ASSISTING ENTRY-LEVEL CONTENT AND COMPETENCIES

CONTENT

- Applications of medical terminology
- Anatomy and physiology for all body systems
- Common pathology and disease
- Diagnostic/treatment modalities
- Asepsis and infection control
- Specimen collection and processing
- Diagnostic testing
- Patient care
- Legal guidelines and requirements for health care
- Medical ethics and related issues
- Risk management
- Basic principles of psychology
- Recognition and response to verbal and nonverbal communication
- Adaptations for individual needs
- Job readiness
- Personal attributes

COMPETENCIES

- All fundamental principles of handwashing, autoclaving, sterilizing, standard precautions
- Prepare and maintain examination and treatment areas
- Prepare patient for and assist with routine and specialty examinations
- Prepare patient for and assist with specialty procedures and treatments
- Recognize of and respond to verbal and nonverbal communication
- Identify and respond to issues of confidentiality
- Document appropriately
- Instruct patients according to needs
- Identify community resources
- Provide instruction for health maintenance and disease prevention
- Instruct patients in collection of specimens
- Perform specialty noninvasive diagnostic tests
- Use methods of quality control
- Screen and follow up test results
- Demonstrate use and care of patient equipment

## 2. MEDICAL ASSISTING ENTRY-LEVEL CURRICULUM INTERFACE

| TEXTBOOK OBJECTIVES | LEARNING SYSTEM LOCATION | MA CURRICULUM |
|---|---|---|
| **Cognitive** | | **Content** |
| 1. Identify the anatomical structures that compose the nervous system | • Text pp. 675–676<br>• Manual Part 1-A | • Applications of medical terminology<br>• Anatomy and physiology for all body systems |
| 2. Explain the functions of the peripheral and central nervous system | • Text p. 676<br>• Manual Part 1-D | • Same as #1 |
| 3. Differentiate between the different layers of the brain's protective covering | • Text p. 677<br>• Manual Part 1-B | • Same as #1 |
| 4. Define a synapse | • Text p. 680<br>• Manual Part 2-B | • Same as #1 |
| 5. Name and describe the functions of the three major sections of the brain | • Text pp. 676-677<br>• Manual Part 1-A | • Same as #1 |
| 6. List the seven symptoms that suggest possible neurological problems | • Text p. 680<br>• Manual Part 2-C | • Common pathology and disease<br>• Patient care<br>• Legal guidelines and requirements for health care<br>• Medical ethics and related issues<br>• Risk management |

| TEXTBOOK OBJECTIVES | LEARNING SYSTEM LOCATION | MA CURRICULUM |
|---|---|---|
| **Cognitive** | | **Content** |
| 6. List the seven symptoms that suggest possible neurological problems (continued) | | • Basic principles of psychology<br>• Recognition of and response to verbal and nonverbal communication<br>• Adaptations for individual needs<br>• Job readiness<br>• Personal attributes |
| 7. Identify three brain disorders that result from injury | • Text pp. 681–685<br>• Manual Part 2-C | • Common pathology and disease<br>• Job readiness |
| 8. Name two disorders that could be work-related injuries | • Text pp. 681–685 | • Common pathology and disease<br>• Job readiness |
| 9. Identify the frequently used diagnostic procedure for nerve disorders | • Text p. 688<br>• Manual Part 2-D | • Diagnostic/treatment modalities<br>• Asepsis and infection control<br>• Specimen collection and processing<br>• Diagnostic testing<br>• Patient care |
| **Performance** | | **Competencies** |
| 1. Describe three tests that might be used during the neurological examination | • Text pp. 688–690<br>• Manual Part 2 | • Instruct patients in collection of specimens<br>• Perform specialty noninvasive diagnostic tests<br>• Use methods of quality control<br>• Screen and follow up test results |
| 2. Prepare a patient for a neurological procedure | • Text pp. 687–690<br>• Manual Part 2<br>• Procedure 35-1 | • Prepare patient and assist with specialty procedures and treatments<br>• Recognize and respond to verbal and nonverbal communication<br>• Provide instruction for health maintenance and disease prevention |

*chart continues on following page*

## MEDICAL ASSISTING ENTRY LEVEL CURRICULUM INTERFACE continued

| TEXTBOOK OBJECTIVES | LEARNING SYSTEM LOCATION | MA CURRICULUM |
|---|---|---|
| Performance | | Competencies |
| 3. Assist with the neurologic examination | • Text pp. 687–690<br>• Manual Part 2<br>• Procedure 35-1 | • All fundamental principles of handwashing, autoclaving, sterilizing, standard precautions<br>• Prepare and maintain examination and treatment areas<br>• Prepare patient for and assist with routine and specialty examinations<br>• Identify and respond to issues of confidentiality<br>• Document appropriately<br>• Instruct patients according to needs<br>• Identify community resources<br>• Demonstrate use and care of patient equipment |

## 3. RESOURCES

1. Neurology-Related Hotlines:
   Alzheimer's disease—1-800-272-3900
   Depressive Illness Foundation—1-800-248-4344
   National Multiple Sclerosis Foundation—1-800-227-3166
   National Parkinsons Foundation—1-800-327-4545 www.parkinson.org
   National Spinal Cord Injury—1-800-526-3456
   Spina Bifida Association—1-800-621-3141
2. Internet Sites

www.aan.com/home.html **This site is the American Academy of Neurology, 1080 Montreal Ave., St. Paul, MN 55116 612-695-1940**

http//cyberactive-1.com **A site for traumatic brain injury via The American Academy of Neurological and Orthopedic Surgeons**

**4. LESSON PLAN Neurology** **TIME 3 hours lecture, 12 hours lab**

**Opening:** Have a 40-watt light bulb burning in a lamp on your desk. Ask students what it represents. The *potential* electrical activity of a brain!

**Pretest:** Copy and enlarge Figure 35-1 in the 8th Edition Textbook. White out structures and make sufficient copies for all students. See if they are able to label major brain structures and subdivisions.

**Objectives:** Put objectives up on flip chart and have students review all responses. Use objectives to provide overview before further discussion.

**Content:** Review anatomy. Have students finish labeling handout you gave them as pretest.

1. Anatomy and Physiology
   a. Peripheral Nervous System
   b. Central Nervous System
   c. Brain
   d. Spinal Cord
   e. Protective Covering of the Brain
2. Diseases and Disorders
   Cerebrovascular Disease (CVD)
   Carpal Tunnel Syndrome (CTS)
   Cerebral Concussion
   Multiple Sclerosis (MS)
   Epilepsy and Seizures
   Brain Tumors
   Cerebrovascular Accident (CVA)
   Migraine Headache
   Encephalitis (Sleeping Sickness)
   Amyotrophic Lateral Sclerosis (ALS)
   Spinal Cord Injuries
3. Medical Assistant's Role in Neurology—Assisting with the Examination
   Lab time.
   Due to the complexity of the subject, the neurologist usually completes a thorough patient history. Emphasizing the medical assistant's role in obtaining the chief complaint and helping the patient relax is essential. The medical assistant also facilitates referrals, testing procedures and reinforcing education.
4. Diagnostic Testing—Students need information to teach and prepare patients
   Electroencephalography (EEG)
   CT
   AFP
   LP
   MRI
5. Patient education, legal and ethical

**Lab:** Obtain a film on brain function and surgery. Some may be obtained from Lifetime TV or the American Health Network. Show film on brain surgery during lab. Have a neurologist come in and demonstrate an EEG. Students cannot prepare patients for an EEG if they do not understand how it is administered. Students may then practice and be evaluated on Procedure 35-1. Use lab time to discuss Parts 2 and 3 in Mastery Manual.

**Assignment:** Have students complete Mastery Manual and Part 2 activities. Then students move to next chapter.

**Posttest:** Choose Examaster testbank questions related to objectives or medical assistant curriculum.

## 5. MASTERY MANUAL ANSWERS

## PART 1 CONTENT MASTERY

### A. Learning Level: Knowledge

Put the correct word in space provided.

1. **anomalies** deformities or deviations from normal from faulty development of the fetus.
2. **syncope** fainting.
3. **gait** the manner of walking.
4. **homeostasis** to maintain constant internal environmental conditions.
5. **malignant** cancerous.
6. **medulloblastoma** a tumor composed of embryonic cells in the medulla oblongata.
7. **remission** a lessening in the severity of a disease or symptoms.
8. **paroxysmal** a sudden recurrent spasm of symptoms.
9. **convulsions** a series of involuntary contractions of the voluntary muscles.
10. **ataxia** failure or irregularity of muscle actions and coordination.
11. **aura** a peculiar sensation preceding the appearance of more definite disturbance.
12. **collodion** type of cellulose nitrate; when applied to skin, dries as a strong, thin, transparent film.
13. **exacerbation** aggravation of symptoms or increased severity of a disease.
14. **atrophy** decrease in the size of a normally developed organ.
15. **glioma** a neoplasm of the supporting structure of nervous tissue in the brain.
16. **stroke** a sudden loss of consciousness and/or paralysis caused by extreme trauma to a brain artery
17. **sheath** the covering surrounding the axon of the nerve cell.
18. **paresthesia** an abnormal sensation of burning, prickling or stinging.
19. **meningioma** a hard vascular tumor invading the dura and skull.
20. **coma** an unconscious state from which the patient cannot be aroused.

Draw a picture or chart of the major structures of the nervous system and include the major subdivisions of each structure.

See text p. 675, 676, and 680: students should include brain figure 35-6 and spinal cord figure 35-2.

### B. Learning Level: Comprehension

1. Give the meaning of the following abbreviations used in the chapter.
   a. CVD—cerebrovascular disease
   b. CVA—cerebrovascular accident
   c. CT—computerized tomography
   d. MRI—magnetic resonance imaging
   e. CNS—central nervous system
   f. CTS—carpal tunnel syndrome
   g. MS—multiple sclerosis
   h. ALS—amyotrophic lateral sclerosis
   i. AFP—alpha-fetoprotein

2. State the point where each neuron contacts another neuron. <u>synapse</u>

3. What is the importance of this area?
   <u>Neurotransmitters released here help transmit impulses along nerves.</u>

### C. Learning Level: Application

1. If there is a blood clot below the outer layer of meninges, what do you think it is called?
   <u>Subdural hematoma</u>

2. Below are listed some neurological symptoms. Choose the disorder you believe is most associated with that group of symptoms. Underline any symptom which by itself points to possible neurologic problems.
   a. inaudible speech, difficulty swallowing, one-sided weakness CVA
   b. pain and paresthesia of radial area CTS
   c. visual disturbance, one-sided headache, aura, N&V Migraine
   d. headache, muscle ache, malaise, fever Encephalitis
   e. diplopia, muscle weakness, paresthesia, ataxia MS
   f. tonic-clonic contraction Epilepsy

## D. Learning Level: Analysis

1. What is the condition called if there is destruction of the spinal cord at C4? quadriplegia
   If destruction is at T7? paraplegia

2. A patient comes in to the office for a yearly checkup. Being an enthusiastic medical assistant, you decide to try a little mental sensory and motor function check.
   Write some specific things you could check and what you would expect for normal function.

| Area | Test Performed | Normal Result |
|---|---|---|
| Mental | Ask date, time, place<br>Ask address | Should answer accurately in a short time |
| Sensory | Have patient close eyes and move cotton swab on arm or leg and see if patient feels it | Should be able to identify area being touched, also heat or cold on an area |
| Motor | Watch patient walk, have patient take something from you, lift something, firmly shake hand | Should be able to walk without limp or stumble or drag, and in straight line |

3. You told physician you were not sure if patient was oriented to time. He did further examination and decided to run some diagnostic imaging tests. What tests might be run to check cerebral function?
   Skull x-ray, cerebral angiogram, myelogram, MRI, CT

## E. Learning Level: Synthesis

Situation: A patient has just been told that her child needs to be evaluated for a possible brain tumor. The physician discussed everything with her, but she is in tears and says she really did not hear anything and is so afraid. The doctor does not want her to go back to her child until she is calm and smiling and asks you to stay with her and talk to her. What are you going to tell her? Go back to patient relations and other areas and draw on the information you learned in this chapter.

Response: Take her to a private room. Ask her about her fears. Tell her you understand the situation is fearful. Have her focus on what child needs. Encourage her to talk a lot and just listen. As she calms down, then point out that her child will react badly if she sees her mom is scared, help her plan to get tests for child ASAP, ask if you can call someone for support and get counseling while the testing goes on, encourage her to take each day one day at a time. Tell her about tests physician has ordered and give her booklets. Encourage her to let it all out before she rejoins child.

## F. Learning Level: Evaluation

1. If someone in your family had to have one of the following diseases, which would you choose and why? CVA, encephalitis, MS, ALS, spinal cord injury, brain tumor.

   These are personal answers only. Hopefully the conversation will be guided to the problems related to daily activities, prognosis, personal feelings about certain types of illness and opportunities to clear up misconceptions.
2. Why would you not choose each of the others? Personal responses
3. Have you become more empathetic by putting yourself in another's place?

   Have students discuss how and why.

## PART 2 COMPETENCY CHALLENGE

1. The procedure on this chapter is for preparing a patient to have an EEG in an EEG lab. Before you attempt this, it is good to talk to someone who has had the procedure and get their ideas about the procedure, its pros and cons. After you have done this, practice the procedure on a classmate. Instructor: When possible, it is wise to prepare students by demonstrating the technique. Many of these procedures are being done in the medical office and students need to be prepared for a variety of assisting tasks.
2. Talk to someone who has had a lumbar puncture. Read the description in the 8th Edition Textbook and write a procedure for preparing the patient to have an LP. These procedures are done both in pediatrics and the neurology office.
3. Write a procedure for preparing the patient for and assisting at a neurological examination. Be sure to explain reflex testing as part of the preparation.

## PART 3 CLINICAL APPLICATIONS

1. Are medical assistants allowed to perform EEGs in your state? ______________________
2. If so, is extra training needed? ______________________
3. Mrs. Soto brought her son in for an examination. You remark to her about the long bus ride. She says she drove! You know she had a seizure 2 months ago and should not be driving. What, if any, action do you take?

   Answers depend upon state laws

# 36

# Assisting in Dermatology

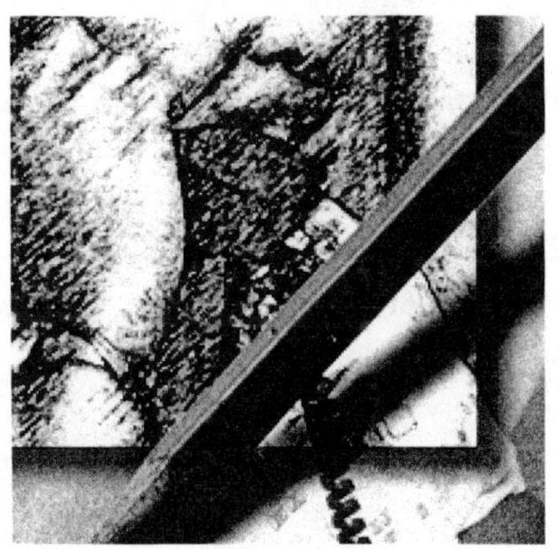

In today's medical practice, more specialty procedures are being performed in the primary care office. Procedures such as skin testing, tissue biopsy, excision of lesions, and treatment of associated disorders may be part of any practice. The medical assistant needs competence in these areas. Medical and surgical asepsis is important when penetrating the skin. When assisting at these procedures, the medical assistant must be aware of procedures from debridement to excision. This requires a firm foundation in the knowledge of structure, function, disorders, and examination techniques. Most neoplasms and chronic disorders are treated in the dermatology office, and this chapter will give the medical assistant student a good foundation.

## USING THE LEARNING SYSTEM

### 1. MEDICAL ASSISTING ENTRY-LEVEL CONTENT AND COMPETENCIES

CONTENT

- Applications of medical terminology
- Anatomy and physiology for all body systems
- Diagnostic/treatment modalities
- Asepsis and infection control
- Specimen collection and processing
- Diagnostic testing
- Patient care
- Common pathology and disease
- Legal guidelines and requirements for health care
- Medical ethics and related issues
- Risk management
- Basic principles of psychology
- Recognition of and response to verbal and nonverbal communication
- Adaptations for individual needs
- Job readiness
- Personal attributes

COMPETENCIES

- All fundamental principles of handwashing, autoclaving, sterilizing, standard precautions
- Prepare and maintain examination and treatment areas
- Prepare patient for and assist with routine and specialty examinations
- Prepare patient for and assist with specialty procedures and treatments
- Recognize and respond to verbal and nonverbal communication
- Identify and respond to issues of confidentiality
- Document appropriately
- Instruct patients according to needs
- Identify community resources
- Provide instruction for health maintenance and disease prevention
- Instruct patients in collection of specimens
- Perform specialty noninvasive diagnostic tests
- Use methods of quality control
- Screen and follow up test results
- Demonstrate use and care of patient equipment

## 2. MEDICAL ASSISTING ENTRY-LEVEL CURRICULUM INTERFACE

| TEXTBOOK OBJECTIVES | LEARNING SYSTEM LOCATION | MA CURRICULUM |
|---|---|---|
| **Cognitive** | | **Content** |
| 1. Identify the anatomical structures of the skin | • Text pp. 694–696<br>• Manual Part 1-A-1 | • Applications of medical terminology<br>• Anatomy and physiology for all body systems |
| 2. Explain the major functions of the skin | • Text p. 695<br>• Manual Part 1-A-2 | • Same as #1 |
| 3. Identify different lesions by name | • Text p. 696<br>• Manual Part 1-B-1 | • Patient care<br>• Common pathology and disease<br>• Legal guidelines and requirements for health care<br>• Medical ethics and related issues<br>• Risk management |
| 4. List and describe types of thermal skin injuries | • Text pp. 696–698<br>• Manual Part 1-C-1 | • Same as #3 |
| 5. Name eight diseases or disorders of the skin | • Text pp. 699–703<br>• Manual Part 1-D-3 | • Same as #3 |
| 6. Discuss your role in assisting with dermatologic testing | • Text pp. 704–706<br>• Manual Part 1-F | • Diagnostic/treatment modalities<br>• Asepsis and infection control<br>• Specimen collection and processing<br>• Diagnostic testing<br>• Patient care |

| TEXTBOOK OBJECTIVES | LEARNING SYSTEM LOCATION | MA CURRICULUM |
|---|---|---|
| **Cognitive** | | **Content** |
| 7. Identify six forms of dermatologic medications | • Text pp. 708–709<br>• Manual Part 1-E | • Diagnostic/treatment modalities<br>• Patient care |
| 8. Analyze your role in patient education | • Text pp. 708–709<br>• Manual Part 3 | • Medical ethics and related issues<br>• Basic principles of psychology<br>• Recognition of and response to verbal and nonverbal communication<br>• Adaptations for individual needs<br>• Job readiness<br>• Personal attributes |
| 9. Discuss legal issues in caring for the dermatology patient | • Text p. 710<br>• Manual Part 3 | • Legal guidelines and requirements for health care<br>• Risk management<br>• Job readiness<br>• Personal attributes |
| **Performance** | | **Competencies** |
| 1. Assist the dermatologist with the examination of the skin | • Manual Part 2 | • All fundamental principles of handwashing, autoclaving, sterilizing, standard precautions<br>• Prepare and maintain examination and treatment areas<br>• Prepare patient and assist with specialty procedures and treatments<br>• Recognize and respond to verbal and nonverbal communication<br>• Identify and respond to issues of confidentiality<br>• Document appropriately |
| 2. Accurately obtain an exudate sample from a wound for laboratory analysis | • Manual Part 2<br>• Procedure 36-1 | • Instruct patients in collection of specimens<br>• Perform specialty noninvasive diagnostic tests<br>• Use methods of quality control<br>• Screen and follow up test results<br>• Demonstrate use and care of patient equipment |

*chart continues on following page*

## MEDICAL ASSISTING ENTRY-LEVEL CURRICULUM INTERFACE continued

| TEXTBOOK OBJECTIVES | LEARNING SYSTEM LOCATION | MA CURRICULUM |
|---|---|---|
| **Performance** | | **Competencies** |
| 3. Prepare patient and assist with a skin biopsy | • Complete as part of externship<br>• Manual Part 3 | • Prepare patient for and assist with routine and specialty examinations |
| 4. Prepare a list of possible skin issues for patient education | • Text p. 709<br>• Manual Part 1-E | • Instruct patients according to needs<br>• Identify community resources<br>• Provide instruction for health maintenance and disease prevention |

## 3. RESOURCES

www.asds-net.org/procderm.htme **Dermatology procedures and pictures**

www.asds-net.org/index.htm **The home page to dermatology society**

http://www.derma.med.uni-erlangen.de/bilddb/index_e.htm **Dermatology atlas on-line**

http://www.aarda.org/ **American Autoimmune Related Diseases Association**

## 4. LESSON PLAN Dermatology Assisting

**TIME 3 hours lecture, 12 hours lab**

**Opening:** Assemble equipment for biopsy and culture. Explain use.

**Pretest:** Students should have studied chapter before class. Use Part 1-A-2 and complete an oral quiz. These pretests are excellent in that they allow the instructor to obtain a feel for actual preparation of class.

**Objectives:** Review with the Role Delineation Study. Talk briefly on each objective and relation to Role Delineation Study.

**Content:** This outline may be enlarged and made into Transparency Masters.

1. Anatomy and Physiology
   Epidermis    Dermis    Subcutaneous Layer Skin
2. Lesions
3. Diseases and Disorders
   a. Thermal Injuries
      First-Degree Burn    Second-Degree Burn    Third-Degree Burn
      Cold Injuries
   b. Acne
   c. Impetigo
   d. Fungal Infections (Dermatophytoses)
   e. Scabies and Pediculosis
   f. Eczema
   g. Psoriasis
   h. Herpes Zoster (Shingles)
   i. Nail Fungus
   j. Benign and Malignant Neoplasms
4. The Role of the Medical Assistant Assisting with the Dermatologic Examination
5. Assisting With Testing Procedures
   Wood's Lamp Examination
   Allergy Skin Testing
   Obtaining a Wound Culture Sample
6. Administration of Dermatology Medications
7. Patient Education
8. Legal and Ethical Issues

**Lab:** Use the lab time to have students write procedures for assisting with a skin examination. Demonstrate and have students practice obtaining exudate samples. Strict aseptic technique must be demanded. Show how skin is mapped and demonstrate how patients can monitor their skin.

**Assignment:** Set a practice and evaluation schedule. Have students draw all the primary and secondary skin lesions. Prepare for next chapter discussion.

**Posttest:** Testbank questions. Use questions addressing Role Delineation Study and objectives.

## 5. MASTERY MANUAL ANSWERS

### PART 1 CONTENT MASTERY

#### A. Learning Level: Knowledge

1. Label skin structure seen on the figure below.
   Figure is in textbook—Figure 36-1, text p. 695
2. Place the medical term for the definition given.

| | |
|---|---|
| 1. **pruritus** | Itching |
| 2. **pallor** | Lack of color; pale skin |
| 3. **palliative** | A substance that alleviates or eases a painful situation without curing |
| 4. **opaque** | Not translucent or transparent |
| 5. **leukoderma** | White patches on the skin |
| 6. **keratin** | A very hard, tough protein found in hair, nails, and epidermal tissue |
| 7. **ecchymosis** | A skin discoloration produced by hemorrhagic areas, bluish-black in color |
| 8. **dermatophytes** | A fungal parasite that grows in or on the skin |
| 9. **debridement** | The removal of foreign material and dead, damaged tissue from a wound |
| 10. **neoplasm** | New growth of cells (used interchangeably with the term cancer) |
| 11. **cyanosis** | Blue discoloration of the skin usually caused by depressed circulation |
| 12. **collagen** | A strong, fibrous, insoluble protein found in connective tissue |
| 13. **cancer** | Any cellular tumor or neoplastic disease in which there is a transformation of normal body cells into malignant cells |
| 14. **electrodesiccation** | The destructive drying of cells and tissue by means of short high-frequency electrical sparks |
| 15. **benign** | Noncancerous (as when describing a mass or tumor) |
| 16. **antipruritic** | Agent that will prevent or relieve itching |

#### B. Learning Level: Comprehension

Describe the following skin conditions with correct medical terms.

| | |
|---|---|
| 1. A mosquito bite on the upper arm | wheal |
| 2. A pimple with pus on the chin | acne |
| 3. White patches on the shin | leukoplakia |
| 4. Fungus on a nail | onychomychosis |
| 5. Redness on hands, palmar | erythema |
| 6. Yellow-colored whites of eyes | conjunctival jaundice |
| 7. Small, purple hemorrhagic spots | petechiae |

8. Dandruff seborrhea
9. Boils furuncle
10. Gives skin its color melanin

11. Differentiate primary from secondary skin lesions.
Primary is the original lesion; secondary is a result of change in primary lesion.

## C. Learning Level: Application

1. Use Figure in Part 1-A-1 and illustrate the degrees of burn depth by separating the areas of first-, second-, and third-degree burns with red lines across the skin. See text p. 698 for depths.
2. Differentiate skin cancers by cell type, appearance and treatment.

| Cell Type | Appearance | Treatment |
|---|---|---|
| Basal Cell | Painless, smooth, waxy translucent, small | Topical liquid nitrogen Cryosurgery |
| Squamous Cell | Firm, red nodule, scales, nay ulcer, non-healing | Cryosurgery or excise |
| Malignant Melanoma | Flat brown or black lesion enlarges, irregular edges, elevates | Biopsy, cryosurgery, electrodesiccation, excision, chemotherapy |

## D. Learning Level: Analysis

1. Name the three methods of obtaining skin biopsy. punch, shave, excision
2. Which method would you rather have and why?
Individual answers will vary. Look at reasoning: solid, based on fact. Is fear of pain a factor? How is this fear answered in patients?
3. The chart below lists symptoms of specific skin diseases. Fill in the disease, cause, tests, and treatments which correspond to the symptoms.

| Symptoms | Diseases | Cause | Tests | Treatments |
|---|---|---|---|---|
| 1. Vessels dilated and skin cold | Hypothermia | Exposure | Observation | Slow warming in hospital |
| 2. Blackheads and pimples | Acne | Heredity, hormonal, sebum attracts bacteria | None | Keratolytics, Retin-A, topical antibiotics |
| 3. Vesicles, pustules, contagious | Impetigo | *Staphylococcus aureus* | Culture | Clean, antibiotic ointment, cover x3 daily |
| 4. Athlete's foot and ringworm | Dermatophytosis | Fungus infection | Wood's lamp—Lesion appearance | Antifungals |
| 5. Itching in hair, nits on hair shaft | Pediculosis | Three louse species | Obtain insect | Medicated shampoo, cream, or lotion; cleaning of house and all furniture |

*chart continues on following page*

*chart continued*

| Symptoms | Disease | Cause | Tests | Treatments |
|---|---|---|---|---|
| 6. Scales, crusts, oozing, itching | Ezcema of many kinds | Inflammatory and allergic reponses | Skin test to specific allergens | Avoid allergic products, apply topical cortico-steroids |
| 7. Pink-red lesions and silvery scales | Psoriasis | Chronic with possible allergic or genetic disorder | Observation, biopsy | Ultraviolet light, coal tar, steroid creams, antihistamines |
| 8. Painful vesicles on torso or face | Herpes zoster | Varicella virus | Observation of lesion pattern, isolate virus in cell culture | Early treatment with antiviral drugs, antipruritics, analgesics |

## E. Learning Level: Synthesis

Instructors—Complete with students in lab a teaching plan.
Activity: Design a teaching plan for one of the chronic skin conditions discussed in the chapter. Refer to Chapter 7 on Patient Communication and the teaching plan guide from Chapter 28 to help plan your presentation. Remember to

—set objectives

—write what patient needs to know

—where you will get the information

—specific resources for patients—pamphlets, books, Internet

## F. Learning Level: Evaluation

Your textbook discusses five major testing procedures that occur in the dermatology office and the primary care office. Which of those procedures carry the greatest responsibility for you, the medical assistant?
Explain your reasoning.
Again, individual answers will vary. Students evaluate types and levels of patient care and knowledge required. Which procedures require greatest depth of comprehension plus technical skill and accuracy?

## PART 2 COMPETENCY CHALLENGE

1. Procedure 36-1 requires obtaining wound exudate for culture.

   Students need this procedure demonstrated before practicing. Manual dexterity and aseptic technique are essential. Students will have to simulate the actual wound. Use gel on an area of skin and draw a circle around it.

   EQUIPMENT AND SUPPLIES NECESSARY

   Sterile culture kit containing tube, swabs, and transport media (for swabbing). Sterile culture kit containing syringe and transport media (for aspirating); gauze flats

2. List the medical assistant's responsibilities when assisting with a tissue (skin) biopsy.
   1. Assemble all supplies using surgical asepsis
   2. Prepare patient by explaining procedure and positioning as directed for biopsy
   3. Prepare biopsy site according to protocol
   4. Assist physician as needed
   5. Label sample container and transport
   6. Clean procedure area and dispose of waste according to regulations

3. Write a competency objective for assisting with a skin biopsy and then simulate assisting the physician with a skin biopsy using the guidelines from #2 above.

## PART 3 CLINICAL APPLICATIONS

1. The patient had a tissue excision after a punch biopsy of a squamous cell carcinoma. After 3 weeks, he returned to the office because it seemed to be growing back. Dr. Healer agreed and then completed a wide and deep excision of the area under local anesthesia. You are the good-bye person, and as the patient leaves he appears upset and says, "It was a big procedure, and I should have been referred to a dermatologist. What if it comes back again? This is cancer and I need a specialist." What do you say and do?

   Answers vary: patient should see physician ASAP.

2. The patient had intradermal skin tests on both forearms. As you say good-bye, the patient opens the door to the outer office and faints. What are you going to do?

   Answer: Go to patient, lay him flat on floor, immediately call physician, call for emergency cart or tray, call for oxygen

3. What are two examples of legal issues related to #1 that you can think of?

   Answer: Examples of legal issues are:

   standard of care
   health care regulations
   adaptation to individual needs
   scope of practice

# 37

# Assisting in Orthopedic Medicine

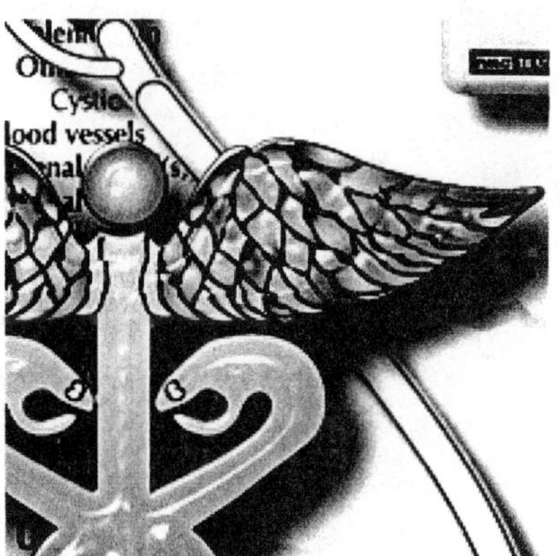

Many types of medical practices in which the medical assistant may find employment encompass orthopedic medicine. Patients appear in various medical settings with complaints related to bones, joints, and muscles due to heredity, trauma or degenerative injuries and changes. The medical assistant instructor will be challenged to observe students and promote education of patients in the proper care of casts, use of crutches, and application of cold. There is much opportunity for the medical assistant student to practice patient education techniques in the Transparency Master to assist.

## USING THE LEARNING SYSTEM

### 1. MEDICAL ASSISTING ENTRY-LEVEL CONTENT AND COMPETENCIES

CONTENT

- Applications of medical terminology
- Anatomy and physiology for all body systems
- Diagnostic/treatment modalities
- Asepsis and infection control
- Patient care
- Common pathology and disease
- Legal guidelines and requirements for health care
- Medical ethics and related issues
- Risk management
- Basic principles of psychology
- Recognition of and response to verbal and nonverbal communication
- Adaptations for individual needs
- Job readiness
- Personal attributes

COMPETENCIES

- Prepare patient for and assist with specialty procedures and treatments
- Instruct patients according to needs
- Identify community resources
- Provide instruction for health maintenance and disease prevention
- Demonstrate use and care of patient equipment
- All fundamental principles of handwashing, autoclaving, sterilizing, standard precautions
- Identify community resources
- Prepare and maintain examination and treatment areas
- Prepare patient for and assist with routine and specialty examinations
- Recognize and respond to verbal and nonverbal communication
- Identify and respond to issues of confidentiality
- Document appropriately
- Instruct patients according to needs
- Provide instruction for health maintenance and disease prevention
- Demonstrate use and care of patient equipment

## 2. MEDICAL ASSISTING ENTRY-LEVEL CURRICULUM INTERFACE

| TEXTBOOK OBJECTIVES | LEARNING SYSTEM LOCATION | MA CURRICULUM |
|---|---|---|
| **Cognitive** | | **Content** |
| 1. Describe the principal structures of the musculoskeletal system | • Text pp. 711–713<br>• Manual Part 1-C | • Applications of medical terminology<br>• Anatomy and physiology for all body systems |
| 2. Identify five types of bones and give an example of each | • Text p. 711<br>• Memory jogger #2 | • Same as #1 |
| 3. Describe three forms of muscles | • Text pp. 712–713<br>• Memory jogger #3<br>• Manual Part 1-D | • Same as #1 |
| 4. Differentiate between tendons, bursae, and ligaments | • Text pp. 713–714<br>• Memory jogger #4 | • Same as #1 |
| 5. List and describe the major disorders of the system | • Text pp. 714–719<br>• Manual Part 1-C | • Common pathology and disease |
| 6. Describe the different types of fractures | • Text pp. 719–720<br>• Manual Part 1-B | • Same as #1 |
| 7. Explain types of diagnostic procedures used | • Text pp. 720–730<br>• Manual Part 1-D-2 | • Patient care<br>• Diagnostic/treatment modalities<br>• Asepsis and infection control<br>• Legal guidelines and requirements for health care<br>• Basic principles of psychology |

| TEXTBOOK OBJECTIVES | LEARNING SYSTEM LOCATION | MA CURRICULUM |
|---|---|---|
| **Cognitive** | | **Content** |
| 8. Explain types of diagnostic procedures used *(continued)* | | • Recognition of and response to verbal and nonverbal communication<br>• Adaptations for individual needs<br>• Personal attributes |
| 9. Describe four types of ambulatory devices | • Text p. 732<br>• Manual Part 1-D | • Medical ethics and related issues<br>• Job readiness<br>• Legal guidelines and requirements for health care |
| 10. Explain the uses for cold applications | • Text pp. 734–735<br>• Manual Part 1-F | • Job readiness<br>• Risk management<br>• Legal guidelines and requirements for health care |
| **Performance** | | **Competencies** |
| 1. Prepare and assist with cast application | • Text p. 726<br>• Manual Part 2<br>• Procedure 37-1 | • Prepare patient for and assist with specialty procedures and treatments<br>• Instruct patients according to needs<br>• Identify community resources<br>• Provide instruction for health maintenance and disease prevention<br>• Demonstrate use and care of patient equipment<br>• All fundamental principles of handwashing, autoclaving, sterilizing, standard precautions<br>• Identify community resources |
| 2. Accurately apply a sling to immobilize an injury | • Text pp. 729–730<br>• Manual Part 2<br>• Procedure 37-2 | • Prepare and maintain examination and treatment areas<br>• Prepare patient for and assist with routine and specialty examinations.<br>• Recognize and respond to verbal and nonverbal communication<br>• Identify and respond to issues of confidentiality<br>• Document appropriately |

*chart continues on following page*

## MEDICAL ASSISTING ENTRY-LEVEL CURRICULUM INTERFACE continued

| TEXTBOOK OBJECTIVES | LEARNING SYSTEM LOCATION | MA CURRICULUM |
|---|---|---|
| **Performance** | | **Competencies** |
| 3. Properly apply an ice bag | • Text p. 735<br>• Manual Part 2<br>• Procedure 37-3 | • Instruct patients according to needs<br>• Provide instruction for health maintenance and disease prevention<br>• Demonstrate use and care of patient equipment |

## 3. RESOURCES

Arthritis Foundation 1-800-283-7800; National Headquarters 404-872-7100; www.arthritis.org

The Muscular Dystrophy Associations of America, 3300 East Sunrise Drive, Tucson, AZ 85718-3802; 1-800-572-1717; www.mdausaa.org

National Association of Rehabilitation Facilities, Box 17675, Washington, DC 20041

1-703-648-9300

Myasthenia Gravis Foundation, Inc. 15 East 26th St, NY, NY 10010

National Genetics Foundation, Inc., 250 W 57th Street, NY, NY 10019

National Organization on Disability, 910 16th St., NW, Suite 600, Washington, DC 20006

1-800-248-able

National Rehabilitation Association, 633 S. Washington St, Alexandria, VA 22314

1-703-836-0850

National Spinal Cord Injury Foundation, 600 W. Cummin Suite 200, Woburn, MA 01801

671-935-2722

## 4. LESSON PLAN Orthopedics — TIME 3 hours lecture, 12 hours lab

**Opening:** If available, have cast equipment out to complete the procedures. Obtain a training film on applying a cast and show it.

**Pretest:** Hold different pieces of orthopedic equipment up. Ask why and how equipment is used and who has experience in using or wearing?

**Objectives:** Before class, put the objectives up on the board and, as discussed, cross them off.

**Content:** Obtain as much of the discussion as possible from the students. Have students draw anatomy and practice teaching the use of equipment as they discuss injuries and disorders. Break class into groups to complete Part 1 of Mastery Manual and develop patient teaching techniques around the activities.

1. Anatomy and Physiology of the Musculoskeletal System
   Bones
   Joints
   Muscles
   Tendons, Bursae, and Ligaments
2. Musculoskeletal Diseases and Disorders—See answers in Part 1-D for chart covering symptoms, cause, and treatment for four diseases. Use as model for students to fill a chart for all diseases.
   a. Bone Disorders
      Spinal Curvatures Fractures Osteomalacia Paget's Disease
   b. Joint Disorders
      Arthritis Osteoarthritis Rheumatoid Arthritis Gout
      Strain
      Herniated Disk
      Dislocation
      Tendinitis
   c. Muscle Disorders
      Muscular Dystrophy
      Muscle Spasms and Tics
      Muscle Sprain
      Myasthenia Gravis
3. The Role of the Medical Assistant in Orthopedic Medicine
   a. Assisting with the General Orthopedic Examination
      Assisting with Range of Motion Evaluation (ROM)
      Assisting with Muscle Strength Evaluation
   b. Radiology and Diagnostic Imaging Evaluation and Procedures
   c. Assisting with Casting Procedure #37-1: Assisting with Cast Application
   d. Placing the Arm in a Sling Procedure #37-2: Application of a Triangular Arm Sling
4. Ambulatory Appliances and Abnormal Gaits
   Fitting and Using Crutches, Walkers and Canes
   Wheelchairs
5. General Principles of Cold Application
   Cold Compresses
   Ice Packs Procedure #37-3: Applying an Ice Bag
6. Patient Education
7. Legal and Ethical Issues

**Lab:** Students may use lab time to become familiar with bones on the skeleton, and to practice procedures after they are demonstrated. Evaluate students' competency when they are ready. Obtain a used bivalved cast that can be used to simulate an applied cast. Students may then simulate Procedure #37-1.

**Assignment:** Students complete Mastery Manual and procedure competency for next class. Make flash cards for bones of arms, legs, torso, and head and flash cards for common muscles of each area. Be prepared to demonstrate one of the crutch walking gaits.

**Posttest:** Use questions from Examaster testbank. Another opportunity for a "walk around" test. Lay bones out on table, number them, and have students write names and identify prominences and depressions. Use the activity in Part 3 for preparing an education plan as part of evaluation. This reinforces the need for patient education.

## 5. MASTERY MANUAL ANSWERS

### PART 1 CONTENT MASTERY

### A. Learning Level: Knowledge

1. Write in the term for the definition given.
   1. reduction: The correction of a fracture, dislocation, or hernia.
   2. luxation: Total dislocation of the bone from the joint.
   3. crepitation: A dry, crackling sound or sensation produced by the grating of the ends of a fractured bone.
   4. gait: The manner or style of walking.
   5. kyphosis: An abnormally increased convex curve of the thoracic spine; also called hunchback.
   6. malaise: A feeling of uneasiness or indisposition.
   7. synovial: Pertaining to a clear fluid found in the joint cavities which facilitates smooth painless movement.
   8. scoliosis: Lateral deviation in the normal vertical curve of the spine.
   9. goniometer: An instrument for measuring joint angles and movement.
   10. diaphysis: The portion of the long bone between the ends enclosing the medullary cavity.
   11. epiphyses: The ends of the long bone that are wider than the shaft of the bone.
   12. medullary cavity: The inner portion of the bone that contains the bone marrow.

### B. Learning Level: Comprehension

1. Label the types of fractures shown below.
   Instructor: figure is on page 720 in textbook

2. Label the types of muscle shown below.
   Instructor: figure is on page 713 in textbook

### C. Learning Level: Application

1. Give the cause, symptoms and treatment of the diseases listed below.

| Disease/Disorder | Cause | Symptoms | Treatment |
|---|---|---|---|
| 1. Herniated disk—the soft nucleus of an intervertebral disk protrudes through a tear or weakened area in the tough outer disk covering | Injury or by sudden straining with the spine in an unnatural position. May come on gradually as a result of a progressive disk deterioration. | Lumbar region: severe lower back pain and difficulty in walking; cervical disk: severe pain in the back of neck radiating down arms into fingers. Positive myelogram or MRI. | Conservative: bed rest on a firm mattress, local application of heat, and muscle relaxant and pain reliever. Chronic: wear a surgical support and/or traction may be applied to the legs; pain, numbness, and progressive weakness of the area may indicate surgery. |
| 2. Osteoarthritis | Usually in older persons; disintegration of the cartilage that covers the ends of bones. | Pain and stiffness and restricted movement of joints. | Rest and therapeutic exercise, prescribe anti-inflammatory medications, intra-articular corticosteroid injections, and the use of a walker or cane when walking. |

| Disease/Disorder | Cause | Symptoms | Treatment |
|---|---|---|---|
| 3. Tendonitis | Inflammation of shoulder or elbow joints | The shoulder pain becomes more profound when affected arm is abducted between 50 and 130 degrees. | Relieving pain and decreasing inflammation for exercise to avoid permanent immobility. Injections of long-acting corticosteroids may be given along with short-acting analgesics. Applications of ice help pain. |
| 4. Muscular dystrophy: Muscle suffers a loss of protein, and muscle fibers are gradually replaced by fat until the voluntary muscle becomes useless. | Hereditary disease | Progressive muscle weakness; muscle biopsy, genetic testing | Activity, supportive, splints, braces, wheelchairs |
| 5. Tendonitis | Overproduction of uric acid within the body | Acute inflammation of great toe | Dietary avoidance of all foods containing purine meats such as liver, certain cold meats, and some forms of sausage. Alcohol-related products and giving drug colchicine or uricosurics |

2. Differentiate a sprain from a strain.

   A sprain is a wrenching or twisting of a joint with partial tearing of its ligaments. There may be damage to the associated blood vessels, muscles, tendons, and nerves, and often the joint is unusable. A sprain is more serious than a muscle strain, which is simply the overstretching of a muscle without swelling.

## D. Learning Level: Analysis

1. Name five tests used in diagnosis of orthopedic disorders. Next to the test, write one specific disease that the test will diagnose.
   a. x-ray — all fractures
   b. arthrogram — joint tears and rips
   c. EMG — muscular dystrophy
   d. goniometry — muscle strength
   e. NVV — nerve conduction disorder
   f. extra biopsy — muscular dysrophy, myasthenia gravis

2. Name three ambulatory appliances and a disorder for which each would be used.
   a. crutches—fractures, sprain, strain
   b. walkers—sprains, stroke, gout, MD
   c. cane—arthritis, gout

## E. Learning Level: Synthesis

1. When a patient comes in to see the physician and is limping, what information must the medical assistant obtain and record before the physician examination?
   a. recording of the patient's description of the circumstances surrounding the onset
   b. what was done to alleviate the problem at time of injury
   c. what are the major concerns right now
   d. where is the pain located
   e. scale of 1 to 10, at what level would the patient put the pain
   f. medication that has been taken, the amount, and the time it was taken.

2. The physician asks you to direct the patient through active ROM of the ankle and knee through range of motion and record the mobility and position. What will you do and how will you do it?

   Direct patient to move first the ankle, then the knee, in all four directions: up, down, internal and external rotation. Use a goniometer and record the angle and pain for each motion in active range. Then assist the physician to complete the activity using passive range to the point of pain and measure each angle. Record readings in degrees, pain, tenderness, etc.

## F. Learning Level: Evaluation

1. Patient comes in being carried by two large men. He just fell from scaffold and cannot walk on right leg. States he thinks he broke his ankle. The men were right across the street and decided to come to the orthopedic office. He is in great pain and asking for medication. What will you do?

   Student answers will vary. According to the 8th Edition Textbook, the patient should be placed on the table with the leg extended and supported. First aid includes preventing movement of the injured part; elevation of the affected extremity; application of ice if ordered; and control of bleeding, if present. Do not attempt to straighten the fracture or move it in any way. If the patient must be moved, give support to the fractured area before moving. Notify physician and obtain order for ice and x-ray. If facility is set up, also prepare for application of cast.
2. Mrs. Alsop is taken in to the examining room. The front of the chart indicates she made the appointment yesterday because she hurt her leg. When she comes into the office, the medical assistant asks what is happening and Mrs. Alsop lifts up her skirt and shows a large hematoma of about 6 inches in length and very swollen and hot on her right thigh. What will you do?

   Answers should include the notification of physician and preparing for ice application.

## PART 2 COMPETENCY CHALLENGE

This chapter has three procedures related to orthopedic medicine. It is important for the medical assistant student to practice each of these procedures until able to perform competently. The procedures and evaluation sheets are located at the end of the chapter in the Mastery Manual. Usually an orthopedist is willing to donate outdated supplies and demonstrate the application of a cast to a doll or a plastic bat so that the student better understands the assisting process before simulating assisting.

PROCEDURE 37-1
PROCEDURE 37-2
PROCEDURE 37-3

## PART 3 CLINICAL APPLICATIONS

A. There are many opportunities for patient education when working in the orthopedic office. Use Practice Activity 1 at the end of Chapter 28 and develop teaching plans for:

1. The patient applying an arm sling at home.
2. Applying and using an ice bag at home.

B. Consider and discuss the following situations

1. The men who brought in the patient in Part 1 activity F call the office near the end of the day and want to know what happened. What are you going to tell them?

   Issues are: confidentiality, risk management, community relationships, legal issues

2. You have applied an ice bag. Then you got busy with other patients and when you return to the examining room the patient complains that the area is numb. When you take off the ice bag the area is very red and cold. How should you proceed?

   Possible solution: Allow area to come to room temperature, have physician look at area and discharge patient with written instructions for application of cold.

# 38

# Assisting in Urology and Male Reproduction

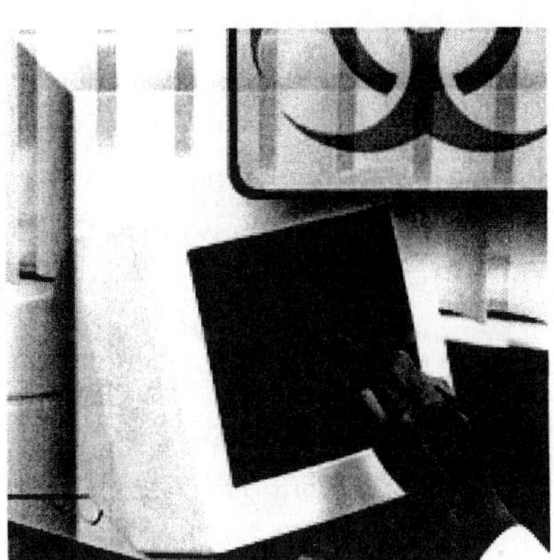

The urinalysis test covered in Chapter 43 is used by the primary care physician to diagnose many urology abnormalities, and the results of that screening test is the reason many patients are referred to the urology specialist. So although the Medical Assistant student may not be working in the urology office, it is essential to learn the techniques for catheterization as it may be used to obtain the urine specimen. In addition, it is important to know the signs of disorders and disease in these areas. Empathy and adequate communication require the medical assistant to be familiar with cancer screening tests, the importance of obtaining accurate samples and of reinforcing physician education and instruction. STDs are reviewed, discussing symptoms particular to the male.

## USING THE LEARNING SYSTEM

### 1. MEDICAL ASSISTING CONTENT AND COMPETENCIES

CONTENT

- Anatomy and physiology for all body systems
- Common pathology and disease
- Diagnostic/treatment modalities
- Applications of medical terminology
- Legal guidelines and requirements for health care
- Medical ethics and related issues
- Risk management
- Basic principles of psychology
- Recognition of and response to verbal and nonverbal communication
- Adaptations for individual needs
- Asepsis and infection control
- Specimen collection and processing
- Diagnostic testing
- Patient care
- Job readiness
- Personal attributes

COMPETENCIES

- All fundamental principles of handwashing, autoclaving, sterilizing, standard precautions
- Prepare and maintain examination and treatment areas
- Prepare patient for and assist with routine and specialty examinations
- Prepare patient for and assist with specialty procedures and treatments
- Recognize and respond to verbal and nonverbal communication
- Identify and respond to issues of confidentiality
- Document appropriately
- Instruct patients according to needs
- Identify community resources
- Provide instruction for health maintenance and disease prevention
- Instruct patients in collection of specimens
- Perform specialty noninvasive diagnostic tests
- Use methods of quality control
- Screen and follow up test results
- Demonstrate use and care of patient equipment
- Perform an inventory of supplies and equipment

## 2. MEDICAL ASSISTING ENTRY-LEVEL CURRICULUM INTERFACE

| TEXTBOOK OBJECTIVES | LEARNING SYSTEM LOCATION | MA CURRICULUM |
|---|---|---|
| Cognitive | | Content |
| 1. List the organs of the urinary system and explain the function of each | • Text p. 740<br>• Manual Part 1-A | • Anatomy and physiology for all body systems<br>• Applications of medical terminology<br>• Job readiness |
| 2. Explain the reasons the urinary system has many occasions for contracting diseases and disorders | • Text p. 741<br>• Manual Part 1-C | • Asepsis and infection control<br>• Patient care<br>• Personal attributes |
| 3. Compare and contrast the diseases and disorders of the urinary system | • Text p. 741<br>• Manual Part 1-D | • Common pathology and disease |
| 4. Identify the primary symptoms of urinary problems | • Text pp. 741–746<br>• Manual Part 1-D | • Common pathology and disease<br>• Applications of medical terminology |
| 5. List the radiologic procedures used to diagnose urinary disorders | • Text p. 745<br>• Manual Part 1-D | • Diagnostic testing<br>• Diagnostic/treatment modalities<br>• Legal guidelines and requirements for health care<br>• Specimen collection and processing |
| 6. List the organs included in male reproduction | • Text pp. 746–747<br>• Manual Part 1-A | • Anatomy and physiology for all body systems<br>• Applications of medical terminology |

| TEXTBOOK OBJECTIVES | LEARNING SYSTEM LOCATION | MA CURRICULUM |
|---|---|---|
| **Cognitive** | | **Content** |
| 7. Trace sperm through the male reproductive tract | • Text pp. 746–747<br>• Manual Part 1-A | • Anatomy and physiology for all body systems<br>• Applications of medical terminology<br>• Job readiness |
| 8. Explain the cause and effects of prostate disorders | • Text pp. 749–750<br>• Manual Part 1-D | • Anatomy and physiology for all body systems<br>• Applications of medical terminology<br>• Job readiness |
| 9. Compare the effects of sexually transmitted diseases in the male with those in the female | • Text pp. 750–751<br>• Manual Part 1-D | • Medical ethics and related issues<br>• Risk management<br>• Recognition of and response to verbal and nonverbal communication<br>• Adaptations for individual needs<br>• Job readiness |
| 10. Understand and demonstrate the medical assistant's role in urology | • Text pp. 751–762<br>• Manual Part 1-B and 2 | • Prepare patient for and assist with routine and specialty examinations<br>• Basic principles of psychology<br>• Recognition of and response to verbal and nonverbal communication<br>• Personal attributes |
| **Performance** | | **Competencies** |
| 1. Demonstrate with accuracy catheterization of both female and male patients | • Manual Part 2<br>• Procedures 38-1, 38-2 | • All fundamental principles of handwashing, autoclaving, sterilizing, standard precautions<br>• Prepare and maintain examination and treatment areas<br>• Prepare patient for and assist with specialty procedures and treatments<br>• Document appropriately<br>• Recognize and respond to verbal and nonverbal communication<br>• Demonstrate use and care of patient equipment<br>• Perform an inventory of supplies and equipment |

*chart continues on following page*

## MEDICAL ASSISTING ENTRY LEVEL CURRICULUM INTERFACE continued

| TEXTBOOK OBJECTIVES | LEARNING SYSTEM LOCATION | MA CURRICULUM |
|---|---|---|
| **Performance** | | **Competencies** |
| 2. Accurately prepare a patient for a vasectomy | • Text p. 759<br>• Manual Part 2 | • Instruct patients according to needs<br>• Identify and respond to issues of confidentiality<br>• Identify community resources |
| 3. Instruct a patient in performing a self-testicular examination | • Manual Part 3<br>• See urology Internet sites | • Provide instruction for health maintenance and disease prevention<br>• Instruct patients in collection of specimens |
| 4. Explain to the patient reasons for a PAP or PSA test | • Manual Part 3 | • Instruct patients according to needs<br>• Perform specialty noninvasive diagnostic tests<br>• Use methods of quality control<br>• Screen and follow up test results |
| 5. Prepare a patient for a tissue biopsy | | • Instruct patients according to needs<br>• Provide instruction for health maintenance and disease prevention |

## 3. RESOURCES

_www.yahoo.com/Health/Medicine/Urology **There are many site links here to male genital pathology images; professional organizations and urology disorders**

www.auanet.com **The direct site for the American Urology Association**

www.aarp.org **Health concerns of seniors**

www.kidney.org

National Kidney Foundation, 30 East 33rd St. NY, New York 10016 1-212-889-2210

**4. LESSON PLAN Urology Assisting** **TIME 3 hours lecture, 12 hours lab**

**Opening:** This little visualization helps students understand simple kidney anatomy. Set up a funnel with a coffee filter in it and a tube on the end that empties into a bottle as a visual method of simulating the filtering mechanism of the glomerulus. Put some yarn in the filter and simulate how the capillaries filter into the capsule. Such an illustration helps students comprehend the anatomy and pathology of common diseases.

**Pretest:** Ask what the average urine output is in a day. Ans: 1000cc average. What is average urine output at each voiding? 300 ml. Most common disorder? Cystitis.

**Objectives:** Write objectives and then discuss each. Use the grid above to locate topics and relate to MA curriculum.

**Content:** Students often are uncomfortable discussing these private matters. Relate their discomfort to the potential patient feelings. Discuss the how's of providing for patient dignity.

**URINARY SYSTEM**

1. Anatomy and Physiology
   Kidney — Ureter
   Urinary Bladder — Urethra
2. Disorders of the Urinary System
   Urinary Incontinence — Glomerulonephritis
   Renal Failure — Kidney Dialysis
   Pyelonephritis — Renal Carcinoma
   Renal Calculi — Cystitis
   Hydronephrosis — Polycystic Kidneys
   Urethritis — Bladder Cancer
   Pediatric Urological Disorders
   Enuresis — Urine Reflux
   Cryptorchidism — Hydrocele
3. Diagnostic Procedures
   Kidney, Ureters, Bladder (KUB)
   Intravenous Pyelogram (IVP)/Urogram
   Angiography
   Computerized Tomography (CT)
   Cystoscopy
   Retrograde Pyelogram
   Voiding Cystourethrogram (VCUG)
   Ultrasound

**MALE REPRODUCTIVE SYSTEM**

4. Anatomy and Physiology of the Male Reproductive System
   Testes — Epididymis
   Vas Deferens — Prostate Gland — Penis
   Hormone Production
5. Disorders of the Male Reproductive System—
   Benign Prostatic Hypertrophy (BPH) — Prostatitis
   Prostate Cancer — Epididymitis
   Balanitis — Testicular Cancer
   Impotence — Infertility
6. Sexually Transmitted Diseases: See Chapter 33 Instructor Curriculum Resource for a chart of STDs:
   Bacterial: Gonorrhea, Chlamydia, Syphilis
   Viral: Genital Herpes, AIDS

*lesson plan continues on following page*

**LESSON PLAN Urology Assisting continued**

7. Medical Assistant's Role in Urology and Male Reproduction Examination
   Text pp. 751–762 Complete an outline on the board as follows:
   - Obtain patient history and vital signs
   - Instruct patient in clean-catch urine (Chapter 43)
   - Obtain a catheterized specimen if ordered
   - Send specimen to lab for immediate urinalysis
   - Prepare patient for examination
   - Explain the procedure and order of physician performance
   - Provide for patient draping and modesty
   - Position patient as required
   - Place equipment and specimen containers as needed
   - Explain diagnostic tests or reinforce explanations
   - Offer to answer questions
   - Provide pamphlets and complete directions
   - Document

   Procedure 38-1: Female Catheterization; Procedure 38-2: Male Catheterization
   Assisting with the Urologic Examination
   Assisting with the Male Reproductive Examination
8. Diagnostic Test Explanations
   Procedure 38-3: Teaching Testicular Self-Examination
   Prostatic Antigen Phosphatase (PAP)
   Prostate-Specific Antigen (PSA)
   Tissue Biopsy
9. Patient Education
10. Legal and Ethical Issues

**Lab:** CD-ROM ⊕ There will be the opportunity to instruct patients or simulate obtaining urine specimens from Mrs. Ferguson. Students should click the main menu and case studies for choices. The Mastery Manual activities vary from matching and labeling to explaining reasons for patient care. Students will be able to complete during lab time and while practicing catheterization.

**Assignment:** Students will complete Mastery Manual Part 1 after learning materials. Study procedures and come to lab prepared to practice as directed in Parts 2 and 3 of Mastery Manual.

**Posttest:** Use the Examaster for multiple-choice questions. Part of grade of posttest will be competency in chapter procedures.

## 5. MASTERY MANUAL ANSWERS

### PART 1 CONTENT MASTERY

#### A. Learning Level: Knowledge

1. Label the parts of the kidney illustrated below.
   See page 740 in textbook for correct labels.
2. Label the structures of the male genitourinary system illustrated below. Use a red pen and trace the passage of sperm through the reproductive tract.
   See page 747 in textbook for answers.

## B. Learning Level: Comprehension

Match structures with function.

1. b; 2. f; 3. g; 4. i; 5. a; 6. j; 7. m; 8. n; 9. c; 10. h; 11. l; 12. k; 13. e; 14. d

## C. Learning Level: Application

1. Name two possible negative consequences of having organs that open to the environment.
   a. more vulnerable to organisms entering, increased number of infections
   b. requires careful cleaning
2. Name and describe three types of catheters.
   a. straight
   b. Coude—has slight bend at end
   c. Foley—has an inflatable bag to keep inside bladder
3. Write three medical assistant responsibilities when assisting the patient and physician for urology examination.
   a. keep patient covered at all times, maintain privacy by leaving if indicated
   b. explain examination or procedure before physician proceeds
   c. maintain patient dignity and be supportive
4. Which tests would you expect to be ordered if a patient was suspected of having prostate cancer?
   PAP, PSA, tissue biopsy

## D. Learning Level: Analysis

1. Complete the charts below which highlight features of common urological diseases. You will need to study the sections carefully before attempting this activity.

| Disease and Causes | Symptoms | Diagnostic Tests | Treatment |
|---|---|---|---|
| 1. Glomerulonephritis | Malaise, edema, albuminuria | U/A, IVP | Antibiotics |
| 2. Renal Failure | Pyuria, hematuria, albuminuria, oliguria, anuria | U/A, RP blood tests | Dialysis: renal or hemodialysis |
| 3. Pyelonephritis | Pyuria, flank pain, fever, hematuria | U/A, ultrasound, IVP | Antibiotics |
| 4. Renal Carcinoma | Flank pain, hematuria, decreased appetite, anemia | IVP, CT, ultrasound; angiography | Nephrectomy |
| 5. Renal Calculi | Renal colic; dysuria, hematuria, leukocytes | IVP, ultrasound | Lithotripsy or surgical crushing |
| 6. Cystitis—most common | Burning, frequency, dysuria, casts leukocytes, bacteria | U/A, IVP | Antibiotics |
| 7. Polycystic kidney | Congenital, flank pain, albuminuria, symptoms of renal failure | U/A, ultrasound | |

2. Complete the chart below.

| Disease and Causes | Symptoms | Diagnostic Tests | Treatment |
|---|---|---|---|
| STDs, bacterial—Chlamydia, GC, Syphilis | Pain on urination, pus discharge<br>Chancre on penis | Smear of discharge | Antibiotic, specific drugs. PCN will not cure most any more |
| STDs, viral—Herpes, HIV, Human Papilloma Virus | Pain, burning, blisters<br>Nonlocal, anorexia, wt. loss, sweats,<br>genital warts | Visual and smear,<br>T cell count, HIV antigen tests, biopsy | Zovirax, cleanliness; combination antivirals and protease inhibitors; excision |
| Cryptorchidism | Testicle not visible | Find level of descent—palpation | Hormones, orchiopexy or laparoscopy |
| Hydrocele | Scrotal swelling, pain | Observation, ultrasound | Surgical correction |
| BPH—Adult | Nocturia, frequency, urgency, retention | Palpation, rectal exam, ultrasound | TURP, laser excision |
| Epididymitis | Painful, enlarged, red, hot scrotum | Observation | Rest, antibiotics, ice packs |
| Testicular Cancer | Felt on TSE—lump | Examination, biopsy | Radiation, chemotherapy or orchiectomy |
| Cancer of Prostate | Same symptoms as BPH, lump on TSE | PAP, PSA, tissue biopsy | TURP, chemotherapy, radiation implants |

## E. Learning Level: Synthesis

Complete the crossword puzzle below. The words are vocabulary and bold print words from the specialty chapters 29–38.

Answers

ACROSS
6. anoscope
7. eczema
9. induration
10. cancer
13. derma
14. neoplasia
15. RAST
20. rales
22. EEG
23. CHF
24. erythema
25. tumor
26. SGOT (Most labs use AST today)
28. staging
29. otitis
30. eustachian tube
31. oto
32. hyperplasia

DOWN
1. colitis
2. scope
3. benign
4. malignant
5. jaundice
6. asthma
8. contraindications
11. CVA
12. neuro
16. melanosis
17. flatus
18. pruritus
19. hemoccult
21. leukoderma
27. ENT

## F. Learning Level: Evaluation

Explain the following physician decisions.

1. The patient is having recurrent bladder infections. You know the physician will want a urine specimen. You think a catheterized specimen will be ordered to get a sterile specimen, but the physician orders a midstream and tells you to prepare the patient carefully before obtaining the specimen.

   A catheter may move a urethral infection retrograde into the bladder; also, catheters may traumatize tissue that is already compromised. Statistics show the midstream can be just as accurate.

2. A male patient has BPH and trouble initiating voiding and emptying the bladder. The physician asks you to catheterize the patient, who seems to have residual urine. You get a small adult #14 catheter. The physician asks you to use a pediatric #10.

   A larger catheter will not pass an obstruction and may cause pain—this size will drain the residual and should easily insert.

3. Mrs. Ari Ben Salam is having continual problems with urinary retention. She has not voided in 12 hours, and the physician tells you to use a Foley catheter and clamp it after 500cc has drained if there is still more draining.

   Taking out more than 500cc at one time may cause bladder spasm and further inability to void.

## PART 2 COMPETENCY CHALLENGE

1. Use Procedures 38-1 and 38-2 and catheterization models. After your instructor's demonstration and your observation of videotape demonstration, proceed to simulate practice of the procedure on the mannequin. Simulate catheterization techniques to perfection. Be very careful to follow strict aseptic techniques. Have someone watch you, as it is easy to contaminate equipment and not be aware of it. The procedures are at the end of this chapter.

   **Instructors:** Students tend to contaminate the procedure easily. It is important to observe all students on their first practice so they become aware of the subtleties of sterile technique. Students will need to review procedures for setting up a sterile field in Chapter 26.

2. Your patient is to have a vasectomy. The physician has explained the procedure and has asked you to reinforce the preparation for the procedure. Use the Internet or any books or periodicals as references with the patient teaching plan from Chapter 28 and prepare a short paper to prepare the patient for the procedure. Look in the reference list in Appendix A for resources. **Note:** See item #4 for this chapter.

3. Write a procedure to prepare the patient for tissue biopsy. Include how tissue is obtained, use of pain medication, length of procedure, aftercare. Use the information from Chapter 36, page 708, to help write the procedure.

## PART 3 CLINICAL APPLICATIONS

1. Is it legal for a medical assistant to perform catheterization in your state?
   Depends upon state—check laws.

2. Explain testicular self-examination to at least two classmates. Use handouts from resource list and Procedure 38-3. Whenever possible, the male medical assistant should explain TSE and the female explain SBE. This is for patient comfort. All medical assistants should be able to explain both without getting red, embarrassed, or nervous. **Note:** This can be easily done on a 3x5 card. Teaching plans do not have to be volumes.

3. Explain the importance of the PAP and PSA examination for a man. Include at what age tests should be started, why, how often, and normal values.

   Usually tests are started at age 50 unless there is a family history, or an indication on physical examination. There is presently some controversy over total PSA versus free PSA testing.

# 39

# Assisting with the Older Patient

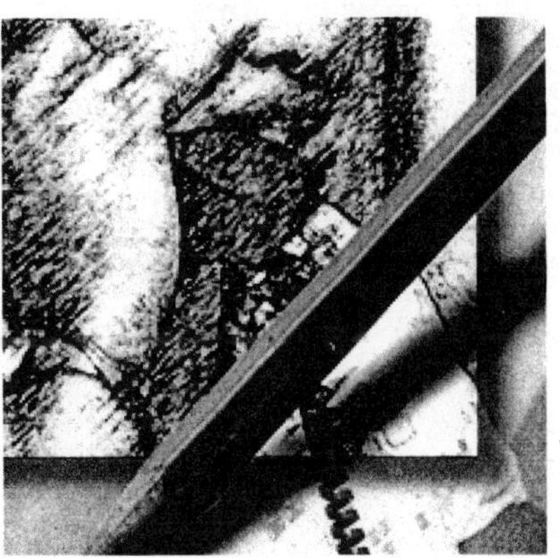

This chapter thoroughly covers elder medical issues, physical changes for all the sytems, and the effects of those changes on behavior. Emphasis is placed on understanding and meeting the needs of the elderly. Patients 60 years and older make up a large percentage of office visits as these people are more likely to visit the physician for preventive care and because they have more health problems as the body gets older. There is a large volume of solid knowledge for the student to apply in the medical office.

## USING THE LEARNING SYSTEM

### 1. MEDICAL ASSISTING CONTENT AND COMPETENCIES

CONTENT

- Anatomy and physiology for all body systems
- Common pathology and disease
- Diagnostic/treatment modalities
- Applications of medical terminology
- Legal guidelines and requirements for health care
- Medical ethics and related issues
- Risk management
- Basic principles of psychology
- Recognition of and response to verbal and nonverbal communication
- Adaptations for individual needs
- Asepsis and infection control
- Specimen collection and processing
- Diagnostic testing
- Patient care
- Job readiness
- Personal attributes

COMPETENCIES

- All fundamental principles of handwashing, autoclaving, sterilizing, standard precautions
- Prepare and maintain examination and treatment areas
- Prepare patient for and assist with routine and specialty examinations
- Prepare patient for and assist with specialty procedures and treatments
- Recognize and respond to verbal and nonverbal communication
- Identify and respond to issues of confidentiality
- Document appropriately
- Instruct patients according to needs
- Identify community resources
- Provide instruction for health maintenance and disease prevention
- Instruct patients in collection of specimens
- Perform specialty noninvasive diagnostic tests
- Use methods of quality control
- Screen and follow up test results
- Demonstrate use and care of patient equipment
- Perform an inventory of supplies and equipment

## 2. MEDICAL ASSISTING ENTRY-LEVEL CURRICULUM INTERFACE

| TEXTBOOK OBJECTIVES | LEARNING SYSTEM LOCATION | MA CURRICULUM |
|---|---|---|
| **Cognitive** | | **Content** |
| 1. Identify the various impacts of an increasing aging population on society | • Text pp. 756–766<br>• Manual Part 1-B | • Legal guidelines and requirements for health care<br>• Medical ethics and related issues<br>• Risk management<br>• Basic principles of psychology<br>• Recognition of and response to verbal and nonverbal communication<br>• Adaptations for individual needs |
| 2. Explain the changes caused by aging in each of the body systems | • Text pp. 766–779<br>• Manual Part 1-D | • Anatomy and physiology for all body systems<br>• Applications of medical terminology<br>• Specimen collection and processing<br>• Diagnostic testing<br>• Personal attributes |
| 3. Identify the major diseases and disorders faced by the elderly | • Text pp. 766–779<br>• Manual Part 1-D | • Common pathology and disease |
| 4. Explain why sleep disorders are a major concern of the elderly | • Text p. 799<br>• Manual Part 1-D | • Patient care<br>• Job readiness |

| TEXTBOOK OBJECTIVES | LEARNING SYSTEM LOCATION | MA CURRICULUM |
|---|---|---|
| **Cognitive** | | **Content** |
| 5. Differentiate between independent, assisted, and skilled nursing facilities | • Text pp. 779–781<br>• Manual Part 1-F | • Diagnostic/treatment modalities<br>• Asepsis and infection control |
| 6. List the basic principles covered in Patient's Rights and Advance Directives | • Text p. 783<br>• Manual Part 3 | • Same as #1 |
| **Performance** | | **Competencies** |
| 1. Demonstrate changes in communication techniques used with elderly patients | • Procedure 39-1, Text p. 768<br>• Procedure 39-2, Text p. 772<br>• ⊕ CD-ROM | • All competencies listed above under MA competencies in preceding grid |

## 3. RESOURCES

http://www.yahoo.com/Health/Geriatrics_and_Aging/ **A site to health subjects, magazines, organizations**

www.aarp.org **American Association of Retired Persons**

www.aol.com/webcenter/health/home.adp **Links to Seniors' Health, National Institute of Aging**

National Institute on Aging Information, PO Box 8057, Gaithersburg, MD 20898-8057,

1-800-222-2225

www.nih.gov.nia **National Institute on Aging**

Alzheimer's Association, 70E Lake #600, Chicago, IL 60601, 1-800-621-0379

Alcohol Rehab for the Elderly, PO Box 267, Hopedale, IL 61747, 1-800-354-7089

See Text p. 783 for more resources.

## 4. LESSON PLAN Elder Care TIME 3 hours lecture, 12 hours lab

**Opening:** In a bowl have 2x2 note paper, each piece having a straight pin and a name of one disability of the elderly. Have students carefully pick out one piece of paper; they must function in school with that disability for ___ days or hours.

**Pretest:** From personal experience, have students list all the changes elderly people experience of which they are aware. Write the changes on board in categories as listed in chapter.

**Objectives:** Use flip chart and review the objectives. Emphasize the number of disabled persons they know.

**Content:** Discuss lesson highlights. Concentrate on physical changes in the elderly that affect their personal safety or their ability to follow directions and care for themselves. As medical assistants, the job will be easier if patients' needs are met.

Instructional goal: To heighten the students' appreciation of and ability to work with the elder patient.

Allow students to talk about their experiences with elderly people and also discuss patience!
This can be a fun and free-flowing chapter.

**Lab:**
1. The CD-ROM ⊕ integrates care of the elderly in the case studies. Case 4 with Mrs. Ferguson requires elder care. Go to the main menu and proceed from there.
2. Have each student complete projects in Procedures 39-1 and 39-2 in the Mastery Manual
3. Have students write a do's: and don'ts list for working with the elderly.
4. Bring an older person into the lab to talk about disabilities, the process of aging, and treatment by medical offices and others.
5. Have students design a procedure with techniques for assisting with the elderly both in administrative and clinical areas. Have students write a procedural step to address medical assisting for each listed competency at beginning of chapter.

**Assignment:** After discussion, allow students to complete all parts in the Mastery Manual and assign preparation for the lab. After lab assign preparation for next topic.

**Posttest:**
1. Set up a role play of an older, difficult patient with an evaluation of techniques as designed by students in Lab activity #5.
2. Use Examaster questions.
3. Ask students what they learned and can apply to the disability they "lived" in 24-hour application of class opening.

## 5 MASTERY MANUAL ANSWERS

### PART 1 CONTENT MASTERY

### A. Learning Level: Knowledge

1. **androgen**—any steroid hormone that promotes male characteristics
2. **autonomy**—the ability to function in an independent fashion
3. **collagen**—primary protein of the skin, tendon, bone, cartilage, and connective tissues
4. **elastin**—the essential part of elastic connective tissue which, when moist, is flexible and elastic.
5. **hot flashes**—flushing of the body caused by blood vessels expanding and then contracting

6. **hypothermia**—greatly reduced body temperature
7. **incontinence**—inability to control excretory functions
8. **lacrimation**—the secretion or discharge of tears
9. **melanin**—a dark, sulfur-containing pigment normally found in hair, skin, ciliary body, choroid of the eye, pigment layer of the retina, and certain nerve cells
10. **menopause**—the phase of life when a woman ceases to menstruate and passes from the reproductive to the non-reproductive stage
11. **mnemonic**—improvement of memory by special methods or techniques
12. **paranoia**—a descriptive term limited to the characterization of behavior that is marked by delusions of persecution or grandeur
13. **senile**—a pronounced loss of mental, physical, or emotional control in aged people, caused by physical or mental deterioration

## B. Learning Level: Comprehension

1. Name three societal impacts of an aging population.
   a. increased need of health services
   b. need more ADL resources to maintain autonomy
   c. others need to improve communication skills
2. List eight resources to help seniors maintain their autonomy.
   a. outreach programs
   b. friendly visitors
   c. senior centers for social and recreation
   d. transportation services
   e. home health agencies
   f. adult day care centers
   g. senior apartments
   h. assisted living facilities

## C. Learning Level: Application

1. Complete the chart below to help you learn to assist those with sensory changes.

| Area | Change | Symptom | Prevention, Care |
|---|---|---|---|
| Taste and Smell | Decreased number of taste buds | More salt and sugar; less appetite; likes different foods | Help plan cooking and shopping, health aide |
| Vision<br>Lens more dense, less elastic and yellows | Decreased acuity, depth perception, color distinction; bright light hurts; cannot focus as well | Needs reading glasses; opacity over lens; decreased visual field; trips on curbs, stairs; seems unstable | Get glasses and magnifier; create contrast at steps and furniture edges; use bright colors, handrails, eyedrops if eyes itchy or dry; get home health aide |
| Hearing | By age 65, 50% loss in high pitch, unable to distinguish sounds in a room; ringing in ears | Appears confused, doesn't follow directions, cannot repeat what's said | Talk in lower pitch, verify that you were heard, speak distinctly and more slowly; encourage new computerized hearing aids which can correct these problems with no feedback! |

## D. Learning Level: Analysis

Summarize the changes in the elderly for each system listed below. Describe symptoms of each change and assistance required at home or by the MA.

| System | Change | Symptom | Assistance Required |
|---|---|---|---|
| Musculoskeletal | Muscle tone, size, strength ⇓; weight loss; fat ⇑; loss of elasticity in joints and ligaments; bones more porous | Change in posture, stooped, pear-shaped, protruding abdomen; Decrease in mobility and motility; joint aches; ⇑ bone fractures; osteoporosis | 30 min walking every day, increase weight-bearing activity, increase calcium intake, HRT, swim for mobility, eat less fat and more vegetables |
| Skin | Cells replace more slowly, collagen decreases, slower regeneration; elastic fibers break; oil glands decrease production | More dry skin, injure easier and slower healing of injury; skin sags and wrinkles; less insulation produces less temperature variance tolerance; sweat less, grey hair | Use moisturizers; exercise; drink plenty of water; wear sufficient clothing; exercise; see dermatologist if fair or history of skin cancer; stay covered in sun |
| Respiratory | Lungs lose elasticity, smaller and flabbier, chest wall stiffens; respiratory muscles weaker | Use accessory muscles, more prone to pneumonia, decreased vital capacity | Encourage deep breathing and shoulders back, stay out of crowds in flu season, stay away from sick children |
| Cardiovascular | Myocardium loses cells; muscle weakens as replaced with fat cells | Cardiac output decreased. Heart rate slower, decreased ability to maintain maximum heart rate, edema of right leg | Encourage consistent exercise; teach signs for possible MI; have yearly physical; low-fat diet |
| Urinary | Sphincter muscles weaken, more water needed to excrete same waste; bladder expands less; medications excreted more slowly | Stress incontinence; urinary retention, urgency, increased bladder infections, up at night to void; medications have prolonged effect | Drink lots of fluid during day; practice emptying bladder totally; encourage open communication, encourage protective padding |
| Gastrointestinal | Decreased tolerance to milk, sugars, fats and protein in large amounts; muscles lose tone and digest slower; gastric secretions and pancreatic enzymes decrease | Foods may cause excessive flatulence or diarrhea; complain of discomfort after large meals, tend to constipation | Nutritional counseling; avoid offending foods; eat smaller meals more often; still need nutrition; eat fibrous foods; medication evaluation for those that have GI effects |
| Neurological | Cells may lose chemicals or die | Parkinsonism, Alzheimer's disease, less sleep | Drugs with dopamine, respite homes for family, may require assisted living |
| Reproductive | Female hormones decrease<br>Male hormones change some | Menopause; hot flashes<br>Prostate enlarges, sexual recovery longer | Some drugs and diseases interfere with sexual functioning. They should be discussed openly with patient |

## E. Learning Level: Synthesis

1. Considering the way to minimize changes that take place with aging, what can you personally do to ensure your own terrific mental functioning for as long as you live?

   Remain mentally and physically stimulated, study, learn to play an instrument, volunteer in the community; paint; write a book; take up a hobby; get on the Internet!!
2. When is it important to emphasize to patients the habits that minimize the effects of aging?

   From childhood on, habits should be directed to caring for the body.

## F. Learning Level: Evaluation

1. It is most impolite to guess a person's age; yet when caring for patients, one must be able to estimate ages. Your instructor will show you a collection of ten persons. Using your knowledge, try to guess their ages. How well did you do? Within 5 years is great!! Some people try to disguise their age. What have you learned about how people age after trying to guess ages?

   Provide a preprinted list to the students and collect when they are finished. Some well-known, more mature actors, politicians, and other famous people are good names for such a list.
2. Explain the difference between assisted living and a skilled nursing facility.
   - Assisted living provides some activities of daily living needed by the person. It may be meals or bathing, ambulation or housekeeping. It is not giving medications unless individual states allow for this. Skilled nursing facilities provide 24-hour care and medical supervision.

   Describe two types of patients you think might be in each.
   - Student's personal response

## PART 2 COMPETENCY CHALLENGE

1. Procedures 39-1 and 39-2 at the end of this chapter contain projects for students' completion to better understand the visually and hearing impaired.
2. Practice using communication techniques described in the textbook. Complete Procedure 39-2 to better understand the hearing impaired older adult.
3. Have students practice talking to each other in a confidential manner. Identify hearing difficulties and solutions which may be applied to the medical office.

   Note: Try to set up small officelike areas. Have music and noise in the background to simulate difficult hearing conditions.

## PART 3 CLINICAL APPLICATIONS

1. Discuss this: Can one honestly teach patients how to prevent degenerative changes with aging when one doesn't role model oneself? Will a patient believe you that it's important not to smoke when they smell smoke on the medical assistant's breath? What about manifesting other self-destructive behaviors when we tell patients to change theirs?
2. Go to an assisted living facility or any residence for seniors and talk to seniors. Obtain their opinions on the changes that are affecting them, how they cope, how they feel mentally. Come back and discuss these answers with your peers.
3. May an adult child obtain information on his or her parent if the parent says no but is also confused at times?

   Unless child is actual court-appointed guardian, legally she or he may not. Some physicians do give out certain amounts of information for the care of the patient.
4. Explain patient rights versus advanced directives. What is the legal implication of each?

   All patients have a right to know about medications, treatments, and side effects. These are included in the 1992 AHA Patient's Bill of Rights, text p. 784. Review with students. Presently this bill of rights has no legal standing. Advance directives are legal instruments if executed correctly. They may be in the form of a living will or a durable power of attorney. See text p. 783.
5. Discuss the loss, loneliness, and isolation older persons may feel as friends and family members die. How might this affect their behavior? Is there anything the medical assistant can do about this?

# 40

# Assisting with Office Emergencies

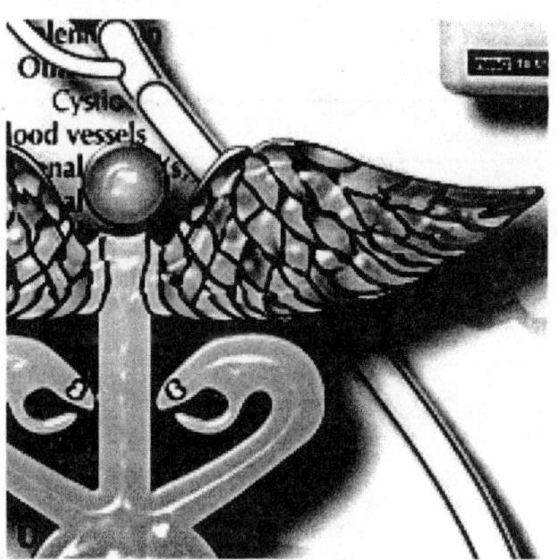

Office emergencies require training in first aid and a clear understanding of the medical assistant's role when an emergency happens. This is true for administrative or clinical assisting. Students must be aware that prevention is the first key in making the office less prone to accidents, and the medical assistant must be involved in helping to maintain a safe office. Having the correct equipment on an emergency cart allows for adequate treatment until medical support arrives. Thinking about potential emergencies and planning ahead will allow the medical assistant some degree of preparation when an emergency develops. Students will find all the information in the competency package. Explain the need for all the competencies listed in the Role Delineation Chart.

## USING THE LEARNING SYSTEM

### 1. MEDICAL ASSISTING CONTENT AND COMPETENCIES

CONTENT

- Medical emergency clinical procedures
- Legal guidelines/requirements for health care
- Risk management
- Diagnostic treatment modalities
- Job readiness
- Workplace dynamics

COMPETENCIES

- Obtain CPR certification and first aid training
- Perform electrocardiogram and respiratory testing
- Apply pharmacology principles to prepare and administer oral and parenteral drugs
- Recognize and respond to verbal and nonverbal communications
- Perform within legal and ethical boundaries
- Identify community resources

## 2. MEDICAL ASSISTING ENTRY-LEVEL CURRICULUM INTERFACE

| TEXTBOOK OBJECTIVES | LEARNING SYSTEM LOCATION | MA CURRICULUM |
|---|---|---|
| **Cognitive** | | **Content** |
| 1. Describe the medical assistant's responsibilities in an emergency | • Text p. 787<br>• Manual Part 1-B | • Medical emergency clinical procedures<br>• Legal guidelines/requirements for health care<br>• Risk management<br>• Diagnostic treatment modalities<br>• Job readiness<br>• Workplace dynamics |
| 2. Recall two resources that can help to make the medical office accident-proof | • Text p. 788<br>• Manual Part 1-B | • Medical emergency clinical procedures<br>• Legal guidelines/requirements for health care<br>• Risk management |
| 3. List the basic items that must be included on an emergency cart | • Text p. 789<br>• Manual Part 1-D | • Diagnostic treatment modalities<br>• Medical emergency clinical procedures<br>• Legal guidelines/requirements for health care |
| 4. Explain the purpose of a defibrillator in an emergency | • Text p. 790<br>• Memory jogger | • Medical emergency clinical procedures<br>• Legal guidelines/requirements for health care |
| 5. Recognize a choking victim | • Text p. 796<br>• Manual Part 1-C | • Medical emergency clinical procedures |
| 6. Recall conditions that necessitate implementation of CPR | • Text p. 794<br>• Manual Part 2 | • Diagnostic treatment modalities<br>• Medical emergency clinical procedures |
| 7. List the major symptoms associated with heart attack | • Text p. 800<br>• Manual Part 1-C | • Same as #6 above |
| 8. Describe the emergency medical care that is usually given to victims of asthma, anaphylactic shock, convulsions, hemorrhagic shock, and other conditions | • Text pp. 800–805<br>• Manual Part 1-C | • Same as #6 above |
| 9. State the functions of a poison control center | • Text p. 800<br>• Manual Part 1-B | • Same as #6 above |

*chart continues on following page*

## MEDICAL ASSISTING ENTRY-LEVEL CURRICULUM INTERFACE continued

| TEXTBOOK OBJECTIVES | LEARNING SYSTEM LOCATION | MA CURRICULUM |
|---|---|---|
| **Performance** | | **Competencies** |
| 1. Demonstrate triage techniques in a simulated emergency situation | • Manual Parts 2 & 3<br>• CD-ROM ⊕ See Cases 1 & 2 and telephone triage | • Recognize and respond to verbal and nonverbal communications<br>• Perform within legal and ethical boundaries |
| 2. Accurately perform CPR using a mannequin | • Manual Part 2 | • Same as #1 above and<br>• Obtain CPR certification and first aid training |

## 3. RESOURCES

www.ahn.com **America's Health Network**

www.yahoo.com/health/Emergency **Sites to health concerns and organizations**

http://www.yahoo.com/Health/Medicine/Emergency Medicine/www.nho.org **Information on hospice and Medicare benefits**

## 4. LESSON PLAN Emergency Assisting TIME 3 hours lecture, 12 hours lab

**Opening:** Simulate an emergency as soon as class is assembled. Usually getting a student to faint works. Pretend you do not see the emergency and observe the students' responses. Note how quickly someone goes to help, whether help is given according to first aid protocols, etc. When over, check out feelings and fears due to lack of knowledge and preparation. Discuss the students' responses and need for education.

**Pretest:** Pass out a sheet asking for a brief response to: What do you do when a patient cannot breathe? When a person seizes?

**Objectives:** Put objectives on a flip chart and review. This is an opportunity to cover the material by discussing each objective. The content outline follows.

**Content:**

1. VOCABULARY: anaphylaxis, ecchymosis, paroxysm, traumatic, triage
2. THE ACCIDENT-PROOF OFFICE
   Planning ahead; using community resources; preventing children's accidents
3. SUPPLIES AND EMERGENCY EQUIPMENT
   Emergency supplies
   Defibrillators
   General emergency rules
   Emergency management
4. COMMON EMERGENCIES

| | |
|---|---|
| Syncope | Choking |
| Chest pain | CVA |
| Poisonings | Insect stings |
| Shock | Asthma attacks |
| Seizure | Abdominal pain |
| Fracture | OB emergency |
| Burns | Lacerations |
| Nosebleed | Head injury |
| Foreign body in eye | CPR |
| Emergency resuscitation | |

5. PATIENT EDUCATION Handouts, aftercare instruction
6. LEGAL AND ETHICAL IMPLICATIONS

**Lab:** The activities in the Mastery Manual chapter cover many of the materials in a first aid course. Students have the opportunity to list symptoms and emergency care and practice CPR. Nationally certified programs require CPR certification for all students. Most medical offices and clinics also require programs to have students certified with BLS certificates. There are activities for telephone triage and simulated emergencies on the CD-ROM ⊕ . Going into the case studies from the main menu will allow students to simulate some office emergencies. Have students complete and discuss all Mastery Manual activities and the CD-ROM ⊕ .

**Assignment:** After discussion, use time to allow students to complete Competency Manual and, if part of the program, practice and certify for CPR (4–8 hours).

**Posttest:** Use questions from the Examaster testbank. CPR certificate must be required.

## 5. MASTERY MANUAL ANSWERS

### PART 1 CONTENT MASTERY

### A. Learning Level: Knowledge

**Definitions**
Write the vocabulary word for each definition:

1. To determine the priority of need for treatment. **triage**
2. Bluish color of the mucous membrane caused by lack of oxygen. **cyanosis**
3. Pulse felt over the base of the heart. **apical**
4. A syrup given to induce vomiting. **ipecac**
5. A bruise. **ecchymosis**
6. An allergic reaction caused by an antigen/antibody reaction. **anaphylaxis**
7. A series of involuntary contractions of the voluntary muscles. **seizure, convulsion**
8. Primary muscle of respiration. **diaphragm**
9. A sudden onset of symptoms. **paroxysm**
10. Loss of consciousness. **syncope**

### B. Learning Level: Comprehension

1. MATCHING: Match the fractures illustrated with the types of fractures listed below. Write the correct letter in the blank provided.

| | | | | | |
|---|---|---|---|---|---|
| E | 1. | Comminuted | I | 8. | Intracapsular |
| K | 2. | Compound | B | 9. | Longitudinal |
| L | 3. | Depressed | N | 10. | Oblique |
| M | 4. | Fracture & Dislocation | J | 11. | Pathologic |
| G | 5. | Extracapsular | A or D | 12. | Simple |
| C | 6. | Greenstick | F | 13. | Spiral |
| H | 7. | Impacted | D or A | 14. | Transverse |

Note: Some diagrams may represent more than one type of fracture. For example, #5: Many of the illustrated fractures are extracapsular. Students may have difficulty seeing differences.

2. State three ways to decrease office accidents.
   a. no scatter rugs or slippery floors
   b. cupboard doors and drawers closed, sharps away
   c. wipe up spills

## C. Learning Level: Application

1. Describe the symptoms and emergency care for the following.

| Condition | Symptoms | Emergency Care |
|---|---|---|
| Asthma | Wheezing, increased shallow resp., coughing, choking | Give inhaler if with patient. Take vital signs. Turn on oxygen, call physician, and get epinephrine. |
| Poisoning | On telephone, ask for name, location, poison taken, how much, when, vomiting? Name, weight, age, do not hang up | Hold on to call; call EMS and poison control, forward directions to caller. Do not induce vomiting unless poison control tells you to. |
| Seizure | Either tic or a stare into space (aura), then general body tremor | Lay in clear space on floor on one side, head also to side, loosen clothing. If in office, physician will see patient. If at home, give 10–15 minutes and then call EMS if not awake. |
| CVA | Headache, confusion, dizziness, one-sided weakness, speech change, memory change | Lie down, cover with warm blanket, keep open airway, take vitals. Call physician and EMS. |
| Heart Attack | Chest pain, across nipple area, radiating up chin & down right arm, sweating, nausea, indigestion, cold clammy skin, apprehension | Put in semi-sitting position, put on ECG, loosen all clothing, take apical pulse and B/P; nitro if patient has. Get physician immediately or call transport. |
| Syncope | Pale, cold, dizzy, nauseated | Lay patient flat, head lower than heart, loosen clothing, maintain airway. Aromatic spirits of ammonia. |

2. List six guidelines for handling and managing emergency situations.
   a. Keep calm and reassure patient
   b. Survey situation and examine the scene
   c. Evaluate patient, injuries, interfering hazards
   d. Take steps to administer aid to remedy situation
   e. Document events and medication
   f. Notify transport and obtain follow-up care

## D. Learning Level: Analysis

1. You are working in your externship. The following is a list of patients who are at the door when you open up at 8 AM. Which patients require immediate intervention? Which can wait? Individually triage and prioritize these patients based on need and number them 1–5 in order of first to last priority. Be prepared to explain your reasons for the order you chose.

A. ____5_ A 70-year-old female with c/o dysuria, frequency and urgency with urination. She has been awake with it since the middle of the night, "and can't wait one more minute to see the doctor."

B. ____3_ A 36-year-old male presents to the waiting area with a blood-soaked rag around his hand. He states he sliced his finger while working in the kitchen. He thinks the bleeding has stopped.

C. ____ 1_ A mother presents with her 2-year-old girl. The baby is very fussy, screaming, and appears very flushed in the face. Mom says the baby's temp. is 105° R.

D. ____ 2_ A 58-year-old male presents with vague complaints of upper abdominal discomfort. He says that he is all right, but his wife insisted he come in. The pain is intermittent and feels "tight." He thinks he has indigestion.

E. ____ 4_ A 32-year-old female comes in with a history of asthma. She is having some audible wheezing on expiration. Her color is pink and her respirations are rapid and shallow.

2. Missing emergency cart equipment is all the medications!! They are listed below but students need to recognize that medications are not on the cart. If possible, go to student health center and set up the cart there as an example.

Amobarbital sodium (Amytal Sodium)
Apomorphine hydrochloride
Atropine
Diazepam (Valium)
Digoxin (Lanoxin)
Epinephrine (Adrenalin)
Furosemide (Lasix)
Isoproterenol hydrochloride aerosol spray (Isuprel)
Metaraminol (Aramine)
Antihistamine, injectable and oral
Dextrose
Disposable syringe and needle units
Glucagon
Lidocaine (Xylocaine)

## E. Learning Level: Synthesis

1. Pick one of the situations and develop a list of telephone triage questions.
   a. Wife calls and says husband can't get his breath
   b. Parent calls and says her child just took some insecticide.
   c. Patient calls and says she was started on penicillin yesterday and today she has hives and welts all over her.

   Questions: Students write questions related to symptoms for triage call

2. How will the medical assistant use a poison control center?

   See text, p. 800. Obtain seven basic sources of information from caller: Location and telephone number; name of poison taken; how much taken; how long ago; whether vomiting occurred; name, weight, and age of victim; first aid if given. Have caller stay on line, get directions from poison control and forward them to caller who is still on phone. Have patient report to physician office or ER.

## F. Learning Level: Evaluation

1. What medications might you expect the physician to order for a patient with:
   a. Possible heart attack—epinephrine, oxygen, atropine, lidocaine, morphine or other narcotic
   b. Severe asthma attack—aminophylline, epinephrine, oxygen, terbutaline, albuterol
   c. Head injuries—None; never with head injury

## Part 2 COMPETENCY CHALLENGE

A. Obtain a CPR mannequin and practice CPR according to Procedure 40-1 at the end of the chapter. When you have all the criteria smooth and are accurate, you will be ready for an evaluation and to test for CPR certification. Often the medical assistant program will assign students to take a certified CPR class and get AHA or Red Cross certification as proof of competence and preparation for the job.

B. Students will have written their responses in the Mastery Manual.

   Situation 1:

   You are assisting the physician with a physical examination. Suddenly, the physician drops what he is holding and falls to the floor. He does not respond when you talk to him. (Remember, you have two people to think about.)

Situation 2

The medical assistant who works with you has been complaining of a severe headache all day. She has taken Tylenol every three hours. It is now 4:00 and you hear a thump in the bathroom. You open the door and find her on the floor having a seizure.

Situation 3

A woman comes in to the office, screaming for help. She is carrying a small infant who looks very cyanotic. She tells you that her other two children were eating peanuts in the car and one of them gave a nut to the baby. The mother fears the nut is caught in the baby's wind-pipe.

## PART 3 CLINICAL APPLICATIONS

The answers will vary depending upon the state laws.

1. What are the Good Samaritan regulations in your state? May you help any person in a true emergency no matter what your training?

   Answer: Usually the law requires the person be trained in first aid but not give care if they have no idea what they are doing. This would not be a reasonable acting person.

2. Make a list of local emergency numbers for your locality.

   Answer: Students need to know these numbers and how to access them.

3. What are your responsibilities and the patient's rights in the following situation? What will you do?

   Answer: The physician must be told immediately. The patient has the right to decide not to go to the hospital.

# 41

# Assisting with Diagnostic Imaging and Therapeutic Modalities

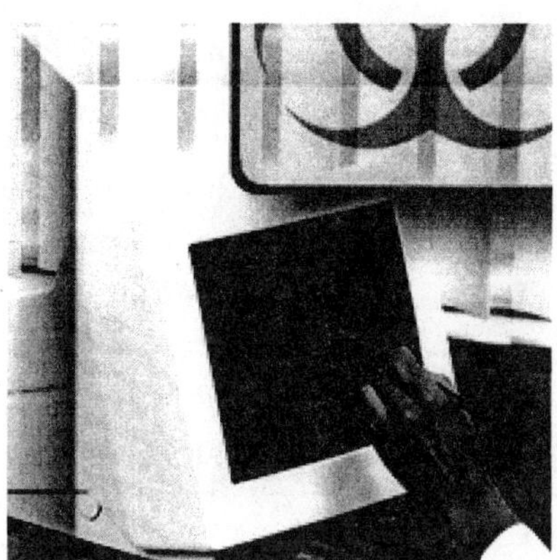

This chapter can be interesting when information is presented in the actual imaging center. It allows the student to question and obtain answers to many questions about these modalities directly from a radiologist or technician. All the knowledge and procedures in this chapter relate to diagnostic and treatment methods with which the medical assistant needs to be familiar. Patients expect answers from personnel who facilitate their care. The medical assistant will be exposed to these tests and modalities daily. Some primary care offices have x-ray and ultrasound in the office. Orthopedic offices often have a physical therapist on staff, and gastroenterologists may have fluoroscopy equipment. Today's medical assistant must be familiar with all the tests and modalities to better serve the physician and patients. Use the AAMA entry-level curriculum below to discuss the medical assistant's role in diagnostic imaging and therapeutic modalities.

## USING THE LEARNING SYSTEM

### 1. MEDICAL ASSISTING CONTENT AND COMPETENCIES

CONTENT

- Anatomy and physiology
- Diagnostic and treatment modalities
- Applications of medical terminology
- Legal guidelines and requirements for health care
- Risk management
- Hereditary, cultural, and environmental influences on behavior
- Adaptations to individual needs
- Diagnostic testing
- Job readiness

COMPETENCIES

- Recognize and respond to verbal and nonverbal communication
- Perform risk management procedures
- Document appropriately
- Provide instruction for health maintenance and disease prevention
- Identify community resources
- Instruct and demonstrate the use and care of patient equipment
- Prepare patient for and assist with procedures, treatments and minor office surgery

## 2. MEDICAL ASSISTING ENTRY LEVEL CURRICULUM INTERFACE

| TEXTBOOK OBJECTIVES | LEARNING SYSTEM LOCATION | MA CURRICULUM |
|---|---|---|
| Cognitive | | Content |
| 1. Explain your role in relation to diagnostic procedures | • Text pp. 817-820<br>• Manual Part 1-E | • Diagnostic and treatment modalities<br>• Legal guidelines and requirements for health care<br>• Risk management<br>• Hereditary, cultural, and environmental influences on behavior<br>• Adaptations to individual needs<br>• Diagnostic testing<br>• Job readiness |
| 2. Identify safety and precautionary measures pertinent to x-ray equipment | • Text pp. 816–817<br>• Manual Part 1-D | • Diagnostic and treatment modalities<br>• Legal guidelines and requirements for health care |
| 3. State the purpose of contrast media in x-ray procedures | • Text p. 810<br>• Manual Part 1-C | • Diagnostic and treatment modalities |
| 4. Discuss the various special x-ray diagnostic procedures | • Text pp. 811–816<br>• Manual Part 1-C | • Diagnostic and treatment modalities |
| 5. Recall the effects of heat on the body and why heat is an important treatment modality | • Text pp. 823–824<br>• Manual Part 1-C | • Anatomy and physiology<br>• Diagnostic and treatment modalities |
| 6. Explain the importance of physical therapy in treatment of physical disabilities | • Text p. 830<br>• Manual Part 1-D | • Anatomy and physiology<br>• Diagnostic and treatment modalities<br>• Legal guidelines and requirements for health care |
| 7. Compare and contrast passive and active exercising | • Text pp. 830–831 | • Diagnostic and treatment modalities<br>• See also Chapter 37 |

| TEXTBOOK OBJECTIVES | LEARNING SYSTEM LOCATION | MA CURRICULUM |
|---|---|---|
| **Cognitive** | | **Content** |
| 8. Recall three theories of pain control | • Text p. 832<br>• Manual Part 1-E | • Anatomy and physiology<br>• Applications of medical terminology |
| 9. Discuss patient teaching activities for x-ray and therapeutic modalities | • Text pp. 811–830<br>• Manual Part 1-F | • Legal guidelines and requirements for health care<br>• Hereditary, cultural, and environmental influences on behavior<br>• Adaptations to individual needs<br>• Diagnostic testing |
| **Performance** | | **Competencies** |
| 1. Accurately prepare and assist with an x-ray procedure on a patient | • Manual Part 2<br>• Procedure 41-1 | • Perform risk management procedures<br>• Document appropriately<br>• Prepare patient for and assist with procedures, treatments and minor office surgery<br>• Recognize and respond to verbal and nonverbal communication |
| 2. Accurately perform a therapeutic ultrasound diathermy on a patient | • Manual Part 2<br>• Procedure 41-2 | • Same as #1 |
| 3. Explain to a patient how to use dry or wet heat therapy at home | • Manual Part 3 | • Instruct and demonstrate the use and care of patient equipment<br>• Provide instruction for health maintenance and disease prevention<br>• Identify community resources |

## 3. RESOURCES

http://www.healthgate.com/HealthGate/free/dph/static/index.html **This source is full of information on almost all procedures. Just click on the alphabet letter and a list of procedures appears.**

## 4. LESSON PLAN Diagnostic Imaging — TIME 3 hours lecture, 12 hours lab

**Opening:** Assign students to read and arrange a field trip (Lab time) to a facility where they can observe at least one x-ray. Usually the radiologist will demonstrate the technique. This is a great time to get a chest x-ray if indicated. Sometimes the school or health center will be able to provide the experience for the students. Bring in some x-rays and have a viewing box. Allow students to guess what the x-rays show.

**Pretest:** If students have read chapter have them complete activity Part 1-B 1, where they can use basic medical terminology to define radiology examinations. Otherwise, ask them to define common x-ray examinations to evaluate current knowledge.

**Objectives:** Post the objectives on a flip chart or on the board and see how many students can discuss without your help. Use the outline below to guide them. Compare objectives with AAMA curriculum.

**Content:**

1. DIAGNOSTIC RADIOLOGY see Part 1-C, p. 362 for answers to discuss these procedures
   a. Contrast Media—types, routes, procedures
   b. Nuclear Medicine—isotopes, scans
   c. Computed Tomography (CT Scan)
   d. Magnetic Resonance Imaging
   e. Fluoroscopy
   f. Mammography
   g. Stereoscopy
   h. Thermography
   i. Ultrasonography
   j. Xeroradiology
   k. Flat Plates
2. X-RAY MACHINE parts—safeguards, tube, table, control panel
3. RADIATION HAZARDS AND SAFEGUARDS—dosimeters, shields, inspections, blood counts, physicist inspections
4. MA ROLE ASSISTING WITH RADIOLOGICAL PROCEDURES
   Preparing the Patient
   Positioning the Patient
   Exposing X-Ray Film
   Processing X-Ray Film
   Filing X-Ray Films and Reports
   Procedure 41-1: Assisting with an X-Ray Examination
5. THERAPEUTIC MODALITIES—heat, water, physical therapy, therapeutic exercise
6. GENERAL PRINCIPLES OF HEAT APPLICATION, See pp 362 and 363 for discussion
   Moist Heat
   Dry Heat
   Heat Application to Deeper Tissues
   Procedure 41-2: Assisting with Ultrasound Therapy
7. THERAPEUTIC EXERCISE
   Joint Mobility
   Muscle Training and Strength
   Relief of Tension and Pain
8. PATIENT EDUCATION
9. LEGAL AND ETHICAL RESPONSIBILITIES

**Lab:** Use the Mastery Manual to achieve all the objectives as noted in item F below. Students need to see radiology equipment if possible and some films of the procedures discussed. Often old films can be obtained from hospitals with all identifiers removed. There are some activities related to preparing Mr. Shapiro and Mr. Johnson for diagnostic testing. Use the main menu to direct students to the CD-ROM ⊕ location..

**Assignment:** Have students complete Mastery Manual. This can be done during lab time and be used as the posttest if collected. Then assign study of the next chapter.

**Posttest:** Use the Examaster questions. Have students write an explanation of a procedure for a patient. Evaluate according to information: who, what, where, when, how, and why.

## 5. MASTERY MANUAL ANSWERS

### PART 1 CONTENT MASTERY

### A. Learning Level: Knowledge

1. Put the medical term next to the definition given. Most of these terms should be familiar.
   a. **extravasation** Bleeding into the tissues.
   b. **rem** Method of measuring the amount of radiation absorbed by a patient exposed to x-rays; similar to rad.
   c. **denervation** A condition in which the nerve supply has been blocked.
   d. **atrophy** Wasting away; decrease in size and substance.
   e. **quackery** Pretense of possessing medical skill.
   f. **roentgen** Unit used to measure x-ray dosage.
   g. **prosthesis** An artificial replacement of a body part.
   h. **rad** A measurement of the actual absorbed dose of radiation.
   i. **claustrophobia** A fear of being trapped in enclosed or narrow places.
   j. **radiation** The transfer through space of any form of energy, such as light, heat, or x-rays.
   k. **scan** The image produced using nuclear medicine and isotopes.

2. Name three kinds of contrast media and three examples of each.

| **Kinds** | **Examples** |
|---|---|
| a. gas | air, oxygen, carbon dioxide |
| b. heavy metals | barium sulfate, bismuth carbonate |
| c. organic iodines | iodine isotopes |

3. How may the above be administered? orally, parenterally, or by enema

### B. Learning Level: Comprehension

1. Name the areas visualized in the following studies. Research and list the kind of contrast medium used for each study.
   angiocardiography—heart and large vessels—organic iodine—organic iodine
   angiography—blood vessels—organic iodine
   arteriography—arteries—organic iodine
   arthrography—joints—air
   barium enema—lower intestinal tract—heavy metal, barium sulfate

bronchography—bronchial tree and lungs—air
cholecystography—gallbladder—organic iodine
hysterosalpingography–uterus and fallopian tubes—organic iodine
intravenous cholangiography— bile ducts—organic iodine
intravenous pyelography—renal pelvis, ureters, and bladder—organic iodine
lymphangiography—lymphatic vessels—organic iodine
myelography—spinal cord—iodine

2. What is the most common contrast medium used in these studies? organic iodine
3. The purpose of using contrast media is to increase visualization of organ, part, or structure.

## C. Learning Level: Application

1. Complete the chart below for diagnostic procedures. Star the procedures not completed using x-rays.

| Procedure | Technique | Areas Studied |
|---|---|---|
| Computed tomography | Cross section x-rays | Tissue structure |
| Flat plate | Plain x-ray film—no media | Usually bones and bony cavities |
| MRI** | Not x-ray—radio waves and a magnetic field | Images of soft tissues |
| Fluoroscopy | Motion of body with structure viewed | Internal hollow body structures |
| Stereoscopy | Three-dimensional image | Primarily inside of skull |
| Xeroradiography | Image produced electrically, not chemically—obtained in 90 seconds | Soft tissue of breast |
| Thermography** | Heat sensing technique | Internal structures, infrared camera |
| Ultrasonography** | High-frequency sound waves echo off body | Internal organs, body parts, eyes, other soft tissues |

2. Complete the chart below for the various heat applications.

| Procedure | Technique /Effects | Areas Studied |
|---|---|---|
| Soaks | Plain water bath of 110°F for 20 min | Extremities |
| Hot moist compresses | Moisten towel, wring it out, warm not hot, cover with plastic, reapply when cool or until time | Increase blood flow to small areas, such as face, hands, upper leg, back |
| Heating pads | Dry heat, do not use near moisture, do not set on high, no longer than prescribed | Small, local areas |

| Procedure | Technique /Effects | Areas Studied |
|---|---|---|
| Ultraviolet radiation | By sun lamps or tanning beds, both penetrating* bactericidal | General body or spot lamps, test for sensitivity, acne, psoriasis, ulcers |
| Hot water bottles | Temp at or below 125°F, less than $^1/_2$ full, flannel cover | Localized areas, used for abdominal discomfort |
| Short wave diathermy | Place plates 1 inch from skin; patients should only feel mild heat, keep controls away from patients | Deep tissue and creates heat, for inflammation; teach patient danger of too much heat from diathermy |
| Ultrasound diathermy | Hold applicator in contact with body area or gel, lotion, or water | Sound waves cause tissue vibration, which speeds up circulation. Penetrates muscle, not bone |

## D. Learning Level: Analysis

1. Differentiate an x-ray view from an x-ray position.
   a. <u>An x-ray view</u> refers to the placement of body part between the film and the tube to direct the x-ray toward a specific part or direction, e.g., anteriorposterior—anterior faces tube and posterior faces the film.
   b. <u>An x-ray position</u> refers to the position the patient is placed in to obtain a view.

2. You learn that the federal government is coming to examine the x-ray equipment. What safety checks and examinations would you expect them to perform? Students may need to be guided to read the descriptions again and then apply the knowledge.
   a. Check protective material around tube for leaks
   b. Make sure control panel is behind lead wall and wall is intact
   c. Ensure that people are wearing monitoring devices measuring rads
   d. Check shields for kind and type and make sure they are worn
   e. Check records for personnel blood counts

## E. Learning Level: Synthesis

1. What types of heat treatment would you expect the physician to prescribe for the following injuries?
   a. an infected sore on the arm **moist compresses, universal precautions**
   b. a slow-healing ulcer on the ankle **soak or diathermy**
   c. an acute sprain **ultrasound diathermy**
   d. a diabetic patient with neuropathy and an ulcer on the lower leg **no heat or cold!!**
   e. chronic sore joints of arthritis **paraffin bath or dry heat**
   f. a patient with acne **ultraviolet radiation**

2. Many techniques of pain control are discussed in the chapter. You are the patient and you pulled a ligament in your ankle 3 days ago. You are in severe pain and the physician has treated you with diathermy and has told you to "go home and rest and take care of yourself." What specific techniques can you use at home to minimize pain without the use of medication? Name at least four.
   a. relaxation, massage
   b. local pain liniments
   c. elevate leg, do not put weight on leg
   d. wrap ankle for support, use crutches
3. What else will you do to take care of yourself? What exactly does this mean?
   Ask physician exactly what you should do not to reinjure the site; generally, this means to use affected area minimally and allow it to heal.
4. One week later, the physician tells you to go to the physical therapist for at least 4 weeks, twice a week. What are the benefits of physical therapy with a physical disability?
   Use of physical measures, devices, and body movements to restore normal function

## F. Learning Level: Evaluation

1. Therapeutic exercise is prescribed for a variety of conditions. Name at least ten conditions or disorders from previous chapters for which the physician might prescribe physical therapy.
   Any condition that would require: joint mobility, active exercise, passive exercise, ROM, muscle training, electronic stimulators, relief of tension and strain; ultraviolet radiation, for example; broken limbs, arthritis, tendonitis, joint injuries, post-op joint replacements or therapy, stroke, MD, MS, etc.
2. Design a patient teaching plan for any two diagnostic procedures. Use the activity at the end of Chapter 28 to design the plan.
   Note: One procedure may be assigned to different students. Then plans can be posted and all students may learn how to prepare patients for most procedures. Be sure to ask a test question or two on this material.

## PART 2 COMPETENCY CHALLENGE

1. Procedure 41-1, Assisting with the X-Ray Examination—This procedure includes preparing the patient and assisting the tech. Have students simulate and practice this procedure in the lab if possible and within the scope of practice in the state.
2. Simulate Procedure 41-2, Assisting with Ultrasound Therapy. This procedure may be practiced, but in many states the medical assistant may not perform such a procedure. First check the state laws. If medical assistants can practice this procedure, instructors may want to bring students to a radiology department in a facility or the school and have them observe patient preparation and assisting before actually practicing the procedure.

## PART 3 CLINICAL APPLICATIONS

1. Research state laws and discuss the medical assistant's role in:
   A. Performing or assisting with x-rays
   B. Performing or assisting with physical therapy procedures
   C. Performing or assisting with heat application procedures
   Answer the following for each A–C above:
   a. Can I legally perform these procedures?
   b. What are my limitations?
   c. What can I do in relation to each of these procedures?
   d. What are my knowledge limitations in performing these procedures?
2. Draw up a short teaching plan to explain to a patient how to use wet or dry heat at home.
   Answers vary according to state law.

# 42

# Assisting in the Clinical Laboratory

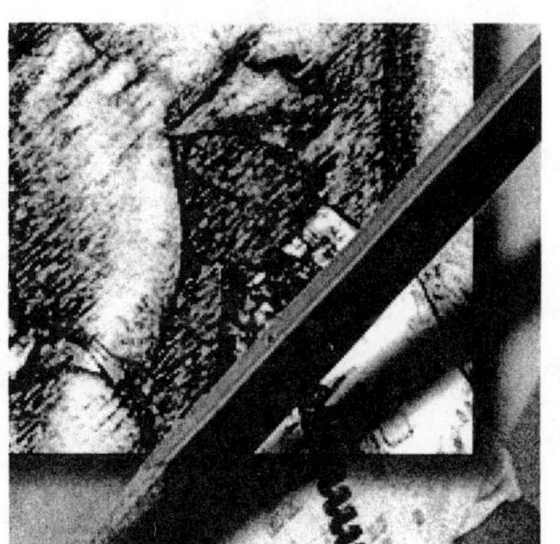

This chapter presents the foundation material for the following four laboratory chapters. It is important to emphasize safety and quality controls. The knowledge will be applied in the coming chapters. This is also a good time to have students get hepatitis B immunizations because externship sites are not required to provide the immunization, but the medical employer is. The lesson plan is expanded and covers location of Transparency Masters for discussion. Instructors should research updated CLIA waived tests because the list has expanded since the 8th Edition Textbook went to print, and is continually changing per HCFA regulations. An Internet site referenced at chapter end will lead you to the information.

## USING THE LEARNING SYSTEM

### 1. MEDICAL ASSISTING CONTENT AND COMPETENCIES

CONTENT

- Anatomy and physiology
- Diagnostic treatment modalities
- Word building and definitions
- Legal guidelines and requirements for health care
- Risk management
- Asepsis infection control
- Specimen collecting and processing
- Adaptation for individual needs
- Patient care
- Job readiness

 

COMPETENCIES

- All fundamental principles
- Use methods of quality control
- Prepare and assist patient with examinations, procedures, and treatments
- Perform risk management procedures
- Identify and respond to issues of confidentiality
- Recognize and respond to verbal and nonverbal communication
- Document accurately
- Perform within legal and ethical boundaries
- Perform an inventory of supplies and equipment

## 2. MEDICAL ASSISTING ENTRY-LEVEL CURRICULUM INTERFACE

| TEXTBOOK OBJECTIVES | LEARNING SYSTEM LOCATION | MA CURRICULUM |
|---|---|---|
| **Cognitive** | | **Content** |
| 1. Discuss your role in coordinating laboratory tests and results | • Text p. 846<br>• Manual Part 1-E | • Legal guidelines and requirements for health care<br>• Risk management<br>• Asepsis infection control<br>• Specimen collecting and processing<br>• Adaptation for individual needs<br>• Patient care<br>• Job readiness |
| 2. List the 12 departments found in most laboratories | • Text p. 835<br>• Manual Part 1-D | • Specimen collecting and processing |
| 3. State the safety rules for the laboratory | • Text p. 836<br>• Manual Part 1-B | • Same as #1 |
| 4. Identify CLIA's three categories of laboratory testing | • Text pp. 837–838<br>• Manual Part 1-B | • Same as #1 |
| 5. Define the objective of quality assurance | • Text p. 837<br>• Manual Part 1-B | • Same as #1 |
| 6. Explain quality control guidelines | • Text p. 839<br>• Manual Part 1-C | • Same as #1 |
| 7. List the elements that are included in every laboratory request form | • Text p. 834<br>• Manual Part 1-C | • Diagnostic treatment modalities |
| 8. Give five reasons that physicians order laboratory tests | • Text p. 844<br>• Manual Part 1-C | • Diagnostic treatment modalities |

| TEXTBOOK OBJECTIVES | LEARNING SYSTEM LOCATION | MA CURRICULUM |
|---|---|---|
| **Cognitive** | | **Content** |
| 9. State the medical assistant's responsibilities in specimen collection | • Text pp. 843, 844–846<br>• Manual Part 1-E | • Anatomy and physiology<br>• Diagnostic treatment modalities<br>• Word building and definitions<br>• All items in # 1 |
| 10. Identify the parts of a microscope | • Text p. 847<br>• Manual Part 1-D | • Diagnostic treatment modalities<br>• Word building and definitions |
| 11. Discuss legal and ethical issues in laboratory testing | • Text pp. 847–848, CLIA regs p. 838, BBP regs, Safety regs, Q and A issues, record keeping, personnel regs, spec collection<br>• Manual Part 3 | • Same as #1 |
| **Performance** | | **Competencies** |
| 1. Focus a microscope under low power, high power, and oil immersion | • Manual Part 2<br>• Procedure 42-1 | • All competencies relate to this procedure when the microscope is used in the laboratory |

## 3. RESOURCES

SAMPLE OSHA and CLIA regulations from the school health facility.

http://www.aap.org/visit/cliaregs.htm **Site to explain regulations; this site is through the American Academy of Pediatricians. It contains a site for almost 30 waived tests as of 9/98.**

http://www.hcfa.gov/medicaid/clia/cliahome.htm **Government site to CLIA regulations, changes, tests, and fee schedules.**

## 4. LESSON PLAN Diagnostic Imaging TIME 3 hours lecture, 12 hours lab

**Opening:** Have a microscope on the desk. Introduce the microscope and its purpose in the medical assistant's life. Review from Chapter 3 the history of the microscope and its meaning today. When was the electron microscope discovered? (1954)

**Pretest:** Ask students purpose of laboratory safety and quality assurance.

**Objectives:** Review each objective. Post the objectives on a flip chart.
It is essential that students understand knowledge expected so they can learn specific tests and perform them according to regulations and standards in this chapter.

**Content:**
Vocabulary

1. The Laboratory: Have students answer Memory Jogger questions as you proceed through materials.
2. Laboratory Safety: physical, chemical and biohazards
   Laboratory rules
   CLIA Mandate waived tests—get updated information from Internet resource
   Quality Assurance—reference values
   Quality Control, i.e., accuracy— guidelines, control samples
3. Personnel Requirements: medical assistant's role
4. Safety Requirements
   OPIM safety guidelines; types of OPIM HBV program
6. Laboratory Requests and Report Components of Request Form
7. Specimen Collection
   Results of Testing
   Achieving Accurate Results
   Using Proper Equipment
   Avoiding Contamination
   Providing Sufficient and True Representative Samples
   Providing Proper Instructions to Patients
   Proper Handling, Processing, and Storage
8. The Microscope
   Procedure 42-1: Using the Microscope
9. PATIENT EDUCATION
10. LEGAL AND ETHICAL RESPONSIBILITIES

**Lab:** Arrange field trips to a clinical lab in your area. Have students observe postings of OSHA regulations; CLIA standards; quality control methods for the tests observed;types of CLIA tests performed.
Have students make a flash card with current low-complexity tests.

**Assignment:** Learn all parts of microscope and be prepared to use it.

**Posttest:** Give multiple choice from Examaster and ask questions from objectives.

## 5. MASTERY MANUAL ANSWERS

## PART 1 CONTENT MASTERY

### A. Learning Level: Knowledge

1. After studying the chapter, fill in the definitions of the given terms.

   Aliquot—A portion of a well-mixed sample that is removed for testing.

   Antibody—An immunoglobulin produced by lymphoid tissue in response to substances interpreted as foreign invaders gaining entry into the body.

   Exudates—fluids with a high concentration of protein and cellular debris that have escaped the blood vessels, usually the result of inflammation.

   Cerebrospinal fluid—Fluid within the subarachnoid space, the central canal of the spinal cord, and the four ventricles of the brain.

   Hematoma—a tumor or sac filled with blood that may be the result of trauma.

   Hemolyzed—A blood sample in which the red cells have been ruptured.

   Preservative—A substance added to a specimen to prevent deterioration of cells or chemicals in the specimen.

   Quality assurance—A law-enforced program that guarantees quality patient care.

   Quality control—The operational procedures used to implement quality assurance.

   Reference values—listings of accepted ranges for normal values for hematology tests.

   Requisition—A formal written request from the physician authorizing a laboratory to perform a procedure.

   Specimen—A sample of body fluid, waste product, or tissue that is collected for analysis.

   Stat—Do immediately (from the Latin word *statin,* meaning "at once").

2. Match the lab test procedures with the descriptions.

   a. 2; b. 3; c. 4 ; d. 1

### B. Learning Level: Comprehension

1. List ten safety rules for the laboratory. Answer: Many are listed below.

   No eating, drinking, or smoking.

   Keep pens, pencils, and fingers away from mouth and eyes.

   Pull long hair back and up.

   Report all accidents to physician or supervisor.

   Wear laboratory coat or apron.

   Wipe spills and splashes immediately.

   Wash hands before and after every procedure.

   Follow manufacturer's instructions for equipment operation.

   Know the location of all safety equipment and supplies and fire escape routes.

   Wear protective gloves and safety glasses.

   Avoid wearing chains, rings, bracelets, and other loose, hanging jewelry.

   Clean work area before and after every procedure.

   Disinfect or sterilize specimens and materials contaminated with blood or microorganisms.

   No storage of food and beverages in laboratory refrigerator.

   Repair malfunctioning equipment immediately.

   Be familiar with appropriate first-aid procedures.

   Properly ground all electric equipment.

   Clearly and accurately label all reagents and solutions.

2. Name three categories of CLIA laboratory testing and list five common tests for the first category.
   a. low-complexity—Common test include: any of the waived tests in textbook, p. 837
   b. moderate-complexity tests
   c. high-complexity tests

3. What are the purposes of quality assurance?
   Assess, verify, and document accuracy of test results

## C. Learning Level: Application

1. List the elements from the list below, which are needed for a laboratory request form.

   Patient's insurance information. | Specific test(s) requested.
   Medications the patient is taking. | Indication of whether test is **stat.**

2. From your personal experience and readings, list five reasons physicians order lab tests.
   a. make a diagnosis
   b. rule out a diagnosis
   c. management of diseases, e.g., diabetic glucose monitor
   d. evaluate medication levels
   e. evaluate untoward reactions to treatments or medications, e.g., Zocor may cause liver damage, x-ray to see if fracture has healed
   f. evaluate patient compliance with treatment

## D. Learning Level: Analysis

1. Larger laboratories have up to 12 departments. Which ones are omitted on the list below? Circle the departments commonly included in the POL.
   Missing departments are hematology, blood bank, histology, cytology, toxicology
   Note: Common POL departments are hematology, serology, chemistry, urinalysis, and a reception collection department.

2. By now you should have handled and looked through the microscope. Label the parts of the microscope pictures below.
   Answer: See Figure 42-13 in textbook.

## E. Learning Level: Synthesis

1. List as many as you can of the medical assistant's responsibilities for obtaining specimens, performing lab tests, and reporting results.
   Assure proper patient preparation
   Know procedure and normal range of each test
   Follow all laboratory instructions for obtaining, labeling, sending specimens
   Alert physicians to abnormal results
   Contact patients concerning reports
   Apply principles of aseptic technique and infection control
   Work as a team member
   Practice within scope of education, training, and personal capabilities
   Document accurately

2. How frequently are controls tested?

   Daily for every test performed.

3. What is the purpose of testing at this frequency?

   Every batch and method must be tested for accuracy. False results may have dire consequences, such as the patient who doesn't get treated or the patient treated for the wrong disease.

## F. Learning Level: Evaluation

You are assigned to assist in the POL today. The medical assistant usually in there needs your help in obtaining specimens. She is obtaining specimens but needs to run tests. She demonstrates on a patient and you have done this before and feel trained and confident, but you notice she is not wearing gloves. You look around and cannot find any. When you ask for gloves, the medical assistant says "You are only drawing blood; you do not need gloves then." Is this true? How do you reply?

Not true. You will need to find a supply. Law requires that you have barrier protection. Ask students how they will handle. How are gloves obtained? Should you report this to anyone?

## PART 2 COMPETENCY CHALLENGE

This chapter introduces students to the medical office laboratory. The role of the medical assistant in the laboratory is clearly defined in the text. The instructor should demonstrate all procedures before the students attempt them. The importance of laboratory rules and following the OSHA requirements for safety when handling body fluids should be strongly stressed. Quality control measures are mandated by law. Refer to Chapter 25 for guidelines pertaining to protective measures when handling blood and body fluids. Students will need to wear gloves for most laboratory procedures. Occasionally goggles will be needed.

PROCEDURE 42-1: USING THE MICROSCOPE

Students should examine two to four items including hair, thread, blood, and yeast cells using different objectives. Have students draw the items as seen at each decreased or increased magnification. Collect and discuss the drawings. Always check to make certain that students have put the microscopes away properly, cleaned and covered, with the low-power objective in the down position.

## PART 3 CLINICAL APPLICATIONS

1. The HMO where you work has sent a memo and your supervisor posted it. It indicated that gloves would only be used in the lab on known AIDS patients or when the lab person has a cut on the hand. Otherwise, the lab personnel are to wash hands with antibacterial soap before and after each test. Is this acceptable procedure? How can you handle the situation?
2. Make a list of teaching points when you are going to take a blood sample of a 6-year-old pediatric patient. Prepare and elicit cooperation. Refer back to Chapter 34.
3. What would you do if you couldn't see through the microscope because the optics were out of alignment?
   - Need to try to adjust eyepieces to eye span and visual acuity if a binocular scope. Give a gentle push inward or pull outward.
   - Check the focus and illumination—start with low power.

# 43

# Urinalysis

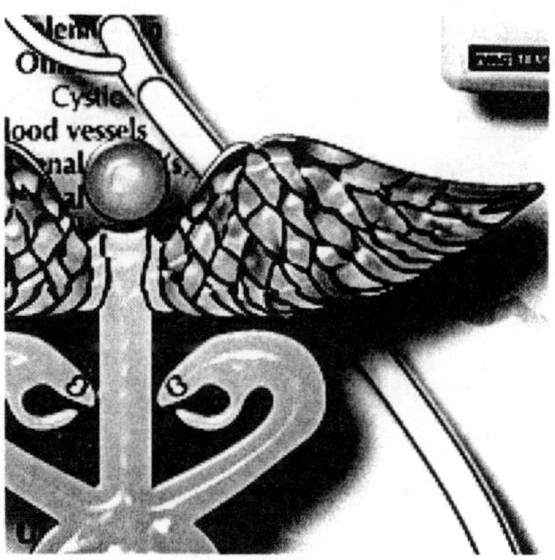

Urinalysis is probably the most commonly performed test in the POL. Students therefore need to gain mastery for determining all the components and completing a microscopic examination on urine. Students need to acquire knowledge of normal and abnormal results, practice to mastery, and be able to teach patients about collection of specimens. Due to unrefrigerated samples or patients not receiving adequate instructions, results are often not accurate. Review of materials in Chapter 26 is important as principles and universal precautions need to be applied in all procedures when handling urine.

## USING THE LEARNING SYSTEM

### 1. MEDICAL ASSISTING CONTENT AND COMPETENCIES

CONTENT

- Anatomy and physiology
- Word building and definitions
- Diagnostic treatment modalities
- Legal guidelines and requirements for health care
- Risk management
- Hereditary, cultural, and environmental influences on behavior
- Adaptations of individual need
- Asepsis and infection control
- Diagnostic testing
- Specimen collecting and processing
- Patient care
- Job readiness

COMPETENCIES

- All fundamental principles
- Use methods of quality control
- Perform urinalysis
- Screen and follow up test results
- Prepare and assist patient with examinations, procedures, and treatments
- Perform risk management procedures
- Recognize and respond to verbal and nonverbal communication
- Instruct a patient in the collection of a clean-catch midstream urine specimen
- Maintain confidentiality
- Document accurately
- Perform within legal and ethical boundaries

## 2. MEDICAL ASSISTING ENTRY-LEVEL CURRICULUM INTERFACE

| TEXTBOOK OBJECTIVES | LEARNING SYSTEM LOCATION | MA CURRICULUM |
|---|---|---|
| **Cognitive** | | **Content** |
| 1. Understand the purpose of routine urinalysis | • Text p. 851<br>• Manual Part 3 | • Diagnostic testing<br>• Patient care<br>• Job readiness |
| 2. State seven types of urine specimens used | • Text p. 851<br>• Manual Part 1-C | • Diagnostic treatment modalities<br>• Hereditary, cultural, and environmental influences on behavior<br>• Adaptations to individual needs<br>• Asepsis and infection control<br>• Patient care<br>• Job readiness |
| 3. Describe the physiology of urine formation | • Text p. 854<br>• Manual Part 1-E | • Anatomy and physiology<br>• Word building and definitions |
| 4. Describe the tests in the physical examination of urine | • Text pp. 855–856<br>• Manual Part 1-B | • Diagnostic testing<br>• Specimen collecting and processing<br>• Patient care<br>• Job readiness |
| 5. Describe the tests in the chemical examination of urine | • Text pp. 860–866<br>• Manual Part 1-A | • Same as #4 above |
| 6. List five materials found in urine sediment microscopically | • Text pp. 866–869<br>• Manual Part 2 | • Diagnostic testing<br>• Specimen collecting and processing |
| 7. Define urinary quality control | • Text p. 874<br>• Manual Part 3 | • Diagnostic testing<br>• Specimen collecting and processing<br>• Legal guidelines and requirements for health care<br>• Risk management |

| TEXTBOOK OBJECTIVES | LEARNING SYSTEM LOCATION | MA CURRICULUM |
|---|---|---|
| **Performance** | | **Competencies** |
| 1. Instruct a patient in the collection of a timed urine specimen | • Text pp. 852–854<br>• Manual Part 2<br>• CD-ROM ⊕ | • Prepare and assist patient with examinations, procedures, and treatments.<br>• Recognize and respond to verbal and nonverbal communication<br>• Maintain confidentiality<br>• Perform within legal and ethical boundaries |
| 2. Instruct a patient in the collection of a clean-catch midstream urine specimen | • Text pp. 852–854<br>• Manual Part 2<br>• CD-ROM ⊕<br>• Procedure 43-7 | • Same as # 1 competencies and<br>• Instruct a patient in the collection of a clean-catch midstream urine specimen |
| 3. Perform a complete urinalysis | • Manual Part 2<br>• CD-ROM ⊕<br>• Procedures 43-1–43-6 | • All fundamental principles<br>• Use methods of quality control<br>• Perform urinalysis<br>• Screen and follow up test results<br>• Perform risk management procedures<br>• Document accurately |
| 4. Describe the proper usage and care of testing equipment | • Manual Part 2<br>• Each procedure | • Perform risk management procedures |
| 5. Demonstrate glucose testing using the Clinitest method | • Text p. 862<br>• Procedure 43-4 | • Same as #3 competencies |
| 6. Demonstrate the use of precipitation testing for protein in urine | • Manual Part 2<br>• Procedure 43-5 | • Same as #3 competencies |
| 7. Demonstrate the methods of pregnancy testing | • Text pp. 874–876<br>• Procedure 43-8 | • Same as #3 competencies |

## 3. RESOURCES

Use previous Chapter 38 resources

**4. LESSON PLAN Urinalysis TIME 3 hours lecture, 12 hours lab**

**Opening:** Set up food coloring jars to mimic various colors of urine. Wear yellow and make yellow the color of the day.

**Pretest:** What do the initials POL mean? What is the most common test performed in the POL? Answer: Urinalysis

**Objectives:** Put up the objectives. Cover each individually. Use MA curriculum interface to explain use of content and competencies in practice.

**Content:** If this is not an area of expertise, try to obtain a lab tech, RMA, or CMA to explain and discuss

1. COLLECTING URINE SPECIMENS
   a. Types of specimens
   b. Catheterization
   c. Instructing Patients to Collect a Urine Specimen Text pp. 852–854. Review with students.
2. PHYSIOLOGY OF URINE FORMATION review A&P, filtration, reabsorption, secretion.
   Bring in a real kidney or a model and explain the process.
   Nephron = afferent arterioles, glomerulus, Bowman's capsule, proximal convoluted tubule, Henle's loop, distal tubule, collecting tubule
3. PHYSICAL EXAMINATION OF URINE—give normal values
   Color and Turbidity
   Volume
   Foam
   Odor
   Specific Gravity
4. CHEMICAL EXAMINATION OF URINE—give normal range
   pH
   Protein
   Glucose
   Ketones
   Blood
   Bilirubin and Urobilinogen
   Nitrite
   Leukocytes
   Specific Gravity
   Phenylketones
   Ascorbic Acid (Vitamin C)
5. MICROSCOPIC EXAMINATION OF URINE SEDIMENT
   Casts
   Cells
   Crystals
   Miscellaneous Findings
   Reporting Findings of a Microscopic Evaluation—explain range reporting
   Interpretation of Urine Cultures
6. QUALITY CONTROL Give methods for each type of testing
7. PREGNANCY TESTING
8. PATIENT EDUCATION Preparation for all tests
9. LEGAL AND ETHICAL ISSUES Reporting results promptly

**Lab:** Demonstrate procedures after reading instructor hints in Part 2 of this Curriculum Guide. Procedures are located in Mastery Manual. Have students complete activities in Mastery Manual Part 2. Students should be able to explain all essential steps in all procedures during evaluation. Some procedures may be completed on CD-ROM before competency is achieved in Lab. Refer to the CD-ROM ⊕ main menu, Clinical Skills, and choose the case study for Mrs. Ferguson and Mr. Shapiro dipstick urine. Students will have the opportunity to interact with these and other urinalysis procedures on the CD-ROM.

**Assignment:** Students may need to be tested for comprehension before they are allowed to practice and be evaluated in urinalysis procedures.

**Posttest:** Give posttest in 2 phases: Cognitive (use Examaster) and then psychomotor (competence in all procedures).

## 5. MASTERY MANUAL ANSWERS

### PART 1 CONTENT MASTERY

#### A. Learning Level: Knowledge

1. Write six terms ending with the suffix -uria and give the meaning of each.
   a. polyuria—excessive urine amounts
   b. hematuria—blood in the urine
   c. anuria—lack of urine output
   d. dysuria—painful urination
   e. oliguria—scant urine production
   f. ketonuria—ketones in urine, bacturia—bacteria in urine

2. Name 10 urinary chemicals measured by dipstick. Students should name 10 of the 12 listed.
   a. proteins
   b. ketones
   c. urobilinogen
   d. phenylketones
   e. acetone
   f. glucose
   g. bilirubins
   h. nitrites
   i. blood
   j. ascorbic acid
   k. pH
   l. specific gravity

#### B. Learning Level: Comprehension

1. Describe the physical properties of urine and state their normal values.
   a. color—light yellow to amber turbidity—-clear
   b. volume—-about 1500 cc per day; 250--300 each voiding
   c. odor—none foam—none
   d. specific gravity—1.010–1.025

2. Explain the indication of the following substances in urine.
   a. blood—infection, trauma, internal bleeding
   b. yeast—infection or vaginal contamination
   c. bacteria—infection or may have sat at room temp. too long
   d. protein—renal disease, sometimes pregnancy, after heavy exercise
   e. WBC casts—seen in pyelonephritis
   f. bilirubin—liver disease

## C. Learning Level: Application

MULTIPLE CHOICE: Circle the *one best* answer to each statement or question.
Note: ✔ = the correct answer

1. A specimen collected over a specific period of time for quantitative analysis is a:
   A. Random specimen.
   B. Timed specimen.
   C. Two-hour postprandial specimen.
   ✔ D. Twenty-four-hour specimen.

2. The odor of urine varies. Some reasons for changes in odor include:
   ✔ A. Disease, infection, foods.
   B. Dehydration, sugar, bacteria.
   C. Drugs, diabetes, foods.
   D. Diabetes, bacteria, urochrome.

3. The refractometer measures specific gravity using only ______ of urine.
   A. 10 ml.
   B. 2 drops.
   ✔ C. 1 drop.
   D. 1 ml.

4. The urine specimen you are testing has a pH of 5.6. This indicates:
   A. Neutral urine.
   B. Alkaline urine.
   ✔ C. Acid urine.
   D. An infection.

5. A specimen collected when more specific information is needed for diagnosis is a
   ✔ A. First morning specimen.
   B. Random specimen.
   C. Timed specimen.
   D. Twenty-four-hour specimen.

6. One of the signs of renal disease is the appearance of ____________ in the urine.
   A. Ketones
   ✔ B. Protein
   C. Glucose
   D. Blood

7. This type of urinary cast means there is damage to the glomerulus.
   A. Hyaline
   B. Granular
   ✔ C. RBC
   D. Epithelial

8. The major parts of a routine urinalysis are:
   A. Chemical, visual, culture.
   ✔ B. Physical, chemical, microscopic.
   C. Visual, analytic, microscopic.
   D. Physical, analytic, chemical.

9. The urinary tract is composed of:
   ✔ A. Paired kidneys, paired ureters, one bladder, one urethra.
   B. Paired kidneys, one ureter, one bladder, paired urethras.
   C. Paired kidneys, paired ureters, one bladder, paired urethras.
   D. One kidney, one ureter, one bladder, one urethra.

10. Water constitutes ____ percent of urine.
    A. 25
    B. 50
    C. 75
    ✔ D. 95

11. Using your text as a reference for the reporting system, calculate the range report results of the microscopic examination as seen below:

| CELLS | NUMBER SEEN | RANGE REPORT |
|---|---|---|
| WBCs | 2–5 | **40–50** |
| RBCs | 0 | **10–20** |
| Casts | 5–10 | **<50** |
| Epithelial | 0–3 | **OCCAS** |

## D. Learning Level: Analysis

1. Explain the changes that take place in the listed physical and chemical properties of urine when left to sit for more than an hour at room temperature.

| | |
|---|---|
| Color and/or turbidity | **turns cloudy** |
| Glucose | **decreases as bacteria phagocytize** |
| Ketones | **decrease** |
| Blood | **may hemolyze—may get false positive** |
| Nitrites | **bacteria may convert to nitrite and give false positive** |
| Bacteria | **multiply frequently** |

2. Complete the report on the routine urinalysis report provided below.
   You may assume that information not provided is normal.
   Add column totals, write in the average and give the final report
   Circle the Abnormal results with red pen in the above chart.
   Jimmy Wong is ill. His mother called your office for an appointment. Dr. Lopez instructed Mrs. Wong to bring a urine specimen to the office with Jimmy at 3:00 pm. Jimmy's fluid intake has been within normal limits. The specimen was collected just before Mrs. Wong and Jimmy left for the appointment about 1/2 hour before arriving at the office. When the physical and chemical analysis was completed, the medical assistant noted a small amount of protein in the specimen. Small amounts of ketones and blood were also noted.
   The microscopic analysis revealed the following:

| | RBC | WBC | Cast | Epithelial | Crystals | Misc | Bacteria |
|---|---|---|---|---|---|---|---|
| | 17 | 4 | 0 | 1 renal | Amorphous | | cocci |
| | 21 | 9 | 0 | 0 | | | |
| | 25 | 7 | 1 hyaline | 0 | Urate | mucus | |
| | 20 | 10 | 1 gran. | 1 | | mucus | |
| | 15 | 1 | 0 | 1 squam. | | | cocci |
| **Answers** | | | | 0 | | | |
| **Total** | **98** | **31** | **2** | **2** | | **few** | **2 cocci** |
| **Average** | **19+** | **6** | **.5** | **Occ.** | | **few** | **few** |
| **Report** | **✔10-20** | **✔ 5-10** | **1-2** | **Occ.** | **Amorphous Urate** | **few** | **few** |

Abnormal results are checked, i.e., RBC and WBC total and report columns.

Are there any explanations for the abnormal results? **The RBCs and WBSs are increased—specimen might have been too warm or patient may have slight infection.**

Is it recommended to have patients bring urine specimens with them when the patient is having an initial evaluation? **Not usually.** Explain your answer. **Want to get accurate fresh specimen for evaluation.**

## E. Learning Level: Synthesis

For the following case studies, write the patient information required.

CASE #1
Phyllis Nelson is seeing Dr. Lopez for low back pain and urinary frequency. The doctor has asked you to obtain a clean-catch midstream specimen. Phyllis tells you she has no idea what that is. Explain the purpose of the test, the proper procedure, and the reasons for specific steps.

**Purpose steps and reasons: Refer to Procedure 43-7**

CASE #2
Daniel Nykata must furnish the laboratory with a twenty-four-hour urinary specimen. Daniel lives at the YMCA and he cannot keep this specimen container in the shared refrigerator. What suggestions could you give him?

**Put in old milk carton on ice. Use a bucket and get ice from the market. Store it under bed or in cool place.**

CASE #3
Mrs. Soto asks you why Robby's urine is so bright yellow in the morning and light yellow in the evening.

**Urine is concentrated and darker in AM because less fluid, same components. More dilute in PM.**

## F. Learning Level: Evaluation

Mr. Moogarian is 86 years old and is suffering from urinary retention. The physician will catheterize him for urinary retention. He asks you to set up the room and prepare the patient for the procedure. Mr. Moogarian' s son tells you that his father has never been catheterized. What equipment will you gather, what factors do you need to consider about this patient, and exactly how are you going to explain the procedure?

**Equipment: Disposable straight catheter set, drapes, pillows for comfort**

| **Factors** | **Explanation of procedure** |
|---|---|
| Patient is old | Purpose to relieve of discomfort—verify that he wants physician to help. |
| Son is with him | Son will stay in room next to him. |
| Patient is male | Physician will do procedure. |
| Patient may be restless | Ask him to hold still, put pillows around so he can lie quietly. |
| Embarrassed about language | Ask son father's terminology for urine and penis. |
| Explain using father's terminology | Physician will put small tube up urethra, empty the bladder, and take away the discomfort. After that his urine will be tested and physician will examine him. |
| Ask if he has questions | Set up catheterization tray on Mayo stand next to patient. Leave sterile cover on top. Call physician. |

## PART 2 COMPETENCY CHALLENGE

Note: Stress 100%-accurate interpretation of test results. Initial all abnormal results completed on students and handle them according to Medical Assistant school health policies. Have the students show all mathematical calculations on the reverse side of their patient report forms. Gloves must be worn during urinalysis procedures. Follow other precaution symbols as given with each procedure in the text. When goggles are indicated for a procedure, the student may remove them to perform the microscopic portion. Be sure to demonstrate every test before allowing students to perform the test.

**Activity:**
There are eight procedures in this chapter for you to master. Some of them may be completed working with the CD-ROM ⊕. Refer to the CD-ROM ⊕ main menu, Clinical Skills, and choose the case study for Mrs. Ferguson, where you will have the opportunity to interact with urinalysis procedures. Your instructor will guide you. In order to be proficient in urinalysis, you need to perform each procedure at least five times. There is a URINALYSIS REPORT form at the end of the chapter, which you may copy and use as often as needed. There is also one in this Instructor Curriculum Resource.

a. The first test may be performed on your own urine. Perform a urinalysis on the first morning specimen. Keep 1/2 refrigerated and 1/2 at room temperature until you get to the lab. Perform a urinalysis on both and record the results on the form for reporting urinalysis at the end of the chapter. Explain the results to your instructor.
b. Drink at least two quarts water, take another specimen later in the day, and record the results. Again, explain the changes. You have already completed three urinalyses. Complete the other two as directed by your instructor.

**Hints:**

**PROCEDURE 43-1 ASSESSING URINE FOR COLOR AND TURBIDITY**
Have students compare urine color with concentration and compare turbidity with amount of sediment when performing this procedure.

**PROCEDURE 43-2 MEASURING SPECIFIC GRAVITY USING A URINOMETER**
Check the standardization at the beginning of each laboratory session. Observe student's technique to be sure that the urinometer floats freely in the specimen and that the meniscus is at eye level when the results are read.

**PROCEDURE 43-3 TESTING URINE WITH CHEMICAL REAGENT STRIPS**
Be certain to have students check the expiration date and the lot numbers of the reagent strips. Stress the importance of keeping the containers closed. Remind students that timing is critical when performing these tests. The instructor should check and initial all abnormal results.

**PROCEDURE 43-4 TESTING URINE FOR GLUCOSE USING CLINITEST TABLETS**
Remind students that Clinitest tablets are poisonous to humans and that they will react in the presence of any moisture. Observe students for technique when removing the tablet from the bottle and reclosing container. Have students correlate the Clinitest results with the chemical reagent strips for quality control.

**PROCEDURE 43-5 TESTING URINE FOR PROTEIN USING THE SSA PRECIPITATION TEST**
The procedure in the text uses the sulfosalicylic acid precipitation testing procedure. SSA is a confirmatory test for protein. Have students correlate the SSA results with the chemical reagent strip test for quality control.

**PROCEDURE 43-6 ANALYZING URINE MICROSCOPICALLY**
Students may remove goggles while using the microscope. Be certain that students properly use a cover slip over the specimen. Students may refer to the identification of sediment chart in the text. Stress proper cleaning of the microscope's objective and stage after completing the analysis.

**PROCEDURE 43-7 OBTAINING A CLEAN-CATCH URINE**
Students will complete this procedure following the patient instruction in the textbook. Emphasize spreading labia or retracting foreskin. Meatus is wiped either forward to back or in circle depending upon sex. All soap removed. Voiding requires voiding a small amount in toilet, placing cup and voiding 50 cc, keeping sterility, and finish voiding in toilet.
Direct patient to maintain sterility of cup and top.

**PROCEDURE 43-8 PERFORMING A PREGNANCY DETECTION TEST**
This procedure is done using the slide agglutination test. Before beginning the procedure, the student should read the manufacturer's directions and procedure recommendations carefully. The instructor should listen to the student while patient instructions are being given for specimen collection. Timing and temperature are important to the accuracy of this test.

### TESTING URINE FOR QUALITY CONTROL

A quality control test should be utilized at every laboratory session. Students should chart the results and the instructor should initial the chart. Students may design a quality control log each year for the clinical laboratory component of the program.

## PART 3 CLINICAL APPLICATIONS

1. Federal regulations require quality controls. Complete a quality control test on your urinalysis. What method did you use? **Depends upon program.**
2. Name two methods of quality control for urinalysis.

   a. **Dual testing with commercial products, check personal procedure performance, check procedure techniques.**

   b. Have students design a quality control log for use in the medical assistant program lab.
3. Mrs. Ferguson is asked to give a clean-catch random specimen because the physician thinks her first one was contaminated. She tells you she just cannot produce one. What can you suggest and do to obtain one for the physician?

   **Discussion—Give water and try again, straight catheter if absolutely necessary**
4. You finally have to catheterize Mrs. Ferguson. After explaining the procedure, setting up the equipment, you begin and contaminate the left pinky on your non-dominant hand. You have no extra gloves. What will you do and why?

   **Nondominant hand becomes contaminated as soon as labia are spread. Wipe with Betadine swab, discard, and continue. This is a safe, realistic approach and prevents contamination.**

## URINALYSIS REPORT

Name ______________________________ Date ______________

Test # and Results Possible Abnormal Indications

### 1. Physical Examination

Color and turbidity ______________________________

Volume and odor ______________________________

Specific gravity ______________________________

### 2. Chemical Examination

pH ______________________________

Protein ______________________________

Glucose ______________________________

Ketone ______________________________

Blood ______________________________

Bilirubin and urobilinogen ______________________________

Leucocytes ______________________________

Phenylketones ______________________________

### 3. Microscopic

| 3. Microscopic | Field Counts | | | | | Total | Average | Report |
|---|---|---|---|---|---|---|---|---|
| RBC/hpf | 1. | 2. | 3. | 4. | 5. | | | |
| WBC/hpf | 1. | 2. | 3. | 4. | 5. | | | |
| Squamous epi. | 1. | 2. | 3. | 4. | 5. | | | |
| Transitional epi. | 1. | 2. | 3. | 4. | 5. | | | |
| Round epi. | 1. | 2. | 3. | 4. | 5. | | | |
| Bacteria | 1. | 2. | 3. | 4. | 5. | | | |
| Crystals | 1. | 2. | 3. | 4. | 5. | | | |
| Casts | 1 | 2. | 3. | 4. | 5. | | | |
| Other | 1. | 2. | 3. | 4. | 5. | | | |

# 44 Venipuncture

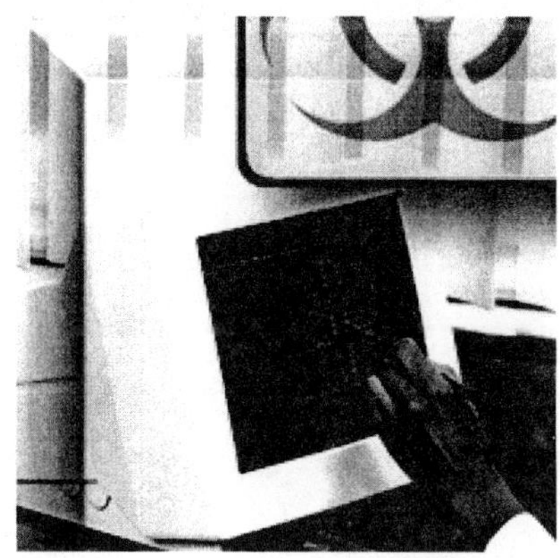

Performing venipuncture involves several skills, which students must practice after they have gained the required knowledge and are able to evaluate and select proper methods for each patient. The chapter presents all the above information for the student. Sites, steps involved, methods, aseptic techniques, and the medical assistant's responsibilities are all included. The instructor must know legal regulations regarding medical assistant's training and scope of practice for this procedure. Should the medical assistant be allowed to perform venipuncture in the state, ethical preparation requires that students be competent and certified before going to an externship for this experience.

## USING THE LEARNING SYSTEM

### 1. MEDICAL ASSISTING CONTENT AND COMPETENCIES

CONTENT

- Anatomy and physiology
- Diagnostic treatment modalities
- Word building and definitions
- Legal guidelines and requirements for health care
- Apply principles of aseptic technique and infection control
- Specimen collecting and processing
- Patient care
- Job readiness
- Adaptations for individual needs
- Recognition of and response to verbal and nonverbal communication

COMPETENCIES

- Prepare and assist patient with examinations, procedures, and treatments
- Perform venipuncture
- Perform capillary puncture
- Instruct according to patient needs
- Recognize and respond to verbal and nonverbal communication
- Maintain confidentiality
- Document accurately
- Perform within legal and ethical boundaries
- Perform an inventory of supplies and equipment

## 2. MEDICAL ASSISTING ENTRY-LEVEL CURRICULUM INTERFACE

| TEXTBOOK OBJECTIVES | LEARNING SYSTEM LOCATION | MA CURRICULUM |
|---|---|---|
| **Cognitive** | | **Content** |
| 1. Explain the medical assistant's responsibility in a venipuncture procedure | • Text p. 882<br>• Manual Part 1-A | • Anatomy and physiology<br>• Word building and definitions<br>• Legal guidelines and requirements for health care<br>• Diagnostic testing<br>• Apply principles of aseptic technique and infection control<br>• Specimen collecting and processing<br>• Patient care<br>• Job readiness |
| 2. Describe the equipment used for obtaining a venous sample by syringe method, evacuated tube method, and butterfly method | • Text pp. 886, 889, and 893<br>• Procedures 44-1—44-3<br>• Manual Part 1 -C | • Diagnostic testing<br>• Apply principles of aseptic technique and infection control<br>• Specimen collecting and processing |
| 3. Identify the anticoagulant that prevents coagulation | • Text p. 881<br>• Manual Part 1-C<br>• Table 44-1 | • Diagnostic testing<br>• Specimen collecting and processing |
| 4. List the color-coded tubes by use and purpose | • Text p. 881<br>• Manual Part 1-C<br>• Table 44-1 | • Diagnostic testing<br>• Specimen collecting and processing |
| 5. Differentiate between a pipette and a Unopette | • Text pp. 896–898 | • Diagnostic testing<br>• Specimen collecting and processing |
| 6. Explain the medical assistant's patient responsibility | • Text pp. 882–884<br>• Manual Part 1-A<br>• Procedures 44-1—44-4 | • Job readiness<br>• Adaptations for individual needs<br>• Recognition of and response to verbal and nonverbal communication |
| **Performance** | | **Competencies** |
| 1. Accurately collect a blood specimen by venipuncture from a patient using a syringe | • Text p. 886<br>• Manual Part 2<br>• Procedure 44-1 | • Prepare and assist patient with examinations, procedures, and treatments<br>• Perform venipuncture<br>• Instruct according to patient needs<br>• Recognition of and response to verbal and nonverbal communication |

| TEXTBOOK OBJECTIVES | LEARNING SYSTEM LOCATION | MA CURRICULUM |
|---|---|---|
| **Performance** | | **Competencies** |
| 1. Accurately collect a blood specimen by venipuncture from a patient using a syringe (*continued*) | | • Maintain confidentiality<br>• Document accurately<br>• Perform within legal and ethical boundaries<br>• Perform an inventory of supplies and equipment |
| 2. Accurately collect a blood specimen by venipuncture from a patient using an evacuated tube | • Text p. 889<br>• Manual Part 2<br>• Procedure 44-2 | • Same as # 1 |
| 3. Accurately collect a blood specimen by hand or wrist venipuncture from a patient using the butterfly needle | • Text p. 893<br>• Manual Part 2<br>• Procedure 44-3 | • Same as # 1 |
| 4. Assemble the appropriate supplies; collect a capillary blood specimen suitable for testing using fingertip puncture technique; and correctly complete each step of the procedure in proper order | • Text p. 897<br>• Manual Part 2<br>• Procedure 44-4 | • Perform capillary puncture<br>• Same as # 1 (except venipuncture) |

## 3. RESOURCES

*THE ROUTINE VENIPUNCTURE* video 26 min. Program #78047
MEDCOM/TRAINEX, Box 3225, Garden Grove, CA 92641

http://www.yahoo.com/Health/Medicine/Hematology/ **The site leading to other sites**

http://www.neosoft.com/~uthman/blood_cells.html **Blood cell and the CBC. Nice 8th Edition Textbook and pictures**

http://www.geocities.com/HotSprings/5340/ **Nice hematology site.**

## 4. LESSON PLAN Venipuncture TIME 3 hours lecture, 12 hours lab

**Opening:** If possible, have an RMA or CMA working in a lab come in, start the class with a demonstration, and have the lab expert explain the technique and procedure. See if the guest will give hints on how to be successful and how not to make errors. Maybe he or she will have a humorous story to start out.

**Pretest:** Ask students to explain the two main purposes of a venipuncture.
*Answer:* Obtain specimen for diagnosis and administer fluids or medication.
Which of these may the medical assistant never perform?
*Answer:* Administer medications or instill any substance in to a vein.

**Objectives:** Place on a flip chart and discuss first.

**Content:**
COLLECTION OF BLOOD SPECIMENS
1. **Venipuncture** cephalic, median cephalic, supplementary cephalic, basilic, median basilic, and median antebrachial veins
   Syringe Method text p. 880
   Evacuated Tube Method, tubes and preservatives, p. 881
   Patient Preparation
   Specimen Collection
   Care of the Puncture Site
   Needle Disposal, OSHA and CLIA Regulations; have containers available
   Specimen Handling
   Glove Removal

Procedure 44-1: Collecting a Venous Blood Sample Using Syringe Method
Procedure 44-2: Collecting a Venous Blood Sample Using Evacuated (Vacutainer) Method
   Using A Butterfly Needle—how and why?
Procedure 44-3: Performing a Butterfly Draw Using a Hand Vein
   Possible Blood Collection Complications—Managing Complications, Table 44-2, p. 895

2. **Microcapillary Blood Collection**
   Patient Preparation
   Collecting the Specimen

Procedure 44-4: Collecting a Capillary Blood Sample
   Pipetting the Blood

PATIENT EDUCATION
LEGAL AND ETHICAL ISSUES

**Lab:** Students will have four procedures in which to develop competence. The Mastery Manual meets all objectives and MA curriculum. There are hints for the instructor in Part 2 answers below. Students should sign waivers and practice on each other when they are ready. Not only does this assure competence; it also develops empathy for patients. Students will be able to complete preparation and follow up activities on the CD-ROM ⊕. They will also apply concepts from the chapter.

**Assignment:** Have students study 8th Edition Textbook, make flash cards for tubes, colors, tests; and complete Mastery Manual Part 1 in preparation for practice in lab. See Part 2 for lab suggestions.

**Posttest:** Use Examaster and competency evaluation for all procedures as testing.

## 5. MASTERY MANUAL ANSWERS

### PART 1 CONTENT MASTERY

### A. Learning Level: Knowledge

1. Fill in the blanks with the defined term.
   - a. bifurcation—the point of forking or separating into two branches.
   - b. heparin—a naturally occurring antithrombin factor that prevents intravascular clotting.
   - c. morphology—the study of the form, structure, and size of organisms, organs, tissues, or cells.
   - d. antecubital—the area in front of and at the bend of the elbow.
   - e. cyanotic—pertaining to a bluish discoloration of the skin and mucous membrane.
   - f. hemolysis—pertaining to the breakdown of red blood cells and the release of hemoglobin into the plasma.
   - g. tourniquet—a device used to compress an artery or a vein.
   - h. lumen—the open space within a blood vessel in which the blood travels.
   - i. invasive—technique that requires entering a body cavity.
   - j. syncope—fainting.

2. Mark the following statements true or false by circling the T or F. Answers are below next to statement.

   F 1. To perform a venipuncture, the needle should be inserted into a deep vein and the blood drawn directly into a syringe or special tube.
   T 2. The puncture site for phlebotomy should be determined only after careful inspection of both arms.
   T 3. Rubber gloves and blood/body-fluid protection barrier devices should be used when collecting a blood specimen from a patient.
   F 4. If the patient's veins are very small or fragile, the Vacutainer method should be used to collect the specimen.
   T 5. The Vacutainer method is most commonly used for the collection of blood specimens because several different specimens can be collected from a single puncture.
   T 6. If too little blood is collected in a tube containing EDTA, the test results may be inaccurate.
   F 7. The capillary puncture is a quick and efficient method for specimen collection when a large amount of blood is required.
   T 8. A capillary puncture site is usually the dominant hand or the earlobe.
   T 9. When blood appears in the tube, immediately withdraw the desired amount.
   T 10. When inserting the needle for venipuncture, the bevel must be up.

### B. Learning Level: Comprehension

1. Locate and list the veins commonly used for venipuncture:

   Answers:

   (a) cephalic
   (b) median cephalic
   (c) supplementary cephalic
   (d) basilic
   (e) median basilic
   (f) median antebrachial

2. Draw a circle on the illustration in #1 above around the most frequently used site for collecting specimens. Answer: Circle around b or d

3. Complete the following.

   In adults and children over 5, the usual capillary puncture site is <u>the ring finger.</u>

   Two alternate sites would be the <u>thumb</u> and <u>heel or earlobe.</u>

   In infants, the usual capillary puncture site is <u>great toe.</u>

   Two alternate sites would be the <u>heel</u> and <u>earlobe.</u>

## C. Learning Level: Application

1. What four physical conditions would make you look for an alternate venipuncture site?
   a. cyanotic
   b. scarred, bruised
   c. edema
   d. burned

2. Explain the specific medical assistant's role in obtaining the venipuncture.
   *Instructors:* Refer to the textbook, pp. 882–884.
   a. Select the proper method for obtaining sample and obtain supplies.
   b. Identify the patient.
   c. Prepare patient for procedure, sit, explain method.
   d. Obtain the specimen, label, and send to lab.
   e. Care of puncture site before discharge.

3. Complete the following chart.

| Venipuncture Method | Equipment | Common Sites | Considerations in Choosing Site |
|---|---|---|---|
| Syringe | Needle syringe, tubes, alcohol, gauze pads, tourniquet, tape, pen | Median cephalic vein, median basilic vein, supplementary cephalic vein | Age of patient, amount of blood needed, size of veins, # blood specimens in 24 hrs, health state |
| Evacuated | Vacutainer needle, adapter and tubes for test, alchohol, gauze pads, tourniquet, tape, pen—permanent | Median cephalic vein, median basilic vein, supplementary cephalic vein | Age of patient, number of tubes needed, size of veins |
| Butterfly | Tourniquet, gauze, alcohol, butterfly set, Luer-Lok syringe, correct pediatric or adult tubes; sharps disposal container, non-allergic bandage, pen | Bifurcation of superficial palmar veins | Used most frequently in children and elderly; condition of veins |

## D. Learning Level: Analysis

1. What color tubes are used in the following tests? If you cannot find the answer in your 8th Edition Textbook, research the answer on the Internet or in a laboratory procedures textbook.
   a. Drug screen **Red**
   b. Most serology tests **Red**
   c. Hematology **Lavender**
   d. Anticoagulant tests **Blue**
   e. Chemistry tests **Red**
   f. Sedimentation rate **Black**
   g. Blood glucose **Gray**

2. Place a number next to the *order* of filling specimen tubes from venipuncture. Number 1 is the first tube filled.

| | |
|---|---|
| Coagulation studies | **2. No additive** |
| Cultures | **1. No additive** |
| Type and crossmatch | **3.** |
| Most serologic tests | **4.** |

Explain your reason for filling tubes in this order.

Must be sure tubes for cultures or without coagulants are filled first in case some of blood gets back into Vacutainer tube, which may affect test results

3. Write the correct name of the capillary collection devices and supplies numbered in the illustration. Put the name in the corresponding blank spaces.

Instructors: The figure is from 8th Edition Textbook. It is Figure 44-16, p. 897, without labels.

## E. Learning Level: Synthesis

1. Without gloves and using a washable blue pen, place marks for veins on a classmate. Put on a tourniquet and find at least two veins and trace them. Take off the tourniquet and then show the area to your instructor. You will have to replace the tourniquet when you show the veins again. Do this at least twice if you can. How long should the tourniquet be safely left on the patient? **1 minute recommended**

2. Why . . .

   a. Is it important not to recap needles? **greatest source of self sticks and contamination**

   b. Is it important to wear gloves? **to prevent any loose blood or fluid getting onto medical assistant**

   c. Is the thumb not used for palpating veins? **You may feel your pulse instead of the patient pulse**

   d. Are butterfly needles inserted at the bifurcation of a hand vein? **To get directly into best vein with small needle size at an easily identified small area**

## F. Learning Level: Evaluation

1. What actions will you take if the following happens when obtaining blood?

   a. You are unable to get into a vein after two tries

      Call the office expert to perform venipuncture

   b. Blood will not flow out of vein

      Try to turn bevel some in case it is against top of vein, and slide it in a little further. Try again to withdraw blood. If you had blood and then none, must presume you went through the vein and need to try once more.

   c. Venipuncture site begins to swell

      Stop, withdraw, take out tourniquet; hold arm at heart level, put pressure on area for two minutes. Use other arm

   d. Patient, at the last moment, withdraws finger and you stab yourself with lancet.

      First stop procedure, have patient wait. Take off glove, wash finger and put on antiseptic cover with Band-Aid and reglove. Ask patient to look away before you resume and to hold still. If child, have parent or other medical assistant restrain arm.

2. What are the basic techniques you want to use to get the most accurate venipuncture?

   Use a large vein, put tourniquet on firmly; have patient hold hand in dependent position and open and close it several times; anchor the vein and make skin taut.

## PART 2 COMPETENCY CHALLENGE

Note: Students often approach this procedure with apprehension. They fear causing the patient pain. They worry they will miss the vein and be unable to collect the specimen. They are afraid of contracting blood-borne diseases. Instructors need to maintain a calm, self-assured manner. Guide the student through the procedure after a thorough demonstration. If the instructor has a problem, it validates the students' concept to be competent, not perfect. Be professional, empathetic, and calm. Students should practice until able to perform without error or in compliance with state law.

**Hints for practice include:**
PRACTICE holding the syringe correctly and tying the tourniquet first. Next practice holding the syringe and needle at the correct angle to the skin. Competence in these parts of the procedure will help students to inject the needle and withdraw blood in a smoother, quicker fashion. Demonstrate everything you are going to do many times before actual practice of the "stick." ALWAYS HAVE STUDENTS PRACTICE USING RUBBER TUBING many times before a real arm is used. If there are mannequin arm models, use them first.

Procedure 44-1: Collecting a Venous Blood Sample Using Syringe Method
Icons: wash hands, gloves, face protection, lab coat, biohazard waste container, sharps container

Procedure 44-2: Collecting a Venous Blood Sample Using the Vacutainer Method
Icons: wash hands, gloves, face protection, lab coat, biohazard waste container, sharps container

Procedure 44-3: Performing a Butterfly Draw
Icons: wash hands, gloves, lab coat, face protection, biohazard waste container, sharps container

STUDENT ACTIVITY
This chapter contains four procedures in which you will develop competency. If this chapter material is part of a certified phlebotomy class, assure yourself of the correct number of state required practice "sticks" and compliance with any other requirements to obtain state certification. The procedures for venipuncture, capillary puncture, butterfly draw and capillary sample collection are at the end of the chapter. There are also many activities in the CD-ROM for using knowledge and competencies. See the case studies for all the patients, especially Mr .Shapiro and Mrs. Ferguson.

## PART 3 CLINICAL APPLICATIONS

1. Research whether medical assistants are allowed to perform phlebotomy in your state. What types of injections or venipuncture are medical assistants allowed to perform in your state?

   ______________________________

2. Mrs. Moseley has asked the physician to draw blood on her 15-year-old pregnant daughter for a drug screen. The physician agreed. What do you say when the girl asks you what the test is for?

   ______________________________

   ______________________________

# 45

# Assisting in Hematology and Serology

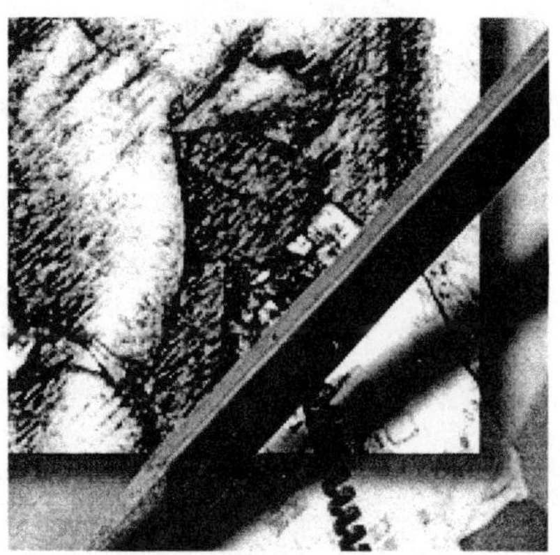

In this chapter, the student learns the purpose and significance of hematologic and serologic testing. Knowledge of the normal values, the significance of results and reporting of those to the physician are essential components of working in the lab. Students will be working with blood and must adhere to standard precautions. As instructors, we must always adhere to these standards and be positive role models. The danger of contamination must be real to students. Obtaining expired blood from the blood bank is a potential source for use in the lab, or students may volunteer to provide samples. Many programs complete only some of the procedures or simulate them using arm mannequins and imitation blood and serum samples. Be sure to have the program director and physician in charge give certificates to students for any procedures in which they have gained mastery.

## USING THE LEARNING SYSTEM

### 1. MEDICAL ASSISTING CONTENT AND COMPETENCIES

CONTENT

- Anatomy and physiology
- Diagnostic treatment modalities
- Word building and definitions
- Legal guidelines and requirements for health care
- Risk management
- Asepsis infection control
- Diagnostic testing
- Specimen collecting and processing
- Patient care
- Job readiness

COMPETENCIES

- All fundamental principles
- Use methods of quality control
- Perform chemistry and immunology testing
- Screen and follow up test results
- Prepare and assist patient with examinations, procedures, and treatments.
- Perform risk management procedures
- Recognize and respond to verbal and nonverbal communication
- Maintain confidentiality
- Document accurately
- Perform within legal and ethical boundaries

## 2. MEDICAL ASSISTING ENTRY-LEVEL CURRICULUM INTERFACE

| TEXTBOOK OBJECTIVES | LEARNING SYSTEM LOCATION | MA CURRICULUM |
|---|---|---|
| **Cognitive** | | **Content** |
| 1. Identify the tests included in a complete blood count | • Text p. 904<br>• Manual Part 1-B | • Anatomy and physiology<br>• Diagnostic treatment modalities<br>• Word building and definitions<br>• Diagnostic testing |
| 2. Describe the composition and function of blood | • Text p. 904<br>• Manual Part 1-B | • Same as # 1 |
| 3. Explain the purpose of a microhematocrit | • Text p. 905<br>• Manual Part 1-D | • Same as # 1 |
| 4. Describe hemoglobin | • Text p. 907<br>• Manual Part 1-D | • Same as # 1 |
| 5. Explain the purpose of a differential cell count | • Text p. 918<br>• Manual Part 1-C | • Anatomy and physiology<br>• Diagnostic treatment modalities<br>• Patient care<br>• Job readiness |
| 6. Explain the methods of evaluating blood cells | • Text pp. 922–925<br>• Manual Part 1-B | • Asepsis infection control<br>• Specimen collecting and processing<br>• Patient care<br>• Job readiness |
| 7. Understand the purpose of an erythrocyte sedimentation rate | • Text p. 926<br>• Manual Part 2 | • Same as # 6 |
| 8. Explain the purpose for lipid testing | • Text p. 929<br>• Manual Part 1-C | • Same as # 6 |
| 9. Describe diabetes mellitus and glucose testing | • Text pp. 931–933<br>• Manual Part 1-C | • Same as # 6 |
| 10. Discuss the Blood Safety Act | • Text p. 939<br>• Manual Part 1-F | • Legal guidelines and requirements for health care<br>• Risk management |

| **TEXTBOOK OBJECTIVES** | **LEARNING SYSTEM LOCATION** | **MA CURRICULUM** |
|---|---|---|
| **Performance** | **All procedures at end of Mastery Manual chapter** | **Competencies** |
| 1. Accurately perform a microhematocrit | • Procedure 45-1 in text p. 906<br>• Manual Part 2<br>• CD-ROM ⊕ | • All fundamental principles<br>• Use methods of quality control<br>• Perform chemistry and immunology testing<br>• Screen and follow up test results<br>• Prepare and assist patient with examinations, procedures and treatments.<br>• Perform risk management procedures<br>• Recognize and respond to verbal and nonverbal communication<br>• Maintain confidentiality<br>• Document accurately<br>• Perform within legal and ethical boundaries |
| 2. Determine the level of hemoglobin present in a given blood sample | • Procedure 45-2 in text p. 908<br>• Manual Part 2<br>• CD-ROM ⊕ | • Same as # 1 above |
| 3. Fill a Unopette capillary pipette transfer to a Unopette reservoir, correctly completing each step in proper order | • Procedure 45-3 in text p. 911<br>• Manual Part 2<br>• CD-ROM ⊕ | • Same as # 1 above |
| 4. Fill a hemacytometer chamber and correctly complete each step of the procedure in the proper sequence | • Procedure 45-4 in text p. 914<br>• Manual Part 2<br>• CD-ROM ⊕ | • Same as # 1 above |
| 5. Using the filled hemacytometer, count and calculate a manual white or red blood cell count to a minimum performance level of 200 WBC/$mm^3$ and 50,000 RBC/$mm^3$ | • Procedure 45-5 in text p. 915<br>• Manual Part 2<br>• CD-ROM ⊕ | • Same as # 1 above |
| 6. Prepare and stain a blood smear, using Wright stain, completing each step in proper sequence | • Procedure 45-6 in text p. 919<br>• Manual Part 2<br>• CD-ROM ⊕ | • Same as # 1 above |
| 7. Perform a differential cell count, red blood cell examination, and platelet estimation to a minimum performance level of 90% accuracy | • Procedure 45-7<br>• Manual Part 2<br>• CD-ROM ⊕ | • Same as # 1 above |

*chart continues on following page*

## MEDICAL ASSISTING ENTRY LEVEL CURRICULUM INTERFACE continued

| TEXTBOOK OBJECTIVES | LEARNING SYSTEM LOCATION | MA CURRICULUM |
|---|---|---|
| **Performance** | **All procedures at end of Mastery Manual chapter** | **Competencies** |
| 8. Using an EDTA blood specimen, determine a sedimentation rate using the Wintrobe method to a minimum performance level of 1 mm | • Procedure 45-8<br>• Manual Part 2<br>• CD-ROM ⊕ | • Same as #1 in competency area |
| 9. Follow manufacturer's directions and accurately determine a patient's cholesterol level | • Procedure 45-9<br>• Manual Part 2<br>• CD-ROM ⊕ | • Same as #1 in competency area |
| 10. Secure a capillary blood sample and determine the ABO and RH grouping of the sample with 100% accuracy | • Procedures 45-11 and 45-12<br>• Manual Part 2<br>• CD-ROM ⊕ | • Same as #1 in competency area |

## 3. RESOURCES

*THE ROUTINE VENIPUNCTURE,* video, 26 min. Program #78047
MEDCOM/TRAINEX
Box 3225, Garden Grove, CA 92641

Internet sites:

http://www.yahoo.com/Health/Medicine/Hematology/ **This site leads to other sites**

http://www.neosoft.com/~uthman/blood_cells.html **Blood cell and the CBC. Nice 8th Edition textbook and pictures.**

http://www.geocities.com/HotSprings/5340/ **Nice hematology site**

## 4. LESSON PLAN Hematology and Serology TIME 3 hours lecture, 12 hours lab

**Opening:** Bring in blood sample, hold it up and ask students to identify substance.

**Pretest:** Ask students what they know about blood. Review the blood types and components of blood. Put up Transparency Master #1 for review.

**Objectives:** Students will complete all cognitive objectives reviewing textbook materials and completing Part 1 in the Mastery Manual. Students need to have comprehension of all concepts. First phase of lab should allow students to become familiar with materials and review OSHA regulations. Performance will be completed as the school lab and program allows; AAMA-accredited programs can call national organization for ideas.

**Content:**
**a. Hematology**
Blood Composition, Function and Formation
Collection of Blood Specimens
  Microhematocrit Procedure 45-1: Performing a Microhematocrit
  Hemoglobin Procedure 45-2: Obtaining a Hemoglobin Count
  Red Blood Cell Count
  White Blood Cell Count
Methods of Counting Red and White Blood Cells
  Manual Counts
  Unopettes
  Hemacytometer
Counting Patterns, Counting Directions
Calculations—RBC, WBC
  Procedure 45-3: Filling a Unopette
  Procedure 45-4: Charging A Hemacytometer
  Procedure 45-5: Counting Cells in the Neubauer Ruled Hemacytometer
Automation
Differential Cell Count
  Preparation of Blood Smears
  Staining of Blood Smears
  Identification of Normal Blood Cells
  Differential Examination
Red Blood Cell Morphology
Platelet Observation
Preparing and Examining Smears
  Procedure 45-6: Preparing a Smear Stained with Wright Stain
  Procedure 45-7: Performing A Differential Examination of a Smear
Erythrocyte Sedimentation Rate
  Procedure 45-8: Determinating a Sedimentation Rate by the Wintrobe Method
Lipid Testing
  Procedure 45-9: Determining Cholesterol Level Using a ProAct Testing Device
Blood Glucose Procedure 45-10: Performing a Blood Glucose Accu-Chek Test

**B. Serology**
Immunohematologic Testing—Strep screen, ABO grouping, Rh factor
Blood Grouping
  Determination of ABO Group
  Procedure 45-11: Determining ABO Group Using a Slide Test
Determination of the Rh Factor
  Procedure 45-12: Determining Rh Factor Using the Slide Method
**Patient Education**
**Legal and Ethical Issues**

**Lab:** Use the Mastery Manual Parts 2 and 3 and the CD-ROM ⊕ to ensure that students know, use, and apply knowledge. Procedures must be demonstrated, discussed and practiced. Problem solving from instructor's past experience is beneficial. New instructors may want a lab person to help with demonstrations. Students obtain demonstration of proper technique in the lab from instructor and then observe under a technologist in a lab facility. Procedures, hints, precautions, and equipment are listed in Part 2 Mastery Manual answers. These procedures will require many more hours than the 12 assigned. Some instructors add hours to this area after subtracting from others.

**Assignment:** Students need to observe demonstration and then practice techniques. The instructor will have to be in the lab supervising at all times. This will require setting up lab times to allow for sufficient practice. If not completing procedures, students move on to next chapter on Microbiology.

**Posttest:** Give test questions from Examaster. For students performing procedures, it is necessary to add procedural questions to the Examaster or have students evaluated with perfect performance criteria. Post competencies from beginning of chapter. Have students write a paper explaining the reasons all competencies apply to all procedures.

## 5. MASTERY MANUAL ANSWERS

### PART 1 CONTENT MASTERY

### A. Learning Level: Knowledge

1. Vocabulary is essential. Match words *used in the chapter* with the meaning given. Place the number of the word next to the definition

   a. **Hormones 10** chemical substances secreted by endocrine glands
   b. **Glucose 7** used as fuel and only substance used by the brain
   c. **Serology 16** tests antigen–antibody reactions
   d. **Centrifuge 3** laboratory machine used to separate particles of different densities
   e. **Enzymes 5** proteins which act as a catalyst
   f. **Agglutinin 1** a substance that causes clumping
   g. **Eosin 6** synthetic dyes used to stain tissues for microscopic identification
   h. **Microhematocrit 12** Measurement of packed RBC volume
   i. **Lipid tests 11** used in assessing triglycerides and cholesterol levels
   j. **Analyte 2** any component in blood or other body fluid that can be measured
   k. **Morphology 13** study of form, structure, and size of organisms
   l. **Hemoglobin 9** rough measurement of oxygen-carrying capacity of blood
   m. **Phagocytosis 14** certain cells ingest microorganisms and cellular debris
   n. **Toxemia 17** poisonous products of bacteria in the bloodstream
   o. **Urea 19** the end product of protein metabolism
   p. **Cholesterol 4** a fat produced by the liver
   q. **Unopette 18** premeasured diluting fluid replacing blood-diluting pipette
   r. **Hemacytometer 8** counts cellular elements of blood
   s. **Sedimentation rate 15** rate at which RBCs separate from plasma

2. Give the meanings of the following abbreviations used in the laboratory.
   a. ESR **erythrocyte sedimentation rate**
   b. POL **physician office laboratory**
   c. % **percent**
   d. cc **cubic centimeter**
   e. mm **millimeter**
   f. g/dl **gram per deciliter**
   g. SIU **system of International Units**
   h. Mg/dl **milligram per deciliter**
   i. Mmol/L **millimol per liter**
   j. mm/h **millimole per hour**
   k. GTT **glucose tolerance test**
   l. FBS **fasting blood sugar**

## B. Learning Level: Comprehension

1. Complete the following chart for the cells in complete blood count and include those in the differential but not the RBC morphology. Use this completed chart as a guide when completing the procedures. Remind students that values vary some from lab to lab. Even the range will be different.

| **Cell and Shape** | **Function** | **Test Method** | **Normal Value** | **Indication**<br>**⇑ = # increase**<br>**⇓ = # decrease** |
|---|---|---|---|---|
| 1. Red blood cell—Biconcave disk, no nucleus stain, pinkish tan | Carry oxygen from lungs to cells | Hemacytometer | Male 4.6–6.1 million/$mm^3$<br>Female 4.0 –5.0 | ⇑ polycythemia,<br>⇓ hemorrhage, anemia, leukemia |
| 2. White blood cell—granular (polymorphonuclear) and agranular, each different shape and stain | Fight allergy, inflammation, infection | Hemacytometer | 5,000–10,000 | ⇑ Acute or chronic infection |
| Differential Cells<br>a. Neutrophil—granules and segmented nuclei stain dark purple | Fight allergy, inflammation, infection | Slide smear and Wright's stain | 50–70% of WBC | ⇑ few granules and acute infection,<br>⇓ rheumatoid arthritis, CML |
| b. Eosinophil—2- or 3-lobed nucleus, stains dark purple and granules stain orange red | Fight allergy, inflammation, infection; phagocytic | Slide smear and Wright's stain | 2-4 % WBC | ⇑ allergy, hay fever, asthma, parasite infection, autoimmune<br>⇓ steroid therapy |

*chart continues on following page*

CHART CONTINUED

| Cell and Shape | Function | Test Method | Normal Value | Indication ⇑ = # increase ⇓ = # decrease |
|---|---|---|---|---|
| c. Basophil—Segmented, stains, light purple, cytoplasm granules stain dark blue | Fight allergy, inflammation, infection | Slide smear and Wright's stain | .5–1 % of WBC | ⇑ inflammation ⇓ hypersensitivity |
| d. Lymphocyte—nucleus oval or round and stains purple, cytoplasm stain blue | Recognize foreign substances, produce circulating antibodies, infection | Slide smear and Wright's stain | 25–35%; may be most numerous cell in children | ⇑ chronic infection, lymphocytic leukemia, viral infections, ⇓ radiation therapy, AIDS, corticosteroid rx |
| e. Monocytes—Largest WBC; nucleus oval, indented, or horseshoe shape; cytoplasm stains gray-blue; vacuoles | Macrophage, ingest bacteria, cell debris | Slide smear and Wright's stain | 2–8% of WBC | ⇑ chronic inflammation, viral infection as hepatitis, mumps, rickettsial infections and TB |
| 3. Platelets—smallest, round, oval, no nucleus, stain blue | Clotting | Slide smear and Wright's stain | 150,000— 400,000/ $mm^3$ danger = <15,000/ $mm^3$ | ⇑ thrombosis, polycythemia v. ⇓ bleeding, leukemias |

2. State the blood component that is not named in the above chart and describe its function.
   Plasma, carries other substances, such as clotting proteins and minerals.
3. State the names by which neutrophils may be known.
   PMNs, polymorphonuclear neutrophils, segmented neutrophils, segs, and polys.

## C. Learning Level: Application

1. Give the indications for (screening) performing the following tests
   a. Differential cell count **evaluate type of infection**
   b. Rh factor **rhesus factor—a blood group found on RBCs of rhesus monkey**
   c. Glucose **evaluate glucose metabolism in diabetics, hypoglycemics**
   d. Lipid tests **atherosclerosis, heart disease, blood vessel blocks**
   e. Sedimentation rate **inflammatory—not infectious disease**

MULTIPLE CHOICE: Directions: More than one number may be correct in each question. Choose one letter which describes the numbers you are choosing for your answer:

| A | B | C | D | E |
|---|---|---|---|---|
| **1, 2, 3 only** | **1, 3 only** | **2, 4 only** | **4 only** | **All are correct** |

2. When preparing the patient for a capillary puncture of the finger: **Ans = B**
   1. Gently massage the finger to increase blood flow.
   2. Apply ice to the finger to decrease the pain.
   3. Place the finger in warm water to increase blood flow.
   4. Squeeze the finger to increase blood flow.

3. Accurate sedimentation rate testing depends on following these guidelines: **Ans = E**
   1. The tube must be totally filled with blood.
   2. The tube must be free of air bubbles.
   3. The tube must rest in an undisturbed vertical position for at least one hour before reading the results.
   4. Testing must be performed within two hours of specimen collection.

4. The microhematocrit (HCT): **Ans = E**
   1. Is frequently performed.
   2. Is a simple procedure.
   3. Requires a small amount of blood.
   4. Valuable procedure patient's progress.

5. The separation of cellular elements from blood plasma can be speeded up by using a centrifuge. After centrifugation: **Ans = A**
   1. The plasma rises to the top.
   2. The red cells fall to the bottom.
   3. The white cells settle to the center.
   4. The platelets dissolve.

6. Automated cell counts have some impressive advantages. They: **Ans = E**
   1. Are more accurate.
   2. Can be done quickly and efficiently.
   3. Reduce the number of times a specimen must be handled.
   4. Decrease the exposure of personnel to hepatitis B and AIDS viruses.

## D. Learning Level: Analysis

1. Differentiate microhematocrit from hemoglobin.

   Microhematocrit measures packed cell volume, which is a reflection of the oxygen-carrying capacity of the blood. Hemoglobin generally measures the oxygen-carrying capacity of the blood.

2. Explain the purpose for the following procedural steps:
   a. Tubes are numbered and placed opposite each other in centrifuge.

      Centrifuge must always be balanced to avoid damage. Procedure 45-1, step 5.

   b. Remove tubes immediately from centrifuge.

      Tubes left in centrifuge will show altered results as layer spreads horizontally. Procedure 45-1, step 10.

   c. Wipe away first drop of blood.

      May have tissue fluid in it and will dilute sample.

   d. Wipe outside of pipette removing all blood traces.

      Blood on the outside will enter reservoir and give inaccurate results. Procedure 45-3, step 7.

e. Expel two drops from well-mixed Unopette before filling hemacytometer.

   Diluent in chamber has no cells and must be expelled to get cells into hemacytometer Procedure 45-4, step 4.

f. Decrease light until cells are easily visible.

   Too much light prevents visualizing cells. Procedure 45-5, step 7.

g. Stand slide with thick end of blood down and let dry.

   Prevent thick end running into thin area of smear and destroying smear. Procedure 45-6, step 10.

h. Place slide on stage with smear facing up

   If the slide is facing down will not be able to focus under oil immersion. Procedure 45-7, step 4.

i. Count 100 consecutive white blood cells in a winding pattern.

   Proceed systematically to avoid missing cells or double counting cells. Procedure 45-7, step 10.

j. Place tube in Wintrobe rack, numbered slot, vertical and free from vibration for 1 hour.

   Jarring will increase ESR and give false result. Procedure 45-8, step 8.

k. Examine test area of CHOL test strip for uneven color development.

   Mottled color indicates invalid test and must be repeated. Procedure 45-9, step 19.

l. Make sure code # on LED display matches code # on testing strip container.

   If code numbers do not match, the device must be reprogrammed to obtain valid results. Procedure 45-10, step 6.

## E. Learning Level: Synthesis

Answer is the illustration 45-6 in Textbook p. 917. Review the counting square methods with students.
Draw a counting square in the counting chamber of the Hemacytometer. As it is difficult to be exact, put the line spaces in and indicate measurements for all areas. Indicate WBC and RBC counting squares. Indicate WBC counting order. Use the frame supplied below.

## F. Learning Level: Evaluation

Consider the following situations and write your responses.

1. Mrs Ferguson's partial CBC comes back with the following results.

   RBC 3.2 million/$mm^3$

   HCT 30

   Hgb 10g/dl

   WBC 8000/$mm^3$

   Platelets 250,000/$mm^3$

   What do these results indicate? **Patient is anemic**

2. A patient comes in to see Dr. Lawler on Monday. He is 24 years old and complains of lower abdominal pain. It was a wild weekend of touch football and eating at a family gathering. He thinks he just ate too much but also took a punch to the gut. He just doesn't feel right. Doctor orders a screening CBC. The patient has abdominal tenderness from the midline to the right side. The CBC comes back and results are

   RBC 4 million/$mm^3$

   HCT 42

   Hgb 15g/dl

   WBC 18,000/$mm^3$

   Platelets 350000/$mm^3$

   What do these results indicate? **An overwhelming infection**

   What further tests might be ordered and why? **Differential, bilirubin and ESR and CT to evaluate possible appendicitis, GB disease**

## PART 2 COMPETENCY CHALLENGE

Demonstrate each procedure to students before practice. When students pass competence evaluation, initial their clinical cards so they may do these procedures in the workplace. Sometimes a hospital, outpatient facility, or clinical laboratory will allow students to rotate through to gain experience under supervision. Information given below will help you prepare for practice by having supplies available.

### PROCEDURE 45-1: PERFORMING A MICROHEMATOCRIT

**Icons:** wash hands, gloves, face protection, biohazard waste container

**Task:** To accurately perform a microhematocrit

**Conditions:** nonsterile gloves, EDTA anticoagulant blood, capillary tubes, sealing clay, centrifuge

Microhematocrit tubes break very easily, so caution students to exercise special care when working with them to avoid breakage and possible injury. Gloves must be worn throughout this procedure.

### PROCEDURE 45-2: OBTAINING A HEMOGLOBIN COUNT

**Icons:** gloves, biohazard waste container, sharps container

**Task:** To accurately determine the level of hemoglobin present in a blood sample using the hemoglobinometer method.

**Conditions:** hemoglobinometer, reagent applicators, Autolet or blood lancet, alcohol preps, gauze squares

### PROCEDURE 45-3: FILLING A UNOPETTE

**Task:** To properly fill a Unopette pipette with blood and to transfer the sample to a Unopette reservoir

**Conditions:** Unopette unit, capillary pipette, pipette shield reservoir, EDTA anticoagulant blood, gauze squares, test tube rack

Be certain that student understands how to choose the appropriate micropipette for the Unopette used. Carefully check student to be certain that this is done. Observe the filling of the micropipette to be certain that it is filled end to end.

### PROCEDURE 45-4: CHARGING (FILLING) A HEMACYTOMETER

**Icons:** wash hands, gloves, face protection, biohazard waste container

**Task:** To fill the hemacytometer for a manual cell count

**Conditions:** Nonsterile gloves, Neubauer ruled hemacytometer, hemacytometer coverslip, lint-free tissue, 70% alcohol, blood-diluting pipette or Unopette

The instructor should carefully check the hemocytometer for proper filling before the student begins to count. Also question the student on the purpose of each step.

### PROCEDURE 45-5: COUNTING CELLS IN THE NEUBAUER RULED HEMACYTOMETER

**Icons:** wash hands, biohazard waste container

**Task:** To properly focus a hemacytometer, to locate the appropriate areas to count, and to direct your field of vision through the chamber in the proper manner while counting cells.

**Conditions:** Properly filled hemacytometer, microscope, hand tally counter

Students may ask you why they are doing this procedure when it is done in an automated machine in the physician's office and in the research laboratory. It is done to help the student to understand the meaning of cell counting and also to aid him or her in learning to identify the different components of the blood.

Students should count 5 RBC squares, and the instructor should count at least 1 square to confirm the count. Students must count 4 WBC squares and the instructor counts 1 square for confirmation. Be sure to check the student's calculations.

### PROCEDURE 45-6 PREPARING A SMEAR STAINED WITH WRIGHT STAIN

**Icons:** wash hands, gloves, face protection, biohazard waste container

**Task:** To prepare and stain a slide that meets the criteria for the performance of a differential examination

**Conditions:** Clean glass slides, transfer pipette or capillary tube, Wright stain materials, EDTA anticoagulant blood specimen

Follow standard laboratory guidelines. Have students use a variety of commercial stains whenever possible. Remind students that this is a dye and it will dye any fabric that it comes in contact with.

### PROCEDURE 45-7 PERFORMING A DIFFERENTIAL EXAMINATION OF A SMEAR

**Icons:** wash hands, biohazard waste container

**Task:** To perform a differential cell count, evaluate the red blood cell morphology, and estimate the number of platelets.

**Conditions:** Microscope, immersion oil, lens tissue, lens cleaner

Observe the students as they begin to learn to count cells. The instructor should confirm and initial each new classification of cell found by the student.

### PROCEDURE 45-8: DETERMINING A SEDIMENTATION RATE BY THE WINTROBE METHOD

**Icons:** wash hands, gloves, face protection

**Task:** To properly fill a Wintrobe tube and observe and record the findings of an erythrocyte sedimentation rate, using the Wintrobe method.

**Conditions:** EDTA anticoagulant blood specimen, Wintrobe tube, Wintrobe rack, timer, Pasteur pipette, bulb

Students must know factors for accurate rate: full tube, no bubbles, vertical position, sit one hour and test within 2 hours of obtaining blood.

### PROCEDURE 45-9: DETERMINING CHOLESTEROL LEVEL USING A PROACT TESTING DEVICE

**Icons:** wash hands, gloves, biohazard waste container, sharps container

**Task:** To accurately perform and and report a ProAct test for cholesterol level

**Conditions:** ProAct testing device, lithium heparin capillary tube and capillary pipettor, lancets and lancet device, sterile gauze, alcohol preps, biohazard waste container, biohazard sharps container

Testing requires accuracy and not touching the strips near recording LED. Capillary tube must not have air bubbles—a tricky technique.

### PROCEDURE 45-10: PERFORMING A BLOOD GLUCOSE ACCU-CHEK TEST

**Icons:** gloves, biohazard waste container, biohazard sharps container.

**Task:** To accurately perform a blood test for possible diabetes mellitus.

**Conditions:** Accu-Chek Glucose Monitor or similar glucose monitoring device,

Accu-Chek Glucose Testing Strip, lancet and autoloading finger puncturing device,

alcohol preps, gauze squares

**Assure that students:**

Do not touch the yellow test pad or round window on the back of the strip when handling the strip.

Do not touch the pad with the patient's finger.

Do not apply a second drop of blood.

Do not smear the blood with finger.

Be certain the yellow test pad is saturated with blood.

All students need to be able to perform this test as it is done very frequently in the physician office.

**PROCEDURE 45-11: DETERMINING ABO GROUP USING A SLIDE TEST**

**Icons:**, gloves, face protection, biohazard waste container, sharps container.

**Task:** To accurately determine patient's ABO group using the slide test technique.

**Conditions:** glass slides with frosted ends, anti-A and anti-B serum, applicator sticks, lancet and automatic finger puncture device, alcohol preps, sterile gauze squares, laboratory marking pen or pencil.

These procedures are done less commonly because the pregnant patient is usually sent to the lab for these and other state mandated screening tests.

**PROCEDURE 45-12: DETERMINING Rh FACTOR USING THE SLIDE METHOD**

**Icons:** gloves, face protection, biohazard waste container, sharps container

**Task:** To accurately determine the presence or absence of anti-D agglutinations

**Conditions:** 2 glass slides with frosted ends, anti-D serum, applicator sticks, lancet and automatic finger puncture device, alcohol preps, sterile gauze squares, laboratory marker or pencil

## PART 3 CLINICAL APPLICATIONS

Note: Use these to develop communication skills, ethical and legal discussions, and educational techniques.

1. Miss Ruby is to have her blood glucose tested using an Accu-Chek. The physician wants you to perform it and role model the correct procedure. As you are doing it she says, "I have so much trouble getting blood that I do not waste it like you do." You ask her to explain and she says that she has to pump her finger so hard that she uses the first drop of blood. What will you respond and teach her?

2. You are medical assistant to a nurse practitioner who is also a trained and certified midwife. Her patient is in for a prenatal visit and the nurse practitioner asks you to draw and test for blood group and Rh typing. The patient asks why you are doing this and why it needs to be done. Explain.

3. Explain to the patient the following CBC test with normal results and why these tests are included in a complete blood count.

   RBC 4.4 mil/mm$^3$ Hct 44% Hg 14 g/dL

   WBC 9000 Polys 55 Lymphs 31 Mono 5 Eos. 3 Baso. 1.

   Platelets 250,000 cells/mm$^3$

4. What are the legal guidelines to remember when drawing blood and testing it in the lab?

   Must have competency certificate from program or qualified instructor.

   Serology and CDC testing must be exactly as described by law.

   Must keep exact documentation of legal specimens.

   Use povidone-iodine for skin preps on venipuncture.

   Follow standard precautions and biohazard waste disposal.

   Follow Blood Safety Act if enacted in your state.

   Must follow federal and state quality control guidelines.

# 46

# Assisting in Microbiology

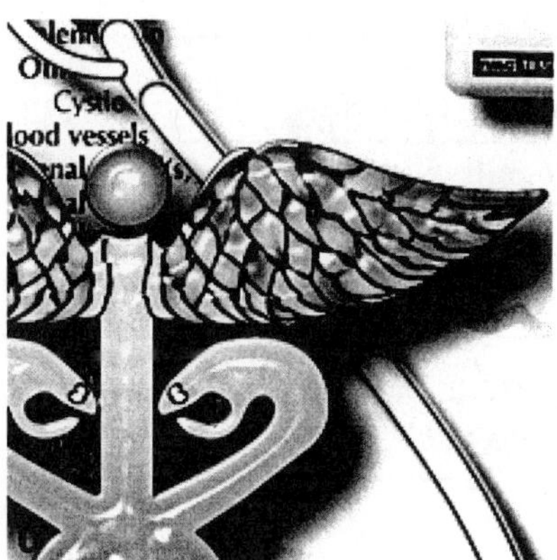

This chapter raises student understanding of the role of microorganisms in causing disease. Students will realize how many microorganisms can be identified in the physician's office, thereby offering rapid treatment. Review the history of medicine in Chapter 2, and discuss discoveries and people involved in microbiology. There are many interesting resources on the Internet. Emphasize the most common diseases caused by microorganisms and seen in the physician office. Seven procedures will prepare the student for many tests done in the family practice office. Students particularly interested in the laboratory area may be able to extern in that setting.

## USING THE LEARNING SYSTEM

### 1. MEDICAL ASSISTING CONTENT AND COMPETENCIES

CONTENT

- Anatomy and physiology
- Diagnostic treatment modalities
- Word building and definitions
- Legal guidelines and requirements for health care
- Medical ethics and related issues
- Risk management
- Asepsis and infection control
- Diagnostic testing
- Specimen collecting and processing
- Patient care
- Job readiness

COMPETENCIES

- All fundamental principles
- Use methods of quality control
- Perform microbiology testing
- Screen and follow-up test results
- Prepare and assist patient with examinations, procedures, and treatments
- Perform risk management procedures
- Recognize and respond to verbal and nonverbal communication
- Maintain confidentiality
- Document accurately
- Perform within legal and ethical boundaries

## 2. MEDICAL ASSISTING ENTRY-LEVEL CURRICULUM INTERFACE

| TEXTBOOK OBJECTIVES | LEARNING SYSTEM LOCATION | MA CURRICULUM |
|---|---|---|
| **Cognitive** | | **Content** |
| 1. List the classifications of microorganisms | • Text p. 942<br>• Manual Part 1-B | • Anatomy and physiology |
| 2. Cite the morphologic differences of bacteria | • Text pp. 942–943<br>• Manual Part 1-B | • Anatomy and physiology<br>• Diagnostic testing |
| 3. Describe the differences between viruses and bacteria | • Text p. 946<br>• Manual Part 1-B | • Anatomy and physiology<br>• Diagnostic testing |
| 4. Cite examples of disease for each of the microorganism classifications | • Tables 46-1–46-6<br>• Manual Part 1-B | • Anatomy and physiology<br>• Diagnostic testing |
| 5. Identify elements needed for microorganism growth | • Text p. 949<br>• Memory Jogger | • Anatomy and physiology<br>• Diagnostic testing |
| 6. Cite the protocols for specimen collection | • Text p. 950<br>• Memory Jogger | • Diagnostic treatment modalities<br>• Asepsis and infection control<br>• Diagnostic testing<br>• Specimen collecting and processing<br>• Patient care<br>• Job readiness |
| 7. Describe the different growth media used for culturing | • Text p. 952<br>• Manual Part 1-D | • Asepsis and infection control<br>• Diagnostic testing<br>• Specimen collecting and processing<br>• Job readiness |
| 8. Compare rapid culture with standard culture growth methods | • Text p. 959<br>• Manual Part 1-D | • Same as # 7 |
| 9. Discuss legal and ethical issues in laboratory testing | • Text p. 966<br>• Manual Part 3 | • Legal guidelines and requirements for health care<br>• Medical ethics and related issues<br>• Risk management |
| 10. Define and spell vocabulary terms | • Text p. 941<br>• Manual Part 1 | • Anatomy and physiology<br>• Word building and definitions |

| TEXTBOOK OBJECTIVES | LEARNING SYSTEM LOCATION | MA CURRICULUM |
|---|---|---|
| **Performance** | | **Competencies** |
| 1. Identify bacteria through microscopic viewing | • Manual Part 2 | • All fundamental principles<br>• Perform microbiology testing |
| 2. Inoculate media for culture | • Manual Part 2<br>• Procedure 46-1 | • Use methods of quality control<br>• Document accurately<br>• Perform risk management procedures<br>• Perform within legal and ethical boundaries |
| 3. Prepare direct smears and indirect smears from culture | • Manual Part 2<br>• Procedures 46-3 and 46-4 | • Same as # 2 |
| 4. Examine stained smears for the presence of microorganisms | • Manual Part 2<br>• Procedure 46-1 | • Same as # 2, and<br>• Screen and follow up test results |
| 5. Perform a rapid culture | • Manual Part 2<br>• Procedure 46-5 | • Same as # 2, and<br>• Screen and follow up test results |
| 6. Secure a collection for pinworms | • Manual Part 2<br>• Procedure 46-6 | • Prepare and assist patient with examinations, procedures, and treatments<br>• Recognize and respond to verbal and nonverbal communication<br>• Maintain confidentiality<br>• Screen and follow up test results |
| 7. Perform slide agglutination testing for infectious mononucleosis | • Manual Part 2<br>• Procedure 46-7 | • Same as # 5 |

## 3. RESOURCES

http://www.yahoo.com/Science/Biology/Microbiology/
http://www.yahoo.com/Science/Biology/Microbiology/Microorganisms
http://www.yahoo.com/Science/Biology/Microbiology/Virology/
http://www.tulane.edu/~dmsander/Big_Virology/BVFamilyGenome.html **The Big Picture Book of Viruses**
Stepp, CA and Woods, M. *Laboratory Procedures for Medical Office Personnel*, Philadelphia, WB Saunders, 1998

## 4. LESSON PLAN Microbiology TIME 3 hours lecture, 12 hours lab

**Opening:** Begin class with an agar plate for each student. When you have their attention, culture 1/2 plate with your fingertips. Do a throat swab and place on the other side. Wait 24 hours—tomorrow during lab, evaluate the results.

**Pretest:** As you swab the plate with your fingers, ask students what you are doing and why. Answer: Trying to grow microorganisms and hoping to show that there are more or as many on your fingers than in your mouth. Medical asepsis is the key to preventing infection.

**Objectives:** Put objectives up on a flip chart and review with students. Have students interrelate objectives to MA curriculum requirements when asked to do so in the Mastery Manual final evaluation.

**Content:**
CHAPTER OUTLINE
1. Classification of Microorganisms
   a. Bacteria
      Chlamydia and Mycoplasms
   b. Fungi
   c. Mycobacteria
   d. Viruses
   e. Parasites
      Helminths, Protozoa, and Rickettsiae
2. Conditions That Favor Microorganism Growth
3. Collection of Microbiology Specimens
   Optimal Collection Times
   Sufficient Sample
   Proper Equipment and Procedures—Try to have items out and organized according to procedure. All procedure supplies are listed in each procedure.
4. Microbiology Procedures
   a. Preparation of Smears
   b. Antimicrobial Sensitivity Testing, Procedures 46-1–46-4
   c. Rapid Culture Methods, Procedures 46-5–46- 7
   d. Interpretation of Throat Culture
   e. Pinworms Testing
   f. Slide Agglutination Test
   g. Collection of Semen
5. Legal and Ethical Issues
6. Patient Education

**Lab:** Have students complete Mastery Manual Parts 2 and 3 in the lab. If possible, demonstrate each procedure. A field trip to a lab would be excellent for students to see these procedures before practicing. Students are given some directions for procedures, but more are included in this Curriculum Guide for the instructor. Lab time can be used for practice of procedures and CD-ROM ⊕ completion. If students are completing both the CD-ROM and lab procedures, it would be good to have the CD-ROM activities completed before practice of procedures.

**Assignment:** Depending upon lab situation and accessibility to supplies, students may complete Mastery Manual or simulate activities lab. Have students make flash cards and procedure cards with important points to remember for each procedure.

**Posttest:** Use Examaster questions. May want to repeat some questions from the Mastery Manual to see if they have learned materials. Set up lab supplies for procedures and have students identify supplies.

## 5. MASTERY MANUAL ANSWERS

### PART 1 CONTENT MASTERY

### A. Learning Level: Knowledge

Fill the terms in next to the correct definitions.

1. **spore** A thick-walled reproductive cell formed within bacteria and capable of withstanding unfavorable environmental conditions.
2. **microorganisms** Microscopic living parasites.
3. **inoculate** To place a specimen in a culture medium to allow it to grow.
4. **hemolysis** The destruction of red blood cells.
5. **asepsis** Absence of contaminated materials.
6. **agglutination** The clumping together of particles.
7. **disease** A definite pathologic process having a descriptive set of signs and symptoms.
8. **nosocomial** Pertaining to the spread of infection among patients, staff, and visitors in hospitals.
9. **pathogens** Disease-causing microorganisms.
10. **toxin** A poisonous protein substance produced by some plants, animals, and pathogenic bacteria.
11. **agar** A substance extracted from algae and used in the laboratory.
12. **antibody** An immunoglobulin produced by lymphoid tissue.
13. **colony** The visible growth on a culture plate, usually resulting from a single bacteria.
14. **infection** Invasion and multiplication of microorganisms in body tissues.
15. **in vitro** Pertaining to a biological reaction that occurs in an artificial environment.
16. **mordant** A chemical (Gram's iodine) used to make the primary stain adhere to the cells it stains.
17. **occult** Hidden; not visible with the eye alone.
18. **reference laboratory** A large laboratory that accepts specimens from smaller laboratories.
19. **screening test** A laboratory test done on large numbers of people to detect occult diseases.
20. **helminth** Animal parasites called *worms.*

21. List the classifications of microorganisms.
    Bacteria, Fungi, Mycobacteria, Viruses, Parasites

### B. Learning Level: Comprehension

1. Complete the chart below using the classifications above in # 21.

| Organism | Transmission | Diagnosis Method | Three Diseases |
|---|---|---|---|
| Bacteria—one-celled plant organisms—cocci, spirilla, bacilli | Direct contact, vectors airborne, indirect—water | Blood test—antibodies, cultures | Pneumonia, meningitis, cystitis<br>Staphylococci, syphilis, gonorrhea |
| Mycobacterium obligate parasites | Must have host, smallest of all bacteria | Smears, x-ray observation | Chlamydia, pneumonia, PID |
| Fungi—larger than bacteria and rigid cell walls | Direct contact, prolonged exposure, inhalation of contaminated dust | Skin tests, x-ray, biopsy | Yeast, molds, tinea, candidiasis, thrush, histoplasmosis, blastomycosis |

*Chart continues on following page*

| Organism | Transmission | Diagnosis Method | Three Diseases |
|---|---|---|---|
| Viruses—smallest organism either RNA or DNA | Only on living host | Antigen-antibody serology tests | Childhood diseases, HIV, encephalitis, shingles |
| Parasites—<br>Helminths<br>Protozoa<br>Rickettsia | Arthropod vectors from animals to humans | Blood test, smears | Worms—roundworm, tapeworm, schistosomiasis<br>Giardia, trichomonas,<br>Lyme disease, Rocky Mountain fever |

2. List the four shapes of bacteria and three forms of disease caused by each. Use the tables in your 8th Edition Textbook and choose common diseases you will remember.

   Use Tables 46-1, 2, and 3, pp. 944-946, and tell students which diseases they must know. The four bacterial shapes are listed in above answer.

## C. Learning Level: Application

1. On the circle below make the pattern you draw on agar when making a culture.

   See textbook p. 952 for examples.

2. Sensitivity testing defines the best antimicrobial agent to use. What is the criteria for choosing the best antimicrobial agent?

   Answer: Demonstrates the most activity against the microbe; least toxicity to patient; least impact on normal body flora; desired pharmaceutical effect; most economical—well, sometimes.

3. Compare rapid culture with standard culture by listing advantages and disadvantages for each.

| Culture Type | Advantages | Disadvantages |
|---|---|---|
| Rapid | Results while patient in office | Patients less likely to follow up |
| | Offer presumptive identification | May need differential or more specific identification |
| Standard | Offers specific diagnosis | Treatment has to be delayed |
| | Specific treatment | Treatment may need changing |

## D. Learning Level: Analysis

1. Differentiate selective and nonselective media and give examples of each.
   a. Selective media allow growth of certain bacteria and prohibit growth of others. Examples are: eosin-methylene blue, MacConkey, and Thayer-Martin.
   b. Nonselective media support the growth of most bacteria. Blood agar of sheep blood and tryptic soy broth are the most common. Expiration dates indicate when these media should be autoclaved and disposed of.
2. What media are used for the following cultures?
   a. throat cultures **blood agar**
   b. urine cultures **2 media—EMB or MacConkey and blood agar**
   c. STD cultures **Thayer-Martin or chocolate agar**

## E. Learning Level: Synthesis

CPT codes from 1998 edition

80061—Lipid panel

81002—Nonautomated, without microscopy (dipstick or tablet reagent urinalysis, nonautomated for bilirubin, glucose, hemoglobin, ketones, leukocytes, nitrate, pH, protein, specific gravity, and urobilinogen)

81025—Urine pregnancy test by visual color comparison methods

82044—Urine, microalbumin, semiquantitative

82770—Blood, occult, feces, 1–3 simultaneous determinations

82273—Other sources qualitative (rapid screening test to detect the presence of gastric occult blood)

82465—Cholesterol, serum, total

82947—Glucose, quantitative

82950—Postglucose dose (includes glucose)

82951—Tolerance test (GTI three specimens (includes glucose))

82952—Tolerance test (GflT), each additional beyond three specimens

82962—Glucose, blood by glucose monitoring device(s) cleared by the FDA specifically for home use

82985—Glycosylated protein (LXN fructosamine test system)

83026—Hemoglobin, by copper sulfate method, nonautomated

83718—Lipoprotein, direct measurement, high-density cholesterol (HDL)

83986—pH, body fluid, except blood

84478—Triglycerides

84830—Ovulation tests, by visual color comparison methods for human luteinizing hormone (This test is not covered by Part B Medicare.)

85013—Blood count; spun hematocrit

85014—Blood count; other than spun hematocrit (Wampole Stat-Crit Hct)

85018—hemoglobin (by single instrument with self-contained or component features to perform specimen/reagent interaction, providing a direct measurement and readout)

85651—Sedimentation rate, erythrocyte, nonautomated

86318—Immunoassay for infectious agent antibody qualitative or semiquantitative single-step method (e.g., reagent strip) (for rapid qualitative detection of IgG antibodies specific to *Helicobacter pylori* in whole blood)

86588 QW—Streptococcus screen direct

87072 QW—Culture or direct bacterial identification method, each organism, by commercial kit, any source except urine

81000—Urinalysis, by dipstick or tablet reagent for bilirubin, glucose, hemoglobin, ketone, leukocytes, nitrite, pH, protein, specific gravity, urobilinogen, any number of these constituents; nonautomated, with microscopy

81020—Urinalysis; two- or three-glass test

89190—Nasal smears for eosinophils

## F. Learning Level: Evaluation

1. When abnormal test results come back to the office, a medical assistant is assigned to notify the physician; then abnormal test results are placed in a basket with all test results. You are helping the medical assistant and notice that for some of these abnormal results, the medical assistant calls the patient and says test results are normal and then files the chart.

   What do you think is happening here? Will you say or do anything? Write your response.

   The medical assistant may be using a set of normal values designated by the physician, not the lab. Ask the medical assistant what values are being used by the office.

## PART 2 COMPETENCY CHALLENGE

**Instructor activity:** Students may culture items used frequently, such as pens, cosmetics, and spoons, and determine types and numbers of microorganisms present. Disinfect items with chemicals and then culture. Finally, have students autoclave the items and make a culture. Neither the chemical nor the sterilized items should grow organisms. If positive, have students problem solve and try again. More hints are with the procedures.

**Suggested activities in Mastery Manual**

1. Take a plain nutrient agar plate and divide it into two halves. Use one half for a culture of your fingers before performing the handwashing procedure, and use the other half for a culture after handwashing.
   - Place four dirty fingers on the first side of the plate.
   - Perform a medical hand wash and inoculate the plate with your fingers on the other side.
   - Incubate for 24 to 48 hours.
   - Compare the two halves to see how successful your handwashing technique was.
2. Compare the microscope and the centrifuge that you are using in class with those at the facility where you do your work experience. What are the differences in how these two instruments are used and how they function? Be prepared to discuss your findings in class.
3. Divide a plain nutrient agar plate into three parts. Obtain media for culture from your shoe, under your fingernail, and a strand of your hair. Incubate the plate and examine it. Compare the growth from the three areas. What conclusions are you able to draw?
4. Complete a throat culture and rapid strep screen on a classmate. Read the rapid test immediately and record. Examine the culture with your instructor. Compare the results and analyze the differences.
5. Complete an ABO grouping and Rh factor agglutination test on yourself. Have a classmate obtain the sample.

**Procedure 46-1: Inoculating a Blood Agar Plate for Strep Throat Culture**

**Icons:** wash hands, gloves, face protection, biohazard waste container

**Task:** To inoculate a blood agar plate for culture of strep throat

**Conditions:** Blood agar plate, Bacitracin disk or strep A disk, Bacti-cinerator, inoculating loop permanent marker, swab from patient's throat, forceps, biohazard waste container

**Note:** Students need to sterilize loop before and after use, be sure to allow 48 hours if first 24 show negative growth

**Procedure 46-2: Streaking Plates for Quantitative Cultures**

**Icons:** wash hands, gloves, face protection, biohazard waste container

**Task:** To inoculate two plates with urine, using quantitative streaking methods

**Conditions:** Urine specimen; Bacti-cinerator; calibrated inoculating loop; blood agar plate or biplates, which are plates having both blood agar and either EMB or MacKintex in a single plate; biohazard waste container

**Note:** Students need to review before starting because it is important to swirl and get specimen promptly before settling. Whenever using the loop, remind students to let it cool—or no growth. Some labs label the bottom of plates before placing the specimen, other labs label the top.

**Procedure 46-3: Preparing a Direct Smear or Culture Smear for Staining**

**Icons:** wash hands, gloves, face protection, biohazard waste container

**Task:** To prepare a smear for staining from a clinical specimen or from a culture medium

**Conditions:** Clean glass slides, permanent marker, Bacti-cinerator, saline solution, specimen

Note: A variety of loops may be used. Students should attempt this 4–5 times. Have them show you their methodology for culture smear.

**Procedure 46-4: Staining a Smear with Gram's Stain**

**Icons:** wash hands, gloves, face protection, biohazard waste container

**Task:** To stain a slide, using Gram's stain, so that the organisms present are colored appropriately (neither overcolorized nor too strongly decolorized)

**Conditions:** Gram's stain reagents, staining rack, forceps, wash, bottle of water, prepared smear for staining, absorbent paper

**Note:** Use a variety of Gram's stains if possible. This takes practice to get the color correct.

**Procedure 46-5: Performing a Rapid Strep Test**

**Icons:** wash hands, gloves, face protection, biohazard waste container

**Task:** To properly prepare a slide for microscopic identification of group A beta-hemolytic streptococci

**Conditions:** Directigen test kit of strep A, timer or wristwatch with sweep second hand,

throat swab specimen, biohazard waste container

**Note:** This procedure uses Directigen group A strep. If a different rapid strep kit is used, follow manufacturer's instructions accurately.

Remind students that with rapid testing, the accuracy is important because the physician is waiting to decide on the treatment.

**Procedure 46-6: Performing a Cellulose Tape Collection for Pinworms**

**Icons:** wash hands, gloves, face protection, biohazard waste container

**Task:** Obtain a rectal sample using cellulose tape for purpose of testing for pinworm eggs

**Conditions:** glass slide, clear cellulose tape, wooden tongue depressor, toluene, microscope, gauze or cotton balls

**Note:** Do not use magic transparent tape; use regular clear cellulose tape.

Often parents insist that the office perform this procedure. If possible, have parent bring in a diaper; if not, the parent has to be taught how to perform the procedure and be given written instructions. If doing collection in the office, parents really need to help hold the child. Teenagers often prefer to complete the sampling themselves.

**Procedure 46-7: Mono-Test for Infectious Mononucleosis**

**Icons:** wash hands, gloves, face protection, biohazard waste container

**Task:** To perform and interpret a slide test for infectious mononucleosis

**Conditions:** Mono-test kit, blood specimen (serum or plasma), biohazard waste container, gloves, face protection

## PART 3 CLINICAL APPLICATIONS

Instructors: Have students discuss situations in small groups and come to a consensus. Discuss each group answer and have class decide best solution.

1. Assess the situations, decide the actions you might take, and be prepared to discuss them with other students in lab. Write comments for discussion.

   SITUATION 1

   Sally Dunn sees the physician for a severe sore throat. The physician orders a "stat" throat culture. You take Sally into the laboratory area and explain the procedure. Sally promptly tells you that she is already nauseated and knows that she will "throw up" if you attempt to obtain the culture. She then begins to cry.

   SITUATION 2

   Joe Garza is seeing the doctor for an infertility problem. The doctor asks him for a semen sample. You explain the procedure and give Joe the necessary supplies. Joe stays in the room for some time, then opens the door and tells you he is so nervous that he just can't fulfill the doctor's request. He asks you if you can give him any "help." What might you suggest to Joe?

SITUATION 3

The office manager sends out a directive to all employees stating that the price of disposable gloves has increased, and gloves will no longer be worn when doing laboratory procedures. You are instructed to be conscious of your technique, avoid spills, and wash your hands with a 10% solution of Clorox after every lab procedure.

2. Discuss and list all the laws relating to the clinical laboratory in your state. Discuss the application to microbiology and the collection, processing, and destruction of specimens and other medical waste.

   Answers vary depending upon state. All states must follow OSHA and CLIA regulations.

# 47

# Applying Nutrition and Exercise Guidelines

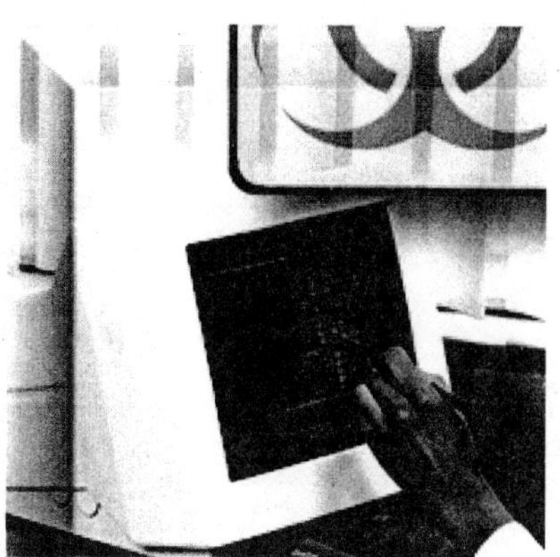

Medical assistants are often asked to discuss nutrition and exercise with patients. The physician has pamphlets and may even train the medical assistant to work with patients needing nutritional counseling. Students need to come to the physician's office prepared with the basics nutrients, the Food Guide Pyramid, vitamins, minerals, and nutrition guidelines. With these basics, students may become involved in planning therapeutic nutrition, understanding federal laws, and assisting the physician in nutritional level assessment. All of this content is presented in the textbook and reviewed in the Mastery Manual.

## USING THE LEARNING SYSTEM

### 1. MEDICAL ASSISTING CONTENT AND COMPETENCIES

CONTENT

- Common pathology/diseases
- Developmental stages of life cycle
- Hereditary, cultural, and environmental influences on behavior
- Basic psychology principles
- Patient care

COMPETENCIES

- Obtain and record patient history
- Prepare and maintain examination areas
- Instruct individuals according to their needs
- Recognize and respond to verbal and nonverbal communications
- Identify community resources

## 2. MEDICAL ASSISTING ENTRY-LEVEL CURRICULUM INTERFACE

| TEXTBOOK OBJECTIVES | LEARNING SYSTEM LOCATION | MA CURRICULUM |
|---|---|---|
| **Cognitive** | | **Content** |
| 1. Describe normal nutrition | • Text p. 971<br>• Manual Part 1-A | • Anatomy and physiology<br>• Patient care |
| 2. List the six areas of the Food Guide Pyramid | • Text p. 973, Figure 47-1<br>• Manual Part 1-A | • Same as # 1 |
| 3. Discuss the meaning of the recommended dietary allowance | • Text p. 971<br>• Manual Part 3 | • Same as # 1 |
| 4. Calculate the caloric value of nutrients | • Text pp. 974–975<br>• Manual Part 1-C | • Same as # 1 |
| 5. Differentiate vitamins and minerals | • Text p. 977<br>• Manual Part 1-C | • Same as # 1 |
| 6. Describe the role of carbohydrates in the diet | • Text p. 974<br>• Manual Part 1-C | • Same as # 1 |
| 7. Explain the need for minerals in the diet | • Text p. 977<br>• Manual Part 1-C | • Same as # 1 |
| 8. Outline the phases in prescribing a diet | • Text p. 984<br>• Manual Part 3 | • Common pathology/diseases<br>• Developmental stages of life cycle<br>• Hereditary, cultural, and environmental influences on behavior<br>• Basic psychology principles |
| 9. Recognize possible eating disorders | • Text p. 933<br>• Manual Part 1-E | • Same as # 9 |
| 10. Understand the role that exercise plays in good health | • Text p. 994<br>• Manual Part 3 | • Developmental stages of life cycle<br>• Hereditary, cultural, and environmental influences on behavior<br>• Basic psychology principles |
| **Performance** | | **Competencies** |
| 1. Read and interpret food labels | • Text pp. 986–987<br>• Manual Part 1-F<br>• Procedure 47-1 | • Instruct individuals according to their needs<br>• Recognize and respond to verbal and nonverbal communications<br>• Identify community resources |

| TEXTBOOK OBJECTIVES | LEARNING SYSTEM LOCATION | MA CURRICULUM |
|---|---|---|
| **Performance** | | **Competencies** |
| 2. Measure body fat using the caliper method | • Manual Part 2<br>• Procedure 47-2 | • Prepare and maintain examination areas<br>• Obtain and record patient history<br>• Instruct individuals according to their needs |

## 3. RESOURCES

www.aadenet.org **American Association of Diabetes Educators 1-800-832-6874**

www.diabetes.org **1-800-342-2383 American Diabetes Association**

www.eatright.org **1-800-366-1655 American Dietetic Association**

www.yahoo.com/ **search by typing in eating disorder treatment centers**

www.eatingdisorder.com

Nutrition teaching materials available through Health Edco. Request the wellness catalog at 1-800-299-3366

## 4. LESSON PLAN Nutrition TIME 3 hours lecture, 12 hours lab

**Opening:** Place foods from the food groups on the desk. Ask who knows what the display represents.

**Pretest:** Put up Food Guide Pyramid text p. 973—Enlarge and make into a transparency. Can anyone explain its use?

**Objectives:** Teach to the objectives. Mastery Manual directs questions to objectives.

**Content:**

1. **Nutrition and Dietetics**—Nutrition versus Nutrients and Food
   Review all words in vocabulary
   Explain energy and a calorie

2. **Food Guide Pyramid**
   Explain six food groups, list foods in each group in pyramid

3. **Nutrients**
   Carbohydrates, Fats, Proteins, Water, Minerals, Vitamins

4. **Therapeutic Nutrition**
   Prescribing a diet

5. **Laws Regulating Food Labels**
   Reading Food Labels, Procedure 47-1
   Calculating Body Fat, Procedure 47-2

**Lab:** Students may complete the Mastery Manual and procedures in the lab time. Students volunteer 8–12 hours in a convalescent facility helping to prepare and set up trays. Observe and make notes of the diets given the elderly, and see if diets meet the Food Guide Pyramid guidelines. This volunteer time is considered a lab assignment. Students should complete the activities in Part 2. Discussion items in Part 3 could be accomplished in lab time. Look in the main menu of the CD-ROM ⊕ for items related to diabetic teaching or teaching of a low-cholesterol diet to Mr. Shapiro.

**Assignment:** Have students complete all activities in Mastery Manual, and arrange for their field experience in a convalescent facility kitchen.

**Posttest:** Construct from Examaster and writing objective questions. Restate the objectives as questions. Have students demonstrate some teaching skills for meeting Food Guide Pyramid guidelines.

## 5. MASTERY MANUAL ANSWERS

### PART 1 CONTENT MASTERY

### A. Learning Level: Knowledge

1. Match the definition with the term. Place the letter of the definition next to the correct term.
   1. f; 2. e; 3. g; 4. a; 5. c; 6. b; 7. d; 8. i; 9. j; 10. h

2. Complete the crossword puzzle below.

| ACROSS answers | | DOWN answers | |
|---|---|---|---|
| 1. | diabetes | 1. | dietitian |
| 2. | diuretic | 2. | digestion |
| 3. | tetany | 4. | peas |
| 6. | endogenous | 5. | cirrhosis |
| 7. | gliadin | 9. | anorexia |
| 8. | goiter | 10. | cellulose |
| 9. | amino | 11. | calorie |
| 11. | carotene | 13. | cholesterol |
| 12. | milk | 15. | biotin |
| 14. | LDL | 17. | exogenous |
| 15. | bulimia | 19. | obesity |
| 16. | choline | 21. | diet |
| 18. | atherosclerosis | 22. | fat |
| 20. | food | | |
| 23. | cretinism | | |
| 24. | sugar | | |
| 25. | PKU | | |
| 26. | glycogen | | |

3. Draw a picture of the Food Guide Pyramid without looking at your textbook.
   Food Guide Pyramid, text p. 973—Enlarge and make into a transparency

### B. Learning Level: Comprehension

1. Indicate the type of food by placing the correct abbreviation in the space provided.
   CHO = carbohydrate, F = fat, P = protein

| | | |
|---|---|---|
| A. | **CHO** | Type of food found in most vegetables. |
| B. | **F** | Furnishes a concentrated form of energy. |
| C. | **P** | Composed of chemical compounds called amino acids. |
| D. | **P** | Only nutrient that makes new cells and rebuilds tissue. |
| E. | **F** | Gives a feeling of satiety because it stays in the stomach longer. |
| F. | **CHO** | Common sources are bread, cereal, and pasta. |
| G. | **F** | Each gram equals 9 calories. |
| H. | **P** | Form may be complete, partially complete, or incomplete. |

2. According to the food groups, what is considered one serving for:

   (1) cooked cereal or pasta **1/2 cup**
   (2) bread **1 slice**
   (3) fruit **1 med. raw or 1/2 cup cooked**
   (4) cantaloupe **1/2 med**
   (5) dry beans **1/2 cup cooked**
   (6) chicken **3 1/2 oz boned**
   (7) egg **1 egg**
   (8) peanut butter **2 Tbsp**
   (9) yogurt **1 cup**
   (10) nuts **1/4 cup**

## C. Learning Level: Application

1. Fill in the chart below.

| Nutrient | Composition or Names | Function | Caloric Value | Examples |
|---|---|---|---|---|
| Protein | C, H, O, and nitrogen | Build and repair tissue, aid in defense against disease, regulate secretions and fluids, energy | 1 gram = 4 Kcal | Complete: meat, fish, dairy<br>Partial: grains<br>Incomplete: corn, gelatin |
| Carbohydrate | Carbon, hydrogen, oxygen | Supply body energy needs | 1 gram = 4 Kcal | Cereal grains, vegetables, sweets |
| Fat | Carbon, hydrogen, oxygen, cholesterol, triglyceride | Source of energy; carry vitamins A & D; supply fatty acids; slow stomach emptying time | 1 gram = 9 Kcal | Animal fats and dairy, vegetable oils |

2. Calculate the number of days for a 150 lb woman to lose 10 pounds. She normally eats 2,200 calories a day and will decrease her calories to 1,500 calories per day.

   Number of days to lose 10 pounds. Answer: It takes 3,400 calories to equal 1 pound, reducing calories by 700 calories per day brings almost five days to lose 1 pound.

   **Fifty days to lose ten pounds**

## D. Learning Level: Analysis

1. When you read a food label, what information will you expect to see in order to meet the USDA legal requirements?

   a. individual serving size
   b. # servings per container
   c. total calories
   d. calories from fat
   e. % of daily nutrient value in serving

2. Name the methods of measuring body fat.
   a. water-body density
   b. electroimpedance
   c. calipers for skin-fold thickness
   d. preprogrammed scale

3. What is the normal range of body fat suggested for men? **15–19 %**
   and women? **22–25 %**

## E. Learning Level: Synthesis

Students will follow Procedure 47-1 and complete the activity. Review page to assure completeness.

Collect five food labels from different types of products. Cereals, meats, cheese, cold drinks, etc. Do labels examined meet legal requirements stated in C-1 above? Place the food name and label information below. Use Procedure 47-1 at the end of the Mastery Manual chapter to assist you in reading the labels.
Review labels and answers with students.

## F. Learning level: Evaluation

Look up the definitions of bulimia and anorexia. Answer the following questions.

What are the similarities in the disorders? **Compulsive behavior, poor self-image, abnormal eating patterns**

How do they differ? **In anorexia, the person does not eat sufficiently and is dangerously thin. In bulimia the person may eat and binge and is usually a little heavy, or the person may just compulsively eat.**

Are these disorders symptoms of addictive behaviors? **According to the experts—yes!**

Go to these sites on the Internet, read about these disorders, and print up information or go to a local treatment center to obtain literature and bring it to class.

www.yahoo.com/ **search by typing in "eating disorder treatment centers"**

www.eatingdisorder.com

## PART 2 COMPETENCY CHALLENGE

There are two procedures in this chapter. Procedure 47-1 was used in Part 1-F. It may be used again to teach about food labels. If the equipment is available for measuring body fat, demonstrate and have students practice.

**Procedure 47-1 : Patient Education: Reading Food Labels**

**Conditions:** Four candy bars, one of each: Snickers, Twix, Healthy Choice, Fat Free Fruit Bar; pencil and paper

**Procedure 47-2** : Determining Fat Fold Measurement

**Task:** To determine and record body fat measurement.

**Conditions:** Fat-fold body calipers, pencil and paper

1. Stop at a fast food restaurant and ask for a caloric and nutritional evaluation of two items. Analyze the content and decide where excesses exist.

2. Students will fill in chart for three days' eating. Collect them and give prizes to the best and worst eating habits.

**Extra activity:** Have students bring food labels from home. Do they indicate a certain style of eating? Discuss which foods are bad for common conditions such as heart disease, diabetes, kidney disease, and celiac disease.

## PART 3 CLINICAL APPLICATIONS

Students are to write some brief responses in preparation for class discussion of the following situations.

1. Mrs. Harris is receiving steroids and her diet is restricted in sodium and carbohydrates as a result of fluid retention. She has a continuous desire for sweets and is emotionally upset and tearful. What might you suggest to help her curb her craving for sweets or how might she satisfy her craving?
2. It is important to individualize the diet of the cancer patient to guard against weight loss because it can lead to poor response to therapy. What are some innovative ways and suggestions you could make that would help this person maintain adequate caloric intake?
3. Sally is a junk food lover. She does not like vegetables and is a very poor cook. She knows she needs nutritional help with her diet, but she also admits that it has to be simple, quick, and easy, or she will never stay with the plan. How could you help her?

# 48

# Applying the Principles of Pharmacology

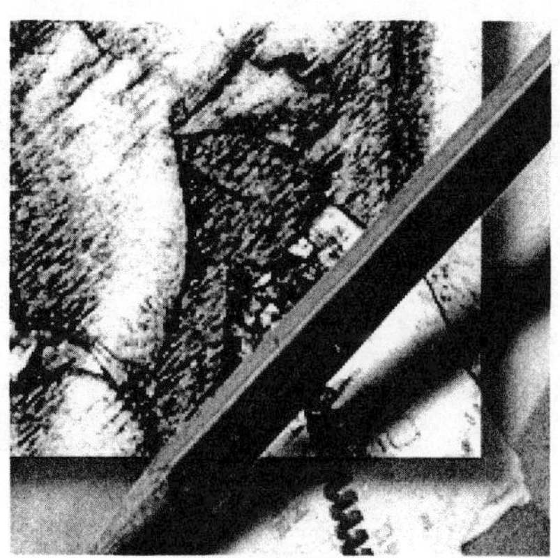

A foundation for assisting in administering medications is essential to the medical assistant. The medical assistant needs to understand the complexity and legal and ethical responsibilities of assisting the physician and patient. Students will learn drug sources, FDA regulations, drug abuse rules and symptoms, drug interactions, routes, distribution, factors influencing the effect of drugs, and classes of drug action. All of this information provides the basic principles to safe, accurate, and error-free administration of medications.

## USING THE LEARNING SYSTEM

### 1. MEDICAL ASSISTING CONTENT AND COMPETENCIES

CONTENT

- Pharmacology content
- All anatomy and physiology, common pathology, diagnostics, and treatment
- All basic medical terminology and applications
- All medical law and ethics guidelines, requirements, related issues
- Hereditary, cultural, and environmental influences on behavior
- Mental health and applied psychology
- Patient care principles
- Personal medical assistant attributes
- Risk management
- Asepsis and infection control
- Adaptations to individual needs
- Recognition of and response to verbal and nonverbal communications

COMPETENCIES

- Apply pharmacology principles to prepare and administer oral and parenteral medications
- Maintain medication and immunization records
- Respond to and initiate written communication
- Instruct individuals according to their needs
- Perform risk management procedures
- Apply principles of aseptic technique and infection control

 

## 2. MEDICAL ASSISTING ENTRY-LEVEL CURRICULUM INTERFACE

| TEXTBOOK OBJECTIVES | LEARNING SYSTEM LOCATION | MA CURRICULUM |
|---|---|---|
| Cognitive | | Content |
| 1. Spell and define words listed in the Vocabulary | • Text p. 997<br>• Manual Part 1-A | • All basic medical terminology and applications |
| 2. Differentiate between a drug's generic and trade name | • Text p. 998<br>• Manual Part 1-D-2 | • Pharmacology content<br>• All anatomy and physiology<br>• Common pathology |
| 3. Cite the dangers of using over-the-counter drugs | • Text p. 998<br>• Manual Part 1-A | • Diagnostics and treatment |
| 4. List information needed in each part of the prescription | • Text p. 1000<br>• Manual Part 1-C | • Recognition of and response to verbal and nonverbal communications<br>• Personal medical assistant attributes<br>• Asepsis and infection control |
| 5. Cite the DEA regulations for the storage of controlled and regulated substances | • Text p. 1002<br>• Manual Part 1-E | • All medical law and ethics guidelines, requirements, related issues<br>• Risk management |
| 6. List DEA regulations for prescription drugs under each of the schedules of the Controlled Substances Act | • Text p. 1002<br>• Manual Part 1-B | • All medical law and ethics guidelines, requirements, related issues<br>• Risk management |
| 7. Define the major types of drug dependency | • Text p. 1003<br>• Manual Part 1-F | • Hereditary, cultural and environmental influences on behavior<br>• Mental health and applied psychology<br>• Patient care principles<br>• Adaptations to individual needs |
| 8. Cite the clinical uses of drugs | • Text p. 1004<br>• Manual Part 1-C | • Diagnostics and treatment<br>• Patient care principles<br>• Adaptations to individual needs |
| 9. Recall the five steps that describe the fate of a drug in the body | • Text p. 1006<br>• Manual Part 1-B | • Diagnostics and treatment<br>• Adaptations to individual needs |
| 10. Cite factors that influence the effect of a drug in the body | • Text pp. 1007–1008<br>• Manual Part 1-F-2 | • Diagnostics and treatment modalities |
| 11. Describe the use of the PDR | • Text p. 1011<br>• Manual Part 1-B | • Diagnostics and treatment modalities |

| TEXTBOOK OBJECTIVES | LEARNING SYSTEM LOCATION | MA CURRICULUM |
|---|---|---|
| **Performance** | | **Competencies** |
| 1. Calculate the correct dosage for administration | • Procedure 48-1<br>• CD-ROM ⊕ | • Apply pharmacology principles to prepare and administer oral and parenteral medications<br>• Perform risk management<br>• Apply principles of aseptic technique and infection control<br>• Respond to and initiate written communication<br>• Maintain medication and immunization records<br>• Instruct individuals according to their needs |
| 2. Calculate the correct dosage for administration using two systems of measurement | • Procedure 48-2 | • Same as # 1 |
| 3. Calculate the correct pediatric dosage when only an adult dose is available | • Procedure 48-3 | • Same as # 1 |
| 4. Calculate the correct pediatric dose using body weight | • Procedure 48-4 | • Same as # 1 |

## 3. RESOURCES

http://www.mayohealth.org/usp/di/usp_aa.htm **Mayo clinic medicine site**

http://www.medicinenet.com/hp.asp?li=MNI **Good resource to Rx and OTC drugs**

http://pharminfo.com/drugdb/db_mnu.html **This is a limited drug database; drugs by generic and trade names**

**4. LESSON PLAN Principles of Pharmacology** **TIME 3 hours lecture, 12 hours lab**

**Opening:** Put some OTC and prescription drugs on your desk. Discuss.

**Pretest:** Ask students to write their opinion on the most important consideration in giving a medication. It is presumed the student has read the chapter. Have students hand this in, so you will better understand their preparation and perspective. Spend 5 minutes discussing possible answers.

**Objectives:** Put up objectives and discuss. These are the lesson. The outline below covers essential concepts that you will expand upon.

**Content:**

1. Drug Sources—Plants, metals, chemistry, soil, rocks
2. Drug Names—Trade, generic
3. Food and Drug Administration Role:: testing before release
   Drug Quality Standards
   Dispensing Regulations (Rx and OTC)
   Prescription Drugs—4 drug parts; also DEA number and MD name and signature
   Guidelines to Pads
4. Drug Use and Abuse
   Regulations—Controlled Substances Act Schedules
   Safety issues and security regulations
   Storage, Rx pads and Form 222; destruction of; dispensing
   Stages of drug abuse: review from 8th Edition Textbook, p. 1003
   Equate to coffee or smoking
5. Use of Drugs
6. Determining the Destiny (fate) of a Drug
7. Drug Routes
8. Drug Distribution
   a. Action—Plasma proteins carry to cells-receptors Blood-brain barrier
      Circulation Placental barrier
   b. Biotransformation
   c. Excretion
9. Factors Influencing Drug Effects
10. Drug Classifications—Use 8th Edition Textbook, pp. 1008–1010 and review; break words into component parts to assist in remembering actions
11. Drug Resources, Learning About and Studying Drugs
12. Medical Assistant's Role in Patient Education
13. Legal and Ethical Issues

**Lab:** Use lab time to explain math concepts for administration of drugs and allow students time to perfect math solving skills. If activities cannot be completed without looking up answers, students should not move on to the next chapter.

**Learning Strategies:**

1. Make flash cards for Tables 48-4 through 48-7 and have students quiz each other on equivalents.
2. Explain the math equivalent Table 48-3 using a circle and cut up the percentages as wedges of a "pie."
3. Use the video "The Metric System" by MEDCOM/TRAINEX 1-800-877-1443. This is an old but accurate film. Use nursing dosage and solutions books to supplement textbook.
4. Call family practitioners and specialists and obtain a list of the most common samples and dosages. Substitute those for dosages in procedures.
5. Discuss the legal and ethical implications of an HMO ordering patients to be given

larger dose pills and instructing the patient to cut them in half, e.g., patient dose is 20 mg Zocor once a day. Pharmacy gives patient 40 mg tabs and a pill cutter. This is done because the 40 mg pill is cheaper than giving two 20 mg pills.

**Assignment:** Students must study and memorize all the principles contained in the objectives. Have them make flash cards of transparencies.

**Posttest:** Suggest that students take test in testing center when ready. Give a little extra time. Choose testbank questions specific to objectives. Put in subjective questions from transparencies, i.e., name the schedules for drugs and list the description for each schedule. What information is necessary for the medical assistant to have before giving any ordered medication? Name all the routes of administration of drugs.

## 5. MASTERY MANUAL ANSWERS

### PART 1 CONTENT MASTERY

### A. Learning Level: Knowledge

1. Write the term next to the definition listed.
   a. **Colloid**—Pertaining to a glue-like substance found within the follicles of the thyroid gland.
   b. **Antidote**—An agent that neutralizes a poison or its effects.
   c. **Enteric-coated**—A drug formulation in which tablets are coated with a special compound that does not dissolve until the tablet is exposed to the fluids of the small intestine.
   d. **Synergism**—Joint action of agents that results in a combined effect that is greater than the effects of the individual components.
   e. **Over-the-counter drugs**—Medications sold without a prescription.
   f. **Psychosomatic**—Disorders that have a physiological component but are thought to originate in the mind of the patient.
   g. **Orphan drugs**—Drugs that once were used in medical treatments, but due to misuse or discovery of side effects, have been removed from USP.
   h. **Alkalosis**—A disorder characterized by excess loss in body fluids.
   i. **Controlled substance**—Drugs that are regulated by the federal government.
   j. **Generic**—Drugs that are not protected by a trademark.
   k. **Lumen**—The space within a vessel or tube.
   l. **Parenteral**—Denoting any medication route other than the gastrointestinal.

2. TRUE or FALSE: Mark the following statements *true* or *false* by circling T or F.
   T a. Each drug manufacturer gives a drug a different trade name.
   T b. Synthetic drugs may have fewer side effects than natural drugs because it is easier to control the final product.
   F c. The medical assistant needs to know the exact chemical names and formulas when administering medications.
   F d. Once a drug is approved by the FDA, it remains on the market as long as patients will buy it.
   T e. Two or more drugs working together for a more advantageous effect are described as having a synergistic effect.
   F f. Most drugs are administered for their local action.
   T g. Tetracyclines are destroyed by milk products and antacids.
   T h. The physician may prescribe medications that can be purchased over-the-counter.
   F i. The medical assistant may administer intravenous medications if directed to do so by the physician.
   F j. Most pain medications are given intradermally.

## B. Learning Level: Comprehension

1. MATCHING: Match the words or expressions in the left column with the definitions in the right column by writing the letters in the blanks. Below the schedule, write two trade names of drugs in the schedule.

   1. E; 2. B; 3. D; 4. A; 5. C

2. Match the drug reference in the first column with the description in the second column. You may need to use the library or the Internet to find the answers.

   1. E; 2. C; 3. D; 4. B; 5. A

## C. Learning Level: Application

1. Describe the information needed for each part of a subscription.

   a. Superscription **Patient name, address, date, and Rx symbol**
   b. Inscription **Names and quantities of drug**
   c. Subscription **Directions for compounding**
   d. Signature **Patient directions—how, when, and what quantities**

2. What is the other information necessary for a prescription to be valid?

   **Also need DEA number, name and address, and physician signature.**

3. Choose the stages of drug dependency in the following story.

   a. When Pat was 15 he started drinking coffee. By the time he was 16, he wanted it every morning. **habituation**
   b. Then he began experimenting with drugs to keep him awake so he could study and felt like he couldn't stay awake past 10 if he did not have his drugs.
   **psychological dependency**
   c. When he woke in the morning, he had to take the drug to get going or he would shake and not function. **physical dependency**
   d. Finally, he took the drug all the time and even though he tried, he couldn't give it up. **drug dependency or addiction**

## D. Learning Level: Analysis

1. Compare over-the-counter and prescription drugs according to categories listed.

| Category | Over-the-Counter | Prescription |
|---|---|---|
| Dosages | Self-determined<br>Uncontrolled | Given by MD<br>Controlled |
| Effect | May or may not be | As prescribed |
| Ingredients | Combinations and mixtures | Usually one or two ingredients always in same amount |
| Supervision | None | By refill # and physician |

2. Differentiate between a trade name drug and generic drug by identifying the type of name listed. If you do not know the drug use a PDR, check it out at a drugstore, or check the Internet sites in Appendix of the manual.

| **Drug** | **Type** |
|---|---|
| a. Advil | **trade** |
| b. Diphenhydramine hydrochloride | **generic** |
| c. Benedryl | **trade** |
| d. Naprosyn | **trade** |
| e. Naproxen sodium | **generic** |
| f. Pseudoephedrine | **generic** |
| g. Digoxin | **generic** |
| h. Nitroglycerin | **generic** |

## E. Learning Level: Synthesis

1. What class of drug would probably be prescribed for patients with the following situations or needs?

| | |
|---|---|
| a. Raised blood pressure | **adrenergic or vasoconstrictor** |
| b. Destroy bacterial infection | **antibiotic** |
| c. Relieve congestion of a cold | **decongestant** |
| d. Stop ovulation | **contraceptive, e.g., birth control pills** |
| e. An asthmatic wheezing | **bronchodilator** |
| f. Constipation | **laxative, cathartic** |
| g. Insomnia—to produce sleep | **hypnotic** |
| h. Headache | **analgesic** |
| i. Increase urine output | **diuretic** |

2. Mary, your friend from another office, calls and tells you a DEA inspector was there checking drug compliance. You tell your office manager, who in turn tells you to check all the compliance items. What are the DEA regulations for drugs in the office, and what must you do?

   Locked cupboard for controlled substances, prescription forms put away, DEA forms put away with controlled substances, limit access to locked cupboard, expired medications need to be flushed. Comply with controlled substances recordkeeping requirements.

## F. Learning Level: Evaluation

1. What do you think is the best way to handle a patient who is loud, boisterous, and smells of alcohol?

   Take patient immediately back to examining room and do not leave alone.

2. Mrs. Nyguen and Mr. Jones each have a kidney infection The physician ordered Septra for both patients, but Mr. Jones is taking twice as much as Mrs. Soto. Why might that be?

   Patient body weight, age, sex, tolerance, degree of infection.

3. Mrs. Nyguen is 6 months pregnant. Obtain drug literature on Septra and Bactrim from your pharmacist or instructor. Are these drugs safe to use for this patient? Where did you find the information?

   Decide the category from the PDR. From the Mayo Clinic Medicine Internet site it appears to be category C.

## PART 2 COMPETENCY CHALLENGE

1. There are four procedures in this chapter. All contain specific activities for you to accomplish. After you have received instruction and demonstration in solving dosage problems, proceed to these procedures and complete them all:
   - Calculate the correct dosage for administration.
   - Calculate the correct dosage for administration using two systems of measurement.
   - Calculate the correct pediatric dosage when only an adult dose is available.
   - Calculate the correct pediatric dose using body weight.
2. Find the trade name drugs listed in the preceding Part 1–D-2 activity. Look three drugs up in the PDR or on the Internet. Complete the information requested for those three drugs. Students have a chart in the Mastery Manual. The information in the left column is needed for each drug every time a person administers a drug.

   Note: When you simulate administration of drugs, students should have drug information in brief form with them.

   You will want to have students turn in the filled-in drug charts with information from PDR to you. Review, return, and discuss. It is important to emphasize patient education for side effects and medical assistant need for knowledge of expected effects. For instance:Benadryl will make most patients sleepy, should not be taken too frequently and patient should not drive. If medication makes patient jumpy, let physician office know. If allergic response does not decrease, let office know.

## PART 3 CLINICAL APPLICATIONS

1. Name six legal and ethical medical assistant considerations in the administration of medications. Students may list any of the following:

   Be informed about the drugs you give.

   Assure correctness of giving medication: the written orders, patient name, drug dosage, route.

   Be exact in following the procedures—no shortcuts.

   Ask patient about allergies.

   Administer correctly.

   Watch patient for adverse effects.

   Provide comfort and encouragment to patients.

   To educate patients for compliance.

   To answer patient questions.
2. Students are to talk about these considerations.
   a. Do you want to give medications? Why or why not?
   b. Have you ever had a painful shot? How can you prevent doing the same to others?
3. Discuss the situation. The police come in to the physician's office. They have with them, and show to the physician, two prescription pads taken from a suspect. All personnel are asked at lunch to review the guidelines and complete a self-evaluation of the office practice to try to determine where the break in controls took effect and how to prevent future breaks. What are the controls they would examine?
4. Have you seen breaks in these controls either as a patient or in externship experience? How can breaks be prevented? List specific steps.

   Collect Rx pads at end of day and place back on physician desk; account for all Rx pads; never put Rx pad in examining room.
5. Discuss the dangers of using OTC drugs; especially when a patient has a chronic illness and is taking other drugs, or when a friend tells the patient what drug to take. Who is the best and most reasonable source for advice on OTC medications?

   The pharmacist

# 49

# Administering Medications

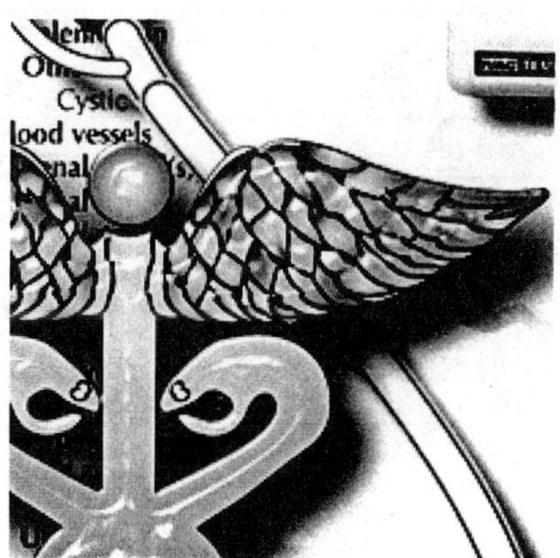

This chapter has many hints throughout for the instructor to help students perfect techniques. After students have studied and completed the Mastery Manual and the CD-ROM activities, it will be time to start demonstrating and practicing techniques. The AAMA curriculum is very important to review as part of the process. Students are expected to know most of the MA required content before developing competencies in the administration of medications. These procedures and those for the medical assistant renewing prescriptions in your particular state must be emphasized.

## USING THE LEARNING SYSTEM

### 1. MEDICAL ASSISTING CONTENT AND COMPETENCIES

CONTENT

- All anatomy and physiology
- All medical terminology
- All psychology
- All communication
- Personal medical assistant attributes
- All pharmacology
- All medical law and ethics
- Asepsis and infection control
- Patient care
- Job readiness

COMPETENCIES

- Apply pharmacology principles to prepare and administer oral and parenteral medications
- Maintain medication and immunization records
- Respond to and initiate written communication
- Instruct individuals according to their needs
- Perform risk management procedures
- Apply principles of aseptic technique and infection control

## 2. MEDICAL ASSISTING ENTRY-LEVEL CURRICULUM INTERFACE

| TEXTBOOK OBJECTIVES | LEARNING SYSTEM LOCATION | MA CURRICULUM |
|---|---|---|
| **Cognitive** | | **Content** |
| 1. Spell and define the words listed in the Vocabulary | • Text p. 1027<br>• Manual Part 1-A-1 | • All medical terminology |
| 2. List six factors of patient assessment that may influence whether you should continue with an order to administer a drug | • Text p. 1028<br>• Manual Part 1-B | • All anatomy and physiology<br>• All medical law and ethics<br>• All psychology |
| 3. State two situations in which it may be your responsibility to further assess an ordered drug before administering it | • Text p. 1029<br>• Manual Part 1-B | • All communication<br>• Personal medical assistant attributes<br>• All pharmacology<br>• Patient care<br>• Job readiness |
| 4. State two environmental factors that would contraindicate the administration of a medication | • Text p. 1029<br>• Manual Part 1-B | • All pharmacology<br>• Patient care<br>• Job readiness |
| 5. Recall the "three befores" and the "six rights" | • Text p. 1029<br>• Manual Part 1-C | • All pharmacology |
| 6. List the basic solid and liquid oral dosage forms and give an example of each | • Text p. 1030<br>• Manual Part 1-D | • All pharmacology |
| 7. For each of five mucous membrane sites, cite methods for administering | • Text pp. 1031–1032<br>• Manual Part 1-D | • All pharmacology |
| 8. Differentiate among the nine types of topical medications | • Text pp. 1033–1034<br>• Manual Part 1-D | • All pharmacology |
| 9. For each parenteral method, list the preferred needle gauges and lengths and the usual syringe size | • Text p. 1039<br>• Table 49-2<br>• Manual Part 1-C | • All pharmacology<br>• Patient care<br>• Job readiness |
| 10. State the risks of using reusable injection equipment and three advantages of disposable injection equipment | • Text p. 1043 | • Asepsis and infection control |
| 11. List contraindications for administering a parenteral drug in any particular site | • Text p. 1040<br>• Manual Part 1-C | • All pharmacology<br>• Patient care<br>• Job readiness |

| TEXTBOOK OBJECTIVES | LEARNING SYSTEM LOCATION | MA CURRICULUM |
|---|---|---|
| **Cognitive** | | **Content** |
| 12. Locate the anatomic landmarks for each intramuscular injection site | • Text pp. 1048–1050<br>• Manual Part 1-B | • Anatomy and physiology<br>• All pharmacology |
| 13. List the special considerations of anatomy when administering injectable medications to infants and small children | • Text p. 1060<br>• Manual Part 1-E | • Anatomy and physiology<br>• All pharmacology |
| 14. Recall the Centers for Disease Control universal precautions | Internet site: www.cdc.gov—send students to this site to get information. | • All medical law and ethics<br>• Asepsis and infection control<br>• Patient care |
| **Performance** | | **Competencies** |
| 1. Fill a syringe using sterile (aseptic) technique | • Manual Part 2<br>• Procedure 49-1<br>• CD-ROM ⊕ | • Apply principles of aseptic technique and infection control<br>• Apply pharmacology principles to prepare and administer oral and parenteral medications |
| 2. Demonstrate giving a intradermal injection | • Manual Part 2<br>• Procedure 49-5<br>• CD-ROM ⊕ | • Apply pharmacology principles to prepare and administer oral and parenteral medications<br>• Maintain medication and immunization records<br>• Respond to and initiate written communication<br>• Instruct individuals according to their needs<br>• Perform risk management procedures |
| 3. Demonstrate giving a subcutaneous injection | • Manual Part 2<br>• Procedure 49-4<br>• CD-ROM ⊕ | • Same as # 2 |
| 4. Demonstrate giving an intramuscular injection | • Manual Part 2<br>• Procedure 49-2<br>• CD-ROM ⊕ | • Same as # 2 |
| 5. Demonstrate giving a Z-track intramuscular injection | • Manual Part 2<br>• Procedure 49-3 | • Same as # 2 |

*chart continues on following page*

## MEDICAL ASSISTING ENTRY-LEVEL CURRICULUM INTERFACE *continued*

| TEXTBOOK OBJECTIVES | LEARNING SYSTEM LOCATION | MA CURRICULUM |
|---|---|---|
| **Performance** | | **Competencies** |
| 6. Demonstrate the application of a transdermal patch | • Text p. 1033<br>• Manual Part 2 | • Same as # 2 |
| 7. Instruct a patient in the use of an oral medication | • Text p. 1032<br>• Manual Part 2 | • Same as # 2 |
| 8. Instruct a patient in the use of a rectal medication | • Text p. 1031<br>• Manual Part 2 | • Same as # 2 |
| 9. Instruct a patient in the use of a vaginal medication | • Text p. 1031<br>• Manual Part 2 | • Same as # 2 |
| 10. Instruct a patient in the use of an inhaler | • Text p. 1032<br>• Manual Part 2 | • Same as # 2 |

## 3. RESOURCES

See previous chapter for Internet sites

MEDCOM/TRAINEX videos # M046 and M045 for injections

MEDCOM/TRAINEX 1-800-877-1443
Box 3225 Garden Grove, CA 92641

*Physicians' Desk Reference*

**4. LESSON PLAN Administering Medications TIME 3 hours lecture, 12 hours lab**

**Opening:** Start with a guest who had an accidental needle stick and have the guest relay the agony of waiting and the number of tests completed before a health clearance was given. Have the person give hints to prevent needle sticks and also tell how the accident happened. This really emphasizes safety and CDC standards.

**Pretest:** The chapter has been assigned to read and study. Hand out a short quiz on the "three befores" and "six rights."

**Objectives:** Integrate objectives, MA curriculum, and procedures in Mastery Manual.

**Content:**

1. **DRUG THERAPY ASSESSMENT**
   Patient assessment
   Drug assessment
   Environment assessment

The "Three Befores"—removing, pouring, returning
The "Six Rights"—patient, drug, dose, time, route, documentation

2. **DRUG FORMS AND ADMINISTRATION**
   a. **Solid Oral Dosage Forms**—describe characteristics
      Tablets and caplets
      Capsules
      Powders
      Lozenges (troches)
      Oral administration
   b. **Liquid and Oral Dosage Forms**
      Oral administration
   c. **Mucous Membrane Forms**
      Rectal administration
      Vaginal administration
      Inhalation
      Oral administration
      Nasal administration
   d. **Topical Forms**
      Lotions
      Liniments
      Ointments
      Soaks, compresses, and wet dressings
      Hot soaks and compresses
      Creams
      The transdermal patch
      Ear drops and irrigations
      Eye drops, ointments, and irrigations
   e. **Parenteral Medication Forms**
      Ampule
      Single-dose vial
      Multi-dose vial
      Prefilled syringe
      Cartridge injection system
   f. **Parenteral Medication Equipment**
      Needle gauge
      Needle length
      Syringes
      Biojector

*chart continues on following page*

g. **Parenteral Administration**
Destruction of used syringes and needles
Reusable syringe Procedure 49-1: Filling a Syringe
Intramuscular injections Procedure 49-2: Giving an Intramuscular Injection
Z-track intramuscular injection Procedure 49-3: Giving a Z-track IM Injection
Subcutaneous injections Procedure 49-4: Giving a Subcutaneous Injection
Intradermal injections Procedure 49-5: Giving an Intradermal Injection
Infants and children

**3. LEGAL AND ETHICAL RESPONSIBILITIES**

**4. PATIENT EDUCATION**

**Lab:** On the CD-ROM ⊕ the Case Studies for Mr. Johnson #3 and Robby Soto #5 will allow the student to develop competency in certain types of medication administration. Have the students practice and be evaluated on all injections after you demonstrate them in the lab. Part of evaluation or testing should include students being asked and stating the purpose for critical steps.

**Assignment:** Have students finish Mastery Manual or CD-ROM and come to lab prepared to practice all Competency Objectives. Make flash cards for "six rights" and other materials to be memorized.

**Posttest:** Testing needs to be in two parts 1. from the Examaster testbank and 2. each student achieving perfect competence for each procedure.

## 5. MASTERY MANUAL ANSWERS

## PART 1 CONTENT MASTERY

### A. Learning Level: Knowledge

1. Put the correct word next to the definition.
   a. **ampule**—A small (usually a single-dose) glass container of medication prepared for parenteral administration.
   b. **radical mastectomy**—The complete surgical removal of the breast, the surrounding muscles, and the lymph glands.
   c. **topical**—Applied to a certain area of the skin and affecting only that area.
   d. **vial**—A small bottle, usually glass.
   e. **volatile**—Referring to an explosive substance's capacity to vaporize at a low temperature.
   f. **sustained or time-released**—Medications that are manufactured to release their action over a period of time.
   g. **viscosity**—The quality of being thick, gluey and lacking the capability of easy movement.
   h. **allergy immunotherapy**—Administering repeated injections of diluted extracts of the substance that caused the allergy.
   i. **hermetically sealed**—Sealed so no air is allowed to enter.
   j. **wheal**—A localized area of edema on the body's surface.
   k. **aspirate**—To withdraw fluid by negative pressure; pulling up on the plunger of the syringe after inserting the needle to check for blood.
   l. **induration**—An abnormally hard spot or place.
   m. **sublingual**—Under the tongue.
   n. **vesiculation**—Formation of blister-like elevations on the skin.

2. TRUE or FALSE: Correct answers are indicated.

T a. The medical assistant must have a thorough understanding of the scientific principles of drug administration and individual state laws.

T b. Most drugs administered in the medical office will be by the oral route.

T c. Drug therapy assessment is never the responsibility of just one person.

T d. If there is any doubt about a drug order, the drug should not be administered until the order has been verified by the physician.

F e. When you have a written order for a medication, it is your professional responsibility to give it whether you understand it or not.

F f. The route of administration usually has little effect upon the patient's responses to the drug.

F g. The medical assistant may schedule appointments for routine medications that can be given by the assistant while the physician is out of the office.

T h. Drugs that stain teeth should be administered through a straw.

F i. Liquid medications should not be given to young children because of the possibility of aspiration of the liquids.

T j. Large amounts of a topical drug that is left on the skin for a long period of time can be absorbed slowly and cause systemic poisoning.

## B. Learning Level: Comprehension

1. Assisting with medications requires that you assess patients before giving a medication because facts are sometimes missed or overlooked. What factors should you assess for each of the following?

   **Patients**—1. Conditions contraindicating drug; 2. Drug use interfering with drug; 3. Allergies to similar drug; 4. Patient's physique correct for dosage; 5. Route acceptable after inspection

   **Environment**—Is physician on site? Patient safe and comfortable; sufficient water and equipment available; emergency cart in office; quiet environment to prepare drugs

   **Drug**—safe route for particular patient, dosage available and appropriate, the order is written; look drug up if unknown, verbalize order and dosage to physician for confirmation

2. Complete the chart for parenteral injections.

| Routes | Site and Angle | Gauge and Length | Indications | Contraindications |
|---|---|---|---|---|
| 1. Intra-muscular | Ventrogluteal, dorsogluteal, vastus lateralis, deltoid, 90° angle | 20–23<br>1–3 in | Drugs irritate subq. spaces<br>More rapid absorption<br>Large volume medication | Drug must be absorbed slowly<br>Heparin<br>Anticoagulant<br>Vaccines, insulin |
| 2. Z-track IM | Gluteus medius only, 90° angle, retract skin | Same as IM | Irritating drugs<br>Prevent oozing | All IM drugs may be given Z-track |
| 3. Subcutaneous | Deltoid, inner aspect arm, thigh, abdomen, back | 25–26<br>1/2 to 5/8<br>2cc insulin, tuberculin | Insulin, heparin, vaccines, toxoids | No heavy medication, e.g., PCN or iron, when rapid onset required |
| 4. Intradermal | Forearm, back | 27–28<br>3/8 in<br>tuberculin | Tuberculin tests, skin tests, allergy tests | Most medications are not given ID |

## C. Learning Level: Application

1. State the importance of the "three befores" and the "six rights."

   Must be able to say yes to all "three befores" and "six rights" before giving any medication. The most common reason for medication errors is due to a break in these two procedures.

2. From memory, complete below.

   The 3 befores are: **before removing, pouring, returning**

   The 6 rights are: **right patient, drug, dosage, route, time, documentation**

3. Draw the syringes indicated below. Indicate the correct increments as lines on the syringe and write the capacity (measurement) that the separation between lines indicates.
   a. 2 cc syringe

      **2 scales calibration cc—calibration in 1/10th increments and minims in one minim increments**
   b. tuberculin syringe

      **1 cc syringe calibrated in tenths and 1/100ths**
   c. U 100 insulin syringe

      **standard syringe is a U 100 syringe for U 100 insulin. Syringe must match insulin strength.**

## D. Learning Level: Analysis

1. State all the sites of absorption that could be used to administer the following medication forms

| | |
|---|---|
| a. Lozenges | **oral** |
| b. Suppositories | **vaginal, rectal** |
| c. Inhalers | **nasal, oral, respiratory membranes** |
| d. Tablets or capsules | **gastric or intestinal mucosa** |
| e. Ointments, liniments, creams | **skin, eyes, vagina, rectum, nose** |
| f. Injections | **IM, subq, ID** |
| g. Lotions | **skin surface** |
| h. Drops | **eyes, ears, nose** |

2. On the figures below, draw all the common intramuscular, subcutaneous, and intradermal sites. Label them according to route and name of site. **The sites are on Figure 40-20 in the textbook**

## E. Learning Level: Synthesis

1. List the preferred specific anatomic sites for injections given to children under 2.

| | |
|---|---|
| IM | **vastus lateralis** |
| SC | **arm** |
| ID | **arm or back depending upon reason** |

2. List the other sites and explain why they are avoided in children under 2. The other sites are the gluteus and deltoid muscles.

   **Blood and nerves are too close to the gluteal IM sites**

   **Deltoid and gluteus are not well developed**

   **Sciatic nerve proportionally larger and in the way than on an adult**

3. What would you do if you were told to give an IM injection to a child and you had never done it before? Panic is not an acceptable answer!
   **Tell the physician and ask if I could get someone to supervise me.**

4. How would you proceed when the patient refuses to allow an injection for penicillin in the vastus lateralis, ventrogluteal, or dorsogluteal muscles?

   **Give it to them in the deltoid if 2 cc or less. Also can split into 2 doses or report to physician.**

## F. Learning Level: Evaluation

Students need to discuss, consider, and respond to the following situations:

1. You gave Mr. Moseley his sensitization shot and returned the antigen to the fridge with the other antigens. Ten minutes later you go to get the antigen for Mr. Johnson. You notice that Mr. Moseley's antigen is not where you placed it in the fridge, but another patient's (Mr. Mosby's) is. What, if anything, do you do? Why?
2. Dr. Lopez orders a medication for his patient. When you get the chart to check the order, you notice that the patient claims an allergy to the medicine.

# PART 2 COMPETENCY CHALLENGE

## Suggested Student Activities

1. There are five procedures in this chapter, all related to filling syringes and giving injections. There is no written procedure for oral medications. Write a competency objective and procedure for administration of oral medications. Turn it in to your instructor. After demonstration of the procedures, practice them on a mattress or orange. Your instructor will decide the standards for your evaluation and competency of each procedure.

2. Medications may only be given under the direct order and supervision of the physician. Explain exactly what this means. **It means physician must be on premises and in the office, have written the order, and have certified that the medical assistant is qualified.**

3. What will you do if Nurse Nan rushes out of the physician's office, hands you a vial, and tells you that the doctor wants you to give it to the patient you just helped him examine. **You must still meet the above criteria and make sure the order is written or ask for the written order.**

4. Make four copies of the patient activity teaching plan form at the end of Chapter 29. As directed by your instructor, make teaching plans for instructing a patient in the use of oral, transdermal patches, rectal, vaginal, and inhaler medications.

   **Note:** Divide the class into five groups and assign each group to develop a teaching plan for patients to self administer each medication form. Have a person in each group teach another group member. This helps students evaluate their plans.

5. **Students are to complete practicing procedures and developing competence**

Instructors need to demonstrate and show videotapes before students practice administering medications. Students should read each step and slowly follow through with each step. Some instructors do not allow syringes to be uncapped until students handle syringes comfortably. Students may practice with oranges, dolls or even mattresses before practicing on each other. Take all precautions to avoid needle sticks due to break in technique. Release forms are needed for practice on each other.

Hints for assisting students to practice and achieve competence follow.

Equipment—syringe and needle appropriate for type of injection, povidone-iodine swab, dry swab, gloves, and needle disposal containers

**Procedure 49-1: Filling a Syringe**

Students should observe strict sterile technique. A reviewer suggests we have students prepare and fill the syringe that will be used on them by their partner. This reduces a chance of "covered-up" contamination. Medical assistants often prepare medications for the physician to administer. Stress the "three befores" and all "six rights." Take necessary precautions to avoid needle sticks.

**Procedure 49-2: Giving an Intramuscular Injection**
Students may fear this injection because of the depth of the needle insertion. Repeated practice with the teaching doll will allow them to refine their technique. Stress the importance of locating the exact anatomical site. The syringe and needle are discarded (without recapping) immediately after administration into a puncture-resistant container.

**Procedure 49-3: Giving a Z-track Intramuscular Injection**
This method is used when irritating medications are injected into the gluteus medius. Have students practice the procedure on a teaching doll. They also can practice on each other, using a needleless syringe, to refine the skills of holding the skin in position while injecting.

**Procedure 49-4: Giving a Subcutaneous Injection**
Because the needle is smaller and shorter and is injected into the subcutaneous tissues only, the instructor may prefer to have the students perform this injection first, then move to the intradermal, intramuscular, and Z-track injections. Stress the importance of careful site selection and observe student to be sure that the needle is injected at the correct angle.

**Procedure 49-5: Giving an Intradermal Injection**
Have students practice on a peach using air in the syringe to obtain the induration, until they have perfected the technique. Site selection should be stressed. Remind students that the injections are given *within* the skin.

## PART 3 CLINICAL APPLICATIONS

1. Students may complete a–e below in small groups and then present to class. Give an assignment that can be reported on by the group.

   Students explain the procedures to a classmate. Write the main points that must be covered for patient teaching. Each patient will have the procedure demonstrated by a student and then written directions will be given.

   a. Application of a transdermal medication
   b. Insertion of vaginal suppository
   c. Using a nasal inhaler
   d. Insertion of a rectal suppository in a baby
   e. Preparing and giving an insulin injection

2. What are the legal and ethical implications of this situation?

   The medical assistant student has given five intramuscular injections in the lab to classmates. The instructor has not signed the certificate of competence yet. In the externship, the student is helping the physician with a patient who needs an immunization. The physician tells the medical assistant to give the patient "this." The student asks what it is, verifies the written order, and then gives the immunization. The patient's mother calls the next day and says the area is red, swollen, and hard and the child is in pain at the site. When the child is brought in, the physician realizes the injection was given IM instead of SQ and has caused a severe and painful tissue and systemic reaction.

   Who is responsible?
   Physician: Student only acts as agent
   Student: Was not properly prepared and practiced outside competence

   What must be done?
   Physician instructs parent in care of child. Student will suffer consequences of program regulations. No charge for visit or care.

# 50

# Preparing for Surgery

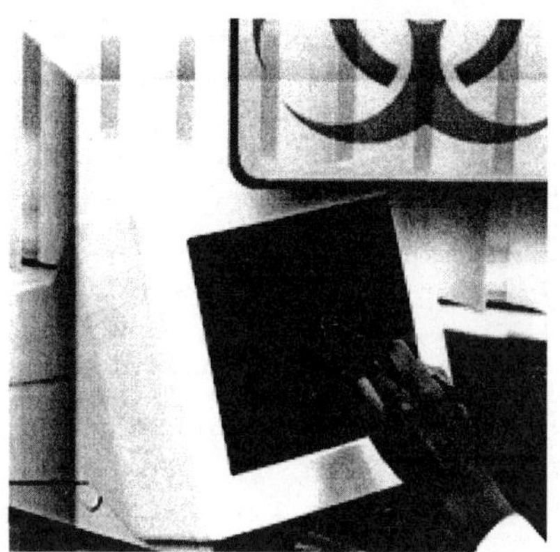

The medical assistant who knows supplies and equipment will be capable of assisting at any minor surgery procedure once aseptic technique and individual physician preferences are understood. This chapter has many instruments for identification and an excellent procedure to guide the student in the identification process.

AAMA Role Delineation is very specific for these skills and does not contain general competencies. Students should continually be evaluated on the general and professional competencies.

## USING THE LEARNING SYSTEM

### 1. MEDICAL ASSISTING CONTENT AND COMPETENCIES

CONTENT

- Applications of medical terminology
- Asepsis and infection control
- Patient care
- Diagnostic testing
- Patient care
- Job readiness

### 2. MEDICAL ASSISTING ENTRY-LEVEL CURRICULUM INTERFACE

| TEXTBOOK OBJECTIVES | LEARNING SYSTEM LOCATION | MA CURRICULUM |
|---|---|---|
| **Cognitive** | | **Content** |
| 1. Define and spell the words in the Vocabulary | • Text p. 1064<br>• Manual Part 1-A | • Applications of medical terminology |
| Extra Objective<br>Identify surgical solutions and medications | • Text p. 1065<br>• Manual Part 1-B | • Asepsis and infection control<br>• Patient care<br>• Diagnostic testing<br>• Patient care<br>• Job readiness |

*chart continues on following page*

## MEDICAL ASSISTING ENTRY-LEVEL CURRICULUM INTERFACE *continued*

| TEXTBOOK OBJECTIVES | LEARNING SYSTEM LOCATION | MA CURRICULUM |
|---|---|---|
| **Cognitive** | | **Content** |
| 2. Identify by name the instruments used in minor surgery procedures | • Text pp. 1067–1079<br>• Manual Part 2 | • Same as # 2 |
| 3. List types of sutures and surgical needles | • Text p. 1080<br>• Manual Part 1-E | • Same as # 2 |

## 3. RESOURCES

www.drkoop.com **Interesting site for procedures and access to many surgical topics**

http://www.yahoo.com/Health/Nursing/Organizations Association of Operating Room Nurses AORN/ **A link to the operating room nurses site with some interesting articles**

**4. LESSON PLAN Preparing for Surgery** **TIME 3 hours lecture, 12 hours lab**

**Opening:** Put out some surgical instruments and a few kitchen ones—such as wiener tongs, a garlic crusher, a small knife, and others; also a needle and thread. Time to have a little fun. See what instruments the students can identify. This serves as an attention-getter and a pretest.

**Pretest:** Use the opening, or ask students to identify different functions of kitchen utensils and identify those as the same as most surgical instruments: cutters and scissors, dissectors, graspers, probes.

**Objectives:** The student will recognize and use the surgical instruments described. Hands-on use and visual imaging are important techniques for this chapter.

**Content:** The lesson plan textbook outline is expanded and may be used with the Transparency Masters to review the essential materials. Students learn and then use the material. They will first classify instruments by grouping them in the four types. When instruments can be identified by class, then proceed to requiring specific identification of the most commonly used office instruments for your locality.

**OUTLINE**

**Preparing for surgery**—knowing the equipment

1. Medical assistant responsibilities are listed in the MA curriculum content above. Notice that this chapter is totally associated with knowledge at a basic level of memorizing instruments.
2. Rooms for Surgical Supplies—changing, separate minor surgery room
3. Surgical Solutions and Medications—sterile water, physiologic saline, Betadine, Duraprep, surgical soap, lidocaine, tincture of benzoin, ethyl chloride, epinephrine, formalin, Vaseline, silver nitrate, iodoform gauze, aromatic ammonia
4. Additional Supplies—electrosurgical unit, fiberoptics, wound drains, surgical sponges, syringes, needles
5. Identifying Surgical Instruments—Use textbook, borrow instruments from hospital, take students to surgical supply rooms, have hospital representative demonstrate instruments.
   a. Classifications of Surgical Instruments: cutting, grasping, retracting, probing, and dilating
   b. Cutting and Dissecting Instruments
   c. Scissors, Scalpels
   d. Grasping and Clamping: Forceps, Retractors
   e. Probes and Dilators
   f. Specialty Instruments

   Gynecology: curette, uterine dressing forceps, dilators, tenaculum forceps
   Ophthalmology and Otolaryngology: nasal speculum, snare, eye spud, ear forceps
   Biopsy
   Genitourinary
   Colon-Rectal
6. Care and Handling of Instruments: examine before use, do not bundle, receiving basin for contaminated instruments in room, immediate cleaning and sterilizing, care with sharps
7. Disposable Surgical Drapes: for surgical sites
8. Sutures
   a. Types of Sutures: absorbable and nonabsorbable—names used
   b. Suture Sizing and Packaging Needles
9. Legal and Ethical Responsibilities

*chart continues on following page*

**Lessson Plan continued**

**Lab:** The Mastery Manual offers activities to meet all the objectives. The case studies are available in Appendix C for students to practice achieving competence when setting out instruments for patient procedures and caring for instruments and sutures. To learn the instruments, intensive study will have to be done in the lab.
⊕ Use the CD-ROM to practice identifying instruments and laying out instruments for specific examinations. Open the main menu and choose clinical skills. If time is available, take students to a hospital supply room and show them instruments. As instructor, photograph common instruments and use photographs in lab for identification and testing.

**Assignment:** Students must memorize the categories and types of instruments. Lots of practice, make flash cards, and learn material in the lab.

**Posttest:** Use the Examaster testbank; for a subjective examination, have students identify pictures of instruments. This is another opportunity to have testing stations and have students move about while testing.

## 5. MASTERY MANUAL ANSWERS

### PART 1 CONTENT MASTERY

### A. Learning Level: Knowledge

Fill in the word that describes the statement.

1. **Biopsy** — A small sample of tissue excised from the body for diagnostic or therapeutic purposes.
2. **Curettage** — The act of scraping a body cavity with a surgical instrument.
3. **Cyst** — A sac of fluid or semisolid material located in or under the skin.
4. **Dilatation** — Opening or widening the circumference of a body orifice with an instrument.
5. **Diluent** — A substance, such as water, that renders a drug or a solution less potent.
6. **Fistula** — An abnormal, tube-like passage within the body tissues.
7. **Lesion** — A wound, sore, ulcer, tumor, or tissue damage that causes a lack of tissue continuity.
8. **Polyps** — Tumors on stems. They are frequently found on mucous membranes.
9. **Abrasion** — Rubbing or scraping of the skin or mucous membrane (e.g., a skinned knee).
10. **Approximation** — The act or process of drawing together skin or wound edges.
11. **Fascia** — A sheet or band of fibrous tissue located deep in the skin that covers muscles and body organs.
12. **Caustic** — A substance that burns or destroys organic tissue by chemical action.
13. **Debridement** — Surgical removal of damaged, diseased, or contaminated tissue until healthy tissue is exposed.
14. **Lumen** — An open space, such as within a blood vessel, the intestine, or an examination instrument.
15. **Suppuration** — Production of purulent material (pus) from a wound.
16. **Patency** — The open condition of a body cavity or canal.
17. **Obturator** — A metal rod with a smooth rounded tip that is placed into hollow instruments to decrease destruction of body tissues during insertion.
18. **Stylus** — A metal probe that is inserted or passed through a catheter, needle, or tube. Used for clearing purposes or to facilitate passage into a body orifice.
19. **Paroxysm** — Sudden turn of symptoms such as a spasm or seizure.
20. **Cannula** — A flexible tube that surrounds a sharp, pointed trocar inserted into the body.

21. **Abscess** A localized collection of pus.
22. **Dissect** To cut or separate tissue with a cutting instrument or scissors.

## B. Learning Level: Comprehension

Match the term with the best definition of the surgical supply described.

1. g; 2. j; 3. i; 4. a; 5. b; 6. h; 7. d; 8. f; 9. c; 10. e

## C. Learning Level: Application

1. Name four other supplies, in addition to those in activity B, that you might need to put on the surgical assisting tray.
   a. electrocautery, fiberoptic lights
   b. headlights, microscope
   c. wound drains, sponges
   d. syringes, needles

2. Complete the following by filling in the blanks. Note: Use textbook to complete work with students by identifying the name, category, and usage of the 15 instruments displayed. The instruments shown are

   1. Plain tissue forceps, 2. Senn retractor, 3. Backhaus towel clamp, 4. Laforce eye foreign body spud, 5. Gauze shears, 6. Krause nasal snare, 7. Lister bandage scissor, 8. Sims uterine curette, 9. Allis tissue forceps, 10. Littauer suture scissors, 11. Plain needle holder, 12. Foerster sponge clamp, 13. Mosquito clamp, 14. Schroeder uterine speculum, 15. Bard-Parker scalpel

## D. Learning Level: Analysis

1. Fill in the missing class of surgical instrument listed below.
   a. Retracting
   b. Cutting
   c. Probing and dilation
   d. Answer: Grasping and clamping

2. Place the number of the classifications above next to the specific instruments listed below.

| Allis tissue forceps 4 | | |
|---|---|---|
| Catheter 3 | Specula 3 | Sounds 3 |
| Elevators 2 | Curettes 2 | Punches, drills, needles 2 |
| Hemostats 4 | Needle holders 4 | Transfer forceps 4 |
| Scissors 2 | Scalpels 2 | Chisels 2 |
| Self-retaining 1 | Weitlander 1 | Crile |
| Trocars 3 | Obdurators 3 | Cystoscope 3 |

## E. Learning Level: Synthesis

Fill in the chart to understand suture types, name, use, care, and removal.

| Type | Name | Use | Care and Removal |
|---|---|---|---|
| Absorbable | 1. Plain catgut | Mucous membrane and subq. tissues | Is not removed, no care |
| | 2. Chromic catgut | Deep tissues that need strength while healing | Up to 80 days to absorb, gives great strength |
| | 3. Vicryl | Deep tissues that need strength while healing | Absorbs in 80–90 days |
| Nonabsorbable | 1. Silk | Strong, easy to tie | Keep covered, remove in 5–8 days |
| | 2. Surgical cotton | Rarely used | Same as above |
| | 3. Polyester fiber | Strong | Large support areas 8–10 days |
| | 4. Stainless steel | Rarely used in office | Easily contaminated Staples most common |
| | 5. Nylon suture | Strong and elastic Allows limited movement | 5–8 days, longer over joints |

## F. Learning Level: Evaluation

Discuss or write how you would evaluate steel instruments to decide if they were of the quality desired and worth the price, i.e., how can one tell a fine steel instrument from a cheap one?

**Check to see if instrument functions perfectly; what is the weight of it? Are there rough areas? Where is it made? German the best, China lighter weight and not as perfect.**

## PART 2 COMPETENCY CHALLENGE

Use Procedure 50-1 Identification of surgical instruments for the CD-ROM or manual activities. Practice identifying surgical instruments until you can identify all the instruments required by your instructor. You will have some form of instruments for this procedure. The CD-ROM may have minor surgical procedures for you to answer questions. Proceed to the main menu and choose clinical skills to find the clinical studies, which have some activities for you.
Instructors: If the CD-ROM and real instruments are not available, make copies of the instruments in the textbook and cut them out. Use them for student practice in identification and for testing.

## PART 3 CLINICAL APPLICATIONS

1. Review care of instruments by setting up an area for receiving, cleaning, and storing instruments in the medical assistant laboratory. What can be used if there are not sufficient storage containers and supplies?
2. Where can the office take shortcuts on caring for instruments? **With asepsis, there is no acceptable area of shortcuts.**
3. **This may bring a lively discussion.** Have you ever seen a procedure where the physician or medical assistant did not wear gloves? Discuss the ethics of this practice and the risk of exposure to patients. What do you think the justification might be for not following standard precautions and aseptic techniques?

# 51

# Surgical Methods

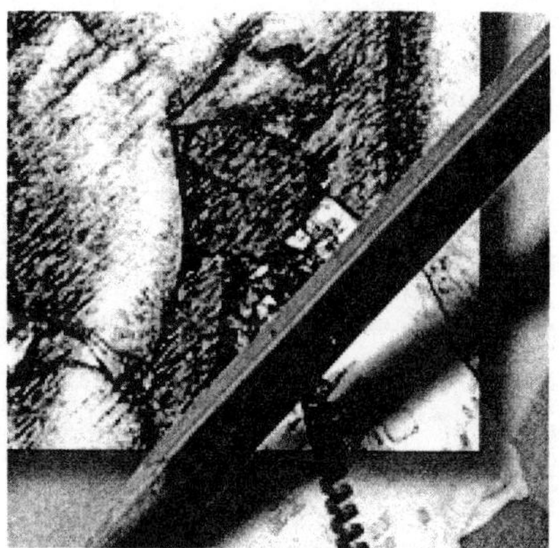

This chapter familiarizes the student with generally acceptable practices in minor surgery. As Medicare and HMOs require more procedures to be performed in the office, medical assistants will become more involved in minor surgery. Once the basics are known, the medical assistant will be able to apply them to a variety of surgical procedures. The procedures for aseptic technique begin with handwashing, gowning, and gloving. The prime emphasis is to learn and practice sterile concepts and to successfully understand the basic process. The next chapter will discuss actual surgical procedures and sterile procedures for assisting.

## USING THE LEARNING SYSTEM

### 1. MEDICAL ASSISTING CONTENT AND COMPETENCIES

CONTENT

- Applications of medical terminology
- Asepsis and infection control
- Patient care
- Risk management
- Legal guidelines and requirements

COMPETENCIES

- Prepare patient for and assist with procedures, treatment, and minor office surgery
- Perform inventory of supplies and equipment
- Perform risk management procedures

## 2. MEDICAL ASSISTING ENTRY-LEVEL CURRICULUM INTERFACE

| TEXTBOOK OBJECTIVES | LEARNING SYSTEM LOCATION | MA CURRICULUM |
|---|---|---|
| **Cognitive** | | **Content** |
| 1. Define and spell the terms in the Vocabulary | • Text p. 1085<br>• Manual Part 1-A | • Applications of medical terminology |
| 2. Define concepts of aseptic technique | • Text pp. 1085–1086<br>• Transparency Master 51-1<br>• Manual Part 1-B | • Asepsis and infection control<br>• Patient care |
| 3. List safety precautions for electrosurgery | • Text p. 1104<br>• Manual Part 1-E | • Risk management<br>• Legal guidelines and requirements |
| 4. List safety precautions for laser surgery | • Text pp. 1105–1106<br>• Manual Part 1-E | • Risk management<br>• Legal guidelines and requirements |
| **Performance** | | **Competencies** |
| 1. Perform surgical hand scrub | • Manual Part 2<br>• Procedure 51-1<br>• Review Transparency Master 51-1 | • Prepare patient for and assist with procedures, treatment, and minor office surgery<br>• Perform inventory of supplies and equipment<br>• Perform risk management procedures |
| 2. Demonstrate the open-glove technique | • Manual Part 2<br>• Procedure 51-2 | • Same as # 1 |
| 3. Demonstrate sterile gowning with closed-glove technique | • Manual Part 2<br>• Procedure 51-4 | • Same as # 1 |

## 3. RESOURCES

For Internet sites, refer to previous chapter resources.

*Fundamentals of Aseptic Technique*, video 21 min
American College of Surgeons

*Instruments and Sterile Technique*, video 26 min
Davis and Geck Surgical Film Library, 1430 Broadway, New York, NY 10018

*Preparing and Monitoring the Sterile Field*, video 22 min
MEDCOM/TRAINEX Box 3225 Garden Grove, CA 92641

*Aseptic Techniques*, W.B. Saunders Medical Assisting video series

## 4. LESSON PLAN Surgical Methods TIME 3 hours lecture, 12 hours lab

**Opening:** A demonstration of the surgical scrub, gowning, and putting on sterile gloves is an interesting way to open this class. Ask students to watch carefully to make sure "white only touches white." After the demonstration, ask the students what was done to keep the gown sterile and any techniques they noticed.

**Pretest:** Ask students to identify the two methods of bacteria removal used in the surgical scrub. Answer*:* mechanical and chemical—explain to students.

**Objectives:** The objectives are more than met in the Mastery Manual. Review them with the students.

**Content:**

1. ASEPTIC TECHNIQUE
   a. Personnel
   b. The Sterile Field and Moisture Considerations
   c. Preparing Sterile Packs
   d. Surgical Asepsis
   e. The Hand Scrub
2. SURGICAL PROCEDURES
   a. Electrosurgery
      Components — Types of Current
      Safety — Patient Care
      Care of the Equipment
   b. Laser Surgery
      Types of Lasers — Components
      Laser Safety and Hazards
      Assisting with Laser Surgery or Microsurgery
   c. Microsurgery: The Microscope
      Components — Care of the Equipment
   d. Endoscopy
      Types of Scopes — Accessory Equipment
      Care of the Equipment
   e. Cystoscopy
      Components — Care of the Equipment
   f. Sigmoidoscopy
      Components — Care of the Equipment
   g. A Minor Surgical Procedure —Excision
3. LEGAL AND ETHICAL RESPONSIBILITIES: PATIENT EDUCATION

**Lab:** Use the CD-ROM ⊕ to identify instruments and interact with surgical situations. Some surgical procedures are available for analysis and practice. Look in the main menu and the Procedures menu. Students need complete demonstrations and video to observe. See the resource list above. Gloves are needed. Demonstrate correct technique and common errors to avoid.

**Assignment:** Students will need to study procedures and begin practicing at home. Hand out examination gloves. Have students fold and wrap gowns to practice sterile gowning at home. This needs to be demonstrated before independent practice.

**Posttest:** Take questions from Examaster testbank. Ask questions about rationale for procedural steps. Students must pass competency objectives in procedures.

## 5. MASTERY MANUAL ANSWERS

### PART 1 CONTENT MASTERY

### A. Learning Level: Knowledge

Write the word for the definition described.

| | |
|---|---|
| 1. **Plume** | Carbon and steam byproducts from electrocautery |
| 2. **Slough** | Shedding of dead tissue |
| 3. **Photocoagulation** | Clotting of blood with light |
| 4. **Pedunculated** | Having a stemlike connecting part |
| 5. **Microsurgery** | Surgery using very small instruments and a form of magnifier |
| 6. **Don** | To put on |
| 7. **Coagulum, or thrombus** | A blood clot |

### B. Learning Level: Comprehension

1. Write the basic analogy of sterile technique.
   Everything that's sterile is white, nonsterile is black, and there are no shades of gray.

2. List five fundamental rules for maintaining sterile technique.
   a. Sterile surfaces must not contact nonsterile surfaces.
   b. Hair must be back and off the shoulders.
   c. Air currents carry bacteria, so talking and motion over field should be kept to a minimum.
   d. Sterile team members face each other.
   e. Never turn your back on sterile field.
   Extra—Nonsterile persons and objects not over sterile field.

### C. Learning Level: Application

Describe eight techniques that must be applied to prepare and maintain sterile fields.

Fanfold sterile towels for easy unfolding at one edge.

Use outer double wrapping as sterile table drape when the package is double wrapped.

Sterile tables are sterile only at table height and not below.

Any item below the waist is considered contaminated.

The first inch around the entire sterile field is considered not sterile and nothing sterile may touch without contamination.

The edges of packs, wraps, and towels are considered not sterile.

Sterile goods may not touch any edges.

When sterility of an item or technique is in question, consider the item or field contaminated.

Do not bring anything unsterile over the field.

Moisture contaminates the field.

A pack without a sterility indicator should not be used.

### D. Learning Level: Analysis

Describe six adaptations made to the medical hand wash to make it a surgical hand wash.

a. Keep hands upright.
b. Use foot or knee lever to turn water on and off.
c. Rinse hand holding upright; clean fingernails and discard file.

d. Lather, wash with surgical soap, and then scrub with brush hands, wrists, and forearms, hold upright.
e. Wash and scrub for 3 minutes, discard brush.
f. Rinse hands, wrists, and forearms holding so water runs off elbows.
g. Sterile towel to dry hands, keep hands and arms upright.

## E. Learning Level: Synthesis

Fill in the following chart to plan assisting techniques when using various equipment.

| Equipment | Types and Components | Safety Concerns and Equipment Care | Patient Care |
|---|---|---|---|
| Electrocautery—high frequency to cut tissue and coagulate | 1. Monopolar tip—use grounding pad<br>2. Bi-polar—electric flows between two tips; no ground needed<br><br>Throw tips away after one use | Know proper grounding, know and do not use any ignitable solutions or alcohol; no moisture near equipment. Read all instructions before using machine; examine all cables before use, electrical examination at least yearly. | Skin always in contact with grounding pad. Place near operative site on fleshy area of skin. Never use oxygen around equipment—especially with face surgery. Anesthesia must be kept away from cautery. Coagulum and skin care taught to patient. |
| Laser light—amplification by simulated emission of radiation | YAG, argon, excimer, and others<br>Components include laser head, excitation source, ancillary components. Control panel, delivery system | Must be trained in use, usually not a medical assistant function. Frequent preventative maintenance; during procedure, have wet sponges nearby, suction plume away, have basin of sterile water. Anticipate physician needs. | Dangers are burns, fire, plume inhalation, and high-wattage burn. Patients need protection from laser, goggles, and reassurance. |
| Microscope—operating microscope | Components include light source, eye pieces, lenses, electric microscope cord, cameras, video lenses, TV, and possibly photo equipment | Inspect cords, clean according to directions, store in padded protective boxes. | Patient needs to maintain stillness, especially in ophthalmic procedures. |
| Endoscope<br>Cystoscope<br>Sigmoidoscope | Fiberoptic light and cable, rigid or flexible, may have cameras, TV etc., may irrigate with water, biopsy tissue, or perform surgery | All equipment expensive and delicate. Fiberoptics must not be dropped, knifed, squashed, or smashed. Lights are hot and must be carefully handled. | Patient must be monitored, observe irrigation returns, take vital signs, allow patient to rest after endoscopic procedures until physician discharges. |

## F. Learning Level: Evaluation

Students should discuss their answers. What are their perceptions of these procedures? Do they have personal experience? Are their perceptions accurate? Can this give them a foundation for planning patient preparation? How would they prepare patients for these procedures? Consider all the surgical procedures listed above. Write the answers to the following.

1. Which procedure would be easiest on the patient and why?
2. Which procedure would be easiest for the medical assistant to assist with and why?
3. Which procedure requires the greatest amount of sterile technique and why?

## PART 2 COMPETENCY CHALLENGE

Chapter procedures are included at the end of the chapter in the student Mastery Manual.

**Procedure 51-1: Hand Scrubbing for Assisting with Surgical Procedures**
Show students the difference in medical and surgical scrub as the technique is demonstrated. Have students observe for a break in technique and then let them practice and observe for breaks. Show students subtle breaks such as brushing against sink or turning away from sink.

**Procedure 51-2: Gloving Using the Open-Glove Method**
This method does not require a gown and may be used to set up a sterile field. Students need to have the skill demonstrated and each student must be observed carefully while they complete at least three perfect gloving practices. Gloves may be powdered and reused.

**Procedure 51-3: Gowning with a Sterile Gown**
The student first gowns and then follows using the closed-glove technique. These procedures are used when the physician needs a scrubbed assistant. It is to the student's benefit to gain competency in these procedures because it makes them more employable.

**Procedure 51-4: Gloving Using the Closed-Glove Technique**
It is suggested that students must practice all the procedures at least five times; then the instructor may evaluate for competence. Part of competence in sterile technique is obtained through repetition.

## PART 3 CLINICAL APPLICATIONS

Students may discuss or write answers.

1. What will you do if you keep contaminating items for gloving? How can you become more proficient?
2. Discuss your handling of a situation in which the physician routinely uses your sterile set-up and trays for excisions but does not wear gloves? How do you feel about this? What are the legal implications? Ethical implications?
3. What would you say to a patient who said she would take out her own stitches because she wasn't going to pay for another visit when "it is easy to do"?

# 52

# Assisting with Surgical Procedures

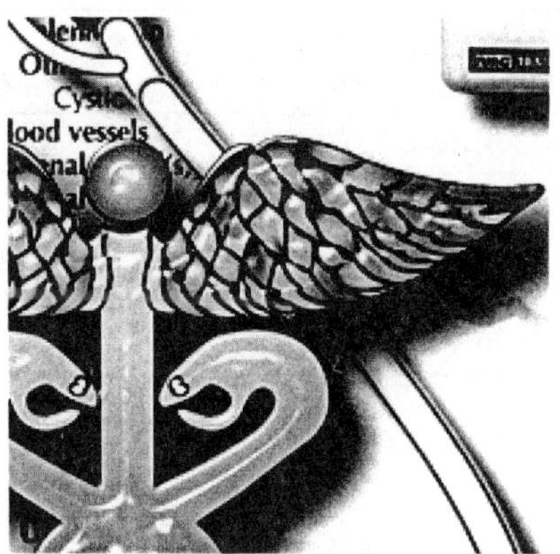

In this chapter the instructor's emphasis is to concentrate on the practice of procedure competence. There are Content Mastery Questions for review. The students will obtain competence in preparing patients, assisting at surgery, and giving post-op instructions. Infection control and standard precautions are essential throughout the process. The knowledge base requires understanding of all MA content as it must be applied to all phases of patient care in the challenge of perfecting aseptic techniques for assisting at surgery. Students will need a lot of guidance, especially in observing for breaks in technique. Often students have one small area where they constantly break technique and instructors need to point these problem areas out.

## USING THE LEARNING SYSTEM

### 1. MEDICAL ASSISTING CONTENT AND COMPETENCIES

CONTENT

- All previous MA basic entry level curriculum for content

COMPETENCIES

- Apply all fundamental principles
- Recognize and respond to verbal and nonverbal communications
- Perform risk management procedures
- Instruct individuals according to their needs
- Provide instruction for health maintenance and disease prevention
- Identify community resources
- Obtain wound specimen for microbiological testing
- Perform inventory of supplies and equipment
- Prepare patient for and assist with procedures, treatment, and minor office surgery

## 2. MEDICAL ASSISTING ENTRY-LEVEL CURRICULUM INTERFACE

| TEXTBOOK OBJECTIVES | LEARNING SYSTEM LOCATION | MA CURRICULUM |
|---|---|---|
| **Cognitive** | | **Content** |
| | | • All previous MA basic entry level curriculum for content |
| **Performance** | | **Competencies** |
| 1. Transfer sterile instruments | • Manual Part 2 | • Apply all fundamental principles<br>• Asepsis and infection control |
| 2. Prepare a patient's skin for minor surgery | • Manual Part 2 | • Apply all fundamental principles<br>• Recognize and respond to verbal and nonverbal communications<br>• Perform risk management procedures<br>• Instruct individuals according to their needs<br>• Perform inventory of supplies and equipment<br>• Prepare patient for and assist with procedures, treatment, and minor office surgery |
| 3. Open a sterile linen pack | • Manual Part 2 | • Prepare patient for and assist with procedures, treatment, and minor office surgery |
| 4. Open and add a sterile pack to a sterile field | • Manual Part 2<br>• Procedure 52-1 | • Prepare patient for and assist with procedures, treatment, and minor office surgery |
| 5. Add sterile items in a peel-back wrapper to a sterile field | • Manual Part 2<br>• Procedure 52-5 | • Prepare patient for and assist with procedures, treatment, and minor office surgery |
| 6. Assist with a minor surgical procedure | • Manual Part 2 | • Same as # 2 and<br>• Obtain wound specimen for microbiological testing |
| 7. Assist with suturing | • Manual Part 2 | • Same as # 2 and # 8 |
| 8. Assist with suture removal | • Manual Part 2 | • Provide instruction for health maintenance and disease prevention |
| 9. Bandage the injured site | • Manual Part 2 | • Same as # 2 |

## 3. RESOURCES

Refer students to health and medical sites from Chapters 29–38 and look for specific operative procedures. Students could use these sites to complete Part 3 activities.

## 4. LESSON PLAN Surgical Procedures TIME 3 hours lecture, 12 hours lab

**Opening:** Have all equipment for all procedures set up. Review some of the common instruments used in excisions.

**Pretest:** Ask students to identify objects: sterile solution, transfer forceps, sterile packs, medication vial, Mayo stand, etc.

**Objectives:** Students need at least 6 hours to practice meeting all the Competency Objectives before being evaluated. All procedures need to be demonstrated at least once. In addition, have videotapes available for review.

**Content:**

1. PROCEDURAL FILE CARD INFORMATION
2. HANDLING EQUIPMENT—MEDICAL ASSISTANT'S ROLE: circulating or scrub or both
   a. Transferring Sterile Instruments —Transfer Forceps
   b. Assisting the Physician Procedure 52-6
3. PREPARATION AND CARE OF THE PATIENT
   a. Preoperative Instructions
   b. Positioning the Patient
   c. The Skin Prep
4. SURGICAL ROUTINES—PROCEDURES 52-1–52-6
   a. Prepare Room, Gather Equipment
   b. Set Up Sterile Field and Packs, Drape the Setup
   c. Drape Patient
   d. Completion of the Surgical Procedure
5. POSTSURGICAL ROUTINES
   Cleaning and Disinfecting after Surgery
6. POSTOPERATIVE INSTRUCTIONS AND CARE—Postoperative Return Visits
   a. Wounds: types of wounds and wound healing
   b. Dressings and Bandages
   c. Procedure 52-7, 8, 9
7. LEGAL AND ETHICAL AND PATIENT TEACHING RESPONSIBILITIES

**Lab:** Demonstrate, Practice, and Evaluate Chapter Procedures. Discuss Mastery Manual Part 3 and complete all Mastery Manual.

**Assignment:** Practice until perfect! Complete all Mastery Manual parts.

**Posttest:** Use testbank questions for unit examination and evaluation of procedures for performance competency.

## 5. MASTERY MANUAL ANSWERS

### PART 1 CONTENT MASTERY

### A. Learning Level: Knowledge

1. Write a sentence using each of the vocabulary words in a patient-related statement that shows you understand the meaning of the term.

   a. Approximate ______________________________

   b. Hematoma ______________________________

   c. Irrigation ______________________________

   d. Lesion ______________________________

   e. Wound ______________________________

2. Match the words with the definitions in the right column. Put the corresponding letter next to the word.

| | | | | |
|---|---|---|---|---|
| **a.** | 2 | **Ace** | 1. | Most commonly used gauze dressing |
| **b.** | 3 | **Band-Aid** | 2. | Elastic roller bandage used for pressure on limbs |
| **c.** | 7 | **Kling** | 3. | Adhesive bandages to fit smaller wounds |
| **d.** | 5 | **Packing** | 4. | Bandage applied with cage-like applicator |
| **e.** | 6 | **Steri-strips** | 5. | Dressing used in open wounds |
| **f.** | 8 | **Telfa** | 6. | Special adhesive tape replaces sutures |
| **g.** | 1 | **Topper sponge** | 7. | Adheres to body and shapes to cover wounds |
| **h.** | 4 | **Tube gauze** | 8. | Nonstick pad used over suture |

### B. Learning Level: Comprehension

1. Give examples of the information needed on the surgical procedural card files.
   a. Preoperative instructions and consent form ready to sign
   b. Preoperative and operative medications
   c. Universal blood and body fluid precautions, listing specific protection barriers (goggles, masks, gowns, aprons, and gloves) to be worn by the surgeon and the assistants
   d. Glove sizes
   e. Prep solution and shaving instructions
   f. Patient position
   g. Sterile packs, instruments, sutures, and equipment
   h. Syringe and needle sizes
   i. Post-operative instructions and the routine number of days for a follow-up appointment

2. List four pre-operative instructions that need to be provided to patients.
   - Medications, special skin cleansing, or other physical preparation.
   - Instruct patients to bring relative or friend to drive them home after surgery.
   - When appropriate, instruct the patient to wear special clothing, easily removed and can be worn over bulky dressings or a cast.
   - Instruct the patient to leave jewelry and other valuables at home.

3. Why should these and all instructions pertaining to surgery be given to the patient in writing and on physician letterhead?

   This protects the physician, allows the patient to refer to directions when home, lessens complications and discomfort for patient, and makes instructions available to caregivers.

## C. Learning Level: Application

1. Mrs. Shapiro has brought her husband home from the medical center where he had quadruple bypass surgery. She calls Blackburn Primary Care Associates to report that he is doing great, and she has all her post-operative care instructions. She tells you he has a chest incision and two leg incisions. What items of care would you expect to be covered in those instructions?
   a. Whether or not to elevate a limb
   b. Limitations of exercise or food intake
   c. Whether or not to bathe
   d. How to apply hot or cold compresses, if needed
   e. How to recognize and care for drainage, if there is a wound drain in place
   f. Whether or not to change dressings
   g. What types of complications necessitate the patient calling the office
   h. The medications prescribed and their purposes
   i. When to return to work or school
   j. The time to call and report in for the next day
   k. The date and time of the next appointment

2. Three days later, Mrs. Shapiro calls and tells you that she does not think the incision looks "right." What should you do?

   Call the cardiac surgeon and make an appointment to be seen immediately and if any problems, call back Blackburn Primary Care Associates.

## D. Learning Level: Analysis

1. Mrs. Ferguson has a small lesion on her right forearm anterior surface that needs to be excised and biopsied. It is 1 centimeter in circumference and will need sutures. The physician tells you to prepare the patient. Which of the listed procedures in this chapter will you need to complete for this surgery?

   All the procedures will need to be completed.

2. The physician has obtained the consent, but you are to do the preoperative teaching. What specific items will you include in the teaching for an excision?
   a. How to clean the skin
   b. Sterile procedure to prevent infection
   c. Local anesthetic given to prevent pain
   d. Cost if she asks
   e. Post-op care

## E. Learning Level: Synthesis

Plan the types of dressings for the wounds used. Give an example of each wound mentioned and the type of bandage that would be considered.

| Wound Type | Example | Dressing and Bandage |
|---|---|---|
| Superficial | An abrasion | May require only an astringent and open-air healing |
| First intention | Sutured laceration | Nonstick pad and topical bandage to keep dry |
| Second intention | Open unsutured wound | Long, thin packing material with lubrication or antibiotic ointment |

## F. Learning Level: Evaluation

1. While gloving for the procedure on Mrs. Ferguson, you contaminate one glove. The physician is impatiently awaiting for you to assist. How do you handle the situation?

   Answers will vary—generally speaking, one needs to explain what's happening and reglove. Do not let anyone dissuade you from protecting yourself and the patient.

2. You need to hold the anesthetic medication vial as described in your 8th Edition Textbook for the physician to withdraw. Practice this and decide what are the three most essential components of this skill.
   a. Hold vial firmly and support with other arm.
   b. Hold label toward physician and let physician read it first.
   c. Hold at 60–75 degree angle so physician can see stopper and fluid can still be withdrawn.

3. What needs to be given to the physician by the scrub nurse when each of the following occurs?
   a. Physician ready to start procedure **hand scalpel**
   b. Lump excised **sterile specimen basin**
   c. Bleeding vessel **topper sponges and hemostat**
   d. Suture handed to physician **scissors to cut**
   e. Sutures completed **dressing and bandage materials**

## PART 2 COMPETENCY CHALLENGE

There are nine procedures at the end of the chapter in the competency package. It is suggested that students proceed in the following order to attain each Competency Objective Learning strategies:

1. Demonstrate each procedure or show on video.
2. Have students practice each one with instructor supervision.
3. Make a list of supplies with students that they can use at home to simulate practice of every procedure.
4. Students use these supplies to practice each procedure at home at least three times.
5. Return to the lab and have classmates observe other classmates and evaluate performance for every procedure.
6. Practice until perfect.
7. Evaluate each student for each procedure.
8. Suggested scenarios to have students complete all procedures in one sitting include:
   a. Excision of a lump on the thigh
   b. Removal of $^1/_2$ the number of steel staples in large wound
   c. Incision and drainage of a carbuncle

## PART 3 CLINICAL APPLICATIONS

Students need to complete this activity to make the chapter applicable to real-life office situations. The more the student is involved with patient teaching, the better an asset they are to the physician employer and the patients.

Choose one of the specialties of Chapters 29–38 in the 8th Edition Textbook.

1. Make a list of commonly performed office procedures or surgeries for that specialty.
2. Write the medical assistant's role in assisting at those specialties.
3. Demonstrate putting a clean bandage over a simulated abrasion approximately 2 inches in diameter.
4. Pick one procedure and complete a pre- and post-op teaching plan for the procedure. For instance, cystoscopy in the urology office. Use the teaching plan guide in Chapter 28.

# Appendix A

## Blank Lesson Plan

**LESSON PLAN**

TOPIC ______________________ TIME __________________

LESSON # ___________________

OPENING: ____________________________________________

______________________________________________________

PRETEST

______________________________________________________

______________________________________________________

CONTENT OBJECTIVES ( At least 1 per 1/2 hour) TIME ____

______________________________________________________

______________________________________________________

______________________________________________________

______________________________________________________

______________________________________________________

______________________________________________________

______________________________________________________

Post objectives on overhead, in syllabus, or on flip chart for each class. Read aloud.

CONTENT OUTLINE *Activities:* Choose from list to right TIME ____

______________________________________________________

______________________________________________________

______________________________________________________

______________________________________________________

______________________________________________________

______________________________________________________

______________________________________________________

______________________________________________________

**Action verbs for writing objectives**

*Knowledge*—define, match, repeat, select

*Comprehension*—express, explain, restate, discuss, demonstrate, describe

*Application*—organize, solve, transfer, classify, choose, illustrate, practice

*Analysis*—distinguish, compare, list, subdivide, contrast, debate

*Synthesis*—design, plan, solve

*Evaluation*—judge, assess, compare, critique, rate

*Classroom Activities*—
Use list below and provide for student learning styles (VAT) and stages (#1-4)

1. *Experiencing*
   a. Laboratories—VAT
   b. Skill Practice—VAT
   c. Observations/transparencies—VT
   d. Games/puzzles —VT
   e. Text reading—V
   f. Simulations—VAT
   g. Fieldwork—VAT
   h. Films—VA
   i. Readings—V, aloud—A
   j. Recall experience—A
   k. Taking notes —VT
2. *Examination*
   a. Logs—T
   b. Journals—VT

| | |
|---|---|
| ASSIGNMENT<br><br>POSTTEST: choose from objectives, give oral and written directions<br><br>LEARNING EQUIPMENT NEEDED<br>LIST forms, activity supplies, clinical supplies | c. Discussion—A<br>d. Brainstorming/Lists—AT<br>e. Thought questions—A<br>f. Rhetorical questions—A<br>g. Drawing pictures—VT<br>h. Designing or graphing—VT<br><br>3. *Explanation*<br>a. Simulations/role play—VTA<br>b. Papers & Homework—VT<br>c. Laboratory & Projects—VAT<br>d. Making videotape for hearing impaired—A<br>e. Making a model of anatomy—VT<br>f. Drawing pictures—VT<br><br>4. *Application*<br>a. Lecture—VAT<br>b. Case study—VT<br>c. Explaining procedure on tape to person—AT<br>d. Making tape for blind person—A<br>e. Describing something to another—AT<br>f. Model building—VT<br>g. Field work—VAT<br>h. Analogies—A |

**NOTES:**

# Appendix B

## Virtual Medical Office Challenge CD-ROM

### ABOUT THE PROGRAM

*Virtual Medical Office Challenge CD-ROM* is designed to be used in conjunction with the 8th Edition of the W.B. Saunders textbook *The Medical Assistant: Administrative and Clinical,* by Mary Kinn and MaryAnn Woods. Through the use of case studies, the program allows students to practice the application of information provided in the textbook, and to use problem-solving, decision-making, and critical thinking skills. In addition, for specific administrative and clinical competencies, the learner's ability to use critical thinking and priority-setting skills during a clinical or administrative procedure can be challenged. This Appendix contains information on how to install and use the program. It also contains materials and forms used throughout the program, should students wish to refer to printed documents or complete any forms manually.

**Minimum System Requirements**

| | | |
|---|---|---|
| PC and PC-Compatible: | Computer: | 80486/66, or Pentium CPU |
| | System: | Windows 95 or 98/Windows NT |
| | Memory: | 24 MB RAM |
| | Other: | 4x CD-ROM Drive<br>256-color mode<br>Sound card/speakers<br>Mouse<br>SVGA, or higher graphics<br>640 x 480 screen resolution |
| Macintosh: | Computer: | Power PC Processor |
| | System: | 7.6x, or higher |
| | Memory: | 24 MB RAM |
| | Other: | 4x CD-ROM Drive<br>256-color mode<br>Mouse<br>640 x 480 screen resolution |

## LOGGING ON TO THE VIRTUAL MEDICAL OFFICE CHALLENGE

### Logging on for the first time

To record the challenges that they complete, students will enter their first initial and last name as a single word (e.g., tsmith). See Figure 1. Students will then click **ENTER**. If students do not wish to record their progress, they will simply click **NEXT** and advance to the **MAIN MENU**.

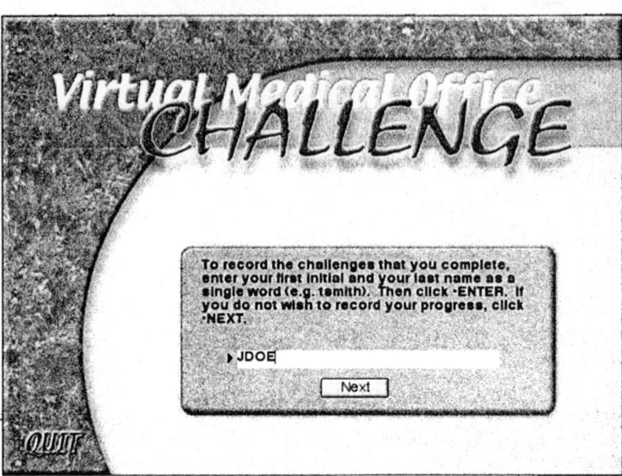


Figure 1

### Logging on after the first time

If students have entered their names during the first log on, the program will keep track of the challenges they have attempted, and those they have completed. If students enter their names the same way every time, the program will recognize them and give them the option to review the status of those challenges they have completed, or attempted, to date. Students can either review this status information or go straight to the **MAIN MENU**.

- **Storing bookmarking to the hard disk.** If the installation is configured to store students' bookmarking on the hard drive, then the students will not need to insert a floppy into the diskette drive and can simply proceed to the **MAIN MENU** after selecting the hard drive option and logging on.
- **Storing bookmarking to a floppy disk.** If the installation is configured to store student bookmarking on data diskettes, the data diskette must be inserted into the diskette drive before logging on. If no diskette is detected, the program will prompt for it. *Note:* The program will accept blank, formatted data diskettes as student data diskettes. After inserting the data diskette into the floppy drive, students can then proceed to the **MAIN MENU** after selecting the A:\drive option and logging on.

## USING THE MAIN MENU

The **MAIN MENU** is the navigational front door to the *Virtual Medical Office Challenge*. Through it, students can select to explore any one of four patient case scenarios, or go directly to either the Clinical or Administrative Skills Building section (see Figure 2). Students also have an option to check Challenge Status, which is a log of what interactions they have either completed or partially explored.

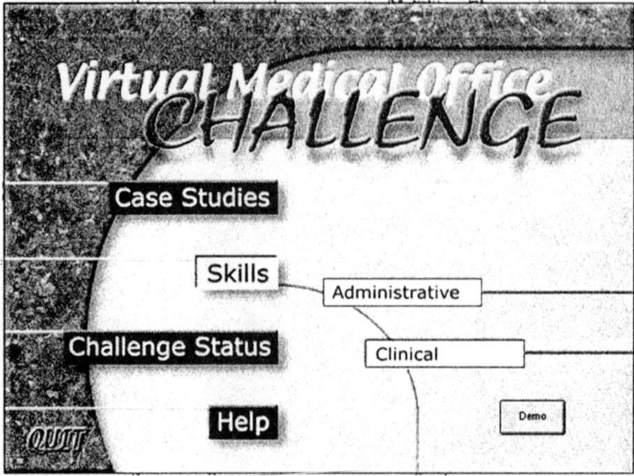


Figure 2

- **Selecting CASE STUDIES**. By selecting **CASE STUDIES** on the **MAIN MENU**, students will be directed to the **Patient Cases** screen, which allows them to select a particular case by patient name (see Figure 3). When the cursor rolls over the patient's name, a description of that case, and the administrative and clinical competencies that are challenged within that case, appears in the dialog box below. Students can then select a case by clicking on a patient case file folder, which will automatically advance them to the beginning of that case. A new case can be accessed at any time from anywhere in the program by first selecting **MAIN MENU**, then selecting **CASE STUDIES**, and a new case folder from the **Patient Cases** screen.

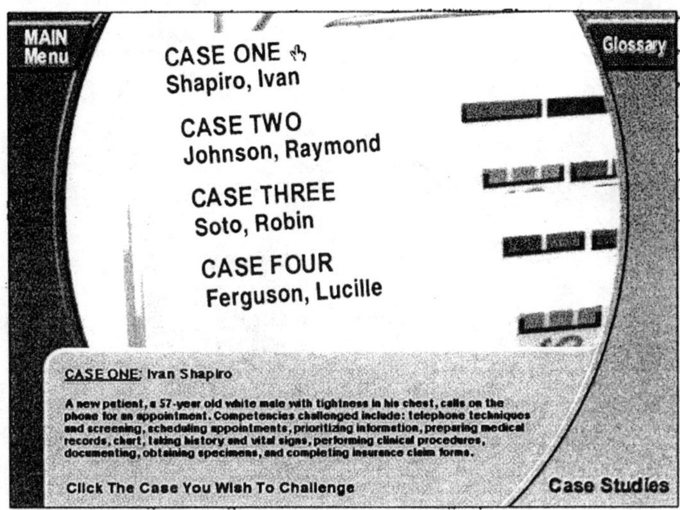


Figure 3

- **Selecting SKILLS.** By selecting **SKILLS** on the **MAIN MENU**, students will be directed to another screen that will then prompt them to select either **Clinical** or **Administrative**, which will take them through all the skills in either skill set, or they can select an individual skill to explore within either skill set. Skills can be selected from anywhere in the program by first selecting **MAIN MENU**, then selecting **SKILLS**.
- **Selecting CHALLENGE STATUS**. The *Virtual Medical Office Challenge* will keep track of where students have been in the program, and what areas are still left to be challenged. Selecting **Challenge Status** on the **MAIN MENU** will bring up a list of what sections of the program have been partially completed and which have been fully completed. Separate screens will then show students what portions of the four patient cases have been completed, or partially completed (see Figure 4), and what portions of the **Clinical** and **Administrative Skills** have been fully, or partially, challenged (see Figure 5). Partially completed sections are marked with a circle that is filled in with color. Fully completed sections are filled in with the same color and marked with an **X** within the circle. The **CHALLENGE STATUS** can be accessed at any point in the program by first selecting **MAIN MENU**, then selecting **CHALLENGE STATUS**.

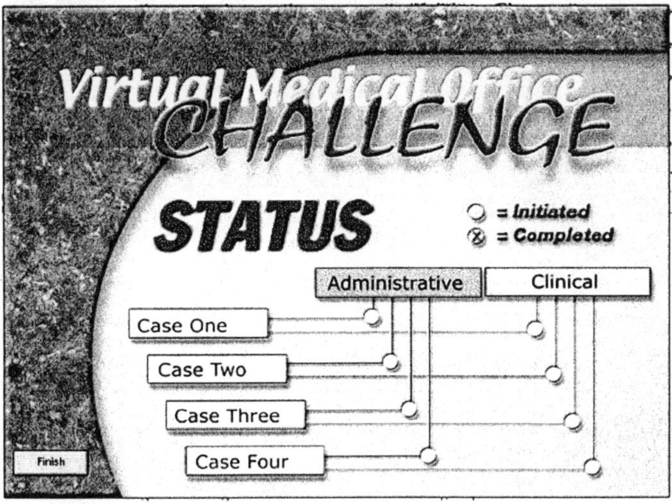


Figure 4

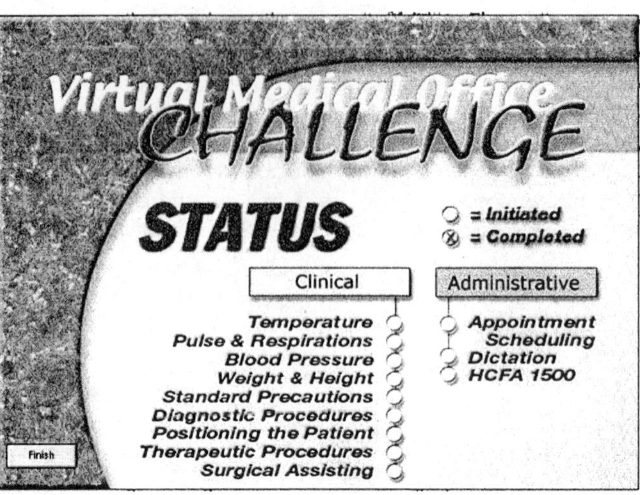


Figure 5

- **Selecting the DEMONSTRATION BUTTON.** It is recommended that all first-time log-on users review the **Demonstration Module** to familiarize themselves with the program before getting into the actual program. The **Demonstration Module** can be accessed from a permanent button on the **MAIN MENU** screen. It is self-running and requires no interaction on the student's part, and runs for approximately three minutes. This **Demonstration Module** will familiarize the first-time user with all program features, including interactions that will be required throughout. This **Demonstration Module** can be accessed at any time from anywhere in the program by selecting **MAIN MENU**, then selecting the **Demo** button.

## PATIENT CASE SCENARIOS

Four patient case scenarios are presented in the *Virtual Medical Office Challenge* (see Table 1). Combined with the **ADMINISTRATIVE** and **CLINICAL** skills sections, they represent most of the key competencies students will need to master, as identified by the American Association of Medical Assistants (AAMA) in their Medical Assisting Curriculum Role Delineation Study. In each of the cases, students will play the role of a certified medical assistant working in either the administrative or clinical area of a busy general practice medical office. The practice, which is called Blackburn Primary Care Associates, has three doctors and a broad mixture of patients with varying situations and needs. Students will be asked to play the role of one of four certified medical assistants, and will be asked to respond to simulated, realistic medical office situations. Students will receive feedback based on the choices they make, and can explore that feedback further to understand the rationale behind their correct or incorrect responses.

When you enter a patient case for the first time, you will start at the beginning of that case. If at any time during that case you wish to return to the main menu, click **MAIN** when you see the icon in the top left corner of the screen. This icon will appear each time you begin a new challenge throughout the case. If you have worked through part of the case previously, the program will bookmark which portion, or portions, you have completed. When you return to that case, it will ask you whether you would like to start at the **BEGINNING**, or your **PREVIOUS LOCATION**, which is the last challenge location you completed the last time you worked in that case.

To make the program as realistic as possible, all the patient situations have been selected from the files of practicing physicians. For confidentiality, all names, dates, places, and any other identifiable characteristics of physicians and patients have been carefully deleted, or changed. All forms are replicas of forms in current use. The four patient cases are described in Table 1.

**Table 1: Patient Case Studies**

### CASE ONE: Ivan Shapiro

A new patient, a 57-year-old white male with tightness in his chest, calls on the phone for an appointment. Competencies challenged include: telephone techniques and screening, scheduling appointments, prioritizing information, preparing medical records, completing insurance claim forms, taking history and vital signs, performing clinical procedures, documenting, obtaining specimens.

### CASE TWO: Raymond Johnson

An established 32-year-old white male patient has an exacerbation of his asthma and calls on the phone for an appointment. Competencies challenged include: telephone screening, responding to emergencies, prioritizing, taking history and vital signs, preparing and giving medications, performing procedures, documenting.

### CASE THREE: Robin Soto

A $4^1/_2$-month-old Hispanic child is brought in for her immunizations after a missed appointment. Also she has not been given her vitamins for a week. Competencies challenged include: taking history and vital signs, performing developmental assessment, giving immunizations and patient instruction, completing insurance claim forms, transcribing.

### CASE FOUR: Lucille Ferguson

A 75-year-old black widow seeks her first appointment in the medical office. Due to her age and state of health, she is having difficulty functioning independently. Competencies challenged include: telephone techniques and confidentiality, scheduling appointments, preparing medical records, taking history and vital signs, positioning, examination procedures, performing diagnostic tests, patient instruction, completing insurance claim forms, transcribing.

## ADMINISTRATIVE AND CLINICAL SKILLS

In addition to the four patient cases, students can select to work on individual skills in either the Administrative or Clinical areas. These can be accessed through the **MAIN MENU** by selecting **SKILLS**, then selecting which skill they wish to explore.

**ADMINISTRATIVE SKILLS.** Individual Administrative skills presented in this part of the program include:

- Schedule and Manage Appointments
- Perform Medical Transcriptions
- Complete Insurance Claim Forms

**CLINICAL SKILLS.** Individual Clinical skills presented in this part of the program include:

- Temperature
- Pulse and Respirations
- Blood Pressure
- Weight and Height
- Diagnostic Procedures
- Standard Precautions
- Positioning the Patient
- Therapeutic Procedures
- Surgical Assisting

## USING THE GLOSSARY

The Glossary can be accessed from all screens in the software once students have selected an activity from the **MAIN MENU**. It can be accessed in one of two ways, either by clicking on any word in red type that appears within a dialog box, or by clicking on the **Glossary** icon button. A word can be selected within the **Glossary** from the alphabetical list provided by scrolling to search for a word. The definition appears in the Definition Box, and students can hear the word pronounced by selecting the **Pronunciation** button (see Figure 6). Clicking on the **RETURN** button on the **Glossary** screen returns students to their previous location.

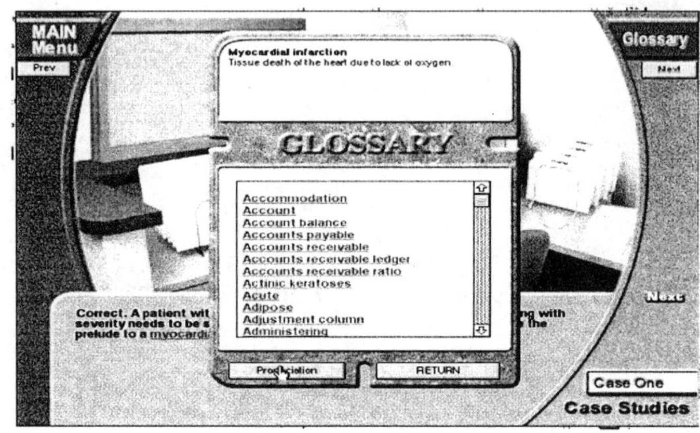


Figure 6

## PATIENT FORMS AND REFERENCE MATERIALS

The following forms are available to students who prefer to reference information or complete any forms manually. These forms and reference materials are exact duplicates of the forms and reference materials used throughout the *Virtual Medical Office Challenge* program. Blank forms are also provided should the instructor wish to use them for additional classroom exercises.

### CASE ONE FORMS:

| | |
|---|---|
| Form 1: | Telephone Message Form |
| Form 2: | Appointment Schedule for Blackburn Primary Care Associates |
| Form 3: | Health History Questionnaire for Ivan Shapiro |
| Form 4: | Patient Information Form for Ivan Shapiro |
| Form 5: | Patient Encounter Form for Ivan Shapiro |
| Form 6: | Blackburn Primary Care Associates Physician's Fee Schedule |
| Form 7: | Blank HCFA-1500 Form for billing Ivan Shapiro's visit |

### CASE TWO FORM:

| | |
|---|---|
| Form 8: | Progress Note Form for documenting Raymond Johnson's visit |

### CASE THREE FORMS:

| | |
|---|---|
| Form 9: | Infant Growth and Development Chart for documenting Robin Soto's Height and Weight |
| Form 10: | Progress Note Form for documenting Robin Soto's visit |
| Form 11: | Patient Information Form for Robin Soto |
| Form 12: | Patient Encounter Form for Robin Soto |
| Form 13: | Blackburn Primary Care Associates Physician's Fee Schedule |
| Form 14: | Blank HCFA-1500 Form for billing Robin Soto's visit |

## CASE FOUR FORMS:

Form 15: Appointment Schedule for Blackburn Primary Care Associates
Form 16: Health History Questionnaire for Lucille Ferguson
Form 17: Patient Information Form for Lucille Ferguson
Form 18: Patient Encounter Form for Lucille Ferguson
Form 19: Blackburn Primary Care Associates Physician's Fee Schedule
Form 20: Blank HCFA-1500 Form for billing Lucille Ferguson's visit

## ADMINISTRATIVE SKILLS FORMS:

Form 21: Patient Information Form for Charles Latham
Form 22: Patient Encounter Form for Charles Latham
Form 23: Blackburn Primary Care Associates Physician's Fee Schedule
Form 24: Blank HCFA-1500 Form for billing Charles Latham's visit
Form 25: Patient Information Form for Marrion Jordon
Form 26: Patient Encounter Form for Marrion Jordon
Form 27: Blackburn Primary Care Associates Physician's Fee Schedule
Form 28: Blank HCFA-1500 Form for billing Marrion Jordon's visit
Form 29: Patient Information Form for Prinnie Minnowitz
Form 30: Patient Encounter Form for Prinnie Minnowitz
Form 31: Blackburn Primary Care Associates Physician's Fee Schedule
Form 32: Blank HCFA-1500 Form for billing Prinnie Minnowitz's visit

## ADDITIONAL BLANK FORMS

Blank Appointment Schedule
Blank Health History Questionnaire
Blank Patient Information Form
Blank Patient Encounter Form
Blank Progress Note Form
Blank Infant Growth and Development Form

Case One, Form 1

# Telephone Message Log

NAME OF CALLER | PATIENT'S NAME | AGE | TEMP. | TIME

TELEPHONE NUMBER | PHARMACY | TELEPHONE | CALLED BY: | DATE

**COMPLAINT / MESSAGE** ☐ PLEASE RETURN THE CALL ☐ WILL CALL AGAIN ☐ RETURNED YOUR CALL ☐ OTHER (SPECIFY) | DOCTOR

INSTRUCTIONS/REPLY:

☐ **URGENT**
☐ **MEDICATION ALLERGY**

**CALLED BACK:** **BY:** **DATE** **OTHER (SPECIFY)**

NAME OF CALLER | PATIENT'S NAME | AGE | TEMP. | TIME

TELEPHONE NUMBER | PHARMACY | TELEPHONE | CALLED BY: | DATE

**COMPLAINT / MESSAGE** ☐ PLEASE RETURN THE CALL ☐ WILL CALL AGAIN ☐ RETURNED YOUR CALL ☐ OTHER (SPECIFY) | DOCTOR

INSTRUCTIONS/REPLY:

☐ **URGENT**
☐ **MEDICATION ALLERGY**

**CALLED BACK:** **BY:** **DATE** **OTHER (SPECIFY)**

NAME OF CALLER | PATIENT'S NAME | AGE | TEMP. | TIME

TELEPHONE NUMBER | PHARMACY | TELEPHONE | CALLED BY: | DATE

**COMPLAINT / MESSAGE** ☐ PLEASE RETURN THE CALL ☐ WILL CALL AGAIN ☐ RETURNED YOUR CALL ☐ OTHER (SPECIFY) | DOCTOR

INSTRUCTIONS/REPLY:

☐ **URGENT**
☐ **MEDICATION ALLERGY**

**CALLED BACK:** **BY:** **DATE** **OTHER (SPECIFY)**



Courtesy of Bibbero Systems, Inc., Petaluma, California.

Case One, Form 2

# Appointment Schedule

DAY | Mon. | Tue. | Wed. | Thu. | Fri. | Sat.

DATE

| Time | HUGHES, M.D. | LAWLER, M.D. | LOPEZ, M.D. |
|---|---|---|---|
| 8 00 | | | |
| 10 | | NO ACUTE | NO NEW |
| 20 | | OR | OB |
| 30 | | NEW PATIENTS | |
| 40 | | | |
| 50 | | | |
| 9 00 | Sx-Blackburn | Johnson, Marvin | |
| 10 | Hosp. | 555-921-3195 | |
| 20 | Smith, | CPE | |
| 30 | Mariano | | |
| 40 | | | |
| 50 | | ↓ | |
| 10 00 | | Seeburn, Kate | Richards, Mary |
| 10 | | INFLUENZA 555-817- | ↓ PAP 619-3191 |
| 20 | | ↓ FLU 3615 | Scheeler, Virginia |
| 30 | | Butler, Carl | ↓ PAP 721-9951 |
| 40 | | NEURO ✓ UP | |
| 50 | ↓ | ↓ 555-331-9195 | |
| 11 00 | Jefferson, Martha | Doyle, Mike 555- | Longfellow, Wilma |
| 10 | NEW OB 555-245-1790 | ↓ PROSTATE ✓ 277- | PAP, PE |
| 20 | | Doyle, Hanah 1965 | 555-317-2198 |
| 30 | | ↓ ✓ UP | |
| 40 | | | |
| 50 | ↓ | | ↓ |
| 12 00 | Davis, Marvin 555- | HOSPITAL | |
| 10 | ↓ ALLERGY 241-9200 | ROUNDS | |
| 20 | Martin, Darlene 555- | | LUNCH MTG |
| 30 | ↓ SUT REM 917-1909 | | |
| 40 | Sorbin, John 555- | | |
| 50 | ↓ VACCINES 914-3190 | | |
| 1 00 | | | Simpson, Lisa |
| 10 | | | 3 MO PRENATAL |
| 20 | | | ↓ 555-129-3190 |
| 30 | | | Schmidt, Cindy |
| 40 | | | STD 555-377- |
| 50 | | | ↓ 2198 |
| 2 00 | Docker, Millie 555-219- | | |
| 10 | CHEST PAIN 7191 | | |
| 20 | ↓ | | |
| 30 | | | |
| 40 | | | |
| 50 | | ↓ | |
| 3 00 | Starvey, Jill 555- | AMA Mtg | Jessup, Carl 719- |
| 10 | ↓ VACCINES 319-2191 | Convention | ↓ STRESS EKG 3307 |
| 20 | | Center | Lawson, Milton 331- |
| 30 | | 3:30 pm | ↓ PROSTATE 9900 |
| 40 | | | |
| 50 | | | |
| 4 00 | HOSPITAL | | Geary, Leon 555- |
| 10 | ROUNDS | | ↓ VACCINE 498-3150 |
| 20 | | | |
| 30 | | | |
| 40 | | | |
| 50 | | | |
| 5 00 | | | MED SOCIETY |
| 10 | | | MTG |
| 20 | | | 5-7 pm |
| 30 | | | |
| 40 | | | |
| 50 | ↓ | ↓ | ↓ |

Case One, Form 3

# ANDRUS/CLINI-REC® HEALTH HISTORY QUESTIONNAIRE

Chart No. ____________

**Identification Information**

Today's Date ____________

Name Shapiro, Ivan    Date of Birth 3/6/45

Occupation Carpenter    Marital Status Married

## PART A – PRESENT HEALTH HISTORY

### I. CURRENT MEDICAL PROBLEMS

Please list the medical problems for which you came to see the doctor. About when did they begin?

| Problems | Date Began |
|---|---|
| Chest pain when exercising | |
| | |
| | |

What concerns you most about these problems?

If you are being treated for any other illness or medical problems by another physician, please describe the problems and write the name of the physician or medical facility treating you.

| Illness or Medical Problem | Physician or Medical Facility | City |
|---|---|---|
| | | |
| | | |

### II. MEDICATIONS

Please list all medications you are now taking, including those you buy without a doctor's prescription (such as aspirin, cold tablets or vitamin supplements).

### III. ALLERGIES AND SENSITIVITIES

List anything that you are allergic to such as certain foods, medications, dust, chemicals or soaps, household items, pollens, bee stings, etc., and indicate how each affects you.

| Allergic To: | Effect | Allergic To: | Effect |
|---|---|---|---|
| Penicillin | Hives | | |
| | | | |

### IV. GENERAL HEALTH, ATTITUDE AND HABITS

| | | |
|---|---|---|
| How is your overall health now? | Health now: | Poor ___ Fair ___ Good X Excellent ___ |
| How has it been most of your life? | Health has been: | Poor ___ Fair ___ Good X Excellent ___ |
| In the past year: | | |
| Has your appetite changed? | Appetite: | Decreased ___ Increased ___ Stayed same X |
| Has your weight changed? | Weight: | Lost ___ lbs. Gained 10 lbs. No change ___ |
| Are you thirsty much of the time? | Thirsty: | No X Yes ___ |
| Has your overall 'pep' changed? | Pep: | Decreased ___ Increased ___ Stayed same X |
| Do you usually have trouble sleeping? | Trouble sleeping: | No ___ Yes X |
| How much do you exercise? | Exercise: | Little or none ___ Less than I need ___ All I need X |
| Do you smoke? | Smokes: | No X Yes ___ If yes, how many years? ___ |
| How many each day? | | ___ Cigarettes ___ Cigars ___ Pipesfull |
| Have you ever smoked? | Smoked: | No ___ Yes X If yes, how many years? 15 |
| How many each day? | | 20 Cigarettes ___ Cigars ___ Pipesfull |
| Do you drink alcoholic beverages? | Alcohol: | No ___ Yes X I drink ___ Beers ___ Glasses of wine ___ Drinks of hard liquor - per day Socially |
| Have you ever had a problem with alcohol? | Prior problem: | No X Yes ___ |
| How much coffee or tea do you usually drink? | Coffee/Tea: | 2 cups of coffee or tea a day |
| Do you regularly wear seatbelts? | Seatbelts: | No ___ Yes X |

| DO YOU: | Rarely/Never | Occasionally | Frequently |
|---|---|---|---|
| Feel nervous? | X | | |
| Feel depressed? | X | | |
| Find it hard to make decisions? | X | | |
| Lose your temper? | | X | |
| Worry a lot? | X | | |
| Tire easily? | | X | |
| Have trouble relaxing? | | X | |
| Have any sexual problems? | X | | |
| Ever feel like committing suicide? | X | | |
| Feel bored with your life? | X | | |
| Use marijuana? | X | | |
| Use "hard drugs"? | X | | |

Do you want to talk to the doctor about a personal matter? No X Yes ___



STOCK NO. 19-742-4 8/95



C O N F I D E N T I A L

# PART A – PRESENT HEALTH HISTORY (continued)

## IV. GENERAL HEALTH, ATTITUDE AND HABITS (continued)

Have you recently had any changes in your: If yes, please explain:

| | No | Yes | If yes, please explain |
|---|---|---|---|
| Marital status? | X | | |
| Job or work? | | X | Self employed |
| Residence? | | X | Moved from LA CA |
| Financial status? | X | | |
| Are you having any legal problems or trouble with the law? | X | | |

# PART B – PAST HISTORY

## I. FAMILY HEALTH

Please give the following information about your immediate family:

| Relationship | Age, if Living | Age At Death | State of Health Or Cause of Death |
|---|---|---|---|
| Father | | 78 | Lung cancer |
| Mother | | 45 | Heart disease |
| Brothers and Sisters | 38 | | good |
| | | | |
| | | | |
| Spouse | 51 | | good |
| Children | 22 | | good |
| | 25 | | good |
| | | | |
| | | | |

Have any **blood relatives** had any of the following illnesses? If so, indicate relationship (mother, brother, etc.)

| Illness | Family Members |
|---|---|
| Asthma | |
| Diabetes | |
| Cancer | Father |
| Blood Disease | |
| Glaucoma | |
| Epilepsy | |
| Rheumatoid Arthritis | Aunt |
| Tuberculosis | |
| Gout | |
| High Blood Pressure | Mother |
| Heart Disease | Mother |
| Mental Problems | |
| Suicide | |
| Stroke | Grandmother |
| Alcoholism | |
| Rheumatic Fever | |

## II. HOSPITALIZATIONS, SURGERIES, INJURIES

Please list all times you have been hospitalized, operated on, or seriously injured.

| Year | Operation, Illness, Injury | Hospital and City |
|---|---|---|
| 1990 | Appendix removed | LA CA |
| | | |
| | | |

## III. ILLNESS AND MEDICAL PROBLEMS

Please mark with an (X) any of the following illnesses and medical problems you have or have had and indicate the year when each started. If you are not certain when an illness started, write down an approximate year.

| Illness | (x) | (Year) | Illness | (x) | (Year) |
|---|---|---|---|---|---|
| Eye or eye lid infection | | | Hernia | | |
| Glaucoma | | | Hemorrhoids | | |
| Other eye problems | | | Kidney or bladder disease | | |
| Ear trouble | | | Prostate problem (male only) | | |
| Deafness or decreased hearing | | | Mental problems | | |
| Thyroid trouble | | | Headaches | | |
| Strep throat | | | Head injury | | |
| Bronchitis | | | Stroke | | |
| Emphysema | | | Convulsions, seizures | | |
| Pneumonia | | | Arthritis | | |
| Allergies, asthma or hay fever | | | Gout | | |
| Tuberculosis | | | Cancer or tumor | | |
| Other lung problems | | | Bleeding tendency | | |
| High blood pressure | | | Diabetes | | |
| Heart attack | | | Measles/Rubeola | | |
| High cholesterol | | | German measles/Rubella | | |
| Arteriosclerosis (Hardening of arteries) | | | Polio | | |
| | | | Mumps | | |
| Heart murmur | | | Scarlet fever | | |
| Other heart condition | | | Chicken pox | | |
| Stomach/duodenal ulcer | | | Mononucleosis | | |
| Diverticulosis | | | Eczema | | |
| Colitis | | | Psoriasis | | |
| Other bowel problems | | | Venereal disease | | |
| Hepatitis | | | Genital herpes | | |
| Liver trouble | | | HIV test | | |
| Gallbladder trouble | | | AIDS | | |

CONFIDENTIAL

## PART C – BODY SYSTEMS REVIEW

Please answer all of the following questions.

Circle any questions you find difficult to answer.

MEN: Please answer questions 1 through 12, then skip to question 18.

WOMEN: Please start on question 6.

MEN ONLY

| | No | Yes |
|---|---|---|
| 1. Have you had or do you have prostate trouble? | X | |
| 2. Do you have any sexual problems or a problem with impotency? | X | |
| 3. Have you ever had sores or lesions on your penis? | X | |
| 4. Have you ever had any discharge from your penis? | X | |
| 5. Do you ever have pain, lumps or swelling in your testicles? | X | |

Check here if you wish to discuss any special problems with the doctor ☐

MEN & WOMEN

|  | Rarely/ Never | Occasionally | Frequently |
|---|---|---|---|
| 6. Is it sometimes hard to start your urine flow? | X | | |
| 7. Is urination ever painful? | X | | |
| 8. Do you have to urinate more than 5 times a day? | X | | |
| 9. Do you get up at night to urinate? | X | | |
| 10. Has your urine ever been bloody or dark colored? | X | | |
| 11. Do you ever lose urine when you strain, laugh, cough or sneeze? | X | | |
| 12. Do you ever lose urine during sleep? | X | | |

WOMEN ONLY

Do you:

|  | Rarely/ Never | Occasionally | Frequently |
|---|---|---|---|
| 13. a. Have any menstrual problems? | | | |
| b. Feel rather tense just before your period? | | | |
| c. Have heavy menstrual bleeding? | | | |
| d. Have painful menstrual periods? | | | |
| e. Have any bleeding between periods? | | | |
| f. Have any unusual vaginal discharge or itching? | | | |
| g. Ever have tender breasts? | | | |
| h. Have any discharge from your nipples? | | | |
| i. Have any hot flashes? | | | |

14. How many times, if any, have you been pregnant? ________

15. How many children born alive? ________

16. Are you taking birth control pills? No____ Yes____

17. Do you examine your breasts monthly for lumps? No____ Yes____

17a. What was the date of your last menstrual period? Date ________

Check here if you wish to discuss any special problem with the doctor ☐

MEN & WOMEN

18. In the past year have you had any:

|  | Rarely/ Never | Occasionally | Frequently |
|---|---|---|---|
| a. Severe shoulder pain? | X | | |
| b. Severe back pain? | X | | |
| c. Muscle or joint stiffness or pain due to sports, exercise or injury? | | X | |
| d. Pain or swelling in any joints not due to sports, exercise or injury? | X | | |

| | No | Yes |
|---|---|---|
| 19. Do you have dry skin or brittle fingernails? | X | |
| 20. Do you bruise easily? | X | |
| 21. Do you have any moles that have changed in color or in size? | X | |
| 22. Do you have any other skin problems? | X | |
| 23. In the last 3 months have you had: | | |
| a. A fever that lasted more than one day? | X | |
| b. Sores or cuts that were hard to heal? | X | |
| c. Any cold sores (fever blisters)? | X | |
| d. Any lumps in your neck, armpits or groin? | X | |
| e. Do you ever have chills or sweat at night? | X | |
| 24. Have you traveled out of the country in the last 2 years? | X | Yes, Traveled in: ________ |

25. Write in the dates for the shots you have had: Measles ____ Mumps ____ Polio ____ Smallpox ____ Tetanus ____ Typhoid ____

26. Have you had a tuberculin (TB) skin test? No____ Yes X Date 2003

If so, was it negative or positive? Neg X Pos____

27. Have you had an HIV test for AIDS? No X Yes____ Date ________

If so, was it negative or positive? Neg____ Pos____

 PLEASE TURN THIS PAGE STOCK NO. 19-742-4 8/95 

CONFIDENTIAL

Case One, Form 3

# BODY SYSTEMS REVIEW

REMOVE THIS PAGE AFTER COMPLETING QUESTIONNAIRE

| | Question | No | Yes | | VISION / HEARING |
|---|---|---|---|---|---|
| 28. | Do you wear eyeglasses? | X | | | Wears eyeglasses |
| 29. | Do you wear contact lenses? | X | | | Wears contacts |
| 30. | Has your vision changed in the last year? | X | | | Vision changes in last year |

| | Question | Rarely/ Never | Occasionally | Frequently | |
|---|---|---|---|---|---|
| 31. | How often do you have: | | | | |
| a. | Double vision? | X | | | Double vision |
| b. | Blurry vision? | X | | | Blurred vision |
| c. | Watery or itchy eyes? | X | | | Watery/itchy eyes |
| 32. | Do you ever see colored rings around lights? | X | | | Sees halos |
| 33. | Do others tell you you have a hearing problem? | X | | | Hearing problem |
| 34. | Do you have trouble keeping your balance? | X | | | Loses balance |
| 35. | Do you have any discharge from your ears? | X | | | Discharge from ears |
| 36. | Do you ever feel dizzy or have motion sickness? | X | | | Dizzy / motion sickness |

| | Question | No | Yes | |
|---|---|---|---|---|
| 37. | Do you have any problems with your hearing? | X | | Hearing Problems |
| 38. | Do you ever have ringing in your ears? | X | | Ringing in ears |

| | Question | Rarely/ Never | Occasionally | Frequently | NOSE / THROAT / RESPIRATORY |
|---|---|---|---|---|---|
| 39. | How often do you have: | | | | |
| a. | Head colds? | | X | | Head colds |
| b. | Chest colds? | | X | | Chest colds |
| c. | Runny nose? | | X | | Runny nose |
| d. | Stuffed up nose? | | X | | Head congestion |
| e. | Sore/hoarse throat? | X | | | Sore / hoarse throat |
| f. | Bad coughing spells? | X | | | Coughing spells |
| g. | Sneezing spells? | X | | | Sneezing spells |
| h. | Trouble breathing? | X | | | Trouble breathing |
| i. | Nose bleeds? | X | | | Nose bleeds |
| j. | Cough blood? | X | | | Cough blood |

| | Question | No | Yes | |
|---|---|---|---|---|
| 40. | Have you ever worked or spent time: | | | |
| a. | On a farm? | | X | Worked on a farm |
| b. | In a mine? | X | | Worked in a mine |
| c. | In a laundry or mill? | X | | Worked in a laundry/mill |
| d. | In very dusty places? | X | | Worked in high dust concentrations |
| e. | With or near toxic chemicals? | X | | Exposed to toxic chemicals |
| f. | With or near radioactive materials? | X | | Exposed to radioactive materials |
| g. | With or near asbestos? | X | | Exposed to asbestos |

| | Question | Rarely/ Never | Occasionally | Frequently | CARDIOVASCULAR |
|---|---|---|---|---|---|
| 41. | Do you get out of breath easily when you are active (like climbing stairs)? | X | | | Out of breath quickly when exercising |
| 42. | Do you ever feel light-headed or dizzy? | | X | | Dizziness |
| 43. | Have you ever fainted or passed out? | X | | | Fainted |
| 44. | Do you sometimes feel your heart is racing or beating too fast? | | X | | Rapid heartbeat |
| 45. | When you exercise do you ever get pains in your chest or shoulders? | | | X | Chest/shoulder pains in exercise |
| 46. | Do you have any leg cramps or pain in your thighs or legs when walking? | X | | | Pain in thighs or legs when walking |
| 47. | Do you ever have to sit up at night to breathe easier? | X | | | Sits up at night to breathe easier |
| 48. | Do you use two pillows at night to help you breathe easier? | X | | | Breathing problems during sleep |
| 49. | Would you say you are a restless sleeper? | | X | | Restless sleeper |
| 50. | Are you bothered by leg cramps at night? | X | | | Leg cramps at night |
| 51. | Do you sometimes have swollen ankles or feet? | X | | | Swollen ankles/feet |

| | Question | Rarely/ Never | Occasionally | Frequently | DIGESTIVE |
|---|---|---|---|---|---|
| 52. | How often, if ever: | | | | |
| a. | Are you nauseated (sick to your stomach)? | X | | | Nauseated |
| b. | Do you have stomach pains? | X | | | Stomach pains |
| c. | Do you burp a lot after eating? | X | | | Burps after eating |
| d. | Do you have heartburn? | | X | | Heartburn |
| e. | Do you have trouble swallowing your food? | X | | | Trouble swallowing food |
| f. | Have you vomited blood? | X | | | Vomited blood |
| g. | Are you constipated? | X | | | Constipated |
| h. | Do you have diarrhea (watery stools)? | X | | | Diarrhea |
| i. | Are your bowel movements painful? | X | | | Painful bowel movements |
| j. | Are your bowel movements bloody? | X | | | Bloody bowel movements |
| k. | Are your bowel movements dark or black? | X | | | Dark bowel movements |

53. Have you ever had a sigmoidoscopy? No X Yes____ Date____ Date of last sigmoidoscopy?

**PLEASE TURN TO BACK PAGE AND COMPLETE QUESTIONS ON NUTRITION.**

Case One, Form 3

Andrus/Clini-Rec®

BIBBERO SYSTEMS, INC.

COMPREHENSIVE
PHYSICAL EXAMINATION
MALE OR FEMALE
NEW OR ESTABLISHED PATIENT
CPT # 99201 - 99215

(For Office Use Only)

NAME Shapiro, Ivan AGE 59 YRS. OLD TODAY'S DATE 1/5/05 DATE OF BIRTH 3/6/45

Key: [O] Neg. Findings [+] Positive Findings [X] Omitted [✔] See Notes/CIRCLE WORDS OF IMPORTANCE & EXPLAIN

| | | |
|---|---|---|
| 1 GEN. APPEARANCE | [ ] | Apparent Age/Nutrition/Development/Mental & Emotional Status/Gait/Posture/Distress/Speech – |
| 2 HEAD / SCALP | [ ] | Size/Shape/Tender over Sinuses/Hair/Alopecia/Eruption/Masses/Bruit – |
| 3 EYES | [ ] | Conjunct/Sclerae/Cornea/Pupils/EOM'S/Arcus/Ptosis/Fundi/Tension/Eyelids/Pallor/Light/Bruit – |
| 4 EARS | [ ] | Ext. Canal/TM's/Perforation/Discharge/Tophi/Hearing Problem/Weber/Rinne – |
| 5 NOSE / SINUSES | [ ] | Septum/Obstruction/Turbinates/Discharge – |
| 6 MOUTH / THROAT | [ ] | Odor/Lips/Tongue/Tonsils/Teeth/Dentures/Gums/Pharynx – |
| 7 NECK | [ ] | Adenopathy/Thyroid/Carotids/Trachea/Veins/Masses/Spine/Motion/Bruit – |
| 8 BACK | [ ] | Kyphosis/Scoliosis/Lordosis/Mobility/CVA/Bone/Tenderness – |
| 9 THORAX | [ ] | Symmetry/Movement/Contour/Tender – |
| 10 BREASTS | [ ] | Size/Size-Consistency/Nipples/Areolar/Palpable Mass/Discharge/Tenderness/Nodes/Scars – |
| 11 HEART | [ ] | Rate/Rhythm/Apical Impulse/Thrills/Quality of Sound/Intensity/Splitting/Extra Sounds/ Murmurs – |
| 12 CHEST / LUNGS | [ ] | Excursion/Dullness or Hyperresonance to Percussion/Quality of Breath Sounds/Rales/Wheezing/ Rhonchi/Diaphragm/Rubs/Bruit – |
| 13 ABDOMEN | [ ] | Bowel Sounds/Appearance/Liver/Spleen/Masses/Hernias/Murmurs/Contour/Tenderness/Bruit/ ING Nodes – |
| 14 GROIN | [ ] | Hernia/Inguinal Nodes/Femoral Pulses – |
| 15 MALE GENITALIA | [ ] | Penis/Testes/Scrotum Epididymis/Varicocele/Scars/Discharge – |
| 16 FEMALE GENITALIA | [ ] | Vuvla/Vagina/Cervix/Uterus/Adnexae/Rectocele/Cystocele/Bartholin Gland/Urethra/ Discharge – Pap Smear (if done ✔) ☐ |
| 17 EXTREMITIES | [ ] | Deformity/Clubbing/Cyanosis/Edema/Nails/Peripheral Pulses/Calf Tenderness/Joints for Swelling/ ROM – |
| 18 SKIN | [ ] | Color/Birthmarks/Scars/Texture/Rash/Eczema/Ulcers – |
| 19 NEUROLOGICAL | [ ] | DTR's/Babinski/Cranial Nerves/Motor Abnormalities/Tremor/Paralysis/Sensory Exam – (touch, pin prick, vibration)/Coordination/Romberg – |
| 20 MUSCULAR SYSTEM | [ ] | Strength/Wasting/Development – |
| 21 RECTAL EXAM | [ ] | Sphincter Tone/Hemorrhoids/Fissures/Masses/Prostate/Stool Guaiac (if done ✔) ☐ Pos ☐ Neg – |

Impression: ☐ Check If Normal Physical Examination

Summary: ______________________

______________________

______________________ Signature ______________________ Date ________

CONFIDENTIAL

Case One, Form 3

## COMPREHENSIVE PHYSICAL EXAMINATION
(continued)

(For Office Use Only)

### PHYSICIAN'S NOTES:

| Body Area Number | REMARKS: |
|---|---|
| | |
| | |
| | |
| | |
| | |

R L L R

R L

| | VISION | AUDIOMETRIC TESTING | BLOOD PRESSURE |
|---|---|---|---|
| HEIGHT______ | Without Glasses<br>Far R 20/ L 20/<br>Near R 20/ L 20/ | 250 500 1000<br>R ____ ____ ____<br>L ____ ____ ____ | Sitting<br>R / L / |
| WEIGHT______ | | | |
| BUILD ______ | With Glasses<br>R 20/ L 20/<br>R 20/ L 20/ | 2000 4000 8000<br>R ____ ____ ____<br>L ____ ____ ____ | Standing<br>R / L / |
| PULSE ______ | | | |
| RESP. ______ | Tonometry R______ L______ | | Lying<br>R / L / |
| TEMP. ______ | Colorvision______<br>Peripheral Fields R____ L____ | Gross Hearing ______ | |

| Diagnostic Test: | Results: |
|---|---|
| | |
| | |
| | |
| | |
| | |

The space below is provided for additional information when these data are being forwarded to a hospital, insurance company, a referral physician, etc.

| Significant Comments / Recommendations: | |
|---|---|
| | Physician's Name ______ |
| | Address ______ |
| | ______ |
| | Telephone (area code) ______ |

CONFIDENTIAL

## NUTRITION AND DIET

1. How many meals do you eat each day? .............................. 3 Meals each day
2. Do you usually eat breakfast? .................................... ☐ No ☒ Yes Breakfast
3. Do you diet frequently and/or are you now dieting? ......................... ☒ No ☐ Yes Diets
4. Do you consider yourself .................. ☐ Underweight ☐ Overweight ☒ Just right? Weight
5. Do you snack? ..................... ☐ More than once a day ☒ Usually daily ☐ Rarely? Snacks
6. Do you add salt to your food at the table? ..... ☐ Almost always ☐ Sometimes ☒ Rarely Salts food
7. Check the frequency you eat the following types of foods:

| | More than once daily | Daily | 3 times weekly | Once weekly | Twice monthly | Less or never |
|---|---|---|---|---|---|---|
| a. Whole grain or enriched bread or cereal | X | | | | | |
| b. Milk, cheese, or other dairy products | | X | | | | |
| c. Eggs | | | | X | | |
| d. Meat, Poultry, Fish | | | X | | | |
| e. Beans, Peas, or other legumes | | X | | | | |
| f. Citrus | X | | | | | |
| g. Dark green or deep yellow vegetables | | X | | | | |

List any food supplements or vitamins you take regularly: One a day vitamins

Additional Patient Comments: ______

Thanks for completing this questionnaire. Please review for skipped questions, sign your name on the space to the right and return it to the physician or assistant. If you wish to add any information, please write it in the spaces provided above.

Patient's Signature ______

Physician's Notes: ______

C O N F I D E N T I A L

Case One, Form 4

Patient Information Sheet

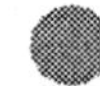 **Blackburn Primary Care Associates** 

1990 Turquoise Drive
Blackburn, WI 54937
(555)555-1234

**REGISTRATION**
(PLEASE PRINT)

Home Phone: 555-297-1349

Today's Date: 1/5/05

## PATIENT INFORMATION

Name SHAPIRO (Last Name) IVAN (First Name) R. (Initial) Soc. Sec.# 591-23-1971

Address 3242 Kentucky Lane

City Blackburn State WI Zip 54938

Single ___ Married ✔ Widowed ___ Separated ___ Divorced ___ Sex M ✔ F ___ Age 59 Birthdate 3/6/45

Patient Employed by SELF Occupation CARPENTER

Business Address as above Business Phone as above

By whom were you referred? ___

In case of emergency who should be notified? MARY ANNE SHAPIRO (Name) (wife) (Relation to Patient) Phone 555-297-1349

## PRIMARY INSURANCE

Person Responsible for Account SHAPIRO (Last Name) IVAN (First Name) R. (Initial)

Relation to Patient SELF Birthdate 3/6/45 Soc. Sec.# 591-23-1971

Address (if different from patient's) same Phone ___

City ___ State ___ Zip ___

Person Responsible Employed by SELF Occupation CARPENTER

Business Address as above Business Phone ___

Insurance Company Blue Cross / Blue Shield

Contract # none Group # none Subscriber # 591-23-1971A

Name of other dependents covered under this plan MARY ANNE SHAPIRO

## ADDITIONAL INSURANCE

Is patient covered by additional insurance? ___ Yes ✔ No

Subscriber Name ___ Relation to Patient ___ Birthdate ___

Address (if different from patient's) ___ Phone ___

City ___ State ___ Zip ___

Subscriber Employed by ___ Business Phone ___

Insurance Company ___ Soc. Sec.# ___

Contract # ___ Group # ___ Subscriber # ___

Name of other dependents covered under this plan ___

## ASSIGNMENT AND RELEASE

I, the undersigned, certify that I (or my dependent) have insurance coverage with *Blue Cross Blue Shield* (Name of Insurance Company(ies)) and assign directly to Dr. Blackburn Primary Care Associates insurance benefits, if any, otherwise payable to me for services rendered. I understand that I am financially responsible for all charges whether or not paid by insurance. I hereby authorize the doctor to release all information necessary to secure the payment of benefits. I authorize the use of this signature on all insurance submissions.

*Ivan Shapiro* (Responsible Party Signature) *self* (Relationship) *01/05/05* (Date)

Case One, Form 5

# Patient Encounter Form

## Blackburn Primary Care Associates

1990 Turquoise Drive
Blackburn, WI 54937
(555) 555-1234

FED. I.D. # 52-1963787

PAT. INFO.

| ACCT. NO. | PATIENT'S LAST NAME | FIRST | M.I. | DATE OF BIRTH | SEX | TODAY'S DATE |
|---|---|---|---|---|---|---|
| | SHAPIRO | IVAN | R | 3/6/45 | ☒ M ☐ F | 01/05/05 |

| INSURANCE | COPAY | DISABILITY RELATED TO: ☐ ACCIDENT ☐ INDUSTRIAL ☐ ILLNESS ☐ OTHER |
|---|---|---|
| BCBS | | DATES SYMPTOMS APPEARED, INCEPTION OF PREGNANCY, OR ACCIDENT OCCURRED: / / |

| ✓ | DESCRIPTION | CPT/MD | FEE | ✓ | DESCRIPTION | CPT/MD | FEE | ✓ | DESCRIPTION | CPT/MD | FEE |
|---|---|---|---|---|---|---|---|---|---|---|---|
| | OFFICE VISITS-NEW PATIENTS | | | | SPECIAL SERVICES | | | | SURGERY | | |
| | Focused | 99201 | | | Drivers Physical | 99214 | | | Toenail Removal | 11750 | |
| | Expanded | 99202 | | | Pelvic/Breast Exam | 99214 | | | Cryosurgery | 17200 | |
| | Detailed | 99203 | | | Industrial | 99214 | | | I & D | 10060 | |
| | Comprehensive | 99204 | | | | | | | Drainage Paronychia | 10060 | |
| X | Complex | 99205 | | | IMMUNIZATIONS | | | | Enucleation Ext. Hemorrhoid | 46320 | |
| | | | | | DtaP | 90700 | | | I & D Abscess/Cyst | 10060 | |
| | | | | | DPT | 90701 | | | Podophyllom | 17100 | |
| | OFFICE VISITS - EST. PATIENTS | | | | DT | 90702 | | | Removal Foreign Body | 10120 | |
| | Minimal | 99211 | | | Td (Tetanus Booster) | 90703 | | | Wart Removal | 17110 | |
| | Focused | 99212 | | | MMR | 90707 | | | Destr. Single Lesion Face | 17000 | |
| | Expanded | 99213 | | | Mumps | 90704 | | | 2nd and 3rd Lesion Face | 17001 | |
| | Detailed | 99214 | | | Pneumococcal | 90732 | | | Destr. Single Lesion Body | 17106 | |
| | Comprehensive | 99215 | | | Rubella | 90706 | | | 2nd and 3rd Lesion Body | 17003 | |
| | | | | | Polio (TOPV) | 90712 | | | Lesion Rem. Excision | | |
| | | | | | PPD | 86580 | | | Anoscopy | 46600 | |
| | PREVENTIVE HEALTH CARE NEW PT. | EST. PT | | | TB Tine Test | 86585 | | | Flex. Scope with Sig. | 45330 | |
| | Eval./Mgmt. > 1 Yr 99381 | 99391 | | | Hib | 90737 | | | Vasectomy | 55250 | |
| | Early Child 1 - 4 Yrs 99382 | 99392 | | | | | | | Therapeutic Abor. | 59840 | |
| | Late Child 5 - 11 Yrs 99383 | 99393 | | | | | | | Removal Foreign Body of Eye | 65205 | |
| | Adolescent 12 - 17 Yrs 99384 | 99394 | | | OFFICE PROCEDURES | | | | | | |
| | Eval./Mgmt. 18 - 39 Yrs 99385 | 99395 | | | Audiometry | 92551 | | | SUPPLIES | | |
| | Eval./Mgmt. 40 - 64 Yrs 99386 | 99396 | | | Diathermy (Ultrasound) | 97024 | | | Ace Wrap | 99070 | |
| | Eval./Mgmt. 65 - Over 99387 | 99397 | | X | EKG Tracing & Interp. | 93000 | | | Cast Material | 99070 | |
| | | | | | Intermed Joint Injection | 20605 | | | Cervical Collar | 99070 | |
| | | | | | Major Joint Injection | 20610 | | | Elastic Bandage | 99070 | |
| | HOSP./SNF/HOME VISITS | | | | Nebulizer TX | 94664 | | | Splint/Sling | 99070 | |
| | House Calls | 99341 | | | Rem. Impact. Cer. | 69210 | | | Sterile Dressing | 99070 | |
| | ER Visit | 9928__ | | | Spirometry | 94010 | | | Surgical Tray | 99070 | |
| | Init. Hosp. Care | 99222 | | | Stress Test | 93015 | | | | | |
| | Sub. Hosp. Care | 99232 | | | Trigger Pt. Inj. | 20550 | | | | | |
| | SNF, Sub. Care | 99312 | | | Eye Wash | 65205* | | | | | |
| | | | | | | | | | | | |
| | | | | | LABORATORY | | | | | | |
| | INJECTIONS | | | | Throat Culture | 87060 | | | | | |
| | Allergy | 95125 | | | Glucose Blood | 82947 | | | | | |
| | B-12 | J3420 | | | Glucose Stick | 82948 | | | | | |
| | Flu Shot | 90724 | | | UA Pregnancy | 81025 | | | | | |
| | Gamma Globulin | 90741 | | | Occult Blood, Stool | 82270 | | | | | |
| | Hormone | | | | Rapid Strep | 86588 | | | | | |
| | Depo Provera | J1055 | | | Smear | 88150 | | | | | |
| | Kenalog 40-60 mg | J3301 | | X | UA Dip | 81002 | | | | | |
| | Morphine/Demerol | J2270 | | | Urinalysis | 81000 | | | | | |
| | Phenergan | J2550 | | | Venipuncture | 36415 | | | | | |
| | Celestone | J0700 | | | Wet Mount, Smear | 87210 | | | | | |
| | Hep B, newborn to 11 years | 90744 | | | Wet Mount KOH | 87220 | | | | | |
| | Hep B, 11 - 19 years | 90745 | | X | Collect/Handing | ~~99000~~ | 36415 | | | | |
| | Hep B, 20 years and above | 90746 | | | | | | | | | |
| | Rocephin/Claforan | J0696 | | | MISCELLANEOUS | | | | | | |
| | Iron | J1760 | | | Pre-OP | 993__ | | | | | |
| | Lidocaine NCL | J2000 | | | After Hours | 99050 | | | | | |
| | Admin of INJ | J0110 | | | Sunday/Holidays | 99054 | | | | | |
| | Unlist INJ | 90782 | | | Cast Removal | 29705 | | | | | |
| | Drug | | | | Norplant Insertion | 11975 | | | | | |
| | Dose | | | | Norplant Kit | 99070 | | | | | |

**DIAGNOSIS:** ICD-9

| | | | | |
|---|---|---|---|---|
| ☐ Abscess Cellulitis . . . 682.9 | ☐ C.T.S. . . . 354.0 | ☐ Flu Shot Only . . . V04.8 | ☐ Internal Derangement Knee . 717.9 | ☐ Prostatitis . . . 601.9 |
| ☐ Abdominal Pain . . . 789.0 | ☐ CAD . . . 746.85 | ☐ Flu Vac . . . V04.8 | ☐ Labyrinthitis . . . 386.30 | ☐ Psoriasis . . . 696.1 |
| ☐ Abrasions . . . 919.0 | ☐ CA-Prostate . . . 185 | ☐ Flu W/Resp. Manifest . . . 487.1 | ☐ Laceration Open Wound . 879.8__ | ☐ Rheumatoid Arthritis . . . 714.0 |
| ☐ Acne . . . 706.1 | ☐ Cardiac Arrhythmia . . . 427.9 | ☐ Folliculitis . . . 704.8 | ☐ Levator Scapular Syndrome 726.90 | ☐ Sciatica . . . 724.3 |
| ☐ ADD . . . 314.00 | ☐ Cataracts . . . 366.9 | ☐ FX ______ | ☐ Menopausal Disorder . . . 627.9 | ☐ Sacroiliac Sprain . . . 846.1 |
| ☐ Alcoholism . . . 303.90 | ☐ Chest Pain . . . 786.50 | ☐ Gallbladder Disease . . . 575.9 | ☐ Metabolic Diff. . . . 277.8 | ☐ Sinusitis, Acute . . . 461.9 |
| ☐ Allergic Rhinitis . . . 477.9 | ☐ Congestive Heart Failure 428.0 | ☐ Ganglion . . . 727.43 | ☐ Migraine . . . 346.90 | ☐ Smoking Cessation . . . 305.10 |
| ☐ Allergy, Unsp . . . 995.3 | ☐ Conjunctivitis . . . 372.30 | ☐ Gastroenteritis . . . 558.9 | ☐ Mitral Valve Disorder . . . 424.0 | ☐ Sprain ______ |
| ☐ Anemia . . . 285.9 | ☐ Constipation . . . 564.0 | ☐ Gout . . . 274.9 | ☐ Myalgia and Myositis . . . 729.1 | ☐ SQ. Cell CA-Face . . . 173.3 |
| ☐ Angina Pectoris . . . 413.9 | ☐ Consult Vasc. . . . V65.8 | ☐ Gyn Exam . . . V72.3 | ☐ Noninf. Gastroenterit. . . . 558.9 | ☐ Sterilization . . . V25.2 |
| ☐ Anxiety Depression . . . 300.4 | ☐ Convulsions . . . 780.3 | ☐ Headache Tension . . . 307.81 | ☐ Obesity . . . 278.0 | ☐ Stye . . . 373.11 |
| ☐ Anxiety State . . . 300.00 | ☐ COPD . . . 496 | ☐ Hemorrhoids Ext. . . . 455.3 | ☐ Osteoarthrosis . . . 715.00 | ☐ TB Exposure . . . V01.1 |
| ☐ ASCVD . . . 429.2 | ☐ Coronary Atherosclerosis . 414.0 | ☐ Hepatitis . . . 573.3 | ☐ Osteoporosis . . . 733.00 | ☐ Tendonitis . . . 726.90 |
| ☐ Asthma W/O Status Asthma 493.90 | ☐ CVA . . . 436 | ☐ Hernia-Inguinal . . . 550.90 | ☐ Otitis Externa . . . 380.10 | ☐ Tinea . . . 110.9 |
| ☐ Atten Surg. Dressing/Suture V58.3 | ☐ Cyst Sebaceous . . . 706.2 | ☐ Herpes Zoster . . . 053.9 | ☐ Otitis Media . . . 382.9 | ☐ Tonsillitis, Acute . . . 463 |
| ☐ BCP Consult . . . V25.9 | ☐ Dermatitis . . . 692.9 | ☐ Hyperlipidemia . . . 272.4 | ☐ P.I.D. . . . 614.9 | ☐ URI, Acute . . . 465.9 |
| ☐ BPH . . . 600 | ☐ Diabetes, Uncomp. Adult 250.00 | ☒ Hypertension . . . 401.9 | ☐ Peptic Ulcer . . . 533.90 | ☐ Urine Tract Infection . . . 599.0 |
| ☐ Bronchitis, Acute . . . 466.0 | ☐ Diabetes, Complicated . . 250.90 | ☐ Hyperthyroidism . . . 242.9 | ☐ Pharyngitis, Acute . . . 462 | ☐ Vaginitis . . . 616.10 |
| ☐ Bronchitis, Chronic . . . 491.9 | ☐ Disc Degeneration . . . 722.6 | ☐ Hypothyroidism . . . 244.9 | ☐ Pneumonia, Viral . . . 480.9 | ☐ Well Adult Medical Exam V70.9 |
| ☐ Burn ______ 949.0 | ☐ Duodenal Ulcer . . . 532.90 | ☐ Impacted Cerumen . . . 380.4 | ☐ Poison Oak . . . 692.6 | ☐ Well Child Health Exam . V20.2 |
| ☐ Bursitis . . . 727.3 | ☐ Dysmenorrhea . . . 625.3 | ☐ Impetigo . . . 684 | ☐ Premarital B-Test . . . V70.3 | |
| | ☐ Fatigue . . . 780.7 | ☐ Ingrown Toenail . . . 703.0 | ☐ Pregnancy Test, Unconf. . V72.4 | |

| DIAGNOSIS (If not checked above) ICD-9 | PHYSICIAN SIGNATURE | TODAY'S FEE | $ |
|---|---|---|---|
| Ischemic heart disease, c̄ Coronary occlusion | | PAYMENT | |
| PLEASE REMEMBER THAT PAYMENT IS YOUR OBLIGATION REGARDLESS OF INSURANCE OR OTHER THIRD PARTY INVOLVEMENT. | PAYMENT BY ☐ CASH ☐ CREDIT CARD ☐ CHECK # ______ | BALANCE DUE | |

Case One, Form 6

# FEE SCHEDULE

## BLACKBURN PRIMARY CARE ASSOCIATES
## 1990 TURQUOISE DRIVE
## BLACKBURN, WI 54937

**Federal Tax ID Number:** **52-1963787**

**BCBS Group Number:** **14982**
**Medicare Group Number:** **14982**

## OFFICE VISIT, NEW PATIENT

| | |
|---|---|
| Focused, 99201 | $ 45.00 |
| Expanded, 99202 | $ 53.00 |
| Detailed, 99203 | $ 60.00 |
| Comprehensive, 99204 | $ 95.00 |
| Complex, 99205 | $195.00 |
| Consultation, 99245 | $250.00 |

## OFFICE VISIT, ESTABLISHED PATIENT

| | |
|---|---|
| Minimal, 99211 | $ 40.00 |
| Focused, 99212 | $ 48.00 |
| Expanded, 99213 | $ 55.00 |
| Detailed, 99214 | $ 65.00 |
| Comprehensive, 99215 | $195.00 |

## OFFICE PROCEDURES

| | |
|---|---|
| EKG, 12 Lead, 93000 | $ 55.00 |
| Stress EKG, Treadmill, 93015 | $295.00 |
| Sigmoidoscopy, Flex., 45330 | $145.00 |
| Spirometry, 94010 | $ 50.00 |
| Cerumen Removal, 69210 | $ 40.00 |
| Collection & Handling | |
| Lab Specimen, 99000 | $ 9.00 |
| Venipuncture, 36415 | $ 9.00 |
| Urinalysis, 81000 | $ 20.00 |
| Urinalysis, 81002 (Dip Only) | $ 12.00 |
| Influenza Injection, 90724 | $ 20.00 |
| Pneumococcal Injection, 90732 | $ 20.00 |
| Oral Polio, 90712 | $ 15.00 |
| DTaP, 90700 | $ 20.00 |
| Tetanus Toxoid, 90703 | $ 15.00 |
| MMR, 90707 | $ 25.00 |
| Hib, 90737 | $ 20.00 |
| Hepatitis B, newborn to age 11 years, 90744 | $ 60.00 |
| Hepatitis B, 11-19 years, 90745 | $ 60.00 |
| Hepatitis B, 20 years and above 90746 | $ 60.00 |
| Intramuscular Injection, 90788 | |
| Penicillin | $ 30.00 |
| Ceftriaxone | $ 25.00 |
| Solu-Medrol | $ 23.00 |
| Vitamin B-12 | $ 13.00 |
| Subcutaneous Injection, 90782 | |
| Epinephrine | $ 18.00 |
| Sus-Pherine | $ 25.00 |
| Insulin, U-100 | $ 15.00 |

## COMMON DIAGNOSIS CODES

| | |
|---|---|
| Ischemic Heart Disease | 414.9 |
| w/o myocardial infarction | 411.89 |
| w/ coronary occlusion | 411.81 |
| Hypertension, Malignant | 401.0 |
| Benign | 401.1 |
| Unspecified | 401.9 |
| w/ congest. heart failure | 402.91 |
| Asthma, Bronchial | 493.9 |
| w/ COPD | 493.2 |
| allergic, w/ S.A. | 493.91 |
| allergic, w/o S.A. | 493.90 |
| Kyphosis | 737.10 |
| w/ osteoporosis | 733.0 |
| Osteoporosis | 733.00 |
| Otitis Media, Acute | 382.9 |
| Chronic | 382.9 |
| Well Child Health Exam | V20.2 |
| Well Adult Medical Exam | V70.9 |

Case One, Form 7

PLEASE DO NOT STAPLE IN THIS AREA

APPROVED OMB-0938-0008

CARRIER

PICA

# HEALTH INSURANCE CLAIM FORM

PICA

1. MEDICARE (Medicare #) MEDICAID (Medicaid #) CHAMPUS (Sponsor's SSN) CHAMPVA (VA File #) GROUP HEALTH PLAN (SSN or ID) FECA BLK LUNG (SSN) OTHER (ID)

1a. INSURED'S I.D. NUMBER (FOR PROGRAM IN ITEM 1)

2. PATIENT'S NAME (Last Name, First Name, Middle Initial)

3. PATIENT'S BIRTHDATE MM DD YY SEX M F

4. INSURED'S NAME (Last Name, First Name, Middle Initial)

5. PATIENT'S ADDRESS (No., Street)

6. PATIENT RELATIONSHIP TO INSURED Self Spouse Child Other

7. INSURED'S ADDRESS (No., Street)

CITY STATE

8. PATIENT STATUS Single Married Other

CITY STATE

ZIP CODE TELEPHONE (Include Area Code) ( )

Employed Full-Time Student Part-Time Student

ZIP CODE TELEPHONE (Include Area Code) ( )

9. OTHER INSURED'S NAME (Last Name, First Name, Middle Initial)

10. IS PATIENT'S CONDITION RELATED TO:

11. INSURED'S POLICY GROUP OR FECA NUMBER

a. OTHER INSURED'S POLICY OR GROUP NUMBER

a. EMPLOYMENT? (CURRENT OR PREVIOUS) YES NO

a. INSURED'S DATE OF BIRTH MM DD YY SEX M F

b. OTHER INSURED'S DATE OF BIRTH MM DD YY SEX M F

b. AUTO ACCIDENT? PLACE (State) YES NO

b. EMPLOYER'S NAME OR SCHOOL NAME

c. EMPLOYER'S NAME OR SCHOOL NAME

c. OTHER ACCIDENT? YES NO

c. INSURANCE PLAN NAME OR PROGRAM NAME

d. INSURANCE PLAN NAME OR PROGRAM NAME

10d. RESERVED FOR LOCAL USE

d. IS THERE ANOTHER HEALTH BENEFIT PLAN? YES NO *If yes, return to and complete item 9a-d.*

**READ BACK OF FORM BEFORE COMPLETING & SIGNING THIS FORM.**

12. PATIENT'S OR AUTHORIZED PERSON'S SIGNATURE I authorize the release of any medical or other information necessary to process this claim. I also request payment of government benefits either to myself or to the party who accepts assignment below.

SIGNED ______ DATE ______

13. INSURED'S OR AUTHORIZED PERSON'S SIGNATURE I authorize payment of medical benefits to the undersigned physician or supplier for services described below.

SIGNED ______

PATIENT AND INSURED INFORMATION

14. DATE OF CURRENT: MM DD YY ILLNESS (First symptom) OR INJURY (Accident) OR PREGNANCY (LMP)

15. IF PATIENT HAS HAD SAME OR SIMILAR ILLNESS, GIVE FIRST DATE MM DD YY

16. DATES PATIENT UNABLE TO WORK IN CURRENT OCCUPATION FROM MM DD YY TO MM DD YY

17. NAME OF REFERRING PHYSICIAN OR OTHER SOURCE

17a. I.D. NUMBER OF REFERRING PHYSICIAN

18. HOSPITALIZATION DATES RELATED TO CURRENT SERVICES FROM MM DD YY TO MM DD YY

19. RESERVED FOR LOCAL USE

20. OUTSIDE LAB? YES NO $ CHARGES

21. DIAGNOSIS OR NATURE OF ILLNESS OR INJURY. (RELATE ITEMS 1,2,3 OR 4 TO ITEM 24E BY LINE)

1. ____ . __ 3. ____ . __

2. ____ . __ 4. ____ . __

22. MEDICAID RESUBMISSION CODE ORIGINAL REF. NO.

23. PRIOR AUTHORIZATION NUMBER

| 24. A DATE(S) OF SERVICE From MM DD YY To MM DD YY | B Place of Service | C Type of Service | D PROCEDURES, SERVICES, OR SUPPLIES (Explain Unusual Circumstances) CPT/HCPCS MODIFIER | E DIAGNOSIS CODE | F $ CHARGES | G DAYS OR UNITS | H EPSDT Family Plan | I EMG | J COB | K RESERVED FOR LOCAL USE |
|---|---|---|---|---|---|---|---|---|---|---|
| 1 | | | | | | | | | | |
| 2 | | | | | | | | | | |
| 3 | | | | | | | | | | |
| 4 | | | | | | | | | | |
| 5 | | | | | | | | | | |
| 6 | | | | | | | | | | |

25. FEDERAL TAX I.D. NUMBER SSN EIN

26. PATIENTS ACCOUNT NUMBER

27. ACCEPT ASSIGNMENT? (For govt. claims, see back) YES NO

28. TOTAL CHARGE $

29. AMOUNT PAID $

30. BALANCE DUE $

31. SIGNATURE OF PHYSICIAN OR SUPPLIER INCLUDING DEGREES OR CREDENTIALS (I certify that the statements on the reverse apply to this bill and are made a part thereof.)

SIGNED DATE

32. NAME AND ADDRESS OF FACILITY WHERE SERVICES WERE RENDERED (If other than home or office)

33. PHYSICIAN'S, SUPPLIER'S BILLING NAME, ADDRESS, ZIP CODE & PHONE #

PIN # GRP#

PHYSICIAN OR SUPPLIER INFORMATION

**(APPROVED BY AMA COUNCIL ON MEDICAL SERVICE 8/88)**

Form 124OLM

***PLEASE PRINT OR TYPE***

FORM HCFA-1500 (12-90) FORM OWCP-1500 FORM RRB-1500

Case Two, Form 8

## OUTLINE FORMAT PROGRESS NOTES

Patient Name Johnson, Raymond

| Prob. No. or Letter | DATE | S Subjective | O Objective | A Assess | P Plans | Page 3 |
|---|---|---|---|---|---|---|

Start each Progress Note (Subjective, Objective, Assessment and Plans) at the appropriate shaded column to create an outline form. Write through the intervening columns to the right margin of the page.

ANDRUS/CLINI-REC® PRIMARY CARE CHARTING SYSTEM FORM NO. 26-7115, ©1976 BIBBERO SYSTEMS, INC., PETALUMA, CA.

Courtesy of Bibbero Systems, Inc., Petaluma, California.

## GIRLS: BIRTH TO 36 MONTHS PHYSICAL GROWTH NCHS PERCENTILES*

Case Three, Form 9

NAME ____________________ RECORD # ____________

AGE (MONTHS)

LENGTH

WEIGHT

MOTHER'S STATURE ____________ GESTATIONAL AGE ________ WEEKS

FATHER'S STATURE ____________

| DATE | AGE | LENGTH | WEIGHT | HEAD CIRC. | COMMENT |
|---|---|---|---|---|---|
| | BIRTH | | | | |
| | | | | | |
| | | | | | |
| | | | | | |
| | | | | | |
| | | | | | |
| | | | | | |
| | | | | | |
| | | | | | |
| | | | | | |

*Adapted from: Hamill PVV, Drizd TA, Johnson CL, Reed RB, Roche AF, Moore WM: Physical growth: National Center for Health Statistics percentiles. AM J CLIN NUTR 32:607-629, 1979. Data from the Fels Longitudinal Study, Wright State University School of Medicine, Yellow Springs, Ohio.

Case Three, Form 10

# OUTLINE FORMAT PROGRESS NOTES

Patient Name Soto, Robin

| Prob. No. or Letter | DATE | S Subjective | O Objective | A Assess | P Plans | Page 2 |
|---|---|---|---|---|---|---|

Start each Progress Note (Subjective, Objective, Assessment and Plans) at the appropriate shaded column to create an outline form. Write through the intervening columns to the right margin of the page.

Case Three, Form 11

# Patient Information Sheet

 **Blackburn Primary Care Associates** 

1990 Turquoise Drive
Blackburn, WI 54937
(555)555-1234

**REGISTRATION**
(PLEASE PRINT)

Home Phone: 555-898-6154

Today's Date: 2/25/00

## PATIENT INFORMATION

Name: Soto (Last Name) Robin (First Name) A (Initial) Soc. Sec.# 765-19-3190

Address: 28 Lakeland Drive APT 308

City: Blackburn State: WI Zip: 54936

Single ✔ Married ___ Widowed ___ Separated ___ Divorced ___ Sex M ___ F ✔ Age 4 1/2 months Birthdate 10-08-99

Patient Employed by: N/A Occupation ___

Business Address ___ Business Phone ___

By whom were you referred? ___

In case of emergency who should be notified? Janet Soto (Name) Mother (Relation to Patient) Phone 555-898-6154

## PRIMARY INSURANCE

Person Responsible for Account: Soto (Last Name) Janet (First Name) M. (Initial)

Relation to Patient: Mother Birthdate 12-11-62 Soc. Sec.# 219-54-3131

Address (if different from patient's): Same Phone ___

City ___ State ___ Zip ___

Person Responsible Employed by: W.B.Saunders Occupation: Editor

Business Address: 3500 Barnum Place 54937 Business Phone: 555-263-3500

Insurance Company: Travelers

Contract #: 31965AR21 Group #: TWB198 Subscriber #: 219543131WB

Name of other dependents covered under this plan: none

## ADDITIONAL INSURANCE

Is patient covered by additional insurance? ___ Yes ✔ No

Subscriber Name ___ Relation to Patient ___ Birthdate ___

Address (if different from patient's) ___ Phone ___

City ___ State ___ Zip ___

Subscriber Employed by ___ Business Phone ___

Insurance Company ___ Soc. Sec.# ___

Contract # ___ Group # ___ Subscriber # ___

Name of other dependents covered under this plan ___

## ASSIGNMENT AND RELEASE

I, the undersigned, certify that I (or my dependent) have insurance coverage with *Travelers* (Name of Insurance Company(ies)) and assign directly to Dr. *Blackburn Primary* insurance benefits, if any, otherwise payable to me for services rendered. I understand that I am financially responsible for all charges whether or not paid by insurance. I hereby authorize the doctor to release all information necessary to secure the payment of benefits. I authorize the use of this signature on all insurance submissions.

*Janet Soto* (Responsible Party Signature) *Mother* (Relationship) *2/25/00* (Date)

Case Three, Form 12

# Patient Encounter Form

## Blackburn Primary Care Associates

1990 Turquoise Drive
Blackburn, WI 54937
(555) 555-1234

FED. I.D. # 52-1963787

**PAT. INFO.**

| ACCT. NO. | PATIENT'S LAST NAME | FIRST | M.I. | DATE OF BIRTH | SEX | TODAY'S DATE |
|---|---|---|---|---|---|---|
| | SOTO | ROBIN | A | 10/8/99 | ☐ M ☒ F | 2/25/00 |

| INSURANCE | COPAY | DISABILITY RELATED TO: ☐ ACCIDENT ☐ INDUSTRIAL ☐ ILLNESS ☐ OTHER |
|---|---|---|
| Travelers | | DATES SYMPTOMS APPEARED, INCEPTION OF PREGNANCY, OR ACCIDENT OCCURRED: / / |

| ✓ | DESCRIPTION | CPT/MD | FEE |
|---|---|---|---|
| | **OFFICE VISITS-NEW PATIENTS** | | |
| | Focused | 99201 | |
| | Expanded | 99202 | |
| | Detailed | 99203 | |
| | Comprehensive | 99204 | |
| | Complex | 99205 | |
| | | | |
| | **OFFICE VISITS - EST. PATIENTS** | | |
| | Minimal | 99211 | |
| | Focused | 99212 | |
| X | Expanded | 99213 | |
| | Detailed | 99214 | |
| | Comprehensive | 99215 | |
| | | | |
| | **PREVENTIVE HEALTH CARE** NEW PT. | EST. PT | |
| | Eval./Mgmt. > 1 Yr 99381 | 99391 | |
| | Early Child 1 - 4 Yrs 99382 | 99392 | |
| | Late Child 5 - 11 Yrs 99383 | 99393 | |
| | Adolescent 12 - 17 Yrs 99384 | 99394 | |
| | Eval./Mgmt. 18 - 39 Yrs 99385 | 99395 | |
| | Eval./Mgmt. 40 - 64 Yrs 99386 | 99396 | |
| | Eval./Mgmt. 65 - Over 99387 | 99397 | |
| | | | |
| | **HOSP./SNF/HOME VISITS** | | |
| | House Calls | 99341 | |
| | ER Visit | 9928___ | |
| | Init. Hosp. Care | 99222 | |
| | Sub. Hosp. Care | 99232 | |
| | SNF, Sub. Care | 99312 | |
| | | | |
| | **INJECTIONS** | | |
| | Allergy | 95125 | |
| | B-12 | J3420 | |
| | Flu Shot | 90724 | |
| | Gamma Globulin | 90741 | |
| | Hormone | | |
| | Depo Provera | J1055 | |
| | Kenalog 40-60 mg | J3301 | |
| | Morphine/Demerol | J2270 | |
| | Phenergan | J2550 | |
| | Celestone | J0700 | |
| | Hep B, newborn to 11 years | 90744 | |
| | Hep B, 11 - 19 years | 90745 | |
| | Hep B, 20 years and above | 90746 | |
| | Rocephin/Claforan | J0696 | |
| | Iron | J1760 | |
| | Lidocaine NCL | J2000 | |
| | Admin of INJ | J0110 | |
| | Unlist INJ | 90782 | |
| | Drug | | |
| | Dose | | |

| ✓ | DESCRIPTION | CPT/MD | FEE |
|---|---|---|---|
| | **SPECIAL SERVICES** | | |
| | Drivers Physical | 99214 | |
| | Pelvic/Breast Exam | 99214 | |
| | Industrial | 99214 | |
| | | | |
| | **IMMUNIZATIONS** | | |
| X | DtaP | 90700 | |
| | DPT | 90701 | |
| | DT | 90702 | |
| | Td (Tetanus Booster) | 90703 | |
| | MMR | 90707 | |
| | Mumps | 90704 | |
| | Pneumococcal | 90732 | |
| | Rubella | 90706 | |
| X | Polio (TOPV) | 90712 | |
| | PPD | 86580 | |
| | TB Tine Test | 86585 | |
| X | Hib | 90737 | |
| | | | |
| | **OFFICE PROCEDURES** | | |
| | Audiometry | 92551 | |
| | Diathermy (Ultrasound) | 97024 | |
| | EKG Tracing & Interp. | 93000 | |
| | Intermed Joint Injection | 20605 | |
| | Major Joint Injection | 20610 | |
| | Nebulizer TX | 94664 | |
| | Rem. Impact. Cer. | 69210 | |
| | Spirometry | 94010 | |
| | Stress Test | 93015 | |
| | Trigger Pt. Inj. | 20550 | |
| | Eye Wash | 65205* | |
| | **LABORATORY** | | |
| | Throat Culture | 87060 | |
| | Glucose Blood | 82947 | |
| | Glucose Stick | 82948 | |
| | UA Pregnancy | 81025 | |
| | Occult Blood, Stool | 82270 | |
| | Rapid Strep | 86588 | |
| | Smear | 88150 | |
| | UA Dip | 81002 | |
| | Urinalysis | 81000 | |
| | Venipuncture | 36415 | |
| | Wet Mount, Smear | 87210 | |
| | Wet Mount KOH | 87220 | |
| | Collect/Handing | 99000 | |
| | **MISCELLANEOUS** | | |
| | Pre-OP | 993___ | |
| | After Hours | 99050 | |
| | Sunday/Holidays | 99054 | |
| | Cast Removal | 29705 | |
| | Norplant Insertion | 11975 | |
| | Norplant Kit | 99070 | |

| ✓ | DESCRIPTION | CPT/MD | FEE |
|---|---|---|---|
| | **SURGERY** | | |
| | Toenail Removal | 11750 | |
| | Cryosurgery | 17200 | |
| | I & D | 10060 | |
| | Drainage Paronychia | 10060 | |
| | Enucleation Ext. Hemorrhoid | 46320 | |
| | I & D Abscess/Cyst | 10060 | |
| | Podophyllom | 17100 | |
| | Removal Foreign Body | 10120 | |
| | Wart Removal | 17110 | |
| | Destr. Single Lesion Face | 17000 | |
| | 2nd and 3rd Lesion Face | 17001 | |
| | Destr. Single Lesion Body | 17106 | |
| | 2nd and 3rd Lesion Body | 17003 | |
| | Lesion Rem. Excision | | |
| | Anoscopy | 46600 | |
| | Flex. Scope with Sig. | 45330 | |
| | Vasectomy | 55250 | |
| | Therapeutic Abor. | 59840 | |
| | Removal Foreign Body of Eye | 65205 | |
| | **SUPPLIES** | | |
| | Ace Wrap | 99070 | |
| | Cast Material | 99070 | |
| | Cervical Collar | 99070 | |
| | Elastic Bandage | 99070 | |
| | Splint/Sling | 99070 | |
| | Sterile Dressing | 99070 | |
| | Surgical Tray | 99070 | |

**DIAGNOSIS:** **ICD-9**

- ☐ Abscess Cellulitis ...... 682.9
- ☐ Abdominal Pain ....... 789.0
- ☐ Abrasions ........... 919.0
- ☐ Acne .............. 706.1
- ☐ ADD .............. 314.00
- ☐ Alcoholism .......... 303.90
- ☐ Allergic Rhinitis ....... 477.9
- ☐ Allergy, Unsp ........ 995.3
- ☐ Anemia ............ 285.9
- ☐ Angina Pectoris ....... 413.9
- ☐ Anxiety Depression .... 300.4
- ☐ Anxiety State ........ 300.00
- ☐ ASCVD ............ 429.2
- ☐ Asthma W/O Status Asthma 493.90
- ☐ Atten Surg. Dressing/Suture V58.3
- ☐ BCP Consult ......... V25.9
- ☐ BPH .............. 600
- ☐ Bronchitis, Acute ...... 466.0
- ☐ Bronchitis, Chronic ..... 491.9
- ☐ Burn ____________ 949.0
- ☐ Bursitis ............ 727.3
- ☐ C.T.S. .............. 354.0
- ☐ CAD ............... 746.85
- ☐ CA-Prostate .......... 185
- ☐ Cardiac Arrhythmia ..... 427.9
- ☐ Cataracts ........... 366.9
- ☐ Chest Pain........... 786.50
- ☐ Congestive Heart Failure 428.0
- ☐ Conjunctivitis ........ 372.30
- ☐ Constipation.......... 564.0
- ☐ Consult Vasc.......... V65.8
- ☐ Convulsions .......... 780.3
- ☐ COPD .............. 496
- ☐ Coronary Atherosclerosis. 414.0
- ☐ CVA................ 436
- ☐ Cyst Sebaceous ....... 706.2
- ☐ Dermatitis ........... 692.9
- ☐ Diabetes, Uncomp. Adult 250.00
- ☐ Diabetes, Complicated .. 250.90
- ☐ Disc Degeneration ..... 722.6
- ☐ Duodenal Ulcer ....... 532.90
- ☐ Dysmenorrhea ........ 625.3
- ☐ Fatigue ............ 780.7
- ☐ Flu Shot Only......... V04.8
- ☐ Flu Vac ............ V04.8
- ☐ Flu W/Resp. Manifest ... 487.1
- ☐ Folliculitis............ 704.8
- ☐ FX ________________
- ☐ Gallbladder Disease .... 575.9
- ☐ Ganglion ............ 727.43
- ☐ Gastroenteritis ........ 558.9
- ☐ Gout .............. 274.9
- ☐ Gyn Exam ........... V72.3
- ☐ Headache Tension ..... 307.81
- ☐ Hemorrhoids Ext. ...... 455.3
- ☐ Hepatitis ........... 573.3
- ☐ Hernia-Inguinal........ 550.90
- ☐ Herpes Zoster ........ 053.9
- ☐ Hyperlipidemia ........ 272.4
- ☐ Hypertension ........ 401.9
- ☐ Hyperthyroidism ....... 242.9
- ☐ Hypothyroidism ....... 244.9
- ☐ Impacted Cerumen ..... 380.4
- ☐ Impetigo ........... 684
- ☐ Ingrown Toenail ....... 703.0
- ☐ Internal Derangement Knee . 717.9
- ☐ Labyrinthitis .......... 386.30
- ☐ Laceration Open Wound . 879.8__
- ☐ Levator Scapular Syndrome 726.90
- ☐ Menopausal Disorder ... 627.9
- ☐ Metabolic Diff. ........ 277.8
- ☐ Migraine ........... 346.90
- ☐ Mitral Valve Disorder ... 424.0
- ☐ Myalgia and Myositis ... 729.1
- ☐ Noninf. Gastroenterit. ... 558.9
- ☐ Obesity ............ 278.0
- ☐ Osteoarthrosis ........ 715.00
- ☐ Osteoporosis ........ 733.00
- ☐ Otitis Externa ........ 380.10
- ☐ Otitis Media ......... 382.9
- ☐ P.I.D. ............. 614.9
- ☐ Peptic Ulcer ......... 533.90
- ☐ Pharyngitis, Acute ..... 462
- ☐ Pneumonia, Viral ...... 480.9
- ☐ Poison Oak ......... 692.6
- ☐ Premarital B-Test ..... V70.3
- ☐ Pregnancy Test, Unconf.. V72.4
- ☐ Prostatitis .......... 601.9
- ☐ Psoriasis ........... 696.1
- ☐ Rheumatoid Arthritis .... 714.0
- ☐ Sciatica ............ 724.3
- ☐ Sacroiliac Sprain ...... 846.1
- ☐ Sinusitis, Acute ....... 461.9
- ☐ Smoking Cessation..... 305.10
- ☐ Sprain ________________
- ☐ SQ. Cell CA-Face...... 173.3
- ☐ Sterilization ......... V25.2
- ☐ Stye............... 373.11
- ☐ TB Exposure ........ V01.1
- ☐ Tendonitis .......... 726.90
- ☐ Tinea.............. 110.9
- ☐ Tonsillitis, Acute ...... 463
- ☐ URI, Acute .......... 465.9
- ☐ Urine Tract Infection .... 599.0
- ☐ Vaginitis............ 616.10
- ☐ Well Adult Medical Exam V70.9
- ☒ Well Child Health Exam . V20.2

| DIAGNOSIS (If not checked above) ICD-9 | PHYSICIAN SIGNATURE | TODAY'S FEE | $ |
|---|---|---|---|
| | | PAYMENT | |
| PLEASE REMEMBER THAT PAYMENT IS YOUR OBLIGATION REGARDLESS OF INSURANCE OR OTHER THIRD PARTY INVOLVEMENT. | PAYMENT BY<br>☐ CASH ☐ CREDIT CARD<br>☐ CHECK # ________ | BALANCE DUE | |

INSUR-A-BILL ® BIBBERO SYSTEMS, INC. • PETALUMA, CA • © 9/94 SB43006.01 (REV. 1/99)

Courtesy of Bibbero Systems, Inc., Petaluma, California.

Case Three, Form 13

# FEE SCHEDULE

## BLACKBURN PRIMARY CARE ASSOCIATES
## 1990 TURQUOISE DRIVE
## BLACKBURN, WI 54937

**Federal Tax ID Number:** **52-1963787**

**BCBS Group Number:** **14982**
**Medicare Group Number:** **14982**

### OFFICE VISIT, NEW PATIENT

| | |
|---|---|
| Focused, 99201 | $ 45.00 |
| Expanded, 99202 | $ 53.00 |
| Detailed, 99203 | $ 60.00 |
| Comprehensive, 99204 | $ 95.00 |
| Complex, 99205 | $195.00 |
| | |
| Consultation, 99245 | $250.00 |

### OFFICE VISIT, ESTABLISHED PATIENT

| | |
|---|---|
| Minimal, 99211 | $ 40.00 |
| Focused, 99212 | $ 48.00 |
| Expanded, 99213 | $ 55.00 |
| Detailed, 99214 | $ 65.00 |
| Comprehensive, 99215 | $195.00 |

### OFFICE PROCEDURES

| | |
|---|---|
| EKG, 12 Lead, 93000 | $ 55.00 |
| Stress EKG, Treadmill, 93015 | $295.00 |
| Sigmoidoscopy, Flex., 45330 | $145.00 |
| Spirometry, 94010 | $ 50.00 |
| Cerumen Removal, 69210 | $ 40.00 |
| | |
| Collection & Handling | |
| Lab Specimen, 99000 | $ 9.00 |
| Venipuncture, 36415 | $ 9.00 |
| Urinalysis, 81000 | $ 20.00 |
| Urinalysis, 81002 (Dip Only) | $ 12.00 |
| | |
| Influenza Injection, 90724 | $ 20.00 |
| Pneumococcal Injection, 90732 | $ 20.00 |
| Oral Polio, 90712 | $ 15.00 |
| DTaP, 90700 | $ 20.00 |
| Tetanus Toxoid, 90703 | $ 15.00 |
| MMR, 90707 | $ 25.00 |
| Hib, 90737 | $ 20.00 |
| Hepatitis B, newborn to age 11 years, 90744 | $ 60.00 |
| Hepatitis B, 11-19 years, 90745 | $ 60.00 |
| Hepatitis B, 20 years and above 90746 | $ 60.00 |
| Intramuscular Injection, 90788 | |
| Penicillin | $ 30.00 |
| Ceftriaxone | $ 25.00 |
| Solu-Medrol | $ 23.00 |
| Vitamin B-12 | $ 13.00 |
| Subcutaneous Injection, 90782 | |
| Epinephrine | $ 18.00 |
| Sus-Pherine | $ 25.00 |
| Insulin, U-100 | $ 15.00 |

### COMMON DIAGNOSIS CODES

| | |
|---|---|
| Ischemic Heart Disease | 414.9 |
| w/o myocardial infarction | 411.89 |
| w/ coronary occlusion | 411.81 |
| Hypertension, Malignant | 401.0 |
| Benign | 401.1 |
| Unspecified | 401.9 |
| w/ congest. heart failure | 402.91 |
| Asthma, Bronchial | 493.9 |
| w/ COPD | 493.2 |
| allergic, w/ S.A. | 493.91 |
| allergic, w/o S.A. | 493.90 |
| Kyphosis | 737.10 |
| w/ osteoporosis | 733.0 |
| Osteoporosis | 733.00 |
| Otitis Media, Acute | 382.9 |
| Chronic | 382.9 |
| Well Child Health Exam | V20.2 |
| Well Adult Medical Exam | V70.9 |

Case Three, Form 14

PLEASE DO NOT STAPLE IN THIS AREA

APPROVED OMB-0938-0008

CARRIER

PICA

# HEALTH INSURANCE CLAIM FORM

PICA

1. MEDICARE (Medicare #) MEDICAID (Medicaid #) CHAMPUS (Sponsor's SSN) CHAMPVA (VA File #) GROUP HEALTH PLAN (SSN or ID) FECA BLK LUNG (SSN) OTHER (ID)

1a. INSURED'S I.D. NUMBER (FOR PROGRAM IN ITEM 1)

2. PATIENT'S NAME (Last Name, First Name, Middle Initial)

3. PATIENT'S BIRTHDATE MM DD YY SEX M F

4. INSURED'S NAME (Last Name, First Name, Middle Initial)

5. PATIENT'S ADDRESS (No., Street)

6. PATIENT RELATIONSHIP TO INSURED Self Spouse Child Other

7. INSURED'S ADDRESS (No., Street)

CITY STATE

8. PATIENT STATUS Single Married Other

CITY STATE

ZIP CODE TELEPHONE (Include Area Code) ( )

Employed Full-Time Student Part-Time Student

ZIP CODE TELEPHONE (Include Area Code) ( )

9. OTHER INSURED'S NAME (Last Name, First Name, Middle Initial)

10. IS PATIENT'S CONDITION RELATED TO:

11. INSURED'S POLICY GROUP OR FECA NUMBER

a. OTHER INSURED'S POLICY OR GROUP NUMBER

a. EMPLOYMENT? (CURRENT OR PREVIOUS) YES NO

a. INSURED'S DATE OF BIRTH MM DD YY SEX M F

b. OTHER INSURED'S DATE OF BIRTH MM DD YY SEX M F

b. AUTO ACCIDENT? YES NO PLACE (State)

b. EMPLOYER'S NAME OR SCHOOL NAME

c. EMPLOYER'S NAME OR SCHOOL NAME

c. OTHER ACCIDENT? YES NO

c. INSURANCE PLAN NAME OR PROGRAM NAME

d. INSURANCE PLAN NAME OR PROGRAM NAME

10d. RESERVED FOR LOCAL USE

d. IS THERE ANOTHER HEALTH BENEFIT PLAN? YES NO *If yes, return to and complete item 9a-d.*

**READ BACK OF FORM BEFORE COMPLETING & SIGNING THIS FORM.**

12. PATIENT'S OR AUTHORIZED PERSON'S SIGNATURE I authorize the release of any medical or other information necessary to process this claim. I also request payment of government benefits either to myself or to the party who accepts assignment below.

SIGNED ______ DATE ______

13. INSURED'S OR AUTHORIZED PERSON'S SIGNATURE I authorize payment of medical benefits to the undersigned physician or supplier for services described below.

SIGNED ______

PATIENT AND INSURED INFORMATION

14. DATE OF CURRENT: MM DD YY ILLNESS (First symptom) OR INJURY (Accident) OR PREGNANCY (LMP)

15. IF PATIENT HAS HAD SAME OR SIMILAR ILLNESS, GIVE FIRST DATE MM DD YY

16. DATES PATIENT UNABLE TO WORK IN CURRENT OCCUPATION FROM MM DD YY TO MM DD YY

17. NAME OF REFERRING PHYSICIAN OR OTHER SOURCE

17a. I.D. NUMBER OF REFERRING PHYSICIAN

18. HOSPITALIZATION DATES RELATED TO CURRENT SERVICES FROM MM DD YY TO MM DD YY

19. RESERVED FOR LOCAL USE

20. OUTSIDE LAB? YES NO $ CHARGES

21. DIAGNOSIS OR NATURE OF ILLNESS OR INJURY. (RELATE ITEMS 1,2,3 OR 4 TO ITEM 24E BY LINE)

1. ___ . ___ 3. ___ . ___

2. ___ . ___ 4. ___ . ___

22. MEDICAID RESUBMISSION CODE ORIGINAL REF. NO.

23. PRIOR AUTHORIZATION NUMBER

| 24. A DATE(S) OF SERVICE From MM DD YY | To MM DD YY | B Place of Service | C Type of Service | D PROCEDURES, SERVICES, OR SUPPLIES (Explain Unusual Circumstances) CPT/HCPCS MODIFIER | E DIAGNOSIS CODE | F $ CHARGES | G DAYS OR UNITS | H EPSDT Family Plan | I EMG | J COB | K RESERVED FOR LOCAL USE |
|---|---|---|---|---|---|---|---|---|---|---|---|
| 1 | | | | | | | | | | | |
| 2 | | | | | | | | | | | |
| 3 | | | | | | | | | | | |
| 4 | | | | | | | | | | | |
| 5 | | | | | | | | | | | |
| 6 | | | | | | | | | | | |

25. FEDERAL TAX I.D. NUMBER SSN EIN

26. PATIENT'S ACCOUNT NUMBER

27. ACCEPT ASSIGNMENT? (For govt. claims, see back) YES NO

28. TOTAL CHARGE $

29. AMOUNT PAID $

30. BALANCE DUE $

31. SIGNATURE OF PHYSICIAN OR SUPPLIER INCLUDING DEGREES OR CREDENTIALS (I certify that the statements on the reverse apply to this bill and are made a part thereof.)

SIGNED DATE

32. NAME AND ADDRESS OF FACILITY WHERE SERVICES WERE RENDERED (If other than home or office)

33. PHYSICIAN'S, SUPPLIER'S BILLING NAME, ADDRESS, ZIP CODE & PHONE #

PIN # GRP#

PHYSICIAN OR SUPPLIER INFORMATION

(APPROVED BY AMA COUNCIL ON MEDICAL SERVICE 8/88) *PLEASE PRINT OR TYPE* FORM HCFA-1500 (12-90) FORM OWCP-1500 FORM RRB-1500

Form 1240LM

Case Four, Form 15

# Appointment Schedule

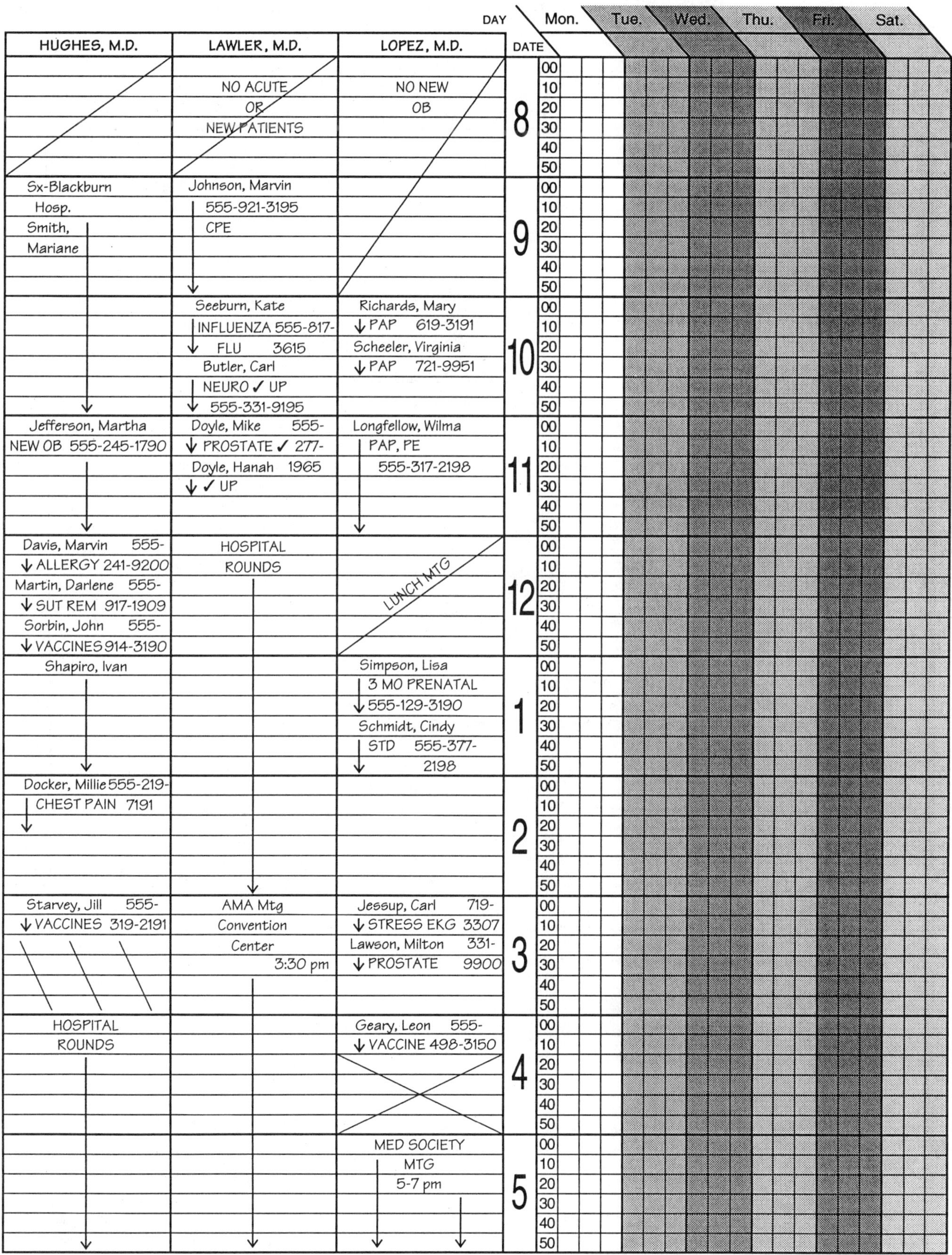

DAY: Mon. | Tue. | Wed. | Thu. | Fri. | Sat.

| DATE | | HUGHES, M.D. | LAWLER, M.D. | LOPEZ, M.D. |
|---|---|---|---|---|
| 8 | 00 | | | |
| | 10 | | NO ACUTE | NO NEW |
| | 20 | | OR | OB |
| | 30 | | NEW PATIENTS | |
| | 40 | | | |
| | 50 | | | |
| 9 | 00 | Sx-Blackburn | Johnson, Marvin | |
| | 10 | Hosp. | 555-921-3195 | |
| | 20 | Smith, | CPE | |
| | 30 | Mariane | | |
| | 40 | | | |
| | 50 | | ↓ | |
| 10 | 00 | | Seeburn, Kate | Richards, Mary |
| | 10 | | INFLUENZA 555-817- | ↓ PAP 619-3191 |
| | 20 | | ↓ FLU 3615 | Scheeler, Virginia |
| | 30 | | Butler, Carl | ↓ PAP 721-9951 |
| | 40 | | NEURO ✓ UP | |
| | 50 | ↓ | ↓ 555-331-9195 | |
| 11 | 00 | Jefferson, Martha | Doyle, Mike 555- | Longfellow, Wilma |
| | 10 | NEW OB 555-245-1790 | ↓ PROSTATE ✓ 277- | PAP, PE |
| | 20 | | Doyle, Hanah 1965 | 555-317-2198 |
| | 30 | | ↓ ✓ UP | |
| | 40 | | | |
| | 50 | ↓ | | ↓ |
| 12 | 00 | Davis, Marvin 555- | HOSPITAL | |
| | 10 | ↓ ALLERGY 241-9200 | ROUNDS | |
| | 20 | Martin, Darlene 555- | | LUNCH MTG |
| | 30 | ↓ SUT REM 917-1909 | | |
| | 40 | Sorbin, John 555- | | |
| | 50 | ↓ VACCINES 914-3190 | | |
| 1 | 00 | Shapiro, Ivan | | Simpson, Lisa |
| | 10 | | | 3 MO PRENATAL |
| | 20 | | | ↓ 555-129-3190 |
| | 30 | | | Schmidt, Cindy |
| | 40 | | | STD 555-377- |
| | 50 | ↓ | | ↓ 2198 |
| 2 | 00 | Docker, Millie 555-219- | | |
| | 10 | CHEST PAIN 7191 | | |
| | 20 | ↓ | | |
| | 30 | | | |
| | 40 | | | |
| | 50 | | ↓ | |
| 3 | 00 | Starvey, Jill 555- | AMA Mtg | Jessup, Carl 719- |
| | 10 | ↓ VACCINES 319-2191 | Convention | ↓ STRESS EKG 3307 |
| | 20 | | Center | Lawson, Milton 331- |
| | 30 | | 3:30 pm | ↓ PROSTATE 9900 |
| | 40 | | | |
| | 50 | | | |
| 4 | 00 | HOSPITAL | | Geary, Leon 555- |
| | 10 | ROUNDS | | ↓ VACCINE 498-3150 |
| | 20 | | | |
| | 30 | | | |
| | 40 | | | |
| | 50 | | | |
| 5 | 00 | | | MED SOCIETY |
| | 10 | | | MTG |
| | 20 | | | 5-7 pm |
| | 30 | | | |
| | 40 | | | |
| | 50 | ↓ | ↓ | ↓ ↓ |

Form No. 56-7310 © 1977 Bibbero Systems, Inc., Petaluma, CA
Courtesy of Bibbero Systems, Inc., Petaluma, California.

Case Four, Form 16

# ANDRUS/CLINI-REC® HEALTH HISTORY QUESTIONNAIRE

Chart No. ________

**Identification Information**

Today's Date 1/15/05

Name Lucille Ferguson　Date of Birth 6/21/30

Occupation ________　Marital Status Widowed

## PART A – PRESENT HEALTH HISTORY

### I. CURRENT MEDICAL PROBLEMS

Please list the medical problems for which you came to see the doctor. About when did they begin?

| Problems | Date Began |
|---|---|
| Pain when urinating | 1 wk ago |
| Fever | Yesterday |
| | |

What concerns you most about these problems?

________

If you are being treated for any other illness or medical problems by another physician, please describe the problems and write the name of the physician or medical facility treating you.

| Illness or Medical Problem | Physician or Medical Facility | City |
|---|---|---|
| Osteoarthritis | | |
| | | |

### II. MEDICATIONS

Please list all medications you are now taking, including those you buy without a doctor's prescription (such as aspirin, cold tablets or vitamin supplements).

________

### III. ALLERGIES AND SENSITIVITIES

List anything that you are allergic to such as certain foods, medications, dust, chemicals or soaps, household items, pollens, bee stings, etc., and indicate how each affects you.

| Allergic To: | Effect | Allergic To: | Effect |
|---|---|---|---|
| None | | | |
| | | | |

### IV. GENERAL HEALTH, ATTITUDE AND HABITS

| | | |
|---|---|---|
| How is your overall health now? | Health now: | Poor ___ Fair ___ Good ✓ Excellent ___ |
| How has it been most of your life? | Health has been: | Poor ___ Fair ___ Good ✓ Excellent ___ |
| In the past year: | | |
| Has your appetite changed? | Appetite: | Decreased ✓ Increased ___ Stayed same ___ |
| Has your weight changed? | Weight: | Lost ___ lbs. Gained ___ lbs. No change ✓ |
| Are you thirsty much of the time? | Thirsty: | No ✓ Yes ___ |
| Has your overall 'pep' changed? | Pep: | Decreased ___ Increased ___ Stayed same ✓ |
| Do you usually have trouble sleeping? | Trouble sleeping: | No ___ Yes ✓ |
| How much do you exercise? | Exercise: | Little or none ___ Less than I need ✓ All I need ___ |
| Do you smoke? | Smokes: | No ✓ Yes ___ If yes, how many years? ___ |
| How many each day? | | ___ Cigarettes ___ Cigars ___ Pipesfull |
| Have you ever smoked? | Smoked: | No ___ Yes ✓ If yes, how many years? 15 |
| How many each day? | | 30 Cigarettes ___ Cigars ___ Pipesfull |
| Do you drink alcoholic beverages? | Alcohol: | No ___ Yes ✓ I drink ___ Beers ✓ Glasses of wine 2 Drinks of hard liquor - per day |
| Have you ever had a problem with alcohol? | Prior problem: | No ✓ Yes ___ |
| How much coffee or tea do you usually drink? | Coffee/Tea: | 1 cups of coffee or tea a day |
| Do you regularly wear seatbelts? | Seatbelts: | No ___ Yes ✓ |

| DO YOU: | Rarely/Never | Occasionally | Frequently |
|---|---|---|---|
| Feel nervous? | X | | |
| Feel depressed? | X | | |
| Find it hard to make decisions? | X | | |
| Lose your temper? | X | | |
| Worry a lot? | X | | |
| Tire easily? | | X | |
| Have trouble relaxing? | X | | |
| Have any sexual problems? | X | | |

| DO YOU: | Rarely/Never | Occasionally | Frequently |
|---|---|---|---|
| Ever feel like committing suicide? | X | | |
| Feel bored with your life? | X | | |
| Use marijuana? | X | | |
| Use "hard drugs"? | X | | |

Do you want to talk to the doctor about a personal matter? No X Yes ___

CONFIDENTIAL



STOCK NO. 19-742-4 8/95



Courtesy of Bibbero Systems, Inc., Petaluma, California.

# PART A – PRESENT HEALTH HISTORY (continued)

## IV. GENERAL HEALTH, ATTITUDE AND HABITS (continued)

Have you recently had any changes in your: — If yes, please explain:

| | No | Yes | If yes, please explain |
|---|---|---|---|
| Marital status? | X | | |
| Job or work? | X | | |
| Residence? | X | | |
| Financial status? | X | | |
| Are you having any legal problems or trouble with the law? | X | | |

# PART B – PAST HISTORY

## I. FAMILY HEALTH

Please give the following information about your immediate family:

| Relationship | Age, if Living | Age At Death | State of Health Or Cause of Death |
|---|---|---|---|
| Father | | 95 | excellent |
| Mother | | unknown | cancer |
| Brothers and Sisters | | | |
| | 68 | | multiple sclerosis |
| | | | |
| Spouse | | | |
| Children | | | |
| | | | |
| | | | |
| | | | |

Have any **blood relatives** had any of the following illnesses? If so, indicate relationship (mother, brother, etc.)

| Illness | Family Members |
|---|---|
| Asthma | Brother |
| Diabetes | — |
| Cancer | Breast cancer-Mom |
| Blood Disease | — |
| Glaucoma | — |
| Epilepsy | — |
| Rheumatoid Arthritis | — |
| Tuberculosis | — |
| Gout | — |
| High Blood Pressure | — |
| Heart Disease | — |
| Mental Problems | — |
| Suicide | — |
| Stroke | — |
| Alcoholism | Uncle |
| Rheumatic Fever | — |

## II. HOSPITALIZATIONS, SURGERIES, INJURIES

Please list all times you have been hospitalized, operated on, or seriously injured.

| Year | Operation, Illness, Injury | Hospital and City |
|---|---|---|
| 1976 | Appendix taken out | Mercy Hospital |
| | | |
| | | |

## III. ILLNESS AND MEDICAL PROBLEMS

Please mark with an (X) any of the following illnesses and medical problems you have or have had and indicate the year when each started. If you are not certain when an illness started, write down an approximate year.

| Illness | (x) | (Year) | Illness | (x) | (Year) |
|---|---|---|---|---|---|
| Eye or eye lid infection | | | Hernia | | |
| Glaucoma | | | Hemorrhoids | X | 1955 |
| Other eye problems | | | Kidney or bladder disease | | |
| Ear trouble | | | Prostate problem (male only) | | |
| Deafness or decreased hearing | | | Mental problems | | |
| Thyroid trouble | | | Headaches | | |
| Strep throat | X | as child | Head injury | | |
| Bronchitis | X | several | Stroke | | |
| Emphysema | | | Convulsions, seizures | | |
| Pneumonia | | | Arthritis | X | now |
| Allergies, asthma or hay fever | | | Gout | | |
| Tuberculosis | | | Cancer or tumor | | |
| Other lung problems | | | Bleeding tendency | | |
| High blood pressure | | | Diabetes | | |
| Heart attack | | | Measles/Rubeola | X | child |
| High cholesterol | X | 1991 | German measles/Rubella | | |
| Arteriosclerosis | | | Polio | X | child |
| (Hardening of arteries) | | | Mumps | X | child |
| Heart murmur | | | Scarlet fever | | |
| Other heart condition | | | Chicken pox | X | child |
| Stomach/duodenal ulcer | | | Mononucleosis | | |
| Diverticulosis | | | Eczema | | |
| Colitis | | | Psoriasis | | |
| Other bowel problems | | | Venereal disease | | |
| Hepatitis | | | Genital herpes | | |
| Liver trouble | | | HIV test | | |
| Gallbladder trouble | | | AIDS | | |

CONFIDENTIAL

Case Four, Form 16

## PART C – BODY SYSTEMS REVIEW

Please answer all of the following questions.

Circle any questions you find difficult to answer.

MEN: Please answer questions 1 through 12, then skip to question 18.
WOMEN: Please start on question 6.

MEN ONLY

1. Have you had or do you have prostate trouble? . . . . . No ______ Yes ______
2. Do you have any sexual problems or a problem with impotency? . . . . . No ______ Yes ______
3. Have you ever had sores or lesions on your penis? . . . . . No ______ Yes ______
4. Have you ever had any discharge from your penis? . . . . . No ______ Yes ______
5. Do you ever have pain, lumps or swelling in your testicles? . . . . . No ______ Yes ______

Check here if you wish to discuss any special problems with the doctor . . . . . ☐

MEN & WOMEN

| | Question | Rarely/ Never | Occasionally | Frequently |
|---|---|---|---|---|
| 6. | Is it sometimes hard to start your urine flow? | X | | |
| 7. | Is urination ever painful? | | | X |
| 8. | Do you have to urinate more than 5 times a day? | X | | |
| 9. | Do you get up at night to urinate? | X | | |
| 10. | Has your urine ever been bloody or dark colored? | X | | |
| 11. | Do you ever lose urine when you strain, laugh, cough or sneeze? | X | | |
| 12. | Do you ever lose urine during sleep? | X | | |

WOMEN ONLY
Do you:

| | | Question | Rarely/ Never | Occasionally | Frequently |
|---|---|---|---|---|---|
| 13. | a. | Have any menstrual problems? | X | | |
| | b. | Feel rather tense just before your period? | X | | |
| | c. | Have heavy menstrual bleeding? | X | | |
| | d. | Have painful menstrual periods? | X | | |
| | e. | Have any bleeding between periods? | X | | |
| | f. | Have any unusual vaginal discharge or itching? | X | | |
| | g. | Ever have tender breasts? | X | | |
| | h. | Have any discharge from your nipples? | X | | |
| | i. | Have any hot flashes? | X | | |

14. How many times, if any, have you been pregnant? . . . . . 3
15. How many children born alive? . . . . . 3
16. Are you taking birth control pills? . . . . . No X Yes ______
17. Do you examine your breasts monthly for lumps? . . . . . No ______ Yes Sometimes
17a. What was the date of your last menstrual period? . . . . . Date 1980

Check here if you wish to discuss any special problem with the doctor . . . . . ☐

MEN & WOMEN

| | | Question | Rarely/ Never | Occasionally | Frequently |
|---|---|---|---|---|---|
| 18. | | In the past year have you had any: | | | |
| | a. | Severe shoulder pain? | X | | |
| | b. | Severe back pain? | X | | |
| | c. | Muscle or joint stiffness or pain due to sports, exercise or injury? | X | | |
| | d. | Pain or swelling in any joints not due to sports, exercise or injury? | X | | |

19. Do you have dry skin or brittle fingernails? . . . . . No X Yes ______
20. Do you bruise easily? . . . . . No X Yes ______
21. Do you have any moles that have changed in color or in size? . . . . . No X Yes ______
22. Do you have any other skin problems? . . . . . No X Yes ______

23. In the last 3 months have you had:
    a. A fever that lasted more than one day? . . . . . No ______ Yes X
    b. Sores or cuts that were hard to heal? . . . . . No X Yes ______
    c. Any cold sores (fever blisters)? . . . . . No X Yes ______
    d. Any lumps in your neck, armpits or groin? . . . . . No X Yes ______
    e. Do you ever have chills or sweat at night? . . . . . No X Yes ______
24. Have you traveled out of the country in the last 2 years? . . . . . No X Yes, Traveled in: ______
25. Write in the dates for the shots you have had: . . . . . Measles ______ Mumps ______ Polio ______ Smallpox ______ Tetanus ______ Typhoid ______
26. Have you had a tuberculin (TB) skin test? . . . . . No X Yes ______ Date ______
    If so, was it negative or positive? . . . . . Neg ______ Pos ______
27. Have you had an HIV test for AIDS? . . . . . No X Yes ______ Date ______
    If so, was it negative or positive? . . . . . Neg ______ Pos ______

C O N F I D E N T I A L

REMOVE THIS PAGE AFTER COMPLETING QUESTIONNAIRE

Case Four, Form 16

# BODY SYSTEMS REVIEW

## VISION / HEARING

| | | | | |
|---|---|---|---|---|
| 28. Do you wear eyeglasses? | No___ | Yes X | | Wears eyeglasses |
| 29. Do you wear contact lenses? | No X | Yes___ | | Wears contacts |
| 30. Has your vision changed in the last year? | No___ | Yes X | | Vision changes in last year |

| Question | Rarely/ Never | Occasionally | Frequently | |
|---|---|---|---|---|
| 31. How often do you have: | | | | |
| a. Double vision? | | X | | Double vision |
| b. Blurry vision? | | X | | Blurred vision |
| c. Watery or itchy eyes? | | | X | Watery/itchy eyes |
| 32. Do you ever see colored rings around lights? | X | | | Sees halos |
| 33. Do others tell you you have a hearing problem? | | X | | Hearing problem |
| 34. Do you have trouble keeping your balance? | X | | | Loses balance |
| 35. Do you have any discharge from your ears? | X | | | Discharge from ears |
| 36. Do you ever feel dizzy or have motion sickness? | X | | | Dizzy / motion sickness |
| 37. Do you have any problems with your hearing? | No X | Yes___ | Hearing Problems | |
| 38. Do you ever have ringing in your ears? | No X | Yes___ | Ringing in ears | |

## NOSE / THROAT / RESPIRATORY

| Question | Rarely/ Never | Occasionally | Frequently | |
|---|---|---|---|---|
| 39. How often do you have: | | | | |
| a. Head colds? | | X | | Head colds |
| b. Chest colds? | | X | | Chest colds |
| c. Runny nose? | | X | | Runny nose |
| d. Stuffed up nose? | | X | | Head congestion |
| e. Sore/hoarse throat? | | X | | Sore / hoarse throat |
| f. Bad coughing spells? | X | | | Coughing spells |
| g. Sneezing spells? | X | | | Sneezing spells |
| h. Trouble breathing? | X | | | Trouble breathing |
| i. Nose bleeds? | X | | | Nose bleeds |
| j. Cough blood? | X | | | Cough blood |
| 40. Have you ever worked or spent time: | | | | |
| a. On a farm? | No___ | Yes X | Worked on a farm | |
| b. In a mine? | No X | Yes___ | Worked in a mine | |
| c. In a laundry or mill? | No X | Yes___ | Worked in a laundry/mill | |
| d. In very dusty places? | No X | Yes___ | Worked in high dust concentrations | |
| e. With or near toxic chemicals? | No X | Yes___ | Exposed to toxic chemicals | |
| f. With or near radioactive materials? | No X | Yes___ | Exposed to radioactive materials | |
| g. With or near asbestos? | No X | Yes___ | Exposed to asbestos | |

## CARDIOVASCULAR

| Question | Rarely/ Never | Occasionally | Frequently | |
|---|---|---|---|---|
| 41. Do you get out of breath easily when you are active (like climbing stairs)? | X | | | Out of breath quickly when exercising |
| 42. Do you ever feel light-headed or dizzy? | X | | | Dizziness |
| 43. Have you ever fainted or passed out? | X | | | Fainted |
| 44. Do you sometimes feel your heart is racing or beating too fast? | X | | | Rapid heartbeat |
| 45. When you exercise do you ever get pains in your chest or shoulders? | X | | | Chest/shoulder pains in exercise |
| 46. Do you have any leg cramps or pain in your thighs or legs when walking? | X | | | Pain in thighs or legs when walking |
| 47. Do you ever have to sit up at night to breathe easier? | X | | | Sits up at night to breathe easier |
| 48. Do you use two pillows at night to help you breathe easier? | X | | | Breathing problems during sleep |
| 49. Would you say you are a restless sleeper? | X | | | Restless sleeper |
| 50. Are you bothered by leg cramps at night? | X | | | Leg cramps at night |
| 51. Do you sometimes have swollen ankles or feet? | X | | | Swollen ankles/feet |

## DIGESTIVE

| Question | Rarely/ Never | Occasionally | Frequently | |
|---|---|---|---|---|
| 52. How often, if ever: | | | | |
| a. Are you nauseated (sick to your stomach)? | X | | | Nauseated |
| b. Do you have stomach pains? | X | | | Stomach pains |
| c. Do you burp a lot after eating? | X | | | Burps after eating |
| d. Do you have heartburn? | X | | | Heartburn |
| e. Do you have trouble swallowing your food? | X | | | Trouble swallowing food |
| f. Have you vomited blood? | X | | | Vomited blood |
| g. Are you constipated? | X | | | Constipated |
| h. Do you have diarrhea (watery stools)? | X | | | Diarrhea |
| i. Are your bowel movements painful? | X | | | Painful bowel movements |
| j. Are your bowel movements bloody? | X | | | Bloody bowel movements |
| k. Are your bowel movements dark or black? | X | | | Dark bowel movements |
| 53. Have you ever had a sigmoidoscopy? | No X | Yes___ | Date___ | Date of last sigmoidoscopy? |

**PLEASE TURN TO BACK PAGE AND COMPLETE QUESTIONS ON NUTRITION.**

Case Four, Form 16

Andrus/Clini-Rec®

BIBBERO SYSTEMS, INC.

COMPREHENSIVE
PHYSICAL EXAMINATION
MALE OR FEMALE
NEW OR ESTABLISHED PATIENT
CPT # 99201 - 99215

(For Office Use Only)

C O N F I D E N T I A L

NAME ______ AGE ______ YRS. OLD TODAY'S DATE ______ DATE OF BIRTH ______

Key: [O] Neg. Findings [+] Positive Findings [X] Omitted [✔] See Notes/CIRCLE WORDS OF IMPORTANCE & EXPLAIN

| | | | |
|---|---|---|---|
| 1 | GEN. APPEARANCE | [ ] | Apparent Age/Nutrition/Development/Mental & Emotional Status/Gait/Posture/Distress/Speech – |
| 2 | HEAD / SCALP | [ ] | Size/Shape/Tender over Sinuses/Hair/Alopecia/Eruption/Masses/Bruit – |
| 3 | EYES | [ ] | Conjunct/Sclerae/Cornea/Pupils/EOM'S/Arcus/Ptosis/Fundi/Tension/Eyelids/Pallor/Light/Bruit – |
| 4 | EARS | [ ] | Ext. Canal/TM's/Perforation/Discharge/Tophi/Hearing Problem/Weber/Rinne – |
| 5 | NOSE / SINUSES | [ ] | Septum/Obstruction/Turbinates/Discharge – |
| 6 | MOUTH / THROAT | [ ] | Odor/Lips/Tongue/Tonsils/Teeth/Dentures/Gums/Pharynx – |
| 7 | NECK | [ ] | Adenopathy/Thyroid/Carotids/Trachea/Veins/Masses/Spine/Motion/Bruit – |
| 8 | BACK | [ ] | Kyphosis/Scoliosis/Lordosis/Mobility/CVA/Bone/Tenderness – |
| 9 | THORAX | [ ] | Symmetry/Movement/Contour/Tender – |
| 10 | BREASTS | [ ] | Size/Size-Consistency/Nipples/Areolar/Palpable Mass/Discharge/Tenderness/Nodes/Scars – |
| 11 | HEART | [ ] | Rate/Rhythm/Apical Impulse/Thrills/Quality of Sound/Intensity/Splitting/Extra Sounds/ Murmurs – |
| 12 | CHEST / LUNGS | [ ] | Excursion/Dullness or Hyperresonance to Percussion/Quality of Breath Sounds/Rales/Wheezing/ Rhonchi/Diaphragm/Rubs/Bruit – |
| 13 | ABDOMEN | [ ] | Bowel Sounds/Appearance/Liver/Spleen/Masses/Hernias/Murmurs/Contour/Tenderness/Bruit/ ING Nodes – |
| 14 | GROIN | [ ] | Hernia/Inguinal Nodes/Femoral Pulses – |
| 15 | MALE GENITALIA | [ ] | Penis/Testes/Scrotum Epididymis/Varicocele/Scars/Discharge – |
| 16 | FEMALE GENITALIA | [ ] | Vuvla/Vagina/Cervix/Uterus/Adnexae/Rectocele/Cystocele/Bartholin Gland/Urethra/ Discharge – Pap Smear (if done ✔) ☐ |
| 17 | EXTREMITIES | [ ] | Deformity/Clubbing/Cyanosis/Edema/Nails/Peripheral Pulses/Calf Tenderness/Joints for Swelling/ ROM – |
| 18 | SKIN | [ ] | Color/Birthmarks/Scars/Texture/Rash/Eczema/Ulcers – |
| 19 | NEUROLOGICAL | [ ] | DTR's/Babinski/Cranial Nerves/Motor Abnormalities/Tremor/Paralysis/Sensory Exam – (touch, pin prick, vibration)/Coordination/Romberg – |
| 20 | MUSCULAR SYSTEM | [ ] | Strength/Wasting/Development – |
| 21 | RECTAL EXAM | [ ] | Sphincter Tone/Hemorrhoids/Fissures/Masses/Prostate/Stool Guaiac (if done ✔) ☐ Pos ☐ Neg – |

Impression: ☐ Check If Normal Physical Examination

Summary: ______

______ Signature ______ Date ______

 

Case Four, Form 16

## COMPREHENSIVE PHYSICAL EXAMINATION
(continued)

(For Office Use Only)

**PHYSICIAN'S NOTES:**

| **Body Area Number** | **REMARKS:** |
|---|---|
| | |
| | |
| | |
| | |
| | |

R L L R

R L

HEIGHT__________

WEIGHT__________

BUILD __________

PULSE __________

RESP. __________

TEMP. __________

**VISION**

Without Glasses

Far R 20/ L 20/

Near R 20/ L 20/

With Glasses

R 20/ L 20/

R 20/ L 20/

Tonometry R______ L______

Colorvision______________

Peripheral Fields R____ L____

**AUDIOMETRIC TESTING**

| | 250 | 500 | 1000 |
|---|---|---|---|
| R | | | |
| L | | | |

| | 2000 | 4000 | 8000 |
|---|---|---|---|
| R | | | |
| L | | | |

Gross Hearing ______________

**BLOOD PRESSURE**

Sitting

R / L /

Standing

R / L /

Lying

R / L /

| **Diagnostic Test:** | **Results:** |
|---|---|
| | |
| | |
| | |
| | |
| | |

**The space below is provided for additional information when these data are being forwarded to a hospital, insurance company, a referral physician, etc.**

**Significant Comments / Recommendations:**

**Physician's Name** ______________

**Address** ______________

**Telephone (area code)** ______________

CONFIDENTIAL

## NUTRITION AND DIET

1. How many meals do you eat each day? .............................. _______ Meals each day
2. Do you usually eat breakfast? .................................... ☐ No ☐ Yes Breakfast
3. Do you diet frequently and/or are you now dieting? ......................... ☐ No ☐ Yes Diets
4. Do you consider yourself .................. ☐ Underweight ☐ Overweight ☐ Just right? Weight
5. Do you snack? .................... ☐ More than once a day ☐ Usually daily ☐ Rarely? Snacks
6. Do you add salt to your food at the table? ..... ☐ Almost always ☐ Sometimes ☐ Rarely Salts food
7. Check the frequency you eat the following types of foods:

| | More than once daily | Daily | 3 times weekly | Once weekly | Twice monthly | Less or never |
|---|---|---|---|---|---|---|
| a. Whole grain or enriched bread or cereal | | | | | | |
| b. Milk, cheese, or other dairy products | | | | | | |
| c. Eggs | | | | | | |
| d. Meat, Poultry, Fish | | | | | | |
| e. Beans, Peas, or other legumes | | | | | | |
| f. Citrus | | | | | | |
| g. Dark green or deep yellow vegetables | | | | | | |

List any food supplements or vitamins you take regularly: ____________________

Additional Patient Comments: ____________________

Thanks for completing this questionnaire. Please review for skipped questions, sign your name on the space to the right and return it to the physician or assistant. If you wish to add any information, please write it in the spaces provided above.

Patient's Signature ____________________

Physician's Notes: ____________________

CONFIDENTIAL





**To order, call or write:**
Bibbero Systems, Inc.
1300 N. McDowell Blvd., Petaluma, CA 94954-1180
Toll Free: 800-BIBBERO (800 242-2376)
Or Fax: 800-242-9330
STOCK NO. 19-742-4 8/95

Case Four, Form 17

# Patient Information Sheet

 **Blackburn Primary Care Associates** 

1990 Turquoise Drive
Blackburn, WI 54937
(555)555-1234

**REGISTRATION**
(PLEASE PRINT)

Home Phone: 555-819-7759

Today's Date: 1/15/00

## PATIENT INFORMATION

Name: FERGUSON (Last Name) LUCILLE (First Name) P (Initial) Soc. Sec.# 576-19-3130

Address: 10 LONGVIEW CIRCLE

City: BLACKBURN State: WI Zip: 54938

Single___ Married___ Widowed ✔ Separated___ Divorced___ Sex M___ F ✔ Age 75 Birthdate 6/21/24

Patient Employed by: Retired Occupation: ———

Business Address___ Business Phone___

By whom were you referred? ___

In case of emergency who should be notified? JAMES FERGUSON (Name) SON (Relation to Patient) Phone 555-811-2191

## PRIMARY INSURANCE

Person Responsible for Account: FERGUSON (Last Name) LUCILLE (First Name) P (Initial)

Relation to Patient: self Birthdate___ Soc. Sec.#___

Address (if different from patient's)___ Phone___

City___ State___ Zip___

Person Responsible Employed by___ Occupation___

Business Address___ Business Phone___

Insurance Company: Medicare

Contract #___ Group #___ Subscriber #: 576193130

Name of other dependents covered under this plan___

## ADDITIONAL INSURANCE

Is patient covered by additional insurance? ___Yes ✔ No

Subscriber Name___ Relation to Patient___ Birthdate___

Address (if different from patient's)___ Phone___

City___ State___ Zip___

Subscriber Employed by___ Business Phone___

Insurance Company___ Soc. Sec.#___

Contract #___ Group #___ Subscriber #___

Name of other dependents covered under this plan___

## ASSIGNMENT AND RELEASE

I, the undersigned, certify that I (or my dependent) have insurance coverage with *Medicare* (Name of Insurance Company(ies)) and assign directly to Dr. *Blackburn Primary* insurance benefits, if any, otherwise payable to me for services rendered. I understand that I am financially responsible for all charges whether or not paid by insurance. I hereby authorize the doctor to release all information necessary to secure the payment of benefits. I authorize the use of this signature on all insurance submissions.

*Lucille Ferguson* (Responsible Party Signature) *Self* (Relationship) *1/15/00* (Date)

Case Four, Form 18

# Patient Encounter Form

## Blackburn Primary Care Associates

1990 Turquoise Drive
Blackburn, WI 54937
(555) 555-1234

FED. I.D. # 52-1963787

**PAT. INFO.**

| ACCT. NO. | PATIENT'S LAST NAME | FIRST | M.I. | DATE OF BIRTH | SEX | TODAY'S DATE |
|---|---|---|---|---|---|---|
| | FERGUSON | LUCILLE | P | 06/21/24 | ☐ M ☒ F | 01/15/00 |

| INSURANCE | COPAY | DISABILITY RELATED TO: ☐ ACCIDENT ☐ INDUSTRIAL ☐ ILLNESS ☐ OTHER |
|---|---|---|
| Medicare | | DATES SYMPTOMS APPEARED, INCEPTION OF PREGNANCY, OR ACCIDENT OCCURRED: / / |

| ✔ | DESCRIPTION | CPT/MD | FEE |
|---|---|---|---|
| | **OFFICE VISITS-NEW PATIENTS** | | |
| | Focused | 99201 | |
| | Expanded | 99202 | |
| | Detailed | 99203 | |
| X | Comprehensive | 99204 | |
| | Complex | 99205 | |
| | | | |
| | **OFFICE VISITS - EST. PATIENTS** | | |
| | Minimal | 99211 | |
| | Focused | 99212 | |
| | Expanded | 99213 | |
| | Detailed | 99214 | |
| | Comprehensive | 99215 | |
| | | | |

| ✔ | PREVENTIVE HEALTH CARE | NEW PT. | EST. PT |
|---|---|---|---|
| | Eval./Mgmt. > 1 Yr | 99381 | 99391 |
| | Early Child 1 - 4 Yrs | 99382 | 99392 |
| | Late Child 5 - 11 Yrs | 99383 | 99393 |
| | Adolescent 12 - 17 Yrs | 99384 | 99394 |
| | Eval./Mgmt. 18 - 39 Yrs | 99385 | 99395 |
| | Eval./Mgmt. 40 - 64 Yrs | 99386 | 99396 |
| | Eval./Mgmt. 65 - Over | 99387 | 99397 |

| ✔ | DESCRIPTION | CPT/MD | FEE |
|---|---|---|---|
| | **HOSP./SNF/HOME VISITS** | | |
| | House Calls | 99341 | |
| | ER Visit | 9928___ | |
| | Init. Hosp. Care | 99222 | |
| | Sub. Hosp. Care | 99232 | |
| | SNF, Sub. Care | 99312 | |
| | **INJECTIONS** | | |
| | Allergy | 95125 | |
| | B-12 | J3420 | |
| | Flu Shot | 90724 | |
| | Gamma Globulin | 90741 | |
| | Hormone | | |
| | Depo Provera | J1055 | |
| | Kenalog 40-60 mg | J3301 | |
| | Morphine/Demerol | J2270 | |
| | Phenergan | J2550 | |
| | Celestone | J0700 | |
| | Hep B, newborn to 11 years | 90744 | |
| | Hep B, 11 - 19 years | 90745 | |
| | Hep B, 20 years and above | 90746 | |
| | Rocephin/Claforan | J0696 | |
| | Iron | J1760 | |
| | Lidocaine NCL | J2000 | |
| | Admin of INJ | J0110 | |
| | Unlist INJ | 90782 | |
| | Drug | | |
| | Dose | | |

| ✔ | DESCRIPTION | CPT/MD | FEE |
|---|---|---|---|
| | **SPECIAL SERVICES** | | |
| | Drivers Physical | 99214 | |
| X | Pelvic/Breast Exam | 99214 | 30.00 |
| | Industrial | 99214 | |
| | **IMMUNIZATIONS** | | |
| | DtaP | 90700 | |
| | DPT | 90701 | |
| | DT | 90702 | |
| | Td (Tetanus Booster) | 90703 | |
| | MMR | 90707 | |
| | Mumps | 90704 | |
| | Pneumococcal | 90732 | |
| | Rubella | 90706 | |
| | Polio (TOPV) | 90712 | |
| | PPD | 86580 | |
| | TB Tine Test | 86585 | |
| | Hib | 90737 | |
| | **OFFICE PROCEDURES** | | |
| | Audiometry | 92551 | |
| | Diathermy (Ultrasound) | 97024 | |
| | EKG Tracing & Interp. | 93000 | |
| | Intermed Joint Injection | 20605 | |
| | Major Joint Injection | 20610 | |
| | Nebulizer TX | 94664 | |
| | Rem. Impact. Cer. | 69210 | |
| | Spirometry | 94010 | |
| | Stress Test | 93015 | |
| | Trigger Pt. Inj. | 20550 | |
| | Eye Wash | 65205* | |
| | **LABORATORY** | | |
| | Throat Culture | 87060 | |
| | Glucose Blood | 82947 | |
| | Glucose Stick | 82948 | |
| | UA Pregnancy | 81025 | |
| | Occult Blood, Stool | 82270 | |
| | Rapid Strep | 86588 | |
| | Smear | 88150 | |
| X | UA Dip | 81002 | |
| | Urinalysis | 81000 | |
| X | Venipuncture | 36415 | |
| | Wet Mount, Smear | 87210 | |
| | Wet Mount KOH | 87220 | |
| | Collect/Handing | 99000 | |
| | **MISCELLANEOUS** | | |
| | Pre-OP | 993___ | |
| | After Hours | 99050 | |
| | Sunday/Holidays | 99054 | |
| | Cast Removal | 29705 | |
| | Norplant Insertion | 11975 | |
| | Norplant Kit | 99070 | |

| ✔ | DESCRIPTION | CPT/MD | FEE |
|---|---|---|---|
| | **SURGERY** | | |
| | Toenail Removal | 11750 | |
| | Cryosurgery | 17200 | |
| | I & D | 10060 | |
| | Drainage Paronychia | 10060 | |
| | Enucleation Ext. Hemorrhoid | 46320 | |
| | I & D Abscess/Cyst | 10060 | |
| | Podophyllom | 17100 | |
| | Removal Foreign Body | 10120 | |
| | Wart Removal | 17110 | |
| | Destr. Single Lesion Face | 17000 | |
| | 2nd and 3rd Lesion Face | 17001 | |
| | Destr. Single Lesion Body | 17106 | |
| | 2nd and 3rd Lesion Body | 17003 | |
| | Lesion Rem. Excision | | |
| | Anoscopy | 46600 | |
| | Flex. Scope with Sig. | 45330 | |
| | Vasectomy | 55250 | |
| | Therapeutic Abor. | 59840 | |
| | Removal Foreign Body of Eye | 65205 | |
| | **SUPPLIES** | | |
| | Ace Wrap | 99070 | |
| | Cast Material | 99070 | |
| | Cervical Collar | 99070 | |
| | Elastic Bandage | 99070 | |
| | Splint/Sling | 99070 | |
| | Sterile Dressing | 99070 | |
| | Surgical Tray | 99070 | |

**DIAGNOSIS:** **ICD-9**

- ☐ Abscess Cellulitis . . . . . . 682.9
- ☐ Abdominal Pain . . . . . . . 789.0
- ☐ Abrasions . . . . . . . . . . . 919.0
- ☐ Acne . . . . . . . . . . . . . . . 706.1
- ☐ ADD . . . . . . . . . . . . . . . 314.00
- ☐ Alcoholism . . . . . . . . . . . 303.90
- ☐ Allergic Rhinitis . . . . . . . 477.9
- ☐ Allergy, Unsp . . . . . . . . . 995.3
- ☐ Anemia . . . . . . . . . . . . . 285.9
- ☐ Angina Pectoris . . . . . . . 413.9
- ☐ Anxiety Depression . . . . 300.4
- ☐ Anxiety State . . . . . . . . . 300.00
- ☐ ASCVD . . . . . . . . . . . . . 429.2
- ☐ Asthma W/O Status Asthma 493.90
- ☐ Atten Surg. Dressing/Suture V58.3
- ☐ BCP Consult . . . . . . . . . V25.9
- ☐ BPH . . . . . . . . . . . . . . . 600
- ☐ Bronchitis, Acute . . . . . . 466.0
- ☐ Bronchitis, Chronic . . . . . 491.9
- ☐ Burn __________ 949.0
- ☐ Bursitis . . . . . . . . . . . . . 727.3
- ☐ C.T.S. . . . . . . . . . . . . . . 354.0
- ☐ CAD . . . . . . . . . . . . . . . 746.85
- ☐ CA-Prostate . . . . . . . . . . 185
- ☐ Cardiac Arrhythmia . . . . . 427.9
- ☐ Cataracts . . . . . . . . . . . . 366.9
- ☐ Chest Pain . . . . . . . . . . . 786.50
- ☐ Congestive Heart Failure 428.0
- ☐ Conjunctivitis . . . . . . . . . 372.30
- ☐ Constipation . . . . . . . . . . 564.0
- ☐ Consult Vasc. . . . . . . . . . V65.8
- ☐ Convulsions . . . . . . . . . . 780.3
- ☐ COPD . . . . . . . . . . . . . . 496
- ☐ Coronary Atherosclerosis. 414.0
- ☐ CVA . . . . . . . . . . . . . . . 436
- ☐ Cyst Sebaceous . . . . . . . 706.2
- ☐ Dermatitis . . . . . . . . . . . 692.9
- ☐ Diabetes, Uncomp. Adult 250.00
- ☐ Diabetes, Complicated . . 250.90
- ☐ Disc Degeneration . . . . . 722.6
- ☐ Duodenal Ulcer . . . . . . . 532.90
- ☐ Dysmenorrhea . . . . . . . . 625.3
- ☐ Fatigue . . . . . . . . . . . . . 780.7
- ☐ Flu Shot Only . . . . . . . . . V04.8
- ☐ Flu Vac . . . . . . . . . . . . . V04.8
- ☐ Flu W/Resp. Manifest . . . 487.1
- ☐ Folliculitis . . . . . . . . . . . 704.8
- ☐ FX __________
- ☐ Gallbladder Disease . . . . 575.9
- ☐ Ganglion . . . . . . . . . . . . 727.43
- ☐ Gastroenteritis . . . . . . . . 558.9
- ☐ Gout . . . . . . . . . . . . . . . 274.9
- ☐ Gyn Exam . . . . . . . . . . . V72.3
- ☐ Headache Tension . . . . . 307.81
- ☐ Hemorrhoids Ext. . . . . . . 455.3
- ☐ Hepatitis . . . . . . . . . . . . 573.3
- ☐ Hernia-Inguinal. . . . . . . . 550.90
- ☐ Herpes Zoster . . . . . . . . 053.9
- ☐ Hyperlipidemia . . . . . . . . 272.4
- ☐ Hypertension . . . . . . . . . 401.9
- ☐ Hyperthyroidism . . . . . . . 242.9
- ☐ Hypothyroidism . . . . . . . 244.9
- ☐ Impacted Cerumen . . . . . 380.4
- ☐ Impetigo . . . . . . . . . . . . 684
- ☐ Ingrown Toenail . . . . . . . 703.0
- ☐ Internal Derangement Knee . 717.9
- ☐ Labyrinthitis . . . . . . . . . . 386.30
- ☐ Laceration Open Wound . 879.8__
- ☐ Levator Scapular Syndrome 726.90
- ☐ Menopausal Disorder . . . 627.9
- ☐ Metabolic Diff. . . . . . . . . 277.8
- ☐ Migraine . . . . . . . . . . . . 346.90
- ☐ Mitral Valve Disorder . . . 424.0
- ☐ Myalgia and Myositis . . . 729.1
- ☐ Noninf. Gastroenterit. . . . 558.9
- ☐ Obesity . . . . . . . . . . . . . 278.0
- ☐ Osteoarthrosis . . . . . . . . 715.00
- ☒ Osteoporosis . . . . . . . . . 733.00
- ☐ Otitis Externa . . . . . . . . . 380.10
- ☐ Otitis Media . . . . . . . . . . 382.9
- ☐ P.I.D. . . . . . . . . . . . . . . 614.9
- ☐ Peptic Ulcer . . . . . . . . . . 533.90
- ☐ Pharyngitis, Acute . . . . . 462
- ☐ Pneumonia, Viral . . . . . . 480.9
- ☐ Poison Oak . . . . . . . . . . 692.6
- ☐ Premarital B-Test . . . . . . V70.3
- ☐ Pregnancy Test, Unconf.. V72.4
- ☐ Prostatitis . . . . . . . . . . . 601.9
- ☐ Psoriasis . . . . . . . . . . . . 696.1
- ☐ Rheumatoid Arthritis . . . . 714.0
- ☐ Sciatica . . . . . . . . . . . . . 724.3
- ☐ Sacroiliac Sprain . . . . . . 846.1
- ☐ Sinusitis, Acute . . . . . . . 461.9
- ☐ Smoking Cessation. . . . . 305.10
- ☐ Sprain __________
- ☐ SQ. Cell CA-Face. . . . . . 173.3
- ☐ Sterilization . . . . . . . . . . V25.2
- ☐ Stye. . . . . . . . . . . . . . . 373.11
- ☐ TB Exposure . . . . . . . . . V01.1
- ☐ Tendonitis . . . . . . . . . . . 726.90
- ☐ Tinea. . . . . . . . . . . . . . . 110.9
- ☐ Tonsillitis, Acute . . . . . . 463
- ☐ URI, Acute . . . . . . . . . . . 465.9
- ☐ Urine Tract Infection . . . . 599.0
- ☐ Vaginitis. . . . . . . . . . . . . 616.10
- ☐ Well Adult Medical Exam V70.9
- ☐ Well Child Health Exam . V20.2

| DIAGNOSIS (If not checked above) ICD-9 | PHYSICIAN SIGNATURE | TODAY'S FEE | $ |
|---|---|---|---|
| Kyphosis | | PAYMENT | |

PLEASE REMEMBER THAT PAYMENT IS YOUR OBLIGATION REGARDLESS OF INSURANCE OR OTHER THIRD PARTY INVOLVEMENT.

PAYMENT BY ☐ CASH ☐ CREDIT CARD ☐ CHECK # ________

**BALANCE DUE**

Case Four, Form 19

# FEE SCHEDULE

## BLACKBURN PRIMARY CARE ASSOCIATES
## 1990 TURQUOISE DRIVE
## BLACKBURN, WI 54937

**Federal Tax ID Number:** **52-1963787**

**BCBS Group Number:** **14982**
**Medicare Group Number:** **14982**

### OFFICE VISIT, NEW PATIENT

| | |
|---|---|
| Focused, 99201 | $ 45.00 |
| Expanded, 99202 | $ 53.00 |
| Detailed, 99203 | $ 60.00 |
| Comprehensive, 99204 | $ 95.00 |
| Complex, 99205 | $195.00 |
| Consultation, 99245 | $250.00 |

### OFFICE VISIT, ESTABLISHED PATIENT

| | |
|---|---|
| Minimal, 99211 | $ 40.00 |
| Focused, 99212 | $ 48.00 |
| Expanded, 99213 | $ 55.00 |
| Detailed, 99214 | $ 65.00 |
| Comprehensive, 99215 | $195.00 |

### OFFICE PROCEDURES

| | |
|---|---|
| EKG, 12 Lead, 93000 | $ 55.00 |
| Stress EKG, Treadmill, 93015 | $295.00 |
| Sigmoidoscopy, Flex., 45330 | $145.00 |
| Spirometry, 94010 | $ 50.00 |
| Cerumen Removal, 69210 | $ 40.00 |
| Collection & Handling | |
| Lab Specimen, 99000 | $ 9.00 |
| Venipuncture, 36415 | $ 9.00 |
| Urinalysis, 81000 | $ 20.00 |
| Urinalysis, 81002 (Dip Only) | $ 12.00 |
| Influenza Injection, 90724 | $ 20.00 |
| Pneumococcal Injection, 90732 | $ 20.00 |
| Oral Polio, 90712 | $ 15.00 |
| DTaP, 90700 | $ 20.00 |
| Tetanus Toxoid, 90703 | $ 15.00 |
| MMR, 90707 | $ 25.00 |
| Hib, 90737 | $ 20.00 |
| Hepatitis B, newborn to age 11 years, 90744 | $ 60.00 |
| Hepatitis B, 11-19 years, 90745 | $ 60.00 |
| Hepatitis B, 20 years and above 90746 | $ 60.00 |
| Intramuscular Injection, 90788 | |
| Penicillin | $ 30.00 |
| Ceftriaxone | $ 25.00 |
| Solu-Medrol | $ 23.00 |
| Vitamin B-12 | $ 13.00 |
| Subcutaneous Injection, 90782 | |
| Epinephrine | $ 18.00 |
| Sus-Pherine | $ 25.00 |
| Insulin, U-100 | $ 15.00 |

### COMMON DIAGNOSIS CODES

| | |
|---|---|
| Ischemic Heart Disease | 414.9 |
| w/o myocardial infarction | 411.89 |
| w/ coronary occlusion | 411.81 |
| Hypertension, Malignant | 401.0 |
| Benign | 401.1 |
| Unspecified | 401.9 |
| w/ congest. heart failure | 402.91 |
| Asthma, Bronchial | 493.9 |
| w/ COPD | 493.2 |
| allergic, w/ S.A. | 493.91 |
| allergic, w/o S.A. | 493.90 |
| Kyphosis | 737.10 |
| w/ osteoporosis | 733.0 |
| Osteoporosis | 733.00 |
| Otitis Media, Acute | 382.9 |
| Chronic | 382.9 |
| Well Child Health Exam | V20.2 |
| Well Adult Medical Exam | V70.9 |

Case Four, Form 20

PLEASE DO NOT STAPLE IN THIS AREA

APPROVED OMB-0938-0008

CARRIER

PICA

# HEALTH INSURANCE CLAIM FORM

PICA

1. MEDICARE (Medicare #) MEDICAID (Medicaid #) CHAMPUS (Sponsor's SSN) CHAMPVA (VA File #) GROUP HEALTH PLAN (SSN or ID) FECA BLK LUNG (SSN) OTHER (ID)

1a. INSURED'S I.D. NUMBER (FOR PROGRAM IN ITEM 1)

2. PATIENT'S NAME (Last Name, First Name, Middle Initial)

3. PATIENT'S BIRTHDATE MM DD YY SEX M F

4. INSURED'S NAME (Last Name, First Name, Middle Initial)

5. PATIENT'S ADDRESS (No., Street)

6. PATIENT RELATIONSHIP TO INSURED Self Spouse Child Other

7. INSURED'S ADDRESS (No., Street)

CITY STATE

8. PATIENT STATUS Single Married Other

CITY STATE

ZIP CODE TELEPHONE (Include Area Code) ( )

Employed Full-Time Student Part-Time Student

ZIP CODE TELEPHONE (Include Area Code) ( )

9. OTHER INSURED'S NAME (Last Name, First Name, Middle Initial)

10. IS PATIENT'S CONDITION RELATED TO:

11. INSURED'S POLICY GROUP OR FECA NUMBER

a. OTHER INSURED'S POLICY OR GROUP NUMBER

a. EMPLOYMENT? (CURRENT OR PREVIOUS) YES NO

a. INSURED'S DATE OF BIRTH MM DD YY SEX M F

b. OTHER INSURED'S DATE OF BIRTH MM DD YY SEX M F

b. AUTO ACCIDENT? YES NO PLACE (State)

b. EMPLOYER'S NAME OR SCHOOL NAME

c. EMPLOYER'S NAME OR SCHOOL NAME

c. OTHER ACCIDENT? YES NO

c. INSURANCE PLAN NAME OR PROGRAM NAME

d. INSURANCE PLAN NAME OR PROGRAM NAME

10d. RESERVED FOR LOCAL USE

d. IS THERE ANOTHER HEALTH BENEFIT PLAN? YES NO *If yes, return to and complete item 9a-d.*

**READ BACK OF FORM BEFORE COMPLETING & SIGNING THIS FORM.**

12. PATIENT'S OR AUTHORIZED PERSON'S SIGNATURE I authorize the release of any medical or other information necessary to process this claim. I also request payment of government benefits either to myself or to the party who accepts assignment below.

SIGNED ____ DATE ____

13. INSURED'S OR AUTHORIZED PERSON'S SIGNATURE I authorize payment of medical benefits to the undersigned physician or supplier for services described below.

SIGNED ____

PATIENT AND INSURED INFORMATION

14. DATE OF CURRENT: MM DD YY ILLNESS (First symptom) OR INJURY (Accident) OR PREGNANCY (LMP)

15. IF PATIENT HAS HAD SAME OR SIMILAR ILLNESS, GIVE FIRST DATE MM DD YY

16. DATES PATIENT UNABLE TO WORK IN CURRENT OCCUPATION FROM MM DD YY TO MM DD YY

17. NAME OF REFERRING PHYSICIAN OR OTHER SOURCE

17a. I.D. NUMBER OF REFERRING PHYSICIAN

18. HOSPITALIZATION DATES RELATED TO CURRENT SERVICES FROM MM DD YY TO MM DD YY

19. RESERVED FOR LOCAL USE

20. OUTSIDE LAB? YES NO $ CHARGES

21. DIAGNOSIS OR NATURE OF ILLNESS OR INJURY. (RELATE ITEMS 1,2,3 OR 4 TO ITEM 24E BY LINE)

1. ____ . __
2. ____ . __
3. ____ . __
4. ____ . __

22. MEDICAID RESUBMISSION CODE ORIGINAL REF. NO.

23. PRIOR AUTHORIZATION NUMBER

| 24. A DATE(S) OF SERVICE From MM DD YY To MM DD YY | B Place of Service | C Type of Service | D PROCEDURES, SERVICES, OR SUPPLIES (Explain Unusual Circumstances) CPT/HCPCS MODIFIER | E DIAGNOSIS CODE | F $ CHARGES | G DAYS OR UNITS | H EPSDT Family Plan | I EMG | J COB | K RESERVED FOR LOCAL USE |
|---|---|---|---|---|---|---|---|---|---|---|
| 1 | | | | | | | | | | |
| 2 | | | | | | | | | | |
| 3 | | | | | | | | | | |
| 4 | | | | | | | | | | |
| 5 | | | | | | | | | | |
| 6 | | | | | | | | | | |

25. FEDERAL TAX I.D. NUMBER SSN EIN

26. PATIENT'S ACCOUNT NUMBER

27. ACCEPT ASSIGNMENT? (For govt. claims, see back) YES NO

28. TOTAL CHARGE $

29. AMOUNT PAID $

30. BALANCE DUE $

31. SIGNATURE OF PHYSICIAN OR SUPPLIER INCLUDING DEGREES OR CREDENTIALS (I certify that the statements on the reverse apply to this bill and are made a part thereof.)

SIGNED DATE

32. NAME AND ADDRESS OF FACILITY WHERE SERVICES WERE RENDERED (If other than home or office)

33. PHYSICIAN'S, SUPPLIER'S BILLING NAME, ADDRESS, ZIP CODE & PHONE #

PIN # GRP#

PHYSICIAN OR SUPPLIER INFORMATION

(APPROVED BY AMA COUNCIL ON MEDICAL SERVICE 8/88)

Form 124OLM

*PLEASE PRINT OR TYPE*

FORM HCFA-1500 (12-90) FORM OWCP-1500 FORM RRB-1500

Administrative Skills, Form 21

# Patient Information Sheet

 **Blackburn Primary Care Associates** 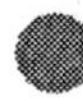

1990 Turquoise Drive
Blackburn, WI 54937
(555)555-1234

**REGISTRATION**
(PLEASE PRINT)

Home Phone: 555-997-1909

Today's Date: 1/15/00

## PATIENT INFORMATION

Name LATHAM (Last Name) CHARLES (First Name) ____ (Initial) Soc. Sec.# 219 61 9002

Address 10971 Clarkbird Road

City Blackburn State WI Zip 54938

Single ____ Married ✔ Widowed ____ Separated ____ Divorced ____ Sex M ✔ F ____ Age 39 Birthdate 7/19/60

Patient Employed by self - LATHAM AUTO Occupation ____

Business Address 10971 Clarkbird Road Business Phone ____

By whom were you referred? ____

In case of emergency who should be notified? PEGGY LATHAM (Name) Wife (Relation to Patient) Phone 555-997-1920

## PRIMARY INSURANCE

Person Responsible for Account Same (Last Name) ____ (First Name) ____ (Initial)

Relation to Patient ____ Birthdate ____ Soc. Sec.# ____

Address (if different from patient's) ____ Phone ____

City ____ State ____ Zip ____

Person Responsible Employed by Self Occupation ____

Business Address ____ Business Phone ____

Insurance Company U.S. Healthcare

Contract # ____ Group # LAT 3600 Subscriber # 1649701

Name of other dependents covered under this plan wife-as above

## ADDITIONAL INSURANCE

Is patient covered by additional insurance? ____ Yes ✔ No

Subscriber Name ____ Relation to Patient ____ Birthdate ____

Address (if different from patient's) ____ Phone ____

City ____ State ____ Zip ____

Subscriber Employed by ____ Business Phone ____

Insurance Company ____ Soc. Sec.# ____

Contract # ____ Group # ____ Subscriber # ____

Name of other dependents covered under this plan ____

## ASSIGNMENT AND RELEASE

I, the undersigned, certify that I (or my dependent) have insurance coverage with *US Healthcare* (Name of Insurance Company(ies))
and assign directly to Dr. *Blackburn Primary* insurance benefits, if any, otherwise payable to me for services rendered. I understand that I am financially responsible for all charges whether or not paid by insurance. I hereby authorize the doctor to release all information necessary to secure the payment of benefits. I authorize the use of this signature on all insurance submissions.

*Charles Latham* (Responsible Party Signature) *self* (Relationship) *1/15/00* (Date)

Administrative Skills, Form 22

# Patient Encounter Form

## Blackburn Primary Care Associates

1990 Turquoise Drive
Blackburn, WI 54937
(555) 555-1234

FED. I.D. # 52-1963787

**PAT. INFO.**

| ACCT. NO. | PATIENT'S LAST NAME | FIRST | M.I. | DATE OF BIRTH | SEX | TODAY'S DATE |
|---|---|---|---|---|---|---|
| | LATHAM | CHARLES | | 07/19/60 | ☒ M ☐ F | 01/15/00 |

| INSURANCE | COPAY | DISABILITY RELATED TO: ☐ ACCIDENT ☐ INDUSTRIAL ☐ ILLNESS ☐ OTHER |
|---|---|---|
| US Healthcare | | DATES SYMPTOMS APPEARED, INCEPTION OF PREGNANCY, OR ACCIDENT OCCURRED: / / |

| ✔ | DESCRIPTION | CPT/MD | FEE |
|---|---|---|---|
| | **OFFICE VISITS-NEW PATIENTS** | | |
| | Focused | 99201 | |
| | Expanded | 99202 | |
| | Detailed | 99203 | |
| X | Comprehensive | 99204 | |
| | Complex | 99205 | |
| | | | |
| | | | |
| | **OFFICE VISITS - EST. PATIENTS** | | |
| | Minimal | 99211 | |
| | Focused | 99212 | |
| | Expanded | 99213 | |
| | Detailed | 99214 | |
| | Comprehensive | 99215 | |
| | | | |
| | | | |
| | **PREVENTIVE HEALTH CARE** NEW PT. | EST. PT | |
| | Eval./Mgmt. > 1 Yr 99381 | 99391 | |
| | Early Child 1 - 4 Yrs 99382 | 99392 | |
| | Late Child 5 - 11 Yrs 99383 | 99393 | |
| | Adolescent 12 - 17 Yrs 99384 | 99394 | |
| | Eval./Mgmt. 18 - 39 Yrs 99385 | 99395 | |
| | Eval./Mgmt. 40 - 64 Yrs 99386 | 99396 | |
| | Eval./Mgmt. 65 - Over 99387 | 99397 | |
| | | | |
| | **HOSP./SNF/HOME VISITS** | | |
| | House Calls | 99341 | |
| | ER Visit | 9928__ | |
| | Init. Hosp. Care | 99222 | |
| | Sub. Hosp. Care | 99232 | |
| | SNF, Sub. Care | 99312 | |
| | | | |
| | **INJECTIONS** | | |
| | Allergy | 95125 | |
| | B-12 | J3420 | |
| X | Flu Shot | 90724 | |
| | Gamma Globulin | 90741 | |
| | Hormone | | |
| | Depo Provera | J1055 | |
| | Kenalog 40-60 mg | J3301 | |
| | Morphine/Demerol | J2270 | |
| | Phenergan | J2550 | |
| | Celestone | J0700 | |
| | Hep B, newborn to 11 years | 90744 | |
| | Hep B, 11 - 19 years | 90745 | |
| | Hep B, 20 years and above | 90746 | |
| | Rocephin/Claforan | J0696 | |
| | Iron | J1760 | |
| | Lidocaine NCL | J2000 | |
| | Admin of INJ | J0110 | |
| | Unlist INJ | 90782 | |
| | Drug | | |
| | Dose | | |

| ✔ | DESCRIPTION | CPT/MD | FEE |
|---|---|---|---|
| | **SPECIAL SERVICES** | | |
| | Drivers Physical | 99214 | |
| | Pelvic/Breast Exam | 99214 | |
| | Industrial | 99214 | |
| | | | |
| | **IMMUNIZATIONS** | | |
| | DtaP | 90700 | |
| | DPT | 90701 | |
| | DT | 90702 | |
| | Td (Tetanus Booster) | 90703 | |
| | MMR | 90707 | |
| | Mumps | 90704 | |
| | Pneumococcal | 90732 | |
| | Rubella | 90706 | |
| | Polio (TOPV) | 90712 | |
| | PPD | 86580 | |
| | TB Tine Test | 86585 | |
| | Hib | 90737 | |
| | | | |
| | | | |
| | **OFFICE PROCEDURES** | | |
| X | Audiometry | 92551 | 35.00 |
| | Diathermy (Ultrasound) | 97024 | |
| | EKG Tracing & Interp. | 93000 | |
| | Intermed Joint Injection | 20605 | |
| | Major Joint Injection | 20610 | |
| | Nebulizer TX | 94664 | |
| | Rem. Impact. Cer. | 69210 | |
| | Spirometry | 94010 | |
| | Stress Test | 93015 | |
| | Trigger Pt. Inj. | 20550 | |
| | Eye Wash | 65205* | |
| | | | |
| | **LABORATORY** | | |
| | Throat Culture | 87060 | |
| | Glucose Blood | 82947 | |
| | Glucose Stick | 82948 | |
| | UA Pregnancy | 81025 | |
| X | Occult Blood, Stool | 82270 | 15.00 |
| | Rapid Strep | 86588 | |
| | Smear | 88150 | |
| | UA Dip | 81002 | |
| X | Urinalysis | 81000 | |
| | Venipuncture | 36415 | |
| | Wet Mount, Smear | 87210 | |
| | Wet Mount KOH | 87220 | |
| | Collect/Handing | 99000 | |
| | | | |
| | **MISCELLANEOUS** | | |
| | Pre-OP | 993__ | |
| | After Hours | 99050 | |
| | Sunday/Holidays | 99054 | |
| | Cast Removal | 29705 | |
| | Norplant Insertion | 11975 | |
| | Norplant Kit | 99070 | |

| ✔ | DESCRIPTION | CPT/MD | FEE |
|---|---|---|---|
| | **SURGERY** | | |
| | Toenail Removal | 11750 | |
| | Cryosurgery | 17200 | |
| | I & D | 10060 | |
| | Drainage Paronychia | 10060 | |
| | Enucleation Ext. Hemorrhoid | 46320 | |
| | I & D Abscess/Cyst | 10060 | |
| | Podophyllom | 17100 | |
| | Removal Foreign Body | 10120 | |
| | Wart Removal | 17110 | |
| | Destr. Single Lesion Face | 17000 | |
| | 2nd and 3rd Lesion Face | 17001 | |
| | Destr. Single Lesion Body | 17106 | |
| | 2nd and 3rd Lesion Body | 17003 | |
| | Lesion Rem. Excision | | |
| | Anoscopy | 46600 | |
| | Flex. Scope with Sig. | 45330 | |
| | Vasectomy | 55250 | |
| | Therapeutic Abor. | 59840 | |
| | Removal Foreign Body of Eye | 65205 | |
| | | | |
| | **SUPPLIES** | | |
| | Ace Wrap | 99070 | |
| | Cast Material | 99070 | |
| | Cervical Collar | 99070 | |
| | Elastic Bandage | 99070 | |
| | Splint/Sling | 99070 | |
| | Sterile Dressing | 99070 | |
| | Surgical Tray | 99070 | |

**DIAGNOSIS: ICD-9**

- ☐ Abscess Cellulitis ...... 682.9
- ☐ Abdominal Pain ........ 789.0
- ☐ Abrasions ........... 919.0
- ☐ Acne ............... 706.1
- ☐ ADD ............... 314.00
- ☐ Alcoholism ........... 303.90
- ☐ Allergic Rhinitis ....... 477.9
- ☐ Allergy, Unsp ......... 995.3
- ☐ Anemia .............. 285.9
- ☐ Angina Pectoris ....... 413.9
- ☐ Anxiety Depression .... 300.4
- ☐ Anxiety State ......... 300.00
- ☐ ASCVD .............. 429.2
- ☐ Asthma W/O Status Asthma 493.90
- ☐ Atten Surg. Dressing/Suture V58.3
- ☐ BCP Consult ......... V25.9
- ☐ BPH ............... 600
- ☐ Bronchitis, Acute ...... 466.0
- ☐ Bronchitis, Chronic ..... 491.9
- ☐ Burn __________ 949.0
- ☐ Bursitis ............. 727.3
- ☐ C.T.S. .............. 354.0
- ☐ CAD ............... 746.85
- ☐ CA-Prostate .......... 185
- ☐ Cardiac Arrhythmia ..... 427.9
- ☐ Cataracts ............ 366.9
- ☐ Chest Pain ........... 786.50
- ☐ Congestive Heart Failure 428.0
- ☐ Conjunctivitis ......... 372.30
- ☐ Constipation .......... 564.0
- ☐ Consult Vasc. ......... V65.8
- ☐ Convulsions .......... 780.3
- ☐ COPD .............. 496
- ☐ Coronary Atherosclerosis. 414.0
- ☐ CVA ............... 436
- ☐ Cyst Sebaceous ....... 706.2
- ☐ Dermatitis ........... 692.9
- ☐ Diabetes, Uncomp. Adult 250.00
- ☐ Diabetes, Complicated .. 250.90
- ☐ Disc Degeneration ..... 722.6
- ☐ Duodenal Ulcer ....... 532.90
- ☐ Dysmenorrhea ........ 625.3
- ☐ Fatigue ............. 780.7
- ☐ Flu Shot Only ......... V04.8
- ☐ Flu Vac ............. V04.8
- ☐ Flu W/Resp. Manifest ... 487.1
- ☐ Folliculitis ........... 704.8
- ☐ FX __________
- ☐ Gallbladder Disease .... 575.9
- ☐ Ganglion ............ 727.43
- ☐ Gastroenteritis ........ 558.9
- ☐ Gout ............... 274.9
- ☐ Gyn Exam ........... V72.3
- ☐ Headache Tension ..... 307.81
- ☐ Hemorrhoids Ext. ...... 455.3
- ☐ Hepatitis ............ 573.3
- ☐ Hernia-Inguinal ....... 550.90
- ☐ Herpes Zoster ........ 053.9
- ☐ Hyperlipidemia ........ 272.4
- ☐ Hypertension ......... 401.9
- ☐ Hyperthyroidism ....... 242.9
- ☐ Hypothyroidism ....... 244.9
- ☐ Impacted Cerumen ..... 380.4
- ☐ Impetigo ............ 684
- ☐ Ingrown Toenail ....... 703.0
- ☐ Internal Derangement Knee . 717.9
- ☐ Labyrinthitis .......... 386.30
- ☐ Laceration Open Wound . 879.8__
- ☐ Levator Scapular Syndrome 726.90
- ☐ Menopausal Disorder ... 627.9
- ☐ Metabolic Diff. ........ 277.8
- ☐ Migraine ............ 346.90
- ☐ Mitral Valve Disorder ... 424.0
- ☐ Myalgia and Myositis ... 729.1
- ☐ Noninf. Gastroenterit. ... 558.9
- ☐ Obesity ............. 278.0
- ☐ Osteoarthrosis ........ 715.00
- ☐ Osteoporosis ......... 733.00
- ☐ Otitis Externa ........ 380.10
- ☐ Otitis Media .......... 382.9
- ☐ P.I.D. .............. 614.9
- ☐ Peptic Ulcer .......... 533.90
- ☐ Pharyngitis, Acute ..... 462
- ☐ Pneumonia, Viral ...... 480.9
- ☐ Poison Oak .......... 692.6
- ☐ Premarital B-Test ...... V70.3
- ☐ Pregnancy Test, Unconf.. V72.4
- ☐ Prostatitis ........... 601.9
- ☐ Psoriasis ............ 696.1
- ☐ Rheumatoid Arthritis .... 714.0
- ☐ Sciatica ............. 724.3
- ☐ Sacroiliac Sprain ...... 846.1
- ☐ Sinusitis, Acute ....... 461.9
- ☐ Smoking Cessation..... 305.10
- ☐ Sprain __________
- ☐ SQ. Cell CA-Face...... 173.3
- ☐ Sterilization .......... V25.2
- ☐ Stye ............... 373.11
- ☐ TB Exposure ......... V01.1
- ☐ Tendonitis ........... 726.90
- ☐ Tinea ............... 110.9
- ☐ Tonsillitis, Acute ....... 463
- ☐ URI, Acute ........... 465.9
- ☐ Urine Tract Infection .... 599.0
- ☐ Vaginitis ............. 616.10
- ☒ Well Adult Medical Exam V70.9
- ☐ Well Child Health Exam . V20.2

| DIAGNOSIS (If not checked above) ICD-9 | PHYSICIAN SIGNATURE | TODAY'S FEE | $ |
|---|---|---|---|
| | *Ralph Lopez, MD* | PAYMENT | |
| PLEASE REMEMBER THAT PAYMENT IS YOUR OBLIGATION REGARDLESS OF INSURANCE OR OTHER THIRD PARTY INVOLVEMENT. | PAYMENT BY ☐ CASH ☐ CREDIT CARD ☐ CHECK # ______ | BALANCE DUE | |

INSUR-A-BILL ® BIBBERO SYSTEMS, INC. • PETALUMA, CA • © 9/94 SB43006.01 (REV. 1/99)

Administrative Skills, Form 23

# FEE SCHEDULE

## BLACKBURN PRIMARY CARE ASSOCIATES
## 1990 TURQUOISE DRIVE
## BLACKBURN, WI 54937

**Federal Tax ID Number:** **52-1963787**

**BCBS Group Number:** **14982**
**Medicare Group Number:** **14982**

## OFFICE VISIT, NEW PATIENT

| | |
|---|---|
| Focused, 99201 | $ 45.00 |
| Expanded, 99202 | $ 53.00 |
| Detailed, 99203 | $ 60.00 |
| Comprehensive, 99204 | $ 95.00 |
| Complex, 99205 | $195.00 |
| Consultation, 99245 | $250.00 |

## OFFICE VISIT, ESTABLISHED PATIENT

| | |
|---|---|
| Minimal, 99211 | $ 40.00 |
| Focused, 99212 | $ 48.00 |
| Expanded, 99213 | $ 55.00 |
| Detailed, 99214 | $ 65.00 |
| Comprehensive, 99215 | $195.00 |

## OFFICE PROCEDURES

| | |
|---|---|
| EKG, 12 Lead, 93000 | $ 55.00 |
| Stress EKG, Treadmill, 93015 | $295.00 |
| Sigmoidoscopy, Flex., 45330 | $145.00 |
| Spirometry, 94010 | $ 50.00 |
| Cerumen Removal, 69210 | $ 40.00 |
| Collection & Handling | |
| Lab Specimen, 99000 | $ 9.00 |
| Venipuncture, 36415 | $ 9.00 |
| Urinalysis, 81000 | $ 20.00 |
| Urinalysis, 81002 (Dip Only) | $ 12.00 |
| Influenza Injection, 90724 | $ 20.00 |
| Pneumococcal Injection, 90732 | $ 20.00 |
| Oral Polio, 90712 | $ 15.00 |
| DTaP, 90700 | $ 20.00 |
| Tetanus Toxoid, 90703 | $ 15.00 |
| MMR, 90707 | $ 25.00 |
| Hib, 90737 | $ 20.00 |
| Hepatitis B, newborn to age 11 years, 90744 | $ 60.00 |
| Hepatitis B, 11-19 years, 90745 | $ 60.00 |
| Hepatitis B, 20 years and above 90746 | $ 60.00 |
| Intramuscular Injection, 90788 | |
| Penicillin | $ 30.00 |
| Ceftriaxone | $ 25.00 |
| Solu-Medrol | $ 23.00 |
| Vitamin B-12 | $ 13.00 |
| Subcutaneous Injection, 90782 | |
| Epinephrine | $ 18.00 |
| Sus-Pherine | $ 25.00 |
| Insulin, U-100 | $ 15.00 |

## COMMON DIAGNOSIS CODES

| | |
|---|---|
| Ischemic Heart Disease | 414.9 |
| w/o myocardial infarction | 411.89 |
| w/ coronary occlusion | 411.81 |
| Hypertension, Malignant | 401.0 |
| Benign | 401.1 |
| Unspecified | 401.9 |
| w/ congest. heart failure | 402.91 |
| Asthma, Bronchial | 493.9 |
| w/ COPD | 493.2 |
| allergic, w/ S.A. | 493.91 |
| allergic, w/o S.A. | 493.90 |
| Kyphosis | 737.10 |
| w/ osteoporosis | 733.0 |
| Osteoporosis | 733.00 |
| Otitis Media, Acute | 382.9 |
| Chronic | 382.9 |
| Well Child Health Exam | V20.2 |
| Well Adult Medical Exam | V70.9 |

PLEASE DO NOT STAPLE IN THIS AREA

APPROVED OMB-0938-0008

CARRIER

PICA

# HEALTH INSURANCE CLAIM FORM

PICA

1. MEDICARE (Medicare #) MEDICAID (Medicaid #) CHAMPUS (Sponsor's SSN) CHAMPVA (VA File #) GROUP HEALTH PLAN (SSN or ID) FECA BLK LUNG (SSN) OTHER (ID)

1a. INSURED'S I.D. NUMBER (FOR PROGRAM IN ITEM 1)

2. PATIENT'S NAME (Last Name, First Name, Middle Initial)

3. PATIENT'S BIRTHDATE MM DD YY SEX M F

4. INSURED'S NAME (Last Name, First Name, Middle Initial)

5. PATIENT'S ADDRESS (No., Street)

6. PATIENT RELATIONSHIP TO INSURED Self Spouse Child Other

7. INSURED'S ADDRESS (No., Street)

CITY STATE

8. PATIENT STATUS Single Married Other

CITY STATE

ZIP CODE TELEPHONE (Include Area Code) ( )

Employed Full-Time Student Part-Time Student

ZIP CODE TELEPHONE (Include Area Code) ( )

9. OTHER INSURED'S NAME (Last Name, First Name, Middle Initial)

10. IS PATIENT'S CONDITION RELATED TO:

11. INSURED'S POLICY GROUP OR FECA NUMBER

a. OTHER INSURED'S POLICY OR GROUP NUMBER

a. EMPLOYMENT? (CURRENT OR PREVIOUS) YES NO

a. INSURED'S DATE OF BIRTH MM DD YY SEX M F

b. OTHER INSURED'S DATE OF BIRTH MM DD YY SEX M F

b. AUTO ACCIDENT? PLACE (State) YES NO

b. EMPLOYER'S NAME OR SCHOOL NAME

c. EMPLOYER'S NAME OR SCHOOL NAME

c. OTHER ACCIDENT? YES NO

c. INSURANCE PLAN NAME OR PROGRAM NAME

d. INSURANCE PLAN NAME OR PROGRAM NAME

10d. RESERVED FOR LOCAL USE

d. IS THERE ANOTHER HEALTH BENEFIT PLAN? YES NO *If yes, return to and complete item 9a-d.*

PATIENT AND INSURED INFORMATION

**READ BACK OF FORM BEFORE COMPLETING & SIGNING THIS FORM.**

12. PATIENT'S OR AUTHORIZED PERSON'S SIGNATURE I authorize the release of any medical or other information necessary to process this claim. I also request payment of government benefits either to myself or to the party who accepts assignment below.

SIGNED ____ DATE ____

13. INSURED'S OR AUTHORIZED PERSON'S SIGNATURE I authorize payment of medical benefits to the undersigned physician or supplier for services described below.

SIGNED ____

14. DATE OF CURRENT: MM DD YY ILLNESS (First symptom) OR INJURY (Accident) OR PREGNANCY (LMP)

15. IF PATIENT HAS HAD SAME OR SIMILAR ILLNESS, GIVE FIRST DATE MM DD YY

16. DATES PATIENT UNABLE TO WORK IN CURRENT OCCUPATION FROM MM DD YY TO MM DD YY

17. NAME OF REFERRING PHYSICIAN OR OTHER SOURCE

17a. I.D. NUMBER OF REFERRING PHYSICIAN

18. HOSPITALIZATION DATES RELATED TO CURRENT SERVICES FROM MM DD YY TO MM DD YY

19. RESERVED FOR LOCAL USE

20. OUTSIDE LAB? YES NO $ CHARGES

21. DIAGNOSIS OR NATURE OF ILLNESS OR INJURY. (RELATE ITEMS 1,2,3 OR 4 TO ITEM 24E BY LINE)

1. ___ . __

2. ___ . __

3. ___ . __

4. ___ . __

22. MEDICAID RESUBMISSION CODE ORIGINAL REF. NO.

23. PRIOR AUTHORIZATION NUMBER

| 24. A DATE(S) OF SERVICE From MM DD YY | To MM DD YY | B Place of Service | C Type of Service | D PROCEDURES, SERVICES, OR SUPPLIES (Explain Unusual Circumstances) CPT/HCPCS MODIFIER | E DIAGNOSIS CODE | F $ CHARGES | G DAYS OR UNITS | H EPSDT Family Plan | I EMG | J COB | K RESERVED FOR LOCAL USE |
|---|---|---|---|---|---|---|---|---|---|---|---|
| 1 | | | | | | | | | | | |
| 2 | | | | | | | | | | | |
| 3 | | | | | | | | | | | |
| 4 | | | | | | | | | | | |
| 5 | | | | | | | | | | | |
| 6 | | | | | | | | | | | |

25. FEDERAL TAX I.D. NUMBER SSN EIN

26. PATIENTS ACCOUNT NUMBER

27. ACCEPT ASSIGNMENT? (For govt. claims, see back) YES NO

28. TOTAL CHARGE $

29. AMOUNT PAID $

30. BALANCE DUE $

31. SIGNATURE OF PHYSICIAN OR SUPPLIER INCLUDING DEGREES OR CREDENTIALS (I certify that the statements on the reverse apply to this bill and are made a part thereof.)

SIGNED DATE

32. NAME AND ADDRESS OF FACILITY WHERE SERVICES WERE RENDERED (If other than home or office)

33. PHYSICIAN'S, SUPPLIER'S BILLING NAME, ADDRESS, ZIP CODE & PHONE #

PIN # GRP#

PHYSICIAN OR SUPPLIER INFORMATION

**(APPROVED BY AMA COUNCIL ON MEDICAL SERVICE 8/88)**

***PLEASE PRINT OR TYPE***

FORM HCFA-1500 (12-90) FORM OWCP-1500 FORM RRB-1500

Form 124OLM

Administrative Skills, Form 25

# Patient Information Sheet

 **Blackburn Primary Care Associates** 

1990 Turquoise Drive
Blackburn, WI 54937
(555)555-1234

**REGISTRATION**
(PLEASE PRINT)

Home Phone: 555-722-1975    Today's Date: 1/20/00

## PATIENT INFORMATION

Name JORDAN (Last Name) MARRION (First Name) (Initial)    Soc. Sec.# 319-21-6115

Address 3242 BOSTON CIRCLE

City BLACKBURN    State WI    Zip 59767

Single __ Married __ Widowed __ Separated __ Divorced ✔    Sex M __ F ✔    Age 29    Birthdate 3/16/70

Patient Employed by UNIVERSITY OF WISCONSIN    Occupation TEACHER

Business Address ____    Business Phone 555-719-0011

By whom were you referred? RAYMOND JOHNSON

In case of emergency who should be notified? CAROL JORDAN (Name) mom (Relation to Patient)    Phone 555-722-1919

## PRIMARY INSURANCE

Person Responsible for Account JORDAN (Last Name) MARRION (First Name) (Initial)

Relation to Patient self    Birthdate 3/16/70    Soc. Sec.# 319216115

Address (if different from patient's) same    Phone ____

City ____    State ____    Zip ____

Person Responsible Employed by as above    Occupation ____

Business Address ____    Business Phone ____

Insurance Company BCBS

Contract # ____    Group # P2170    Subscriber # 319216115

Name of other dependents covered under this plan ____

## ADDITIONAL INSURANCE

Is patient covered by additional insurance? __ Yes ✔ No

Subscriber Name ____    Relation to Patient ____    Birthdate ____

Address (if different from patient's) ____    Phone ____

City ____    State ____    Zip ____

Subscriber Employed by ____    Business Phone ____

Insurance Company ____    Soc. Sec.# ____

Contract # ____    Group # ____    Subscriber # ____

Name of other dependents covered under this plan ____

## ASSIGNMENT AND RELEASE

I, the undersigned, certify that I (or my dependent) have insurance coverage with BCBS (Name of Insurance Company(ies)) and assign directly to Dr. Blackburn Primary insurance benefits, if any, otherwise payable to me for services rendered. I understand that I am financially responsible for all charges whether or not paid by insurance. I hereby authorize the doctor to release all information necessary to secure the payment of benefits. I authorize the use of this signature on all insurance submissions.

Marrion Jordan (Responsible Party Signature)    self (Relationship)    1/20/00 (Date)

Administrative Skills, Form 26

# Patient Encounter Form

## Blackburn Primary Care Associates

1990 Turquoise Drive
Blackburn, WI 54937
(555) 555-1234

FED. I.D. # 52-1963787

**PAT. INFO.**

| ACCT. NO. | PATIENT'S LAST NAME | FIRST | M.I. | DATE OF BIRTH | SEX | TODAY'S DATE |
|---|---|---|---|---|---|---|
| | JORDAN | MARRION | | 03/16/70 | ☐ M ☒ F | 01/20/00 |

| INSURANCE | COPAY | DISABILITY RELATED TO: ☐ ACCIDENT ☐ INDUSTRIAL ☐ ILLNESS ☐ OTHER |
|---|---|---|
| BCBS | | DATES SYMPTOMS APPEARED, INCEPTION OF PREGNANCY, OR ACCIDENT OCCURRED: / / |

| ✔ | DESCRIPTION | CPT/MD | FEE |
|---|---|---|---|
| | **OFFICE VISITS-NEW PATIENTS** | | |
| | Focused | 99201 | |
| | Expanded | 99202 | |
| X | Detailed | 99203 | |
| | Comprehensive | 99204 | |
| | Complex | 99205 | |
| | **OFFICE VISITS - EST. PATIENTS** | | |
| | Minimal | 99211 | |
| | Focused | 99212 | |
| | Expanded | 99213 | |
| | Detailed | 99214 | |
| | Comprehensive | 99215 | |
| | **PREVENTIVE HEALTH CARE** (NEW PT. / EST. PT) | | |
| | Eval./Mgmt. > 1 Yr — 99381 | 99391 | |
| | Early Child 1 - 4 Yrs — 99382 | 99392 | |
| | Late Child 5 - 11 Yrs — 99383 | 99393 | |
| | Adolescent 12 - 17 Yrs — 99384 | 99394 | |
| | Eval./Mgmt. 18 - 39 Yrs — 99385 | 99395 | |
| | Eval./Mgmt. 40 - 64 Yrs — 99386 | 99396 | |
| | Eval./Mgmt. 65 - Over — 99387 | 99397 | |
| | **HOSP./SNF/HOME VISITS** | | |
| | House Calls | 99341 | |
| | ER Visit | 9928__ | |
| | Init. Hosp. Care | 99222 | |
| | Sub. Hosp. Care | 99232 | |
| | SNF, Sub. Care | 99312 | |
| | **INJECTIONS** | | |
| | Allergy | 95125 | |
| | B-12 | J3420 | |
| | Flu Shot | 90724 | |
| | Gamma Globulin | 90741 | |
| | Hormone | | |
| X | Depo Provera | J1055 | 30.00 |
| | Kenalog 40-60 mg | J3301 | |
| | Morphine/Demerol | J2270 | |
| | Phenergan | J2550 | |
| | Celestone | J0700 | |
| | Hep B, newborn to 11 years | 90744 | |
| | Hep B, 11 - 19 years | 90745 | |
| | Hep B, 20 years and above | 90746 | |
| | Rocephin/Claforan | J0696 | |
| | Iron | J1760 | |
| | Lidocaine NCL | J2000 | |
| | Admin of INJ | J0110 | |
| | Unlist INJ | 90782 | |
| | Drug | | |
| | Dose | | |

| ✔ | DESCRIPTION | CPT/MD | FEE |
|---|---|---|---|
| | **SPECIAL SERVICES** | | |
| | Drivers Physical | 99214 | |
| | Pelvic/Breast Exam | 99214 | |
| | Industrial | 99214 | |
| | **IMMUNIZATIONS** | | |
| | DtaP | 90700 | |
| | DPT | 90701 | |
| | DT | 90702 | |
| | Td (Tetanus Booster) | 90703 | |
| | MMR | 90707 | |
| | Mumps | 90704 | |
| | Pneumococcal | 90732 | |
| | Rubella | 90706 | |
| | Polio (TOPV) | 90712 | |
| | PPD | 86580 | |
| | TB Tine Test | 86585 | |
| | Hib | 90737 | |
| | **OFFICE PROCEDURES** | | |
| | Audiometry | 92551 | |
| | Diathermy (Ultrasound) | 97024 | |
| | EKG Tracing & Interp. | 93000 | |
| | Intermed Joint Injection | 20605 | |
| | Major Joint Injection | 20610 | |
| | Nebulizer TX | 94664 | |
| | Rem. Impact. Cer. | 69210 | |
| | Spirometry | 94010 | |
| | Stress Test | 93015 | |
| | Trigger Pt. Inj. | 20550 | |
| | Eye Wash | 65205* | |
| | **LABORATORY** | | |
| | Throat Culture | 87060 | |
| | Glucose Blood | 82947 | |
| | Glucose Stick | 82948 | |
| X | UA Pregnancy | 81025 | 22.00 |
| | Occult Blood, Stool | 82270 | |
| | Rapid Strep | 86588 | |
| | Smear | 88150 | |
| | UA Dip | 81002 | |
| | Urinalysis | 81000 | |
| | Venipuncture | 36415 | |
| | Wet Mount, Smear | 87210 | |
| | Wet Mount KOH | 87220 | |
| | Collect/Handing | 99000 | |
| | **MISCELLANEOUS** | | |
| | Pre-OP | 993__ | |
| | After Hours | 99050 | |
| | Sunday/Holidays | 99054 | |
| | Cast Removal | 29705 | |
| | Norplant Insertion | 11975 | |
| | Norplant Kit | 99070 | |

| ✔ | DESCRIPTION | CPT/MD | FEE |
|---|---|---|---|
| | **SURGERY** | | |
| | Toenail Removal | 11750 | |
| | Cryosurgery | 17200 | |
| | I & D | 10060 | |
| | Drainage Paronychia | 10060 | |
| | Enucleation Ext. Hemorrhoid | 46320 | |
| | I & D Abscess/Cyst | 10060 | |
| | Podophyllom | 17100 | |
| | Removal Foreign Body | 10120 | |
| | Wart Removal | 17110 | |
| | Destr. Single Lesion Face | 17000 | |
| | 2nd and 3rd Lesion Face | 17001 | |
| | Destr. Single Lesion Body | 17106 | |
| | 2nd and 3rd Lesion Body | 17003 | |
| | Lesion Rem. Excision | | |
| | Anoscopy | 46600 | |
| | Flex. Scope with Sig. | 45330 | |
| | Vasectomy | 55250 | |
| | Therapeutic Abor. | 59840 | |
| | Removal Foreign Body of Eye | 65205 | |
| | **SUPPLIES** | | |
| | Ace Wrap | 99070 | |
| | Cast Material | 99070 | |
| | Cervical Collar | 99070 | |
| | Elastic Bandage | 99070 | |
| | Splint/Sling | 99070 | |
| | Sterile Dressing | 99070 | |
| | Surgical Tray | 99070 | |

**DIAGNOSIS: ICD-9**

- ☐ Abscess Cellulitis . . . . . . 682.9
- ☐ Abdominal Pain . . . . . . . 789.0
- ☐ Abrasions . . . . . . . . . . . 919.0
- ☐ Acne . . . . . . . . . . . . . . . 706.1
- ☐ ADD . . . . . . . . . . . . . . . 314.00
- ☐ Alcoholism . . . . . . . . . . . 303.90
- ☐ Allergic Rhinitis . . . . . . . 477.9
- ☐ Allergy, Unsp . . . . . . . . . 995.3
- ☐ Anemia . . . . . . . . . . . . . 285.9
- ☐ Angina Pectoris . . . . . . . 413.9
- ☐ Anxiety Depression . . . . 300.4
- ☐ Anxiety State . . . . . . . . . 300.00
- ☐ ASCVD . . . . . . . . . . . . . 429.2
- ☐ Asthma W/O Status Asthma 493.90
- ☐ Atten Surg. Dressing/Suture V58.3
- ☐ BCP Consult . . . . . . . . . V25.9
- ☐ BPH . . . . . . . . . . . . . . . 600
- ☐ Bronchitis, Acute . . . . . . 466.0
- ☐ Bronchitis, Chronic . . . . . 491.9
- ☐ Burn ____________ 949.0
- ☐ Bursitis . . . . . . . . . . . . . 727.3
- ☐ C.T.S. . . . . . . . . . . . . . . 354.0
- ☐ CAD . . . . . . . . . . . . . . . 746.85
- ☐ CA-Prostate . . . . . . . . . . 185
- ☐ Cardiac Arrhythmia . . . . . 427.9
- ☐ Cataracts . . . . . . . . . . . . 366.9
- ☐ Chest Pain . . . . . . . . . . . 786.50
- ☐ Congestive Heart Failure 428.0
- ☐ Conjunctivitis . . . . . . . . . 372.30
- ☐ Constipation . . . . . . . . . . 564.0
- ☐ Consult Vasc. . . . . . . . . . V65.8
- ☐ Convulsions . . . . . . . . . . 780.3
- ☐ COPD . . . . . . . . . . . . . . 496
- ☐ Coronary Atherosclerosis. 414.0
- ☐ CVA . . . . . . . . . . . . . . . 436
- ☐ Cyst Sebaceous . . . . . . . 706.2
- ☐ Dermatitis . . . . . . . . . . . 692.9
- ☐ Diabetes, Uncomp. Adult 250.00
- ☐ Diabetes, Complicated . . 250.90
- ☐ Disc Degeneration . . . . . 722.6
- ☐ Duodenal Ulcer . . . . . . . 532.90
- ☒ Dysmenorrhea . . . . . . . . 625.3
- ☐ Fatigue . . . . . . . . . . . . . 780.7
- ☐ Flu Shot Only . . . . . . . . . V04.8
- ☐ Flu Vac . . . . . . . . . . . . . V04.8
- ☐ Flu W/Resp. Manifest . . . 487.1
- ☐ Folliculitis . . . . . . . . . . . 704.8
- ☐ FX ____________
- ☐ Gallbladder Disease . . . . 575.9
- ☐ Ganglion . . . . . . . . . . . . 727.43
- ☐ Gastroenteritis . . . . . . . . 558.9
- ☐ Gout . . . . . . . . . . . . . . . 274.9
- ☐ Gyn Exam . . . . . . . . . . . V72.3
- ☐ Headache Tension . . . . . 307.81
- ☐ Hemorrhoids Ext. . . . . . . 455.3
- ☐ Hepatitis . . . . . . . . . . . . 573.3
- ☐ Hernia-Inguinal . . . . . . . . 550.90
- ☐ Herpes Zoster . . . . . . . . . 053.9
- ☐ Hyperlipidemia . . . . . . . . 272.4
- ☐ Hypertension . . . . . . . . . 401.9
- ☐ Hyperthyroidism . . . . . . . 242.9
- ☐ Hypothyroidism . . . . . . . 244.9
- ☐ Impacted Cerumen . . . . . 380.4
- ☐ Impetigo . . . . . . . . . . . . 684
- ☐ Ingrown Toenail . . . . . . . 703.0
- ☐ Internal Derangement Knee . 717.9
- ☐ Labyrinthitis . . . . . . . . . . 386.30
- ☐ Laceration Open Wound . 879.8__
- ☐ Levator Scapular Syndrome 726.90
- ☐ Menopausal Disorder . . . 627.9
- ☐ Metabolic Diff. . . . . . . . . 277.8
- ☒ Migraine . . . . . . . . . . . . 346.90
- ☐ Mitral Valve Disorder . . . 424.0
- ☐ Myalgia and Myositis . . . 729.1
- ☐ Noninf. Gastroenterit. . . . 558.9
- ☐ Obesity . . . . . . . . . . . . . 278.0
- ☐ Osteoarthrosis . . . . . . . . 715.00
- ☐ Osteoporosis . . . . . . . . . 733.00
- ☐ Otitis Externa . . . . . . . . . 380.10
- ☐ Otitis Media . . . . . . . . . . 382.9
- ☐ P.I.D. . . . . . . . . . . . . . . 614.9
- ☐ Peptic Ulcer . . . . . . . . . . 533.90
- ☐ Pharyngitis, Acute . . . . . 462
- ☐ Pneumonia, Viral . . . . . . 480.9
- ☐ Poison Oak . . . . . . . . . . 692.6
- ☐ Premarital B-Test . . . . . . V70.3
- ☐ Pregnancy Test, Unconf.. V72.4
- ☐ Prostatitis . . . . . . . . . . . 601.9
- ☐ Psoriasis . . . . . . . . . . . . 696.1
- ☐ Rheumatoid Arthritis . . . . 714.0
- ☐ Sciatica . . . . . . . . . . . . . 724.3
- ☐ Sacroiliac Sprain . . . . . . 846.1
- ☐ Sinusitis, Acute . . . . . . . 461.9
- ☐ Smoking Cessation. . . . . 305.10
- ☐ Sprain ____________
- ☐ SQ. Cell CA-Face. . . . . . 173.3
- ☐ Sterilization . . . . . . . . . . V25.2
- ☐ Stye. . . . . . . . . . . . . . . . 373.11
- ☐ TB Exposure . . . . . . . . . V01.1
- ☐ Tendonitis . . . . . . . . . . . 726.90
- ☐ Tinea . . . . . . . . . . . . . . . 110.9
- ☐ Tonsillitis, Acute . . . . . . 463
- ☐ URI, Acute . . . . . . . . . . . 465.9
- ☐ Urine Tract Infection . . . . 599.0
- ☐ Vaginitis. . . . . . . . . . . . . 616.10
- ☐ Well Adult Medical Exam V70.9
- ☐ Well Child Health Exam . V20.2

| DIAGNOSIS (If not checked above) ICD-9 | PHYSICIAN SIGNATURE | TODAY'S FEE | $ |
|---|---|---|---|
| | | PAYMENT | |
| PLEASE REMEMBER THAT PAYMENT IS YOUR OBLIGATION REGARDLESS OF INSURANCE OR OTHER THIRD PARTY INVOLVEMENT. | PAYMENT BY ☐ CASH ☐ CREDIT CARD ☐ CHECK # ______ | BALANCE DUE | |

INSUR-A-BILL ® BIBBERO SYSTEMS, INC. • PETALUMA, CA • © 9/94 SB43006.01 (REV. 1/99)

Courtesy of Bibbero Systems, Inc., Petaluma, California.

Administrative Skills, Form 27

# FEE SCHEDULE

## BLACKBURN PRIMARY CARE ASSOCIATES
## 1990 TURQUOISE DRIVE
## BLACKBURN, WI 54937

**Federal Tax ID Number:** **52-1963787**

**BCBS Group Number:** **14982**
**Medicare Group Number:** **14982**

### OFFICE VISIT, NEW PATIENT

| | |
|---|---|
| Focused, 99201 | $ 45.00 |
| Expanded, 99202 | $ 53.00 |
| Detailed, 99203 | $ 60.00 |
| Comprehensive, 99204 | $ 95.00 |
| Complex, 99205 | $195.00 |
| Consultation, 99245 | $250.00 |

### OFFICE PROCEDURES

| | |
|---|---|
| EKG, 12 Lead, 93000 | $ 55.00 |
| Stress EKG, Treadmill, 93015 | $295.00 |
| Sigmoidoscopy, Flex., 45330 | $145.00 |
| Spirometry, 94010 | $ 50.00 |
| Cerumen Removal, 69210 | $ 40.00 |
| Collection & Handling | |
| Lab Specimen, 99000 | $ 9.00 |
| Venipuncture, 36415 | $ 9.00 |
| Urinalysis, 81000 | $ 20.00 |
| Urinalysis, 81002 (Dip Only) | $ 12.00 |
| Influenza Injection, 90724 | $ 20.00 |
| Pneumococcal Injection, 90732 | $ 20.00 |
| Oral Polio, 90712 | $ 15.00 |
| DTaP, 90700 | $ 20.00 |
| Tetanus Toxoid, 90703 | $ 15.00 |
| MMR, 90707 | $ 25.00 |
| Hib, 90737 | $ 20.00 |
| Hepatitis B, newborn to age 11 years, 90744 | $ 60.00 |
| Hepatitis B, 11-19 years, 90745 | $ 60.00 |
| Hepatitis B, 20 years and above 90746 | $ 60.00 |
| Intramuscular Injection, 90788 | |
| Penicillin | $ 30.00 |
| Ceftriaxone | $ 25.00 |
| Solu-Medrol | $ 23.00 |
| Vitamin B-12 | $ 13.00 |
| Subcutaneous Injection, 90782 | |
| Epinephrine | $ 18.00 |
| Sus-Pherine | $ 25.00 |
| Insulin, U-100 | $ 15.00 |

### OFFICE VISIT, ESTABLISHED PATIENT

| | |
|---|---|
| Minimal, 99211 | $ 40.00 |
| Focused, 99212 | $ 48.00 |
| Expanded, 99213 | $ 55.00 |
| Detailed, 99214 | $ 65.00 |
| Comprehensive, 99215 | $195.00 |

### COMMON DIAGNOSIS CODES

| | |
|---|---|
| Ischemic Heart Disease | 414.9 |
| w/o myocardial infarction | 411.89 |
| w/ coronary occlusion | 411.81 |
| Hypertension, Malignant | 401.0 |
| Benign | 401.1 |
| Unspecified | 401.9 |
| w/ congest. heart failure | 402.91 |
| Asthma, Bronchial | 493.9 |
| w/ COPD | 493.2 |
| allergic, w/ S.A. | 493.91 |
| allergic, w/o S.A. | 493.90 |
| Kyphosis | 737.10 |
| w/ osteoporosis | 733.0 |
| Osteoporosis | 733.00 |
| Otitis Media, Acute | 382.9 |
| Chronic | 382.9 |
| Well Child Health Exam | V20.2 |
| Well Adult Medical Exam | V70.9 |

PLEASE DO NOT STAPLE IN THIS AREA

APPROVED OMB-0938-0008

CARRIER

PICA

# HEALTH INSURANCE CLAIM FORM

PICA

1. MEDICARE (Medicare #) MEDICAID (Medicaid #) CHAMPUS (Sponsor's SSN) CHAMPVA (VA File #) GROUP HEALTH PLAN (SSN or ID) FECA BLK LUNG (SSN) OTHER (ID)

1a. INSURED'S I.D. NUMBER (FOR PROGRAM IN ITEM 1)

2. PATIENT'S NAME (Last Name, First Name, Middle Initial)

3. PATIENT'S BIRTHDATE MM DD YY SEX M F

4. INSURED'S NAME (Last Name, First Name, Middle Initial)

5. PATIENT'S ADDRESS (No., Street)

6. PATIENT RELATIONSHIP TO INSURED Self Spouse Child Other

7. INSURED'S ADDRESS (No., Street)

CITY STATE

8. PATIENT STATUS Single Married Other

CITY STATE

ZIP CODE TELEPHONE (Include Area Code) ( )

Employed Full-Time Student Part-Time Student

ZIP CODE TELEPHONE (Include Area Code) ( )

9. OTHER INSURED'S NAME (Last Name, First Name, Middle Initial)

10. IS PATIENT'S CONDITION RELATED TO:

11. INSURED'S POLICY GROUP OR FECA NUMBER

a. OTHER INSURED'S POLICY OR GROUP NUMBER

a. EMPLOYMENT? (CURRENT OR PREVIOUS) YES NO

a. INSURED'S DATE OF BIRTH MM DD YY SEX M F

b. OTHER INSURED'S DATE OF BIRTH MM DD YY SEX M F

b. AUTO ACCIDENT? YES NO PLACE (State)

b. EMPLOYER'S NAME OR SCHOOL NAME

c. EMPLOYER'S NAME OR SCHOOL NAME

c. OTHER ACCIDENT? YES NO

c. INSURANCE PLAN NAME OR PROGRAM NAME

d. INSURANCE PLAN NAME OR PROGRAM NAME

10d. RESERVED FOR LOCAL USE

d. IS THERE ANOTHER HEALTH BENEFIT PLAN? YES NO *If yes, return to and complete item 9a-d.*

**READ BACK OF FORM BEFORE COMPLETING & SIGNING THIS FORM.**

12. PATIENT'S OR AUTHORIZED PERSON'S SIGNATURE I authorize the release of any medical or other information necessary to process this claim. I also request payment of government benefits either to myself or to the party who accepts assignment below.

SIGNED ______ DATE ______

13. INSURED'S OR AUTHORIZED PERSON'S SIGNATURE I authorize payment of medical benefits to the undersigned physician or supplier for services described below.

SIGNED ______

PATIENT AND INSURED INFORMATION

14. DATE OF CURRENT: MM DD YY ILLNESS (First symptom) OR INJURY (Accident) OR PREGNANCY (LMP)

15. IF PATIENT HAS HAD SAME OR SIMILAR ILLNESS, GIVE FIRST DATE MM DD YY

16. DATES PATIENT UNABLE TO WORK IN CURRENT OCCUPATION FROM MM DD YY TO MM DD YY

17. NAME OF REFERRING PHYSICIAN OR OTHER SOURCE

17a. I.D. NUMBER OF REFERRING PHYSICIAN

18. HOSPITALIZATION DATES RELATED TO CURRENT SERVICES FROM MM DD YY TO MM DD YY

19. RESERVED FOR LOCAL USE

20. OUTSIDE LAB? YES NO $ CHARGES

21. DIAGNOSIS OR NATURE OF ILLNESS OR INJURY. (RELATE ITEMS 1,2,3 OR 4 TO ITEM 24E BY LINE)

1. ___ . __

2. ___ . __

3. ___ . __

4. ___ . __

22. MEDICAID RESUBMISSION CODE ORIGINAL REF. NO.

23. PRIOR AUTHORIZATION NUMBER

| 24. | A DATE(S) OF SERVICE From MM DD YY To MM DD YY | B Place of Service | C Type of Service | D PROCEDURES, SERVICES, OR SUPPLIES (Explain Unusual Circumstances) CPT/HCPCS MODIFIER | E DIAGNOSIS CODE | F $ CHARGES | G DAYS OR UNITS | H EPSDT Family Plan | I EMG | J COB | K RESERVED FOR LOCAL USE |
|---|---|---|---|---|---|---|---|---|---|---|---|
| 1 | | | | | | | | | | | |
| 2 | | | | | | | | | | | |
| 3 | | | | | | | | | | | |
| 4 | | | | | | | | | | | |
| 5 | | | | | | | | | | | |
| 6 | | | | | | | | | | | |

25. FEDERAL TAX I.D. NUMBER SSN EIN

26. PATIENTS ACCOUNT NUMBER

27. ACCEPT ASSIGNMENT? (For govt. claims, see back) YES NO

28. TOTAL CHARGE $

29. AMOUNT PAID $

30. BALANCE DUE $

31. SIGNATURE OF PHYSICIAN OR SUPPLIER INCLUDING DEGREES OR CREDENTIALS (I certify that the statements on the reverse apply to this bill and are made a part thereof.)

SIGNED DATE

32. NAME AND ADDRESS OF FACILITY WHERE SERVICES WERE RENDERED (If other than home or office)

33. PHYSICIAN'S, SUPPLIER'S BILLING NAME, ADDRESS, ZIP CODE & PHONE #

PIN # GRP#

PHYSICIAN OR SUPPLIER INFORMATION

(APPROVED BY AMA COUNCIL ON MEDICAL SERVICE 8/88)

Form 124OLM

*PLEASE PRINT OR TYPE*

FORM HCFA-1500 (12-90) FORM OWCP-1500 FORM RRB-1500

Administrative Skills, Form 29

# Patient Information Sheet

 **Blackburn Primary Care Associates** 

1990 Turquoise Drive
Blackburn, WI 54937
(555)555-1234

**REGISTRATION**
(PLEASE PRINT)

Home Phone: 555-219-7676

Today's Date: 1/15/00

## PATIENT INFORMATION

Name MINNOWITZ (Last Name) PRINNIE (First Name) ____ (Initial) Soc. Sec.# 197-24-6119

Address 16 A PARKTON ROAD

City BLACKBURN State WI Zip 54938

Single ____ Married ____ Widowed X Separated ____ Divorced ____ Sex M ____ F X Age 89 Birthdate 1/30/10

Patient Employed by ———— Occupation ____

Business Address ____ Business Phone ____

By whom were you referred? ____

In case of emergency who should be notified? Janice Selleman (Name) Daughter (Relation to Patient) Phone 555-219-7821

## PRIMARY INSURANCE

Person Responsible for Account as above (Last Name) ____ (First Name) ____ (Initial)

Relation to Patient self Birthdate ____ Soc. Sec.# ____

Address (if different from patient's) ____ Phone ____

City ____ State ____ Zip ____

Person Responsible Employed by ____ Occupation ____

Business Address ____ Business Phone ____

Insurance Company Medicare

Contract # ____ Group # ____ Subscriber # 197246119 A

Name of other dependents covered under this plan ____

## ADDITIONAL INSURANCE

Is patient covered by additional insurance? ____ Yes X No

Subscriber Name ____ Relation to Patient ____ Birthdate ____

Address (if different from patient's) ____ Phone ____

City ____ State ____ Zip ____

Subscriber Employed by ____ Business Phone ____

Insurance Company ____ Soc. Sec.# ____

Contract # ____ Group # ____ Subscriber # ____

Name of other dependents covered under this plan ____

## ASSIGNMENT AND RELEASE

I, the undersigned, certify that I (or my dependent) have insurance coverage with *Medicare* (Name of Insurance Company(ies))

and assign directly to Dr. *Blackburn Primary Care* insurance benefits, if any, otherwise payable to me for services rendered. I understand that I am financially responsible for all charges whether or not paid by insurance. I hereby authorize the doctor to release all information necessary to secure the payment of benefits. I authorize the use of this signature on all insurance submissions.

*Prinnie Minnowitz* (Responsible Party Signature) *self* (Relationship) *1/15/00* (Date)

Administrative Skills, Form 30

# Patient Encounter Form

## Blackburn Primary Care Associates

1990 Turquoise Drive
Blackburn, WI 54937
(555) 555-1234

FED. I.D. # 52-1963787

**PAT. INFO.**

| ACCT. NO. | PATIENT'S LAST NAME | FIRST | M.I. | DATE OF BIRTH | SEX | TODAY'S DATE |
|---|---|---|---|---|---|---|
| | MINNOWITZ | PRINNIE | | 01/30/10 | ☐ M ☒ F | 01/15/00 |

| INSURANCE | COPAY | DISABILITY RELATED TO: ☐ ACCIDENT ☐ INDUSTRIAL ☐ ILLNESS ☐ OTHER |
|---|---|---|
| Medicare | | DATES SYMPTOMS APPEARED, INCEPTION OF PREGNANCY, OR ACCIDENT OCCURRED: / / |

| ✔ | DESCRIPTION | CPT/MD | FEE |
|---|---|---|---|
| | **OFFICE VISITS-NEW PATIENTS** | | |
| | Focused | 99201 | |
| | Expanded | 99202 | |
| X | Detailed | 99203 | |
| | Comprehensive | 99204 | |
| | Complex | 99205 | |
| | | | |
| | | | |
| | **OFFICE VISITS - EST. PATIENTS** | | |
| | Minimal | 99211 | |
| | Focused | 99212 | |
| | Expanded | 99213 | |
| | Detailed | 99214 | |
| | Comprehensive | 99215 | |
| | | | |
| | | | |
| | **PREVENTIVE HEALTH CARE** NEW PT. | EST. PT | |
| | Eval./Mgmt. > 1 Yr 99381 | 99391 | |
| | Early Child 1 - 4 Yrs 99382 | 99392 | |
| | Late Child 5 - 11 Yrs 99383 | 99393 | |
| | Adolescent 12 - 17 Yrs 99384 | 99394 | |
| | Eval./Mgmt. 18 - 39 Yrs 99385 | 99395 | |
| | Eval./Mgmt. 40 - 64 Yrs 99386 | 99396 | |
| | Eval./Mgmt. 65 - Over 99387 | 99397 | |
| | | | |
| | **HOSP./SNF/HOME VISITS** | | |
| | House Calls | 99341 | |
| | ER Visit | 9928___ | |
| | Init. Hosp. Care | 99222 | |
| | Sub. Hosp. Care | 99232 | |
| | SNF, Sub. Care | 99312 | |
| | | | |
| | | | |
| | **INJECTIONS** | | |
| | Allergy | 95125 | |
| | B-12 | J3420 | |
| | Flu Shot | 90724 | |
| | Gamma Globulin | 90741 | |
| | Hormone | | |
| | Depo Provera | J1055 | |
| | Kenalog 40-60 mg | J3301 | |
| | Morphine/Demerol | J2270 | |
| | Phenergan | J2550 | |
| | Celestone | J0700 | |
| | Hep B, newborn to 11 years | 90744 | |
| | Hep B, 11 - 19 years | 90745 | |
| | Hep B, 20 years and above | 90746 | |
| | Rocephin/Claforan | J0696 | |
| | Iron | J1760 | |
| | Lidocaine NCL | J2000 | |
| | Admin of INJ | J0110 | |
| | Unlist INJ | 90782 | |
| | Drug | | |
| | Dose | | |

| ✔ | DESCRIPTION | CPT/MD | FEE |
|---|---|---|---|
| | **SPECIAL SERVICES** | | |
| | Drivers Physical | 99214 | |
| | Pelvic/Breast Exam | 99214 | |
| | Industrial | 99214 | |
| | | | |
| | **IMMUNIZATIONS** | | |
| | DtaP | 90700 | |
| | DPT | 90701 | |
| | DT | 90702 | |
| | Td (Tetanus Booster) | 90703 | |
| | MMR | 90707 | |
| | Mumps | 90704 | |
| | Pneumococcal | 90732 | |
| | Rubella | 90706 | |
| | Polio (TOPV) | 90712 | |
| | PPD | 86580 | |
| | TB Tine Test | 86585 | |
| | Hib | 90737 | |
| | | | |
| | | | |
| | **OFFICE PROCEDURES** | | |
| | Audiometry | 92551 | |
| | Diathermy (Ultrasound) | 97024 | |
| X | EKG Tracing & Interp. | 93000 | |
| | Intermed Joint Injection | 20605 | |
| | Major Joint Injection | 20610 | |
| | Nebulizer TX | 94664 | |
| | Rem. Impact. Cer. | 69210 | |
| | Spirometry | 94010 | |
| | Stress Test | 93015 | |
| | Trigger Pt. Inj. | 20550 | |
| | Eye Wash | 65205* | |
| | | | |
| | **LABORATORY** | | |
| | Throat Culture | 87060 | |
| X | Glucose Blood | 82947 | 10.00 |
| | Glucose Stick | 82948 | |
| | UA Pregnancy | 81025 | |
| | Occult Blood, Stool | 82270 | |
| | Rapid Strep | 86588 | |
| | Smear | 88150 | |
| X | UA Dip | 81002 | |
| | Urinalysis | 81000 | |
| | Venipuncture | 36415 | |
| | Wet Mount, Smear | 87210 | |
| | Wet Mount KOH | 87220 | |
| | Collect/Handing | 99000 | |
| | | | |
| | **MISCELLANEOUS** | | |
| | Pre-OP | 993___ | |
| | After Hours | 99050 | |
| | Sunday/Holidays | 99054 | |
| | Cast Removal | 29705 | |
| | Norplant Insertion | 11975 | |
| | Norplant Kit | 99070 | |

| ✔ | DESCRIPTION | CPT/MD | FEE |
|---|---|---|---|
| | **SURGERY** | | |
| | Toenail Removal | 11750 | |
| | Cryosurgery | 17200 | |
| | I & D | 10060 | |
| | Drainage Paronychia | 10060 | |
| | Enucleation Ext. Hemorrhoid | 46320 | |
| | I & D Abscess/Cyst | 10060 | |
| | Podophyllom | 17100 | |
| | Removal Foreign Body | 10120 | |
| | Wart Removal | 17110 | |
| | Destr. Single Lesion Face | 17000 | |
| | 2nd and 3rd Lesion Face | 17001 | |
| | Destr. Single Lesion Body | 17106 | |
| | 2nd and 3rd Lesion Body | 17003 | |
| | Lesion Rem. Excision | | |
| | Anoscopy | 46600 | |
| | Flex. Scope with Sig. | 45330 | |
| | Vasectomy | 55250 | |
| | Therapeutic Abor. | 59840 | |
| | Removal Foreign Body of Eye | 65205 | |
| | | | |
| | **SUPPLIES** | | |
| | Ace Wrap | 99070 | |
| | Cast Material | 99070 | |
| | Cervical Collar | 99070 | |
| | Elastic Bandage | 99070 | |
| | Splint/Sling | 99070 | |
| | Sterile Dressing | 99070 | |
| | Surgical Tray | 99070 | |

**DIAGNOSIS: ICD-9**

- ☐ Abscess Cellulitis . . . . . . 682.9
- ☐ Abdominal Pain . . . . . . . 789.0
- ☐ Abrasions . . . . . . . . . . . 919.0
- ☐ Acne . . . . . . . . . . . . . . . 706.1
- ☐ ADD . . . . . . . . . . . . . . . 314.00
- ☐ Alcoholism . . . . . . . . . . . 303.90
- ☐ Allergic Rhinitis . . . . . . . 477.9
- ☐ Allergy, Unsp . . . . . . . . . 995.3
- ☐ Anemia . . . . . . . . . . . . . 285.9
- ☐ Angina Pectoris . . . . . . . 413.9
- ☐ Anxiety Depression . . . . 300.4
- ☐ Anxiety State . . . . . . . . . 300.00
- ☐ ASCVD . . . . . . . . . . . . . 429.2
- ☐ Asthma W/O Status Asthma 493.90
- ☐ Atten Surg. Dressing/Suture V58.3
- ☐ BCP Consult . . . . . . . . . V25.9
- ☐ BPH . . . . . . . . . . . . . . . 600
- ☐ Bronchitis, Acute . . . . . . 466.0
- ☐ Bronchitis, Chronic . . . . . 491.9
- ☐ Burn ______________ 949.0
- ☐ Bursitis . . . . . . . . . . . . . 727.3
- ☐ C.T.S. . . . . . . . . . . . . . . 354.0
- ☐ CAD . . . . . . . . . . . . . . . 746.85
- ☐ CA-Prostate . . . . . . . . . . 185
- ☐ Cardiac Arrhythmia . . . . . 427.9
- ☐ Cataracts . . . . . . . . . . . . 366.9
- ☐ Chest Pain . . . . . . . . . . . 786.50
- ☐ Congestive Heart Failure 428.0
- ☐ Conjunctivitis . . . . . . . . . 372.30
- ☐ Constipation . . . . . . . . . . 564.0
- ☐ Consult Vasc. . . . . . . . . . V65.8
- ☐ Convulsions . . . . . . . . . . 780.3
- ☐ COPD . . . . . . . . . . . . . . 496
- ☐ Coronary Atherosclerosis. 414.0
- ☐ CVA . . . . . . . . . . . . . . . 436
- ☐ Cyst Sebaceous . . . . . . . 706.2
- ☐ Dermatitis . . . . . . . . . . . 692.9
- ☒ Diabetes, Uncomp. Adult 250.00
- ☐ Diabetes, Complicated . . 250.90
- ☐ Disc Degeneration . . . . . 722.6
- ☐ Duodenal Ulcer . . . . . . . 532.90
- ☐ Dysmenorrhea . . . . . . . . 625.3
- ☐ Fatigue . . . . . . . . . . . . . 780.7
- ☐ Flu Shot Only . . . . . . . . . V04.8
- ☐ Flu Vac . . . . . . . . . . . . . V04.8
- ☐ Flu W/Resp. Manifest . . . 487.1
- ☐ Folliculitis . . . . . . . . . . . 704.8
- ☐ FX ______________
- ☐ Gallbladder Disease . . . . 575.9
- ☐ Ganglion . . . . . . . . . . . . 727.43
- ☐ Gastroenteritis . . . . . . . . 558.9
- ☐ Gout . . . . . . . . . . . . . . . 274.9
- ☐ Gyn Exam . . . . . . . . . . . V72.3
- ☐ Headache Tension . . . . . 307.81
- ☐ Hemorrhoids Ext. . . . . . . 455.3
- ☐ Hepatitis . . . . . . . . . . . . 573.3
- ☐ Hernia-Inguinal . . . . . . . . 550.90
- ☐ Herpes Zoster . . . . . . . . 053.9
- ☐ Hyperlipidemia . . . . . . . . 272.4
- ☐ Hypertension . . . . . . . . . 401.9
- ☐ Hyperthyroidism . . . . . . . 242.9
- ☐ Hypothyroidism . . . . . . . 244.9
- ☐ Impacted Cerumen . . . . . 380.4
- ☐ Impetigo . . . . . . . . . . . . 684
- ☐ Ingrown Toenail . . . . . . . 703.0
- ☐ Internal Derangement Knee . 717.9
- ☐ Labyrinthitis . . . . . . . . . . 386.30
- ☐ Laceration Open Wound . 879.8__
- ☐ Levator Scapular Syndrome 726.90
- ☐ Menopausal Disorder . . . 627.9
- ☐ Metabolic Diff. . . . . . . . . 277.8
- ☐ Migraine . . . . . . . . . . . . 346.90
- ☐ Mitral Valve Disorder . . . 424.0
- ☐ Myalgia and Myositis . . . 729.1
- ☐ Noninf. Gastroenterit. . . . 558.9
- ☐ Obesity . . . . . . . . . . . . . 278.0
- ☐ Osteoarthrosis . . . . . . . . 715.00
- ☐ Osteoporosis . . . . . . . . . 733.00
- ☐ Otitis Externa . . . . . . . . . 380.10
- ☐ Otitis Media . . . . . . . . . . 382.9
- ☐ P.I.D. . . . . . . . . . . . . . . 614.9
- ☐ Peptic Ulcer . . . . . . . . . . 533.90
- ☐ Pharyngitis, Acute . . . . . 462
- ☐ Pneumonia, Viral . . . . . . 480.9
- ☐ Poison Oak . . . . . . . . . . 692.6
- ☐ Premarital B-Test . . . . . . V70.3
- ☐ Pregnancy Test, Unconf.. V72.4
- ☐ Prostatitis . . . . . . . . . . . 601.9
- ☐ Psoriasis . . . . . . . . . . . . 696.1
- ☐ Rheumatoid Arthritis . . . . 714.0
- ☐ Sciatica . . . . . . . . . . . . . 724.3
- ☐ Sacroiliac Sprain . . . . . . 846.1
- ☐ Sinusitis, Acute . . . . . . . 461.9
- ☐ Smoking Cessation. . . . . 305.10
- ☐ Sprain ______________
- ☐ SQ. Cell CA-Face. . . . . . 173.3
- ☐ Sterilization . . . . . . . . . . V25.2
- ☐ Stye. . . . . . . . . . . . . . . . 373.11
- ☐ TB Exposure . . . . . . . . . V01.1
- ☐ Tendonitis . . . . . . . . . . . 726.90
- ☐ Tinea . . . . . . . . . . . . . . . 110.9
- ☐ Tonsillitis, Acute . . . . . . 463
- ☐ URI, Acute . . . . . . . . . . . 465.9
- ☒ Urine Tract Infection . . . . 599.0
- ☐ Vaginitis . . . . . . . . . . . . . 616.10
- ☐ Well Adult Medical Exam V70.9
- ☐ Well Child Health Exam . V20.2

| DIAGNOSIS (If not checked above) ICD-9 | PHYSICIAN SIGNATURE | TODAY'S FEE | $ |
|---|---|---|---|
| | | PAYMENT | |
| PLEASE REMEMBER THAT PAYMENT IS YOUR OBLIGATION REGARDLESS OF INSURANCE OR OTHER THIRD PARTY INVOLVEMENT. | PAYMENT BY ☐ CASH ☐ CREDIT CARD ☐ CHECK # ______ | BALANCE DUE | |

Administrative Skills, Form 31

# FEE SCHEDULE

## BLACKBURN PRIMARY CARE ASSOCIATES
## 1990 TURQUOISE DRIVE
## BLACKBURN, WI 54937

**Federal Tax ID Number:** **52-1963787**

**BCBS Group Number:** **14982**
**Medicare Group Number:** **14982**

### OFFICE VISIT, NEW PATIENT

| | |
|---|---|
| Focused, 99201 | $ 45.00 |
| Expanded, 99202 | $ 53.00 |
| Detailed, 99203 | $ 60.00 |
| Comprehensive, 99204 | $ 95.00 |
| Complex, 99205 | $195.00 |
| Consultation, 99245 | $250.00 |

### OFFICE VISIT, ESTABLISHED PATIENT

| | |
|---|---|
| Minimal, 99211 | $ 40.00 |
| Focused, 99212 | $ 48.00 |
| Expanded, 99213 | $ 55.00 |
| Detailed, 99214 | $ 65.00 |
| Comprehensive, 99215 | $195.00 |

### OFFICE PROCEDURES

| | |
|---|---|
| EKG, 12 Lead, 93000 | $ 55.00 |
| Stress EKG, Treadmill, 93015 | $295.00 |
| Sigmoidoscopy, Flex., 45330 | $145.00 |
| Spirometry, 94010 | $ 50.00 |
| Cerumen Removal, 69210 | $ 40.00 |
| Collection & Handling | |
| Lab Specimen, 99000 | $ 9.00 |
| Venipuncture, 36415 | $ 9.00 |
| Urinalysis, 81000 | $ 20.00 |
| Urinalysis, 81002 (Dip Only) | $ 12.00 |
| Influenza Injection, 90724 | $ 20.00 |
| Pneumococcal Injection, 90732 | $ 20.00 |
| Oral Polio, 90712 | $ 15.00 |
| DTaP, 90700 | $ 20.00 |
| Tetanus Toxoid, 90703 | $ 15.00 |
| MMR, 90707 | $ 25.00 |
| Hib, 90737 | $ 20.00 |
| Hepatitis B, newborn to age 11 years, 90744 | $ 60.00 |
| Hepatitis B, 11-19 years, 90745 | $ 60.00 |
| Hepatitis B, 20 years and above 90746 | $ 60.00 |
| Intramuscular Injection, 90788 | |
| Penicillin | $ 30.00 |
| Ceftriaxone | $ 25.00 |
| Solu-Medrol | $ 23.00 |
| Vitamin B-12 | $ 13.00 |
| Subcutaneous Injection, 90782 | |
| Epinephrine | $ 18.00 |
| Sus-Pherine | $ 25.00 |
| Insulin, U-100 | $ 15.00 |

### COMMON DIAGNOSIS CODES

| | |
|---|---|
| Ischemic Heart Disease | 414.9 |
| w/o myocardial infarction | 411.89 |
| w/ coronary occlusion | 411.81 |
| Hypertension, Malignant | 401.0 |
| Benign | 401.1 |
| Unspecified | 401.9 |
| w/ congest. heart failure | 402.91 |
| Asthma, Bronchial | 493.9 |
| w/ COPD | 493.2 |
| allergic, w/ S.A. | 493.91 |
| allergic, w/o S.A. | 493.90 |
| Kyphosis | 737.10 |
| w/ osteoporosis | 733.0 |
| Osteoporosis | 733.00 |
| Otitis Media, Acute | 382.9 |
| Chronic | 382.9 |
| Well Child Health Exam | V20.2 |
| Well Adult Medical Exam | V70.9 |

PLEASE DO NOT STAPLE IN THIS AREA

APPROVED OMB-0938-0008

CARRIER

PICA

# HEALTH INSURANCE CLAIM FORM

PICA

1. MEDICARE (Medicare #) MEDICAID (Medicaid #) CHAMPUS (Sponsor's SSN) CHAMPVA (VA File #) GROUP HEALTH PLAN (SSN or ID) FECA BLK LUNG (SSN) OTHER (ID)

1a. INSURED'S I.D. NUMBER (FOR PROGRAM IN ITEM 1)

2. PATIENT'S NAME (Last Name, First Name, Middle Initial)

3. PATIENT'S BIRTHDATE MM DD YY SEX M F

4. INSURED'S NAME (Last Name, First Name, Middle Initial)

5. PATIENT'S ADDRESS (No., Street)

6. PATIENT RELATIONSHIP TO INSURED Self Spouse Child Other

7. INSURED'S ADDRESS (No., Street)

CITY STATE

8. PATIENT STATUS Single Married Other; Employed Full-Time Student Part-Time Student

CITY STATE

ZIP CODE TELEPHONE (Include Area Code) ( )

ZIP CODE TELEPHONE (Include Area Code) ( )

9. OTHER INSURED'S NAME (Last Name, First Name, Middle Initial)

10. IS PATIENT'S CONDITION RELATED TO:

11. INSURED'S POLICY GROUP OR FECA NUMBER

a. OTHER INSURED'S POLICY OR GROUP NUMBER

a. EMPLOYMENT? (CURRENT OR PREVIOUS) YES NO

a. INSURED'S DATE OF BIRTH MM DD YY SEX M F

b. OTHER INSURED'S DATE OF BIRTH MM DD YY SEX M F

b. AUTO ACCIDENT? PLACE (State) YES NO

b. EMPLOYER'S NAME OR SCHOOL NAME

c. EMPLOYER'S NAME OR SCHOOL NAME

c. OTHER ACCIDENT? YES NO

c. INSURANCE PLAN NAME OR PROGRAM NAME

d. INSURANCE PLAN NAME OR PROGRAM NAME

10d. RESERVED FOR LOCAL USE

d. IS THERE ANOTHER HEALTH BENEFIT PLAN? YES NO *If yes, return to and complete item 9a-d.*

**READ BACK OF FORM BEFORE COMPLETING & SIGNING THIS FORM.**

12. PATIENT'S OR AUTHORIZED PERSON'S SIGNATURE I authorize the release of any medical or other information necessary to process this claim. I also request payment of government benefits either to myself or to the party who accepts assignment below.

SIGNED ______ DATE ______

13. INSURED'S OR AUTHORIZED PERSON'S SIGNATURE I authorize payment of medical benefits to the undersigned physician or supplier for services described below.

SIGNED ______

PATIENT AND INSURED INFORMATION

14. DATE OF CURRENT: MM DD YY ILLNESS (First symptom) OR INJURY (Accident) OR PREGNANCY (LMP)

15. IF PATIENT HAS HAD SAME OR SIMILAR ILLNESS, GIVE FIRST DATE MM DD YY

16. DATES PATIENT UNABLE TO WORK IN CURRENT OCCUPATION FROM MM DD YY TO MM DD YY

17. NAME OF REFERRING PHYSICIAN OR OTHER SOURCE

17a. I.D. NUMBER OF REFERRING PHYSICIAN

18. HOSPITALIZATION DATES RELATED TO CURRENT SERVICES FROM MM DD YY TO MM DD YY

19. RESERVED FOR LOCAL USE

20. OUTSIDE LAB? YES NO $ CHARGES

21. DIAGNOSIS OR NATURE OF ILLNESS OR INJURY. (RELATE ITEMS 1,2,3 OR 4 TO ITEM 24E BY LINE)

1. ___ . __ 3. ___ . __

2. ___ . __ 4. ___ . __

22. MEDICAID RESUBMISSION CODE ORIGINAL REF. NO.

23. PRIOR AUTHORIZATION NUMBER

| 24. A DATE(S) OF SERVICE From MM DD YY To MM DD YY | B Place of Service | C Type of Service | D PROCEDURES, SERVICES, OR SUPPLIES (Explain Unusual Circumstances) CPT/HCPCS MODIFIER | E DIAGNOSIS CODE | F $ CHARGES | G DAYS OR UNITS | H EPSDT Family Plan | I EMG | J COB | K RESERVED FOR LOCAL USE |
|---|---|---|---|---|---|---|---|---|---|---|
| 1 | | | | | | | | | | |
| 2 | | | | | | | | | | |
| 3 | | | | | | | | | | |
| 4 | | | | | | | | | | |
| 5 | | | | | | | | | | |
| 6 | | | | | | | | | | |

25. FEDERAL TAX I.D. NUMBER SSN EIN

26. PATIENTS ACCOUNT NUMBER

27. ACCEPT ASSIGNMENT? (For govt. claims, see back) YES NO

28. TOTAL CHARGE $

29. AMOUNT PAID $

30. BALANCE DUE $

31. SIGNATURE OF PHYSICIAN OR SUPPLIER INCLUDING DEGREES OR CREDENTIALS (I certify that the statements on the reverse apply to this bill and are made a part thereof.)

SIGNED DATE

32. NAME AND ADDRESS OF FACILITY WHERE SERVICES WERE RENDERED (If other than home or office)

33. PHYSICIAN'S, SUPPLIER'S BILLING NAME, ADDRESS, ZIP CODE & PHONE #

PIN # GRP#

PHYSICIAN OR SUPPLIER INFORMATION

**(APPROVED BY AMA COUNCIL ON MEDICAL SERVICE 8/88)**

**Form 124OLM**

***PLEASE PRINT OR TYPE***

FORM HCFA-1500 (12-90)
FORM OWCP-1500 FORM RRB-1500

# Telephone Message Log

NAME OF CALLER | PATIENT'S NAME | AGE | TEMP. | TIME

TELEPHONE NUMBER | PHARMACY | TELEPHONE | CALLED BY: | DATE

**COMPLAINT / MESSAGE** ☐ PLEASE RETURN THE CALL ☐ WILL CALL AGAIN ☐ RETURNED YOUR CALL ☐ OTHER (SPECIFY) | DOCTOR

INSTRUCTIONS/REPLY:

☐ **URGENT**
☐ **MEDICATION ALLERGY**

**CALLED BACK:** **BY:** **DATE** **OTHER (SPECIFY)**

---

NAME OF CALLER | PATIENT'S NAME | AGE | TEMP. | TIME

TELEPHONE NUMBER | PHARMACY | TELEPHONE | CALLED BY: | DATE

**COMPLAINT / MESSAGE** ☐ PLEASE RETURN THE CALL ☐ WILL CALL AGAIN ☐ RETURNED YOUR CALL ☐ OTHER (SPECIFY) | DOCTOR

INSTRUCTIONS/REPLY:

☐ **URGENT**
☐ **MEDICATION ALLERGY**

**CALLED BACK:** **BY:** **DATE** **OTHER (SPECIFY)**

---

NAME OF CALLER | PATIENT'S NAME | AGE | TEMP. | TIME

TELEPHONE NUMBER | PHARMACY | TELEPHONE | CALLED BY: | DATE

**COMPLAINT / MESSAGE** ☐ PLEASE RETURN THE CALL ☐ WILL CALL AGAIN ☐ RETURNED YOUR CALL ☐ OTHER (SPECIFY) | DOCTOR

INSTRUCTIONS/REPLY:

☐ **URGENT**
☐ **MEDICATION ALLERGY**

**CALLED BACK:** **BY:** **DATE** **OTHER (SPECIFY)**



Courtesy of Bibbero Systems, Inc., Petaluma, California.

# Appointment Schedule

| | | | DAY / DATE | | Mon. | Tue. | Wed. | Thu. | Fri. | Sat. |
|---|---|---|---|---|---|---|---|---|---|---|
| | | | 8 | 00 | | | | | | |
| | | | | 10 | | | | | | |
| | | | | 20 | | | | | | |
| | | | | 30 | | | | | | |
| | | | | 40 | | | | | | |
| | | | | 50 | | | | | | |
| | | | 9 | 00 | | | | | | |
| | | | | 10 | | | | | | |
| | | | | 20 | | | | | | |
| | | | | 30 | | | | | | |
| | | | | 40 | | | | | | |
| | | | | 50 | | | | | | |
| | | | 10 | 00 | | | | | | |
| | | | | 10 | | | | | | |
| | | | | 20 | | | | | | |
| | | | | 30 | | | | | | |
| | | | | 40 | | | | | | |
| | | | | 50 | | | | | | |
| | | | 11 | 00 | | | | | | |
| | | | | 10 | | | | | | |
| | | | | 20 | | | | | | |
| | | | | 30 | | | | | | |
| | | | | 40 | | | | | | |
| | | | | 50 | | | | | | |
| | | | 12 | 00 | | | | | | |
| | | | | 10 | | | | | | |
| | | | | 20 | | | | | | |
| | | | | 30 | | | | | | |
| | | | | 40 | | | | | | |
| | | | | 50 | | | | | | |
| | | | 1 | 00 | | | | | | |
| | | | | 10 | | | | | | |
| | | | | 20 | | | | | | |
| | | | | 30 | | | | | | |
| | | | | 40 | | | | | | |
| | | | | 50 | | | | | | |
| | | | 2 | 00 | | | | | | |
| | | | | 10 | | | | | | |
| | | | | 20 | | | | | | |
| | | | | 30 | | | | | | |
| | | | | 40 | | | | | | |
| | | | | 50 | | | | | | |
| | | | 3 | 00 | | | | | | |
| | | | | 10 | | | | | | |
| | | | | 20 | | | | | | |
| | | | | 30 | | | | | | |
| | | | | 40 | | | | | | |
| | | | | 50 | | | | | | |
| | | | 4 | 00 | | | | | | |
| | | | | 10 | | | | | | |
| | | | | 20 | | | | | | |
| | | | | 30 | | | | | | |
| | | | | 40 | | | | | | |
| | | | | 50 | | | | | | |
| | | | 5 | 00 | | | | | | |
| | | | | 10 | | | | | | |
| | | | | 20 | | | | | | |
| | | | | 30 | | | | | | |
| | | | | 40 | | | | | | |
| | | | | 50 | | | | | | |

# ANDRUS/CLINI-REC® HEALTH HISTORY QUESTIONNAIRE

Chart No. ___________

**Identification Information**

Today's Date _______________

Name_______________________________ Date of Birth_______________________________

Occupation _______________________________ Marital Status _______________________________

## PART A – PRESENT HEALTH HISTORY

### I. CURRENT MEDICAL PROBLEMS

Please list the medical problems for which you came to see the doctor. About when did they begin?

Problems ______________________________ Date Began ____________

What concerns you most about these problems?

If you are being treated for any other illness or medical problems by another physician, please describe the problems and write the name of the physician or medical facility treating you.

Illness or Medical Problem | Physician or Medical Facility | City

### II. MEDICATIONS

Please list all medications you are now taking, including those you buy without a doctor's prescription (such as aspirin, cold tablets or vitamin supplements).

### III. ALLERGIES AND SENSITIVITIES

List anything that you are allergic to such as certain foods, medications, dust, chemicals or soaps, household items, pollens, bee stings, etc., and indicate how each affects you.

Allergic To: | Effect | Allergic To: | Effect

### IV. GENERAL HEALTH, ATTITUDE AND HABITS

How is your overall health now? .................... Health now: Poor ______ Fair ______ Good ______ Excellent ______

How has it been most of your life? .................... Health has been: Poor ______ Fair ______ Good ______ Excellent ______

In the past year:

Has your appetite changed? .................... Appetite: Decreased ______ Increased ______ Stayed same ______

Has your weight changed? .................... Weight: Lost _______lbs. Gained _______lbs. No change ______

Are you thirsty much of the time? .................... Thirsty: No _______ Yes _______

Has your overall 'pep' changed? .................... Pep: Decreased ______ Increased ______ Stayed same ______

Do you usually have trouble sleeping? .................... Trouble sleeping: No ______ Yes ______

How much do you exercise? .................... Exercise: Little or none _____ Less than I need _____ All I need _____

Do you smoke? .................... Smokes: No ______ Yes ______ If yes, how many years? ______

How many each day? .................... ______ Cigarettes ______ Cigars ______ Pipesfull

Have you ever smoked? .................... Smoked: No ______ Yes ______ If yes, how many years? ______

How many each day? .................... ______ Cigarettes ______ Cigars ______ Pipesfull

Do you drink alcoholic beverages? .................... Alcohol: No ____ Yes ____ I drink ____ Beers ____ Glasses of wine ______ Drinks of hard liquor - per day

Have you ever had a problem with alcohol? .................... Prior problem: No ______ Yes ______

How much coffee or tea do you usually drink? .................... Coffee/Tea: ______ cups of coffee or tea a day

Do you regularly wear seatbelts? .................... Seatbelts: No ______ Yes ______

| DO YOU: | Rarely/ Never | Occasionally | Frequently |
|---|---|---|---|
| Feel nervous? | ______ | ______ | ______ |
| Feel depressed? | ______ | ______ | ______ |
| Find it hard to make decisions? | ______ | ______ | ______ |
| Lose your temper? | ______ | ______ | ______ |
| Worry a lot? | ______ | ______ | ______ |
| Tire easily? | ______ | ______ | ______ |
| Have trouble relaxing? | ______ | ______ | ______ |
| Have any sexual problems? | ______ | ______ | ______ |

| DO YOU: | Rarely/ Never | Occasionally | Frequently |
|---|---|---|---|
| Ever feel like committing suicide? | ______ | ______ | ______ |
| Feel bored with your life? | ______ | ______ | ______ |
| Use marijuana? | ______ | ______ | ______ |
| Use "hard drugs"? | ______ | ______ | ______ |

Do you want to talk to the doctor about a personal matter? No _____ Yes _____

C O N F I D E N T I A L



STOCK NO. 19-742-4 8/95

## PART A – PRESENT HEALTH HISTORY (continued)

### IV. GENERAL HEALTH, ATTITUDE AND HABITS (continued)

Have you recently had any changes in your: | If yes, please explain:

| | No | Yes | If yes, please explain |
|---|---|---|---|
| Marital status? | No______ | Yes______ | ______ |
| Job or work? | No______ | Yes______ | ______ |
| Residence? | No______ | Yes______ | ______ |
| Financial status? | No______ | Yes______ | ______ |
| Are you having any legal problems or trouble with the law? | No______ | Yes______ | ______ |

## PART B – PAST HISTORY

### I. FAMILY HEALTH

Please give the following information about your immediate family:

| Relationship | Age, if Living | Age At Death | State of Health Or Cause of Death |
|---|---|---|---|
| Father | ______ | ______ | ______ |
| Mother | ______ | ______ | ______ |
| Brothers and Sisters | ______ | ______ | ______ |
| | ______ | ______ | ______ |
| | ______ | ______ | ______ |
| Spouse | ______ | ______ | ______ |
| Children | ______ | ______ | ______ |
| | ______ | ______ | ______ |
| | ______ | ______ | ______ |
| | ______ | ______ | ______ |

Have any **blood relatives** had any of the following illnesses? If so, indicate relationship (mother, brother, etc.)

| Illness | Family Members |
|---|---|
| Asthma | ______ |
| Diabetes | ______ |
| Cancer | ______ |
| Blood Disease | ______ |
| Glaucoma | ______ |
| Epilepsy | ______ |
| Rheumatoid Arthritis | ______ |
| Tuberculosis | ______ |
| Gout | ______ |
| High Blood Pressure | ______ |
| Heart Disease | ______ |
| Mental Problems | ______ |
| Suicide | ______ |
| Stroke | ______ |
| Alcoholism | ______ |
| Rheumatic Fever | ______ |

### II. HOSPITALIZATIONS, SURGERIES, INJURIES

Please list all times you have been hospitalized, operated on, or seriously injured.

| Year | Operation, Illness, Injury | Hospital and City |
|---|---|---|
| ______ | ______ | ______ |
| ______ | ______ | ______ |
| ______ | ______ | ______ |

### III. ILLNESS AND MEDICAL PROBLEMS

Please mark with an (X) any of the following illnesses and medical problems you have or have had and indicate the year when each started. If you are not certain when an illness started, write down an approximate year.

| Illness | (x) | (Year) | Illness | (x) | (Year) |
|---|---|---|---|---|---|
| Eye or eye lid infection | ___ | ___ | Hernia | ___ | ___ |
| Glaucoma | ___ | ___ | Hemorrhoids | ___ | ___ |
| Other eye problems | ___ | ___ | Kidney or bladder disease | ___ | ___ |
| Ear trouble | ___ | ___ | Prostate problem (male only) | ___ | ___ |
| Deafness or decreased hearing | ___ | ___ | Mental problems | ___ | ___ |
| Thyroid trouble | ___ | ___ | Headaches | ___ | ___ |
| Strep throat | ___ | ___ | Head injury | ___ | ___ |
| Bronchitis | ___ | ___ | Stroke | ___ | ___ |
| Emphysema | ___ | ___ | Convulsions, seizures | ___ | ___ |
| Pneumonia | ___ | ___ | Arthritis | ___ | ___ |
| Allergies, asthma or hay fever | ___ | ___ | Gout | ___ | ___ |
| Tuberculosis | ___ | ___ | Cancer or tumor | ___ | ___ |
| Other lung problems | ___ | ___ | Bleeding tendency | ___ | ___ |
| High blood pressure | ___ | ___ | Diabetes | ___ | ___ |
| Heart attack | ___ | ___ | Measles/Rubeola | ___ | ___ |
| High cholesterol | ___ | ___ | German measles/Rubella | ___ | ___ |
| Arteriosclerosis (Hardening of arteries) | ___ | ___ | Polio | ___ | ___ |
| Heart murmur | ___ | ___ | Mumps | ___ | ___ |
| Other heart condition | ___ | ___ | Scarlet fever | ___ | ___ |
| Stomach/duodenal ulcer | ___ | ___ | Chicken pox | ___ | ___ |
| Diverticulosis | ___ | ___ | Mononucleosis | ___ | ___ |
| Colitis | ___ | ___ | Eczema | ___ | ___ |
| Other bowel problems | ___ | ___ | Psoriasis | ___ | ___ |
| Hepatitis | ___ | ___ | Venereal disease | ___ | ___ |
| Liver trouble | ___ | ___ | Genital herpes | ___ | ___ |
| Gallbladder trouble | ___ | ___ | HIV test | ___ | ___ |
| | | | AIDS | ___ | ___ |

CONFIDENTIAL



To Order Call:800-BIBBERO (800 242-2376) Or Fax: (800 242-9330)

STOCK NO. 19-742-4 8/95

## PART C – BODY SYSTEMS REVIEW

Please answer all of the following questions.

Circle any questions you find difficult to answer.

MEN: Please answer questions 1 through 12, then skip to question 18.
WOMEN: Please start on question 6.

MEN ONLY

1. Have you had or do you have prostate trouble? ........ No ______ Yes ______
2. Do you have any sexual problems or a problem with impotency? ........ No ______ Yes ______
3. Have you ever had sores or lesions on your penis? ........ No ______ Yes ______
4. Have you ever had any discharge from your penis? ........ No ______ Yes ______
5. Do you ever have pain, lumps or swelling in your testicles? ........ No ______ Yes ______

Check here if you wish to discuss any special problems with the doctor ........ ☐

| MEN & WOMEN | Rarely/ Never | Occasionally | Frequently |
|---|---|---|---|
| 6. Is it sometimes hard to start your urine flow? | ______ | ______ | ______ |
| 7. Is urination ever painful? | ______ | ______ | ______ |
| 8. Do you have to urinate more than 5 times a day? | ______ | ______ | ______ |
| 9. Do you get up at night to urinate? | ______ | ______ | ______ |
| 10. Has your urine ever been bloody or dark colored? | ______ | ______ | ______ |
| 11. Do you ever lose urine when you strain, laugh, cough or sneeze? | ______ | ______ | ______ |
| 12. Do you ever lose urine during sleep? | ______ | ______ | ______ |

| WOMEN ONLY<br>Do you: | Rarely/ Never | Occasionally | Frequently |
|---|---|---|---|
| 13. a. Have any menstrual problems? | ______ | ______ | ______ |
| b. Feel rather tense just before your period? | ______ | ______ | ______ |
| c. Have heavy menstrual bleeding? | ______ | ______ | ______ |
| d. Have painful menstrual periods? | ______ | ______ | ______ |
| e. Have any bleeding between periods? | ______ | ______ | ______ |
| f. Have any unusual vaginal discharge or itching? | ______ | ______ | ______ |
| g. Ever have tender breasts? | ______ | ______ | ______ |
| h. Have any discharge from your nipples? | ______ | ______ | ______ |
| i. Have any hot flashes? | ______ | ______ | |

14. How many times, if any, have you been pregnant? ........ ______________
15. How many children born alive? ........ ______________
16. Are you taking birth control pills? ........ No______ Yes ______
17. Do you examine your breasts monthly for lumps? ........ No______ Yes ______
17a. What was the date of your last menstrual period? ........ Date ______________

Check here if you wish to discuss any special problem with the doctor ........ ☐

| MEN & WOMEN | Rarely/ Never | Occasionally | Frequently |
|---|---|---|---|
| 18. In the past year have you had any: | | | |
| a. Severe shoulder pain? | ______ | ______ | ______ |
| b. Severe back pain? | ______ | ______ | ______ |
| c. Muscle or joint stiffness or pain due to sports, exercise or injury? | ______ | ______ | ______ |
| d. Pain or swelling in any joints not due to sports, exercise or injury? | ______ | ______ | ______ |

19. Do you have dry skin or brittle fingernails? ........ No______ Yes ______
20. Do you bruise easily? ........ No______ Yes ______
21. Do you have any moles that have changed in color or in size? ........ No______ Yes ______
22. Do you have any other skin problems? ........ No______ Yes ______

23. In the last 3 months have you had:
    a. A fever that lasted more than one day? ........ No______ Yes ______
    b. Sores or cuts that were hard to heal? ........ No______ Yes ______
    c. Any cold sores (fever blisters)? ........ No______ Yes ______
    d. Any lumps in your neck, armpits or groin? ........ No______ Yes ______
    e. Do you ever have chills or sweat at night? ........ No______ Yes ______
24. Have you traveled out of the country in the last 2 years? ........ No______ Yes, Traveled in: ______________
25. Write in the dates for the shots you have had: ........ Measles ______ Smallpox ______ Mumps ______ Tetanus ______ Polio ______ Typhoid ______
26. Have you had a tuberculin (TB) skin test? ........ No______ Yes ______ Date ______________
    If so, was it negative or positive? ........ Neg ____ Pos ______
27. Have you had an HIV test for AIDS? ........ No ____ Yes ______ Date ______________
    If so, was it negative or positive? ........ Neg ____ Pos ______

CONFIDENTIAL


PLEASE TURN THIS PAGE
STOCK NO. 19-742-4 8/95

REMOVE THIS PAGE AFTER COMPLETING QUESTIONNAIRE

# BODY SYSTEMS REVIEW

| | Question | | | | VISION / HEARING |
|---|---|---|---|---|---|
| 28. | Do you wear eyeglasses? | No______ | Yes______ | | Wears eyeglasses |
| 29. | Do you wear contact lenses? | No______ | Yes______ | | Wears contacts |
| 30. | Has your vision changed in the last year? | No______ | Yes______ | | Vision changes in last year |

| | Question | Rarely/ Never | Occasionally | Frequently | |
|---|---|---|---|---|---|
| 31. | How often do you have: | | | | |
| a. | Double vision? | ______ | ______ | ______ | Double vision |
| b. | Blurry vision? | ______ | ______ | ______ | Blurred vision |
| c. | Watery or itchy eyes? | ______ | ______ | ______ | Watery/itchy eyes |
| 32. | Do you ever see colored rings around lights? | ______ | ______ | ______ | Sees halos |
| 33. | Do others tell you you have a hearing problem? | ______ | ______ | ______ | Hearing problem |
| 34. | Do you have trouble keeping your balance? | ______ | ______ | ______ | Loses balance |
| 35. | Do you have any discharge from your ears? | ______ | ______ | ______ | Discharge from ears |
| 36. | Do you ever feel dizzy or have motion sickness? | ______ | ______ | ______ | Dizzy / motion sickness |
| 37. | Do you have any problems with your hearing? | No______ | Yes______ | Hearing Problems | |
| 38. | Do you ever have ringing in your ears? | No______ | Yes______ | Ringing in ears | |

| | Question | Rarely/ Never | Occasionally | Frequently | NOSE / THROAT / RESPIRATORY |
|---|---|---|---|---|---|
| 39. | How often do you have: | | | | |
| a. | Head colds? | ______ | ______ | ______ | Head colds |
| b. | Chest colds? | ______ | ______ | ______ | Chest colds |
| c. | Runny nose? | ______ | ______ | ______ | Runny nose |
| d. | Stuffed up nose? | ______ | ______ | ______ | Head congestion |
| e. | Sore/hoarse throat? | ______ | ______ | ______ | Sore / hoarse throat |
| f. | Bad coughing spells? | ______ | ______ | ______ | Coughing spells |
| g. | Sneezing spells? | ______ | ______ | ______ | Sneezing spells |
| h. | Trouble breathing? | ______ | ______ | ______ | Trouble breathing |
| i. | Nose bleeds? | ______ | ______ | ______ | Nose bleeds |
| j. | Cough blood? | ______ | ______ | ______ | Cough blood |
| 40. | Have you ever worked or spent time: | | | | |
| a. | On a farm? | No______ | Yes______ | Worked on a farm | |
| b. | In a mine? | No______ | Yes______ | Worked in a mine | |
| c. | In a laundry or mill? | No______ | Yes______ | Worked in a laundry/mill | |
| d. | In very dusty places? | No______ | Yes______ | Worked in high dust concentrations | |
| e. | With or near toxic chemicals? | No______ | Yes______ | Exposed to toxic chemicals | |
| f. | With or near radioactive materials? | No______ | Yes______ | Exposed to radioactive materials | |
| g. | With or near asbestos? | No______ | Yes______ | Exposed to asbestos | |

| | Question | Rarely/ Never | Occasionally | Frequently | CARDIOVASCULAR |
|---|---|---|---|---|---|
| 41. | Do you get out of breath easily when you are active (like climbing stairs)? | ______ | ______ | ______ | Out of breath quickly when exercising |
| 42. | Do you ever feel light-headed or dizzy? | ______ | ______ | ______ | Dizziness |
| 43. | Have you ever fainted or passed out? | ______ | ______ | ______ | Fainted |
| 44. | Do you sometimes feel your heart is racing or beating too fast? | ______ | ______ | ______ | Rapid heartbeat |
| 45. | When you exercise do you ever get pains in your chest or shoulders? | ______ | ______ | ______ | Chest/shoulder pains in exercise |
| 46. | Do you have any leg cramps or pain in your thighs or legs when walking? | ______ | ______ | ______ | Pain in thighs or legs when walking |
| 47. | Do you ever have to sit up at night to breathe easier? | ______ | ______ | ______ | Sits up at night to breathe easier |
| 48. | Do you use two pillows at night to help you breathe easier? | ______ | ______ | ______ | Breathing problems during sleep |
| 49. | Would you say you are a restless sleeper? | ______ | ______ | ______ | Restless sleeper |
| 50. | Are you bothered by leg cramps at night? | ______ | ______ | ______ | Leg cramps at night |
| 51. | Do you sometimes have swollen ankles or feet? | ______ | ______ | ______ | Swollen ankles/feet |

| | Question | Rarely/ Never | Occasionally | Frequently | DIGESTIVE |
|---|---|---|---|---|---|
| 52. | How often, if ever: | | | | |
| a. | Are you nauseated (sick to your stomach)? | ______ | ______ | ______ | Nauseated |
| b. | Do you have stomach pains? | ______ | ______ | ______ | Stomach pains |
| c. | Do you burp a lot after eating? | ______ | ______ | ______ | Burps after eating |
| d. | Do you have heartburn? | ______ | ______ | ______ | Heartburn |
| e. | Do you have trouble swallowing your food? | ______ | ______ | ______ | Trouble swallowing food |
| f. | Have you vomited blood? | ______ | ______ | ______ | Vomited blood |
| g. | Are you constipated? | ______ | ______ | ______ | Constipated |
| h. | Do you have diarrhea (watery stools)? | ______ | ______ | ______ | Diarrhea |
| i. | Are your bowel movements painful? | ______ | ______ | ______ | Painful bowel movements |
| j. | Are your bowel movements bloody? | ______ | ______ | ______ | Bloody bowel movements |
| k. | Are your bowel movements dark or black? | ______ | ______ | ______ | Dark bowel movements |
| 53. | Have you ever had a sigmoidoscopy? | No______ | Yes______ | Date__________ | Date of last sigmoidoscopy? |

**PLEASE TURN TO BACK PAGE AND COMPLETE QUESTIONS ON NUTRITION.**

Andrus/Clini-Rec®
BIBBERO SYSTEMS, INC.

# COMPREHENSIVE PHYSICAL EXAMINATION

MALE OR FEMALE
NEW OR ESTABLISHED PATIENT
CPT # 99201 - 99215

(For Office Use Only)

C O N F I D E N T I A L

NAME ______________________ AGE ________ YRS. OLD TODAY'S DATE ____________ DATE OF BIRTH ____________

Key: [O] Neg. Findings [+] Positive Findings [X] Omitted [✔] See Notes/CIRCLE WORDS OF IMPORTANCE & EXPLAIN

| | | |
|---|---|---|
| 1 GEN. APPEARANCE | [ ] | Apparent Age/Nutrition/Development/Mental & Emotional Status/Gait/Posture/Distress/Speech – |
| 2 HEAD / SCALP | [ ] | Size/Shape/Tender over Sinuses/Hair/Alopecia/Eruption/Masses/Bruit – |
| 3 EYES | [ ] | Conjunct/Sclerae/Cornea/Pupils/EOM'S/Arcus/Ptosis/Fundi/Tension/Eyelids/Pallor/Light/Bruit – |
| 4 EARS | [ ] | Ext. Canal/TM's/Perforation/Discharge/Tophi/Hearing Problem/Weber/Rinne – |
| 5 NOSE / SINUSES | [ ] | Septum/Obstruction/Turbinates/Discharge – |
| 6 MOUTH / THROAT | [ ] | Odor/Lips/Tongue/Tonsils/Teeth/Dentures/Gums/Pharynx – |
| 7 NECK | [ ] | Adenopathy/Thyroid/Carotids/Trachea/Veins/Masses/Spine/Motion/Bruit – |
| 8 BACK | [ ] | Kyphosis/Scoliosis/Lordosis/Mobility/CVA/Bone/Tenderness – |
| 9 THORAX | [ ] | Symmetry/Movement/Contour/Tender – |
| 10 BREASTS | [ ] | Size/Size-Consistency/Nipples/Areolar/Palpable Mass/Discharge/Tenderness/Nodes/Scars – |
| 11 HEART | [ ] | Rate/Rhythm/Apical Impulse/Thrills/Quality of Sound/Intensity/Splitting/Extra Sounds/ Murmurs – |
| 12 CHEST / LUNGS | [ ] | Excursion/Dullness or Hyperresonance to Percussion/Quality of Breath Sounds/Rales/Wheezing/ Rhonchi/Diaphragm/Rubs/Bruit – |
| 13 ABDOMEN | [ ] | Bowel Sounds/Appearance/Liver/Spleen/Masses/Hernias/Murmurs/Contour/Tenderness/Bruit/ ING Nodes – |
| 14 GROIN | [ ] | Hernia/Inguinal Nodes/Femoral Pulses – |
| 15 MALE GENITALIA | [ ] | Penis/Testes/Scrotum Epididymis/Varicocele/Scars/Discharge – |
| 16 FEMALE GENITALIA | [ ] | Vuvla/Vagina/Cervix/Uterus/Adnexae/Rectocele/Cystocele/Bartholin Gland/Urethra/ Discharge – Pap Smear (if done ✔) ☐ |
| 17 EXTREMITIES | [ ] | Deformity/Clubbing/Cyanosis/Edema/Nails/Peripheral Pulses/Calf Tenderness/Joints for Swelling/ ROM – |
| 18 SKIN | [ ] | Color/Birthmarks/Scars/Texture/Rash/Eczema/Ulcers – |
| 19 NEUROLOGICAL | [ ] | DTR's/Babinski/Cranial Nerves/Motor Abnormalities/Tremor/Paralysis/Sensory Exam – (touch, pin prick, vibration)/Coordination/Romberg – |
| 20 MUSCULAR SYSTEM | [ ] | Strength/Wasting/Development – |
| 21 RECTAL EXAM | [ ] | Sphincter Tone/Hemorrhoids/Fissures/Masses/Prostate/Stool Guaiac (if done ✔) ☐ Pos ☐ Neg – |

Impression: ☐ Check If Normal Physical Examination

Summary: ________________________________________________

________________________________________________

________________________ Signature ________________________ Date ____________

 

## COMPREHENSIVE PHYSICAL EXAMINATION (continued)

(For Office Use Only)

**PHYSICIAN'S NOTES:**

| Body Area Number | REMARKS: |
|---|---|
| | |
| | |
| | |
| | |
| | |

R L L R

R L

CONFIDENTIAL

HEIGHT__________

WEIGHT__________

BUILD __________

PULSE __________

RESP. __________

TEMP. __________

**VISION**

Without Glasses

Far R 20/ L 20/

Near R 20/ L 20/

With Glasses

R 20/ L 20/

R 20/ L 20/

Tonometry R______ L______

Colorvision__________

Peripheral Fields R____ L____

**AUDIOMETRIC TESTING**

| | 250 | 500 | 1000 |
|---|---|---|---|
| R | | | |
| L | | | |
| | **2000** | **4000** | **8000** |
| R | | | |
| L | | | |

Gross Hearing __________

**BLOOD PRESSURE**

Sitting

R / L /

Standing

R / L /

Lying

R / L /

| Diagnostic Test: | Results: |
|---|---|
| | |
| | |
| | |
| | |
| | |

The space below is provided for additional information when these data are being forwarded to a hospital, insurance company, a referral physician, etc.

**Significant Comments / Recommendations:**

**Physician's Name** __________

**Address** __________

**Telephone (area code)** __________

## NUTRITION AND DIET

1. How many meals do you eat each day? . . . . . . . . . . . . . . . . . . . . . . . . . . . . . . . ________ Meals each day
2. Do you usually eat breakfast? . . . . . . . . . . . . . . . . . . . . . . . . . . . . . . . . . . . . . ☐ No ☐ Yes Breakfast
3. Do you diet frequently and/or are you now dieting? . . . . . . . . . . . . . . . . . . . . . . . . . ☐ No ☐ Yes Diets
4. Do you consider yourself . . . . . . . . . . . . . . . . . . . ☐ Underweight ☐ Overweight ☐ Just right? Weight
5. Do you snack? . . . . . . . . . . . . . . . . . . . . . ☐ More than once a day ☐ Usually daily ☐ Rarely? Snacks
6. Do you add salt to your food at the table? . . . . . ☐ Almost always ☐ Sometimes ☐ Rarely Salts food
7. Check the frequency you eat the following types of foods:

| | More than once daily | Daily | 3 times weekly | Once weekly | Twice monthly | Less or never |
|---|---|---|---|---|---|---|
| a. Whole grain or enriched bread or cereal | | | | | | |
| b. Milk, cheese, or other dairy products | | | | | | |
| c. Eggs | | | | | | |
| d. Meat, Poultry, Fish | | | | | | |
| e. Beans, Peas, or other legumes | | | | | | |
| f. Citrus | | | | | | |
| g. Dark green or deep yellow vegetables | | | | | | |

List any food supplements or vitamins you take regularly: ________________________________

Additional Patient Comments: ________________________________

Thanks for completing this questionnaire. Please review for skipped questions, sign your name on the space to the right and return it to the physician or assistant. If you wish to add any information, please write it in the spaces provided above.

Patient's Signature ________________________________

Physician's Notes: ________________________________

CONFIDENTIAL

**To order, call or write:**
Bibbero Systems, Inc.
1300 N. McDowell Blvd., Petaluma, CA 94954-1180
Toll Free: 800-BIBBERO (800 242-2376)
Or Fax: 800-242-9330
STOCK NO. 19-742-4 8/95

Patient Information Sheet

 **Blackburn Primary Care Associates** 
1990 Turquoise Drive
Blackburn, WI 54937
(555)555-1234

**REGISTRATION**
(PLEASE PRINT)

Home Phone: ____________ Today's Date: ____________

## PATIENT INFORMATION

Name ____________ (Last Name) ____________ (First Name) ____ (Initial) Soc. Sec.# ____________

Address ____________

City ____________ State ____________ Zip ____________

Single ___ Married ___ Widowed ___ Separated ___ Divorced ___ Sex M ___ F ___ Age ___ Birthdate ____________

Patient Employed by ____________ Occupation ____________

Business Address ____________ Business Phone ____________

By whom were you referred? ____________

In case of emergency who should be notified? ____________ (Name) ____________ (Relation to Patient) Phone ____________

## PRIMARY INSURANCE

Person Responsible for Account ____________ (Last Name) ____________ (First Name) ____ (Initial)

Relation to Patient ____________ Birthdate ____________ Soc. Sec.# ____________

Address (if different from patient's) ____________ Phone ____________

City ____________ State ____________ Zip ____________

Person Responsible Employed by ____________ Occupation ____________

Business Address ____________ Business Phone ____________

Insurance Company ____________

Contract # ____________ Group # ____________ Subscriber # ____________

Name of other dependents covered under this plan ____________

## ADDITIONAL INSURANCE

Is patient covered by additional insurance? ___ Yes ___ No

Subscriber Name ____________ Relation to Patient ____________ Birthdate ____________

Address (if different from patient's) ____________ Phone ____________

City ____________ State ____________ Zip ____________

Subscriber Employed by ____________ Business Phone ____________

Insurance Company ____________ Soc. Sec.# ____________

Contract # ____________ Group # ____________ Subscriber # ____________

Name of other dependents covered under this plan ____________

## ASSIGNMENT AND RELEASE

I, the undersigned, certify that I (or my dependent) have insurance coverage with ____________ (Name of Insurance Company(ies))

and assign directly to Dr. ____________ insurance benefits, if any, otherwise payable to me for services rendered. I understand that I am financially responsible for all charges whether or not paid by insurance. I hereby authorize the doctor to release all information necessary to secure the payment of benefits. I authorize the use of this signature on all insurance submissions.

____________ (Responsible Party Signature) ____________ (Relationship) ____________ (Date)

# Patient Encounter Form

## Blackburn Primary Care Associates

1990 Turquoise Drive
Blackburn, WI 54937
(555) 555-1234

FED. I.D. # 52-1963787

**PAT. INFO.**

| ACCT. NO. | PATIENT'S LAST NAME | FIRST | M.I. | DATE OF BIRTH | SEX ☐ M ☐ F | TODAY'S DATE |
|---|---|---|---|---|---|---|
| | | | | | | |

| INSURANCE | COPAY | DISABILITY RELATED TO: ☐ ACCIDENT ☐ INDUSTRIAL ☐ ILLNESS ☐ OTHER<br>DATES SYMPTOMS APPEARED, INCEPTION OF PREGNANCY, OR ACCIDENT OCCURRED: / / |
|---|---|---|
| | | |

| ✔ | DESCRIPTION | CPT/MD | FEE |
|---|---|---|---|
| | **OFFICE VISITS-NEW PATIENTS** | | |
| | Focused | 99201 | |
| | Expanded | 99202 | |
| | Detailed | 99203 | |
| | Comprehensive | 99204 | |
| | Complex | 99205 | |
| | | | |
| | | | |
| | **OFFICE VISITS - EST. PATIENTS** | | |
| | Minimal | 99211 | |
| | Focused | 99212 | |
| | Expanded | 99213 | |
| | Detailed | 99214 | |
| | Comprehensive | 99215 | |
| | | | |
| | | | |
| | **PREVENTIVE HEALTH CARE** NEW PT. | EST. PT | |
| | Eval./Mgmt. > 1 Yr 99381 | 99391 | |
| | Early Child 1 - 4 Yrs 99382 | 99392 | |
| | Late Child 5 - 11 Yrs 99383 | 99393 | |
| | Adolescent 12 - 17 Yrs 99384 | 99394 | |
| | Eval./Mgmt. 18 - 39 Yrs 99385 | 99395 | |
| | Eval./Mgmt. 40 - 64 Yrs 99386 | 99396 | |
| | Eval./Mgmt. 65 - Over 99387 | 99397 | |
| | | | |
| | | | |
| | **HOSP./SNF/HOME VISITS** | | |
| | House Calls | 99341 | |
| | ER Visit | 9928___ | |
| | Init. Hosp. Care | 99222 | |
| | Sub. Hosp. Care | 99232 | |
| | SNF, Sub. Care | 99312 | |
| | | | |
| | | | |
| | **INJECTIONS** | | |
| | Allergy | 95125 | |
| | B-12 | J3420 | |
| | Flu Shot | 90724 | |
| | Gamma Globulin | 90741 | |
| | Hormone | | |
| | Depo Provera | J1055 | |
| | Kenalog 40-60 mg | J3301 | |
| | Morphine/Demerol | J2270 | |
| | Phenergan | J2550 | |
| | Celestone | J0700 | |
| | Hep B, newborn to 11 years | 90744 | |
| | Hep B, 11 - 19 years | 90745 | |
| | Hep B, 20 years and above | 90746 | |
| | Rocephin/Claforan | J0696 | |
| | Iron | J1760 | |
| | Lidocaine NCL | J2000 | |
| | Admin of INJ | J0110 | |
| | Unlist INJ | 90782 | |
| | Drug | | |
| | Dose | | |

| ✔ | DESCRIPTION | CPT/MD | FEE |
|---|---|---|---|
| | **SPECIAL SERVICES** | | |
| | Drivers Physical | 99214 | |
| | Pelvic/Breast Exam | 99214 | |
| | Industrial | 99214 | |
| | | | |
| | **IMMUNIZATIONS** | | |
| | DtaP | 90700 | |
| | DPT | 90701 | |
| | DT | 90702 | |
| | Td (Tetanus Booster) | 90703 | |
| | MMR | 90707 | |
| | Mumps | 90704 | |
| | Pneumococcal | 90732 | |
| | Rubella | 90706 | |
| | Polio (TOPV) | 90712 | |
| | PPD | 86580 | |
| | TB Tine Test | 86585 | |
| | Hib | 90737 | |
| | | | |
| | | | |
| | **OFFICE PROCEDURES** | | |
| | Audiometry | 92551 | |
| | Diathermy (Ultrasound) | 97024 | |
| | EKG Tracing & Interp. | 93000 | |
| | Intermed Joint Injection | 20605 | |
| | Major Joint Injection | 20610 | |
| | Nebulizer TX | 94664 | |
| | Rem. Impact. Cer. | 69210 | |
| | Spirometry | 94010 | |
| | Stress Test | 93015 | |
| | Trigger Pt. Inj. | 20550 | |
| | Eye Wash | 65205* | |
| | | | |
| | **LABORATORY** | | |
| | Throat Culture | 87060 | |
| | Glucose Blood | 82947 | |
| | Glucose Stick | 82948 | |
| | UA Pregnancy | 81025 | |
| | Occult Blood, Stool | 82270 | |
| | Rapid Strep | 86588 | |
| | Smear | 88150 | |
| | UA Dip | 81002 | |
| | Urinalysis | 81000 | |
| | Venipuncture | 36415 | |
| | Wet Mount, Smear | 87210 | |
| | Wet Mount KOH | 87220 | |
| | Collect/Handing | 99000 | |
| | | | |
| | **MISCELLANEOUS** | | |
| | Pre-OP | 993___ | |
| | After Hours | 99050 | |
| | Sunday/Holidays | 99054 | |
| | Cast Removal | 29705 | |
| | Norplant Insertion | 11975 | |
| | Norplant Kit | 99070 | |

| ✔ | DESCRIPTION | CPT/MD | FEE |
|---|---|---|---|
| | **SURGERY** | | |
| | Toenail Removal | 11750 | |
| | Cryosurgery | 17200 | |
| | I & D | 10060 | |
| | Drainage Paronychia | 10060 | |
| | Enucleation Ext. Hemorrhoid | 46320 | |
| | I & D Abscess/Cyst | 10060 | |
| | Podophyllom | 17100 | |
| | Removal Foreign Body | 10120 | |
| | Wart Removal | 17110 | |
| | Destr. Single Lesion Face | 17000 | |
| | 2nd and 3rd Lesion Face | 17001 | |
| | Destr. Single Lesion Body | 17106 | |
| | 2nd and 3rd Lesion Body | 17003 | |
| | Lesion Rem. Excision | | |
| | Anoscopy | 46600 | |
| | Flex. Scope with Sig. | 45330 | |
| | Vasectomy | 55250 | |
| | Therapeutic Abor. | 59840 | |
| | Removal Foreign Body of Eye | 65205 | |
| | | | |
| | **SUPPLIES** | | |
| | Ace Wrap | 99070 | |
| | Cast Material | 99070 | |
| | Cervical Collar | 99070 | |
| | Elastic Bandage | 99070 | |
| | Splint/Sling | 99070 | |
| | Sterile Dressing | 99070 | |
| | Surgical Tray | 99070 | |

**DIAGNOSIS: ICD-9**

☐ Abscess Cellulitis . . . . . . 682.9
☐ Abdominal Pain . . . . . . . 789.0
☐ Abrasions . . . . . . . . . . . 919.0
☐ Acne . . . . . . . . . . . . . . . 706.1
☐ ADD . . . . . . . . . . . . . . . 314.00
☐ Alcoholism . . . . . . . . . . . 303.90
☐ Allergic Rhinitis . . . . . . . 477.9
☐ Allergy, Unsp . . . . . . . . . 995.3
☐ Anemia . . . . . . . . . . . . . 285.9
☐ Angina Pectoris . . . . . . . 413.9
☐ Anxiety Depression . . . . 300.4
☐ Anxiety State . . . . . . . . . 300.00
☐ ASCVD . . . . . . . . . . . . . 429.2
☐ Asthma W/O Status Asthma 493.90
☐ Atten Surg. Dressing/Suture V58.3
☐ BCP Consult . . . . . . . . . V25.9
☐ BPH . . . . . . . . . . . . . . . 600
☐ Bronchitis, Acute . . . . . . 466.0
☐ Bronchitis, Chronic . . . . . 491.9
☐ Burn ______________ 949.0
☐ Bursitis . . . . . . . . . . . . . 727.3

☐ C.T.S. . . . . . . . . . . . . . . 354.0
☐ CAD . . . . . . . . . . . . . . . 746.85
☐ CA-Prostate . . . . . . . . . . 185
☐ Cardiac Arrhythmia . . . . . 427.9
☐ Cataracts . . . . . . . . . . . . 366.9
☐ Chest Pain . . . . . . . . . . . 786.50
☐ Congestive Heart Failure 428.0
☐ Conjunctivitis . . . . . . . . . 372.30
☐ Constipation . . . . . . . . . . 564.0
☐ Consult Vasc. . . . . . . . . . V65.8
☐ Convulsions . . . . . . . . . . 780.3
☐ COPD . . . . . . . . . . . . . . 496
☐ Coronary Atherosclerosis. 414.0
☐ CVA . . . . . . . . . . . . . . . 436
☐ Cyst Sebaceous . . . . . . . 706.2
☐ Dermatitis . . . . . . . . . . . 692.9
☐ Diabetes, Uncomp. Adult 250.00
☐ Diabetes, Complicated . . 250.90
☐ Disc Degeneration . . . . . 722.6
☐ Duodenal Ulcer . . . . . . . 532.90
☐ Dysmenorrhea . . . . . . . . 625.3
☐ Fatigue . . . . . . . . . . . . . 780.7

☐ Flu Shot Only . . . . . . . . . V04.8
☐ Flu Vac . . . . . . . . . . . . . V04.8
☐ Flu W/Resp. Manifest . . . 487.1
☐ Folliculitis . . . . . . . . . . . 704.8
☐ FX ______________
☐ Gallbladder Disease . . . . 575.9
☐ Ganglion . . . . . . . . . . . . 727.43
☐ Gastroenteritis . . . . . . . . 558.9
☐ Gout . . . . . . . . . . . . . . . 274.9
☐ Gyn Exam . . . . . . . . . . . V72.3
☐ Headache Tension . . . . . 307.81
☐ Hemorrhoids Ext. . . . . . . 455.3
☐ Hepatitis . . . . . . . . . . . . 573.3
☐ Hernia-Inguinal . . . . . . . . 550.90
☐ Herpes Zoster . . . . . . . . 053.9
☐ Hyperlipidemia . . . . . . . . 272.4
☐ Hypertension . . . . . . . . . 401.9
☐ Hyperthyroidism . . . . . . . 242.9
☐ Hypothyroidism . . . . . . . 244.9
☐ Impacted Cerumen . . . . . 380.4
☐ Impetigo . . . . . . . . . . . . 684
☐ Ingrown Toenail . . . . . . . 703.0

☐ Internal Derangement Knee . 717.9
☐ Labyrinthitis . . . . . . . . . . 386.30
☐ Laceration Open Wound . 879.8__
☐ Levator Scapular Syndrome 726.90
☐ Menopausal Disorder . . . 627.9
☐ Metabolic Diff. . . . . . . . . 277.8
☐ Migraine . . . . . . . . . . . . 346.90
☐ Mitral Valve Disorder . . . 424.0
☐ Myalgia and Myositis . . . 729.1
☐ Noninf. Gastroenterit. . . . 558.9
☐ Obesity . . . . . . . . . . . . . 278.0
☐ Osteoarthrosis . . . . . . . . 715.00
☐ Osteoporosis . . . . . . . . . 733.00
☐ Otitis Externa . . . . . . . . . 380.10
☐ Otitis Media . . . . . . . . . . 382.9
☐ P.I.D. . . . . . . . . . . . . . . 614.9
☐ Peptic Ulcer . . . . . . . . . . 533.90
☐ Pharyngitis, Acute . . . . . 462
☐ Pneumonia, Viral . . . . . . 480.9
☐ Poison Oak . . . . . . . . . . 692.6
☐ Premarital B-Test . . . . . . V70.3
☐ Pregnancy Test, Unconf.. V72.4

☐ Prostatitis . . . . . . . . . . . 601.9
☐ Psoriasis . . . . . . . . . . . . 696.1
☐ Rheumatoid Arthritis . . . . 714.0
☐ Sciatica . . . . . . . . . . . . . 724.3
☐ Sacroiliac Sprain . . . . . . 846.1
☐ Sinusitis, Acute . . . . . . . 461.9
☐ Smoking Cessation. . . . . 305.10
☐ Sprain ______________
☐ SQ. Cell CA-Face. . . . . . 173.3
☐ Sterilization . . . . . . . . . . V25.2
☐ Stye. . . . . . . . . . . . . . . . 373.11
☐ TB Exposure . . . . . . . . . V01.1
☐ Tendonitis . . . . . . . . . . . 726.90
☐ Tinea . . . . . . . . . . . . . . . 110.9
☐ Tonsillitis, Acute . . . . . . 463
☐ URI, Acute . . . . . . . . . . . 465.9
☐ Urine Tract Infection . . . . 599.0
☐ Vaginitis . . . . . . . . . . . . . 616.10
☐ Well Adult Medical Exam V70.9
☐ Well Child Health Exam . V20.2

| DIAGNOSIS (If not checked above) ICD-9 | PHYSICIAN SIGNATURE | TODAY'S FEE | $ |
|---|---|---|---|
| | PAYMENT BY | PAYMENT | |
| PLEASE REMEMBER THAT PAYMENT IS YOUR OBLIGATION REGARDLESS OF INSURANCE OR OTHER THIRD PARTY INVOLVEMENT. | ☐ CASH ☐ CREDIT CARD<br>☐ CHECK # ________ | BALANCE DUE | |

PLEASE DO NOT STAPLE IN THIS AREA

APPROVED OMB-0938-0008

CARRIER

PICA

# HEALTH INSURANCE CLAIM FORM

PICA

1. MEDICARE (Medicare #) MEDICAID (Medicaid #) CHAMPUS (Sponsor's SSN) CHAMPVA (VA File #) GROUP HEALTH PLAN (SSN or ID) FECA BLK LUNG (SSN) OTHER (ID)

1a. INSURED'S I.D. NUMBER (FOR PROGRAM IN ITEM 1)

2. PATIENT'S NAME (Last Name, First Name, Middle Initial)

3. PATIENT'S BIRTHDATE MM DD YY SEX M F

4. INSURED'S NAME (Last Name, First Name, Middle Initial)

5. PATIENT'S ADDRESS (No., Street)

6. PATIENT RELATIONSHIP TO INSURED Self Spouse Child Other

7. INSURED'S ADDRESS (No., Street)

CITY STATE

8. PATIENT STATUS Single Married Other

CITY STATE

ZIP CODE TELEPHONE (Include Area Code) ( )

Employed Full-Time Student Part-Time Student

ZIP CODE TELEPHONE (Include Area Code) ( )

9. OTHER INSURED'S NAME (Last Name, First Name, Middle Initial)

10. IS PATIENT'S CONDITION RELATED TO:

11. INSURED'S POLICY GROUP OR FECA NUMBER

a. OTHER INSURED'S POLICY OR GROUP NUMBER

a. EMPLOYMENT? (CURRENT OR PREVIOUS) YES NO

a. INSURED'S DATE OF BIRTH MM DD YY SEX M F

b. OTHER INSURED'S DATE OF BIRTH MM DD YY SEX M F

b. AUTO ACCIDENT? YES NO PLACE (State)

b. EMPLOYER'S NAME OR SCHOOL NAME

c. EMPLOYER'S NAME OR SCHOOL NAME

c. OTHER ACCIDENT? YES NO

c. INSURANCE PLAN NAME OR PROGRAM NAME

d. INSURANCE PLAN NAME OR PROGRAM NAME

10d. RESERVED FOR LOCAL USE

d. IS THERE ANOTHER HEALTH BENEFIT PLAN? YES NO *If yes, return to and complete item 9a-d.*

**READ BACK OF FORM BEFORE COMPLETING & SIGNING THIS FORM.**

12. PATIENT'S OR AUTHORIZED PERSON'S SIGNATURE I authorize the release of any medical or other information necessary to process this claim. I also request payment of government benefits either to myself or to the party who accepts assignment below.

SIGNED ______ DATE ______

13. INSURED'S OR AUTHORIZED PERSON'S SIGNATURE I authorize payment of medical benefits to the undersigned physician or supplier for services described below.

SIGNED ______

PATIENT AND INSURED INFORMATION

14. DATE OF CURRENT: MM DD YY ILLNESS (First symptom) OR INJURY (Accident) OR PREGNANCY (LMP)

15. IF PATIENT HAS HAD SAME OR SIMILAR ILLNESS, GIVE FIRST DATE MM DD YY

16. DATES PATIENT UNABLE TO WORK IN CURRENT OCCUPATION FROM MM DD YY TO MM DD YY

17. NAME OF REFERRING PHYSICIAN OR OTHER SOURCE

17a I.D. NUMBER OF REFERRING PHYSICIAN

18. HOSPITALIZATION DATES RELATED TO CURRENT SERVICES FROM MM DD YY TO MM DD YY

19. RESERVED FOR LOCAL USE

20. OUTSIDE LAB? YES NO $ CHARGES

21. DIAGNOSIS OR NATURE OF ILLNESS OR INJURY. (RELATE ITEMS 1,2,3 OR 4 TO ITEM 24E BY LINE)

1. ___ . __
2. ___ . __
3. ___ . __
4. ___ . __

22. MEDICAID RESUBMISSION CODE ORIGINAL REF. NO.

23. PRIOR AUTHORIZATION NUMBER

| 24. A DATE(S) OF SERVICE From MM DD YY To MM DD YY | B Place of Service | C Type of Service | D PROCEDURES, SERVICES, OR SUPPLIES (Explain Unusual Circumstances) CPT/HCPCS MODIFIER | E DIAGNOSIS CODE | F $ CHARGES | G DAYS OR UNITS | H EPSDT Family Plan | I EMG | J COB | K RESERVED FOR LOCAL USE |
|---|---|---|---|---|---|---|---|---|---|---|
| 1 | | | | | | | | | | |
| 2 | | | | | | | | | | |
| 3 | | | | | | | | | | |
| 4 | | | | | | | | | | |
| 5 | | | | | | | | | | |
| 6 | | | | | | | | | | |

25. FEDERAL TAX I.D. NUMBER SSN EIN

26. PATIENTS ACCOUNT NUMBER

27. ACCEPT ASSIGNMENT? (For govt. claims, see back) YES NO

28. TOTAL CHARGE $

29. AMOUNT PAID $

30. BALANCE DUE $

31. SIGNATURE OF PHYSICIAN OR SUPPLIER INCLUDING DEGREES OR CREDENTIALS (I certify that the statements on the reverse apply to this bill and are made a part thereof.)

SIGNED DATE

32. NAME AND ADDRESS OF FACILITY WHERE SERVICES WERE RENDERED (If other than home or office)

33. PHYSICIAN'S, SUPPLIER'S BILLING NAME, ADDRESS, ZIP CODE & PHONE #

PIN # GRP#

PHYSICIAN OR SUPPLIER INFORMATION

**(APPROVED BY AMA COUNCIL ON MEDICAL SERVICE 8/88)**

***PLEASE PRINT OR TYPE***

FORM HCFA-1500 (12-90) FORM OWCP-1500 FORM RRB-1500

Form 124OLM

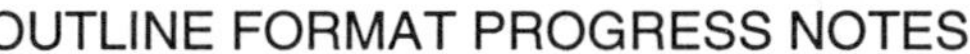

# OUTLINE FORMAT PROGRESS NOTES

Patient Name ______________________________

| Prob. No. or Letter | DATE | S Subjective | O Objective | A Assess | P Plans | Page______ |
|---|---|---|---|---|---|---|
| | | | | | | |

Start each Progress Note (Subjective, Objective, Assessment and Plans) at the appropriate shaded column to create an outline form. Write through the intervening columns to the right margin of the page.

ANDRUS/CLINI-REC® PRIMARY CARE CHARTING SYSTEM FORM NO. 26-7115, ©1976 BIBBERO SYSTEMS, INC., PETALUMA, CA.

Courtesy of Bibbero Systems, Inc., Petaluma, California.

## GIRLS: BIRTH TO 36 MONTHS PHYSICAL GROWTH NCHS PERCENTILES*

NAME ____________________ RECORD # ____________

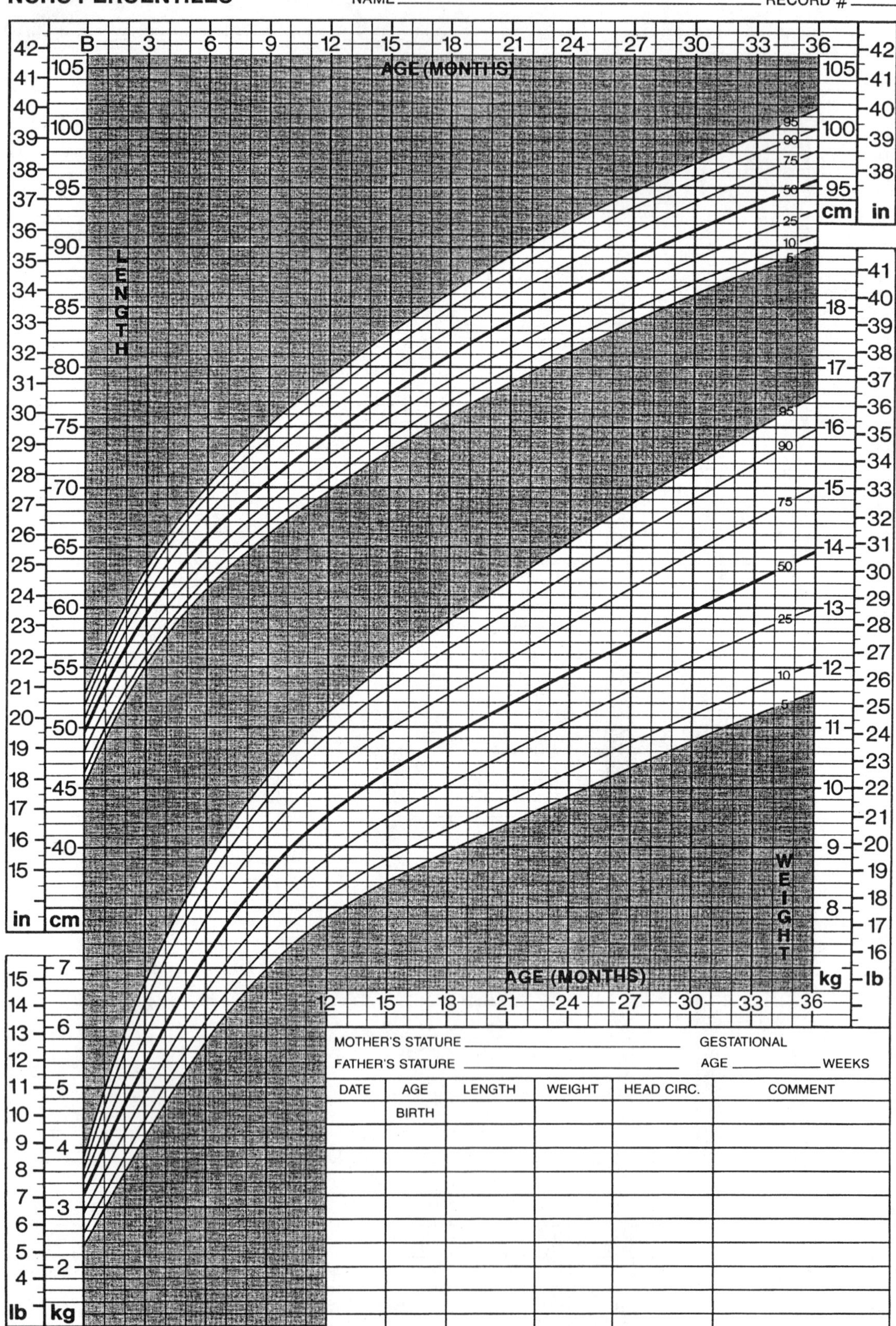


MOTHER'S STATURE ____________ GESTATIONAL

FATHER'S STATURE ____________ AGE ________ WEEKS

| DATE | AGE | LENGTH | WEIGHT | HEAD CIRC. | COMMENT |
|---|---|---|---|---|---|
| | BIRTH | | | | |
| | | | | | |
| | | | | | |
| | | | | | |
| | | | | | |
| | | | | | |
| | | | | | |
| | | | | | |
| | | | | | |

* Adapted from: Hamill PVV, Drizd TA, Johnson CL, Reed RB, Roche AF, Moore WM: Physical growth: National Center for Health Statistics percentiles. AM J CLIN NUTR 32:607-629, 1979. Data from the Fels Longitudinal Study, Wright State University School of Medicine, Yellow Springs, Ohio.